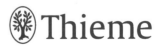

Clinical Case Studies Across the Medical Continuum for Physical Therapists

Julie M. Skrzat, PT, DPT, PhD
Board Certified Clinical Specialist in Cardiovascular &
    Pulmonary Physical Therapy
Assistant Professor
Physical Therapy Program, Murphy Deming College of Health Sciences
Mary Baldwin University
Fishersville, Virginia, USA

Sean F. Griech, PT, DPT, PhD, COMT
Board Certified Clinical Specialist in Orthopaedic Physical Therapy
Associate Professor
Doctor of Physical Therapy Program
DeSales University
Center Valley, Pennsylvania, USA

119 illustrations

Thieme
New York • Stuttgart • Delhi • Rio de Janeiro

Library of Congress Cataloging-in-Publication Data is available from the publisher.

Important note: Medicine is an ever-changing science undergoing continual development. Research and clinical experience are continually expanding our knowledge, in particular our knowledge of proper treatment and drug therapy. Insofar as this book mentions any dosage or application, readers may rest assured that the authors, editors, and publishers have made every effort to ensure that such references are in accordance with **the state of knowledge at the time of production of the book.**

Nevertheless, this does not involve, imply, or express any guarantee or responsibility on the part of the publishers in respect to any dosage instructions and forms of applications stated in the book. **Every user is requested to examine carefully** the manufacturers' leaflets accompanying each drug and to check, if necessary in consultation with a physician or specialist, whether the dosage schedules mentioned therein or the contraindications stated by the manufacturers differ from the statements made in the present book. Such examination is particularly important with drugs that are either rarely used or have been newly released on the market. Every dosage schedule or every form of application used is entirely at the user's own risk and responsibility. The authors and publishers request every user to report to the publishers any discrepancies or inaccuracies noticed. If errors in this work are found after publication, errata will be posted at www.thieme.com on the product description page.

Some of the product names, patents, and registered designs referred to in this book are in fact registered trademarks or proprietary names even though specific reference to this fact is not always made in the text. Therefore, the appearance of a name without designation as proprietary is not to be construed as a representation by the publisher that it is in the public domain.

Thieme addresses people of all gender identities equally. We encourage our authors to use gender-neutral or gender-equal expressions wherever the context allows.

Thieme Publishers New York
333 Seventh Avenue, 18th Floor
New York, NY 10001, USA
www.thieme.com
+1 800 782 3488, customerservice@thieme.com

Cover design: © Thieme
Cover image source: © Thieme
Typesetting by TNQ Technologies, India

Printed in Germany by Beltz Grafische Betriebe   5 4 3 2 1

ISBN: 978-1-68420-187-7

Also available as an e-book:
eISBN (PDF): 978-1-68420-188-4
eISBN (epub): 978-1-63853-692-5

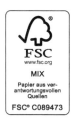

FSC
www.fsc.org
MIX
Papier aus ver-
antwortungsvollen
Quellen
FSC® C089473

This book is dedicated to our students. Thank you for trusting us with your education. We hope that you continue to critically think, ask thoughtful questions, and never "regress to the mean." Thank you for continuing to advance the profession.

Contents

Videos

Preface

The world's population is aging, with developing countries seeing an increase in the 65 years of age and older population by 140% by 2030; however with aging may come chronic diseases. The Global Burden of Disease, a study conducted by the World Health Organization and the World Bank, with partial support from the U.S. National Institute on Aging, predicts a very large increase in disability caused by age-related chronic diseases in all regions of the world.

As a result, individuals are coming to health care providers with much more complex presentations and medical histories. Health care providers must be prepared to not only manage their trained specialty but also understand the integration of multiple body systems to develop a comprehensive plan of care. This includes collaborating with an interprofessional health care team to optimize patients' care and quality of life. This is true for physical therapists, especially since the implementation of direct access. Direct access refers to the removal of the physician referral mandated by state law to access physical therapist services for evaluation and treatment. As of January 2015, all the 50 states, the District of Columbia, and the US Virgin Islands have some form of direct access to physical therapist services. With this, the number of individuals with medical complexities presenting to physical therapy is likely to increase.

To accommodate this change in clinical practice, it is imperative that physical therapists be prepared to evaluate and treat individuals with medical complexities. Physical therapists must know how to critically think and solve problem to synthesize medical data and execute an appropriate plan of care regardless of practice setting.

To ensure physical therapy, students must be utmost prepared to enter the demanding workforce, and academic educators must provide clinical experiences that match the clinical demands. When not available, clinical case studies tend to be presented. It is important that these case studies mimic the clinical environment to promote clinical thinking and problem solving. This textbook was developed to help meet this need.

This textbook includes 20 medically complex case studies, all of which have three standalone parts in three distinct clinical settings across the continuum of care. By designing the cases this way, learners are able to appreciate disease evolution, progression of medical management, and subsequent changes in physical therapy plan of care. At the end of each case, questions are offered through all levels of Bloom's Taxonomy to promote critical thinking and problem solving. Additionally, this textbook promotes interprofessional education by requiring the learners to consider elements beyond physical therapy plan of care in a single episode. Current medical data, past medical data, social history, home environment, and discharge location (including where the past was discharged from and where the patient is being discharged to) are examples of such elements. By stating and requiring the integration of these elements, the learners are forced to consider comprehensive medical and therapeutic plans of care, providing a more authentic preparation for clinical practice.

With that, it is our goal that this textbook will become a companion throughout the physical therapist curriculum to encourage critical thinking and problem solving. We hope that it acts as a guide to promote synthesis of information, including disease evolution and medical management, to give a multi-dimensional representation of the patient which in turn will allow the learners to optimize the physical therapy plans of care, both in the classroom and clinic.

Julie M. Skrzat, PT, DPT, PhD, CCS
Sean F. Griech, PT, DPT, PhD, OCS, COMT

Acknowledgments

We would like to acknowledge the chapter authors. Little did we know that this textbook would be written during a global pandemic. Despite the personal and professional changes and challenges, the authors' commitment never wavered. They were able to write rigorous, and comprehensive case studies. We sincerely thank you for all your work to facilitate the growth of the next generation of physical therapists.

Julie M. Skrzat, PT, DPT, PhD, CCS
Sean F. Griech, PT, DPT, PhD, OCS, COMT

Contributors

Pamela Bartlo, PT, DPT
Board Certified Clinical Specialist in Cardiovascular
    & Pulmonary Physical Therapy
Clinical Associate Professor
Department of Physical Therapy, D'Youville College
Buffalo, New York, USA

Melissa Bednarek, PT, DPT, PhD
Board Certified Clinical Specialist in Cardiovascular
    & Pulmonary Physical Therapy
Associate Professor
Doctor of Physical Therapy Program
Chatham University
Pittsburgh, Pennsylvania, USA

Karen Blood, PT, DPT
Board Certified Clinical Specialist in Geriatrics
    Physical Therapy
Clinical Assistant Professor
Department of Physical Therapy
Quinnipiac University
Hamden, Connecticut, USA

Melissa Brown, MSPAS, PA-C
Assistant Professor
Master of Physician Assistant Studies Program
DeSales University
Center Valley, Pennsylvania, USA

Stephen J. Carp, PT, PhD
Board Certified Clinical Specialist in Geriatrics
    Physical Therapy
Assistant Professor
Doctor of Physical Therapy Program
DeSales University
Center Valley, Pennsylvania, USA

Aubree Colorito, PT, DPT, COS-C
Board Certified Clinical Specialist in Oncologic
    Physical Therapy
Manager of Innovation and Onboarding
Allegheny Health Network Healthcare at Home
Pittsburgh, Pennsylvania, USA

Todd Davenport, PT, DPT, MPH
Board Certified Clinical Specialist in Orthopaedic
    Physical Therapy
Professor
Department of Physical Therapy
University of the Pacific
Stockton, California, USA

Brian Eckenrode, PT, DPT
Board Certified Clinical Specialist in Orthopaedic
    Physical Therapy
Associate Professor
Department of Physical Therapy
Arcadia University
Glenside, Pennsylvania, USA

Kathleen Ehrhardt, MMS, PA-C, DFAAPA
Assistant Professor
Master of Physician Assistant Studies Program
DeSales University
Center Valley, Pennsylvania, USA

Josh Fede, PT, DPT, MTC, CSCS, USATF-L1
Clinician
Holy Cross Orthopedic Institute
Pompano Beach, Florida, USA

Sarah Ferrero, PT, DPT
Board Certified Clinical Specialist in Geriatrics
    Physical Therapy
Clinical Associate Professor
Department of Physical Therapy
Quinnipiac University
Hamden, Connecticut, USA

Mike Fletcher, PT, DPT
Outpatient Staff Physical Therapist
Allegheny Health Network
Pittsburgh, Pennsylvania, USA

Aaron S. Frey, DO
Clinical Instructor
Emergency Medicine
University of Virginia
Charlottesville, Virginia, USA

Laura Friedman, PT, DPT
Board Certified Clinical Specialist in Cardiovascular
    & Pulmonary Physical Therapy
Assistant Professor
Department of Physical Therapy
Rosalind Franklin University of Medicine and Science
North Chicago, Illinois, USA

David Gillette, PT, DPT
Board Certified Clinical Specialist in Geriatrics
    Physical Therapy
Assistant Professor
Department of Physical Therapy
University of the Pacific
Stockton, California, USA

Melissa Gilroy, DC, MSPAS, PA-C
Assistant Professor
Master of Physician Assistant Studies Program
DeSales University
Center Valley, Pennsylvania, USA

Brian Goonan, PT, DPT
Board Certified Clinical Specialist in Orthopaedic
    Physical Therapy
Advanced Clinician
Hospital for Special Surgery
New York, New York, USA

Sean F. Griech, PT, DPT, PhD, COMT
Board Certified Clinical Specialist in Orthopaedic
    Physical Therapy
Associate Professor
Doctor of Physical Therapy Program
DeSales University
Center Valley, Pennsylvania, USA

Carolyn Haggerty, PT, DPT
Clinician
Department of Therapy Services
Penn State Milton S. Hershey Medical Center
Hershey, Pennsylvania, USA

Ethan Hood, PT, DPT, MBA
Board Certified Clinical Specialist in Geriatrics
    Physical Therapy, Board Certified Clinical
    Specialist in Neurologic Physical Therapy
Assistant Professor
Doctor of Physical Therapy Program
DeSales University
Center Valley, Pennsylvania, USA

Kevin Jenney, PT, DPT
Board Certified Clinical Specialist in Neurologic
    Physical Therapy
Clinical Specialist
Department of Rehabilitation Services
Erie County Medical Center
Buffalo, New York, USA

Ari Kaplan PT, DPT, CSCS, COMT, Cert MDT
Board Certified Clinical Specialist in Sports
    Physical Therapy
CEO and Lead Instructor
Association of Clinical Excellence
Middletown, Delaware, USA

Erin Lampron, PT, DPT
Board Certified Clinical Specialist in Neurologic
    Physical Therapy
Clinical Assistant Professor
Department of Physical Therapy
Quinnipiac University
Hamden, Connecticut, USA

Kelly Lindenberg, PT, MSPT, PhD, CSCS
Associate Professor
Graduate School of Physical Therapy
Slippery Rock University
Slippery Rock, Pennsylvania, USA

Sheena MacFarlane, PT, DPT
Board Certified Clinical Specialist in Cardiovascular
    & Pulmonary Physical Therapy
Assistant Professor
Department of Rehabilitation and Movement
    Sciences, Doctor of Physical Therapy Program
Rutgers University
Blackwood, New Jersey, USA

Rebecca Maidansky, PT, DPT
Clinician
Lady Bird Physical Therapy
Austin, Texas, USA

Kala Markel, PT, DPT
Clinician
Lifeline Physical Therapy
Pittsburgh, Pennsylvania, USA

Suzanne F. Migliore, PT, DPT, MS
Board Certified Clinical Specialist in Pediatric
    Physical Therapy
Assistant Professor
Doctor of Physical Therapy Program
DeSales University
Center Valley, Pennsylvania, USA

Margot Miller, PT, DPT
Clinician
Department of Therapy Services
Loyola University Medical Center
Maywood, Illinois, USA

Rachel Pata, PT, DPT, CHSE
Board Certified Clinical Specialist in Cardiovascular
    & Pulmonary Physical Therapy
Clinical Associate Professor
Department of Physical Therapy
Quinnipiac University
Hamden, Connecticut, USA

Bhavana Raja, PT, PhD
Assistant Professor
Department of Physical Therapy
University of the Pacific
Stockton, California, USA

Judith Schaad, PT, DPT, CWS, CLT-LANA
Board Certified Clinical Specialist in Oncology
    Physical Therapy
Director
Allegheny Health Network Oncology Rehab Program
Pittsburgh, Pennsylvania, USA

Jessica Schwartz, MSPAS, PA-C
Assistant Professor
Master of Physician Assistant Studies Program
DeSales University
Center Valley, Pennsylvania, USA

Scott Siverling, PT, DPT
Board Certified Clinical Specialist in Orthopaedic
    Physical Therapy, Fellow of the American
    Academy of Orthopedic Physical Therapy
Clinical Lead
Paramus Outpatient Center, Hospital for
Special Surgery
New York, New York, USA

Julie M. Skrzat, PT, DPT, PhD
Board Certified Clinical Specialist in Cardiovascular
    & Pulmonary Physical Therapy
Assistant Professor
Physical Therapy Program, Murphy Deming College
    of Health Sciences
Mary Baldwin University
Fishersville, Virginia, USA

Karen Snowden, PT, DPT
Board Certified Clinical Specialist in Women's Health
    Physical Therapy
Clinical Specialist
Rehabilitation Services, Lehigh Valley Health Network
Allentown, Pennsylvania, USA

Brian Stagno, PT
Senior Physical Therapist
Allegheny Health Network
West Penn Hospital
Pittsburgh, Pennsylvania, USA

Christopher Tumminello PT, DPT, EP-C
Clinic Director and Clinician
ATI Physical Therapy at Abessinio Stadium
Wilmington, Delaware, USA

Tracy Wall, PT, PhD
Clinical Professor
Department of Physical Therapy
Quinnipiac University
Hamden, Connecticut, USA

Karen Warenius, PT, DPT, C/NDT
Clinician
Children's Hospital of Philadelphia
Philadelphia, Pennsylvania, USA

1 Adolescent Sports Injury

General Information	
Case no.	1.A Adolescent Sports Injury
Authors	Christopher Tumminello, PT, DPT, EP-C Brian Eckenrode, PT, DPT, Board Certified Clinical Specialist in Orthopaedic Physical Therapy Ari Kaplan, PT, DPT, CSCS, COMT, Cert MDT, Board Certified Clinical Specialist in Sports Physical Therapy
Diagnosis	Knee dislocation with multiligamentous knee injury (KD III-MC)
Setting	On-field assessment and emergency room management
Learner expectations	☑ Initial evaluation ☐ Re-evaluation ☐ Treatment session
Learner objectives	1. Describe the management of an acute on-field knee injury. 2. Determine the need for immediate medical attention of a patient with an acute on-field knee injury. 3. Describe the appropriate tests and measures considered for this patient in the acute phase of injury.

Pre-case clarification	
Physical therapy scope of practice	It should be noted that all physical therapists are not qualified to provide coverage of athletic events. The highest qualification physical therapists can obtain in order to be able to provide athletic venue coverage is through becoming a board-certified sports clinical specialist (SCS) offered through the American Board of Physical Therapy Specialties (ABPTS). Additional credentials for physical therapists to be able to provide on-field coverage include the certified athletic trainer (ATC) or emergency medical responder (EMR) certification.

Medical	
Chief complaint	Instability and pain in left knee
History of present illness	While assisting with on-field coverage of a high school football game with an athletic trainer and sports medicine physician, a 16-year-old, right-handed male, who plays quarterback, sustained a traumatic left knee injury. The quarterback was dropping back to attempt a pass, when he transitioned his weight to his front leg (left leg) and sustained a hit from an opposing player to the anterolateral aspect of his left knee.
Past medical history	Asthma
Past surgical history	None
Allergies	Peanuts
Medications	Albuterol inhaler as needed
Precautions/Orders	N/A—on-field assessment

Social history	
Home setup	• Lives with his parents, younger sister, and dog in a two-story home. • Four steps to enter, with right handrail when ascending. • Bedroom is on the second floor. • Half bathroom on the first floor, and full bathroom on the second floor. • Indoor stairs have handrails on both sides.
Occupation	• Full-time high school student. • Busses tables at a local restaurant on the weekends.
Prior level of function	• Independent with all activities of daily living.
Recreational activities	• Starting high school quarterback in the fall. • Starting shortstop for baseball in the spring.

Physical Examination: On-Field Assessment	
Subjective	
"My knee bent backward, and I definitely heard a pop. Pretty sure everyone heard it."	
Objective	
Observation	• No head or neck trauma noted with injury. • Player is alert and oriented to person, place, and time. • No blood or open wound present. • No obvious deformity to the left lower extremity. • Effusion absent to the left lower extremity.
Neurovascular assessment	• Unable to detect a left popliteal artery, posterior tibial artery, or dorsalis pedis pulse. (▶ Fig. 1.1). • No temperature change noted to the distal left lower extremity. • No complaints of numbness or tingling at this time to the left leg.
Musculoskeletal assessment	• Knee special testing was deferred due to acuity of injury, combined with the loss of pulses to the left lower extremity.
Treatment	• Given the current presentation and inability to bear weight through the left leg, and undetectable pulses, the left knee was immobilized on field. • An ambulance was called for immediate transportation to the hospital.

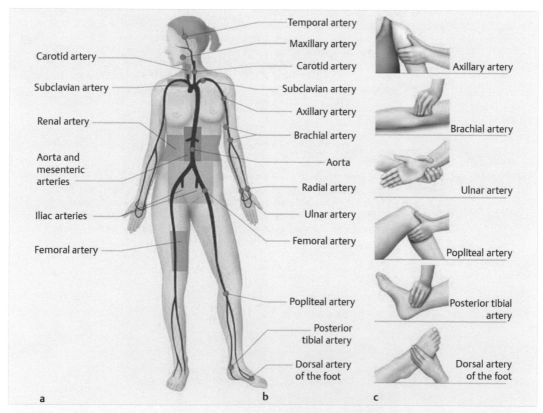

Fig. 1.1 Areas of auscultation and palpation of the peripheral arterial pulses. **(a)** Auscultation areas. **(b)** Palpation points. **(c)** Palpation techniques. (Source: Vascular diagnosis. In: Steffers G, Credner S, eds. General Pathology and Internal Medicine for Physical Therapists. 1st ed. Thieme; 2012.)

Pause points
Based on the above information, what is the priority • Diagnostic tests and measures? • Outcome measures? • Treatment interventions?

Vital signs	Hospital day 0: emergency department
Blood pressure (mmHg)	132/80
Heart rate (beats/min)	92
Respiratory rate (breaths/min)	16
Pulse oximetry on room air (SpO$_2$)	98%
Temperature (°F)	98.6

Hospital Day 0, Emergency Room: Physical Examination			
Subjective			
"I got hit, and my left knee got bent backward and popped. It's really hurting now."			
Objective			
General	Observation	• Well-nourished fit high school male. • Appears to have left knee pain, cognitively intact and answering questions appropriately. • Left lower extremity pallor, right lower extremity was unremarkable.	
	Pain (left knee)	• 8/10 currently	
	Palpation	• Left lower extremity slightly colder to touch compared to the right lower extremity.	
Head, ears, eyes, nose, and throat (HEENT)	• (−) Congestion, sore throat or otalgia, denies head injury with hit during the game.		
Cardiovascular and pulmonary	• (−) Chest pain, palpitations, dyspnea on exertion, edema, syncope, aspiration, shortness of breath, orthopnea • (−) Cough, congestion, wheezing, or sputum production • Lower extremity pulses: Right: 2 + throughout Left: femoral artery, 4 +; popliteal artery, 0; posterior tibial, 0; dorsalis pedis, 0		
Gastrointestinal	• (−) Abdominal pain, hematemesis, melena, nausea, vomiting, diarrhea		
Genitourinary	• (−) Dysuria, frequency, urgency, blood in urine		
Musculoskeletal	Range of motion	Right	Left
		Unremarkable	Limited knee flexion and extension due to pain/ acuteness of injury.
	Strength (manual muscle testing)	• 5/5 ankle dorsiflexion • 5/5 ankle plantar flexion • 5/5 ankle inversion • 5/5 ankle eversion	• 1/5 ankle dorsiflexion • 1/5 ankle plantar flexion • 1/5 ankle inversion • 1/5 ankle eversion
	Other	• Special tests (including ligamentous testing) of the left lower extremity were deferred due to loss of pulses and findings from diagnostic imaging.	

(Continued)

(Continued)

Hospital Day 0, Emergency Room: Physical Examination		
Neurological	Balance	• Not assessed due to lower extremity injury.
	Cognition	• Alert and oriented x four.
	Coordination	• Not assessed at this time.
	Cranial nerves	• II–XII: intact
	Reflexes	• Not assessed at this time.
	Sensation	• Right lower extremity: unremarkable • Left lower extremity: diminished below the knee

Imaging/Diagnostic tests	Hospital Day 1, Emergency Room: Emergency Department
Radiographs	Trauma series (AP and lateral views): negative for fractures on left lower extremity. No signs of growth plate injury or disruption.
Magnetic resonance	Magnetic resonance angiography (MRA): presence of popliteal arterial occlusion in left leg.

Medical management	Hospital Day 1, Postoperative Day 0: Medical Ward
Surgical intervention	• Under general anesthesia, the patient underwent exploration of the popliteal artery via a medial approach. An intimal flap disruption was discovered in the popliteal artery, leading to a thrombectomy via catheter with suturing of the intimal flap. To avoid restenosis, the repair utilized a saphenous vein patch from the contralateral leg.
Postoperative	• Restoration of normal popliteal, posterior tibialis, and dorsalis pedis pulses.
Additional imaging	• Magnetic resonance imaging (MRI): tear of the left posterior cruciate ligament (PCL), anterior cruciate ligament (ACL), medial collateral ligament (MCL), and lateral meniscus. These findings meet the diagnostic criteria of a KD III-MC via anatomic (Schenck) classification of knee dislocations.

Assessment	
☑ Physical therapist's	*Assessment left blank for learner to develop.*
Goals	
Patient's	"To play football again."
Short term	1. *Goals left blank for learner to develop.* 2.
Long term	1. *Goals left blank for learner to develop.* 2.

Plan	
☐ Physician's ☑ Physical therapist's ☐ Other's	Provide single visit for crutch training along with written instructions for home exercise program and wound management for safe discharge home with supervision from parents.

Bloom's Taxonomy Level	Case 1.A Questions
Create	1. Synthesizing the medical data and physical examination findings, develop an appropriate physical therapy assessment of the patient.
	2. Develop two short-term physical therapy goals, including an appropriate timeframe.
	3. Develop two long-term physical therapy goals, including an appropriate timeframe.
Evaluate	4. Which findings decrease suspicion for a catastrophic spine injury?
Analyze	5. After an artery injury, how many hours can pass before there is an increased risk of limb amputation?
	6. If a vascular injury is present with a knee dislocation, how often is surgery indicated?
	7. What is the hierarchy of an on-field assessment?
Apply	8. What are the proper procedures for applying a splint to the patient on the field prior to transportation to the hospital?
	9. In the initial plan of care as the treating physical therapist in the acute care hospital, what exercises could safely be implemented upon discharge from the hospital?
Understand	10. What are the common nerve and artery injuries associated with a knee dislocation?
	11. What knee structures are involved in the diagnosis of KD III—MC, and what knee structures are involved in the other KD classifications?
	12. What are the 6 Ps of acute ischemia?
Remember	13. What must be ruled out when there is a complaint of extremity numbness following a traumatic on-field injury?

Bloom's Taxonomy Level	Case 1.A Answers
Create	1. The patient is a 16-year-old male who underwent surgery after sustaining a traumatic left knee dislocation, involving tears of his ACL, PCL, and MCL (KD III—MC). Upon his in-hospital postoperative physical therapy evaluation, pulses and capillary refill were intact in his left lower extremity. He demonstrates the physical ability to ambulate with axillary crutches independently and understands importance of utilizing a locked knee brace or immobilizer with mobility activities. Poor quadriceps muscle activation was observed by having the patient attempt an isometric quadriceps contraction. His home exercise program should focus on frequent application of ice, compression, and elevation, In addition to beginning quadriceps isometrics, gluteal isometrics, ankle pumps, and knee range of motion (ROM) ahead of a consult with an orthopaedic surgeon.
	2. Short-term goals:
	• The patient will ambulate 150 feet using bilateral axillary crutches independently while maintaining non–weight-bearing status within 3 days to be independent at home.
	• The patient will ascend/descend a flight of steps using bilateral axillary crutches while maintaining a non–weight-bearing status independently within 3 days to be independent at home.
	• The patient will demonstrate the ability to properly don and doff his knee immobilizer brace independently within 3 days to be independent at home.
	3. Long-term goals:
	• The patient will perform a left straight leg raise without a quadriceps lag to improve LLE strength and allow for safe functional transfers and bed mobility within 4 weeks.
	• The patient will demonstrate left knee active ROM from 0 to at least 90 degrees of flexion within 4 weeks, prior to his scheduled knee reconstruction, in order to maximize a favorable postoperative outcome. (*It should be noted that patients may be immobilized in 20 degrees of flexion to prevent posterior subluxation of the tibia, which could endanger the popliteal artery after popliteal artery repair.*)
Evaluate	4. Possible findings of catastrophic spine injury would include unconsciousness or altered level of consciousness, bilateral neurologic findings or complaints, significant midline spine pain with or without palpation, and obvious spinal column deformity.
Analyze	5. Without an early diagnosis of vascular changes (within 8 hours), the risk of required amputation increases.
	6. Of patients who sustained a vascular injury with a knee dislocation, 80% required vascular surgery and 12% resulted in amputation.

(Continued)

(Continued)

Bloom's Taxonomy Level	Case 1.A Answers
	7. Prevent further injury, minimize the zone of injury, decrease pain, promote healing, and allow a safe return to athletic competition if appropriate is the hierarchy of an on-field assessment.
Apply	8. A splint for a knee dislocation should be applied so that it adequately supports the joint at, above, and below the injury. In this case, splinting of the hip and ankle may be excessive, but a posterior knee splint or long leg immobilizer should be applied to prevent additional injuries.
	9. Straight leg raises, side lying hip abduction, and prone hip extension can be initiated with the knee in an immobilizer or locked brace. Additionally, ankle and knee passive/active assist ROM should be included for this patient. The patient should avoid active hip adduction, to minimize stress to the healing MCL. Knee flexion beyond 90 degrees of flexion and 0 degrees of extension should be avoided at this stage to minimize tension on the vascular repair.
Understand	10. The popliteal artery and common peroneal nerve are the most commonly associated injuries with knee dislocations, occurring in 19 and 20% of knee dislocations, respectively.
	11. See ▶ Table 1.1.
	12. Pain, pallor, paralysis, pulse deficit, paresthesia, and poikilothermia
Remember	13. Cervical and lumbar spine injuries must be cleared prior to transporting or moving a patient with complaints of numbness, tingling, or weakness after sustaining a traumatic on-field injury.

Table 1.1 Anatomic classification of knee dislocations

Class[a]	Injury
KD I	PCL or ACL intact knee dislocation Variable collateral involvement
KD II	Both cruciate ligaments torn, collaterals intact
KD III	Both cruciate ligaments torn, one collateral torn. Subset M (medial) or L (lateral)
KD IV	All four ligaments torn.
KD V	Knee fracture dislocation
KD V.1	Fracture dislocation with a single cruciate injury.
KD V.2	Fracture dislocation with both cruciate ligaments torn, collaterals/corners intact.
KD V.3	Fracture dislocation with both cruciate ligaments and one collateral/corner torn. Subset M (medial) or L (lateral)
KD V.4	Fracture dislocation with both cruciate ligaments and both collaterals/corners torn.

Abbreviations: ACL, anterior cruciate ligament; KD, knee dislocation; PCL, posterior cruciate ligament.
[a]Subtypes may include: C, arterial injury; N, neurologic injury.

Key points
1. The hierarchies for on-field injury assessments include preventing further injury, minimizing the zone of injury, decreasing pain, promoting healing, and allowing for a safe return to athletic competition if appropriate. The athlete's safety should always be the first concern.
2. Being aware of the patient's orientation level, clearing spine injuries, and understanding indications for orthopaedic special tests are all necessary. In this case, specific skills including pulse palpation and sensation testing were needed for appropriate triage of the patient. Since his knee reduced on its own, as no obvious deformity was present, appropriate management to ensure he did not bear weight on his leg was key.
3. Understanding the mechanism of injury for this case and possible anatomical structures that could be involved helps determine the immediate need for medical attention. Furthermore, clinician knowledge of the six Ps of acute ischemia

(Continued)

(Continued)

Key points
and clinical understanding of orthopaedic special tests will promote optimal patient safety in this scenario. For these reasons, additional educational training and certifications are required for those physical therapists interested in the ability to provide field coverage at athletic events.

General Information	
Case no.	1.B
Authors	Christopher Tumminello, PT, DPT, EP-C Brian Eckenrode, PT, DPT, Board Certified Clinical Specialist in Orthopaedic Physical Therapy Ari Kaplan, PT, DPT, CSCS, COMT, Cert MDT, Board Certified Clinical Specialist in Sports Physical Therapy
Diagnosis	Knee dislocation with multiligamentous knee injury (KD III–MC), postoperative knee reconstruction
Setting	Outpatient clinic
Learner expectations	☑ Initial evaluation ☐ Re-evaluation ☑ Treatment session
Learner objectives	1. Determine the evidence-based physical therapy interventions for the management of a patient following multiple ligamentous surgical reconstruction of the knee. 2. Understand the associated musculoskeletal impairments on a patient with a multiligamentous knee injury. 3. Understand the progression of the early to intermediate phases of a plan of care for a knee dislocation.

Medical	
Chief complaint	Left knee pain and limited mobility s/p arthroscopic knee surgery.
History of present illness	Four weeks after the initial on-field knee injury (see below), a 16-year-old male underwent reconstruction of his left ACL and PCL, along with a lateral partial meniscectomy. He presents to clinic 1-week post-op, non–weight-bearing on his left lower extremity with bilateral axillary crutches and with his knee in an immobilizer. During the assessment, the patient reports that his knee is painful, stiff, and weak.
Past medical history	Asthma
Past surgical history	ACL and PCL reconstruction with partial lateral meniscectomy—left knee (1 week ago) See below for further information.
Allergies	Peanuts
Medications	Albuterol inhaler as needed
Precautions/Orders	Begin physical therapy per the ACL/PCL protocol. WBAT LLE

Medical management	
Surgical intervention (vascular surgery—4 weeks ago)	The patient underwent a thrombectomy via catheter with suturing of the intimal flap. To avoid restenosis, the repair utilized a saphenous vein patch from the contralateral leg.
Surgical intervention (orthopaedic surgery—1 week ago)	A review of the patient's postoperative report shows that he underwent a hamstring tendon autograft for reconstruction of the ACL and patella tendon autograft for reconstruction of the PCL arthroscopically.

Social history	
Home setup	Prior to accident: • Lives with his parents, younger sister, and dog in a two-story home. • Four steps to enter, with right handrail when ascending. • Bedroom is on the second floor. • Half bathroom on the first floor, and full bathroom on the second floor. • Indoor stairs have handrails on both sides. Upon hospital discharge: • Modified independent with bilateral axillary crutches for transfers, gait, and stair negotiation. • Modified independent for activities of daily living—sits to dress.
Occupation	• Full-time high school student. • Busses tables at a local restaurant on the weekends
Prior level of function	• Independent with all activities of daily living.
Recreational activities	• Starting high school quarterback in the fall. • Starting shortstop for baseball in the spring.

Physical Therapy Examination		
Subjective		
"My knee is stiff and swollen." "It's hard to get around school on crutches."		
Objective		
General	Observation	• Well-nourished fit high school male. Presents ambulating with bilateral axillary crutches and post-op knee brace.
	Pain level (left knee)	4/10 at rest. 7/10 when trying to bend knee.
	Effusion (sweep test) ▶ Fig. 1.2	Right knee: 0 Left knee: 3+
	Medications:	Naproxen as needed
Cardiovascular and pulmonary	Blood pressure (mmHg)	115/76
	Heart rate (beats/min)	68
	Respiratory rate (breaths/min)	14
	Pulse oximetry on room air (SpO$_2$)	99%
Integumentary	• Three arthroscopic portal incisions and a small 4-cm incision were noted. • Wounds were intact and sealed with skin glue. • No outward sign for infection or excessive drainage.	
Musculoskeletal	Range of motion (knee flexion)	Right	Left
		4–0–136 degrees	6–58 degrees
	Strength (MMT)	5/5 hip flexion 4+/5 hip abduction 4+/5 hip extension 5/5 knee flexion 5/5 knee extension 5/5 ankle dorsiflexion 5/5 ankle plantar flexion 5/5 ankle inversion 5/5 ankle eversion	4+/5 hip flexion 3+/5 hip abduction 3+/5 hip extension Not tested knee flexion 2+/5 knee extension 4+/5 ankle dorsiflexion 4–/5 ankle plantar flexion 4–/5 ankle inversion 4–/5 ankle eversion
	Other	Straight leg raise: 16-degree knee extension lag with left knee. Quadriceps setting: normal superior patellar glide on the right. Phasic shaking of quadriceps on the left, with no observable superior patella glide.	
Neurological	Cognition	• Alert and oriented x four

(Continued)

(Continued)

Physical Therapy Examination		
	Reflexes	• Not assessed at this time.
	Sensation	• Right lower extremity: unremarkable. • Left lower extremity: absent sensation medial to the incision at the patella tendon.

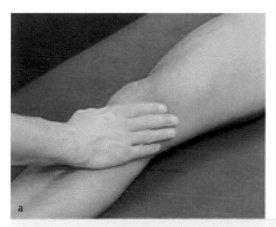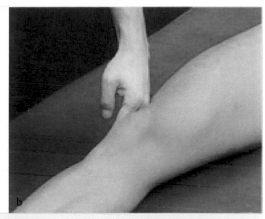

Fig. 1.2 (a, b) Sweep test. (Source: Reichert B, ed. Palpation Techniques. 1st ed. Thieme; 2010.)

Pause points
Based on the above information: • Which treatment interventions would the physical therapist start with on day 1? • Is weight bearing contraindicated for this patient? • How does a physical therapist plan to progress this patient from non–weight-bearing to normal ambulation?

Functional status	
Transfers	• Sit to/from stand: modified independent using bilateral axillary crutches while maintaining non–weight-bearing on left lower extremity.
Ambulation	• Ambulates 50 feet with modified independence using bilaterally axillary crutches while maintaining non–weight-bearing on left lower extremity.
Stairs	• Ascend/descend flight of stairs with modified independence using bilateral axillary crutches while maintaining non–weight-bearing on left lower extremity.
Sport specific	• Deferred at this time.

Assessment	
☑ Physical therapist's	*Assessment left blank for learner to develop*
Goals	
Patient's	"To walk without crutches"
Short term	1. *Goals left blank for learner to develop.* 2.
Long term	1. *Goals left blank for learner to develop.* 2.

Plan	
☐ Physician's ☑ Physical therapist's ☐ Other's	Appropriately progress patient off of crutches and normalize gait pattern as quadriceps activation, ROM, and general lower extremity strength improve.

Bloom's Taxonomy Level	Case 1.B Questions
Create	1. Synthesizing the medical data and physical examination findings, develop an appropriate physical therapy assessment of the patient. 2. Develop 2 short-term physical therapy goals, including an appropriate timeframe. 3. Develop 2 long-term physical therapy goals, including an appropriate timeframe.
Evaluate	4. Review protocols for ACL and PCL reconstructions to evaluate similarities and differences in precautions. Which protocol is most limiting?
Analyze	5. Distinguish the differences in joint effusion grading using the sweep test. 6. Describe the effects of joint effusion in the knee on recovery time. 7. Describe the knee joint arthrokinematics during ROM activities including the potential risk on the PCL graft. 8. Analyze the mechanics of a third-class lever as seen with the quadriceps during open-chain exercises and the possible effects on the ACL graft.
Apply	9. Design a progression of quadriceps strengthening exercises for this patient as he progresses from the early to intermediate phases of his postoperative recovery. 10. What precautions need to be considered in the implementation of quadriceps strengthening with regard to the arthrokinematics?
Understand	11. Based on the patient's knee effusion, ROM, surgical precautions, and quadriceps strength at his initial evaluation, should he be cleared to weight bear through his involved lower extremity?
Remember	12. What objectives and goals should be met prior to discharging the use of crutches in this patient?

Bloom's Taxonomy Level	Case 1.B Answers
Create	1. The patient is a 16-year-old male who presents to outpatient physical therapy status-post ACL and PCL reconstructions with a partial lateral meniscectomy of his left knee 1-week postoperatively. He ambulates with bilateral axillary crutches and non–weight-bearing on the involved limb. The initial evaluation reveals limitations in left knee ROM, patellofemoral mobility, quadriceps activation, and general lower extremity strength. At this time, it is likely that the limited quadriceps isometric and straight leg raise ability is partially due to the findings of 3 + effusion in his left knee. The patient will benefit from a progressive quadriceps' strengthening program to improve his ability to perform straight leg raises without a knee extension lag to wean off of crutches and normalize his gait. 2. Short-term goals: • The patient will demonstrate active left knee ROM from 0 to 110 degrees in 2 weeks (3 weeks postoperatively) to allow for improved functional mobility with activities of daily living (ADLs). • The patient will perform 20 consecutive straight leg raises without a knee extension lag in 2 weeks (3 weeks postoperatively) to safely progress weight-bearing through the left lower extremity. 3. Long-term goals • The patient will demonstrate left knee active ROM which is symmetrical to the right knee in 12 weeks to allow for full functional mobility for transfers and stairs. • The patient will demonstrate left quadriceps strength ratio of 80% compared to the uninvolved limb in 12 weeks.
Evaluate	4. The postoperative limitation which would be most restrictive for this patient would be for the PCL reconstruction, followed by the ACL reconstructions. In general, the PCL rehabilitative protocol should become the primary plan of care to be followed, while considering the precautions of the ACL rehabilitative protocol.

(Continued)

(Continued)

Bloom's Taxonomy Level	Case 1.B Answers
Analyze	5. Grades: zero, trace, 1+, 2+, and 3+ Respective test results: 0, no wave produced on downstroke; trace, small wave on medial side with downstroke; 1+, larger bulge on medial side with downstroke; 2+, effusion spontaneously returns to medial side after upstroke (no downstroke needed); 3+, so much fluid present that it is not possible to move the effusion out of the medial aspect of the knee. 6. Knee joint effusion may lead to arthrogenic muscle inhibition (AMI) of the quadriceps, causing atrophy and prolonged recovery times with acute, chronic, and postoperative injuries. This can cause secondary effects of limited quadriceps strength, whereby the effusion may contribute to the measurable weakness. 7. For a PCL reconstruction, knee flexion ROM should be limited to 60 degrees for the first 2 weeks and gradually progressed to 110 degrees from weeks 3 to 5, prior to achieving pain-free active ROM within 10 degrees of contralateral limb by week 12 and full ROM compared to contralateral limb by week 16. This helps preserve the PCL reconstruction and popliteal artery repair and prevent damage by compressive popliteal artery or overstretching the PCL. It is important to also protect the healing PCL graft during passive knee motion exercises. Any knee position which may cause posterior tibial translation should be avoided including isolated active hamstring activation, passive knee flexion where the tibia may passively translate posteriorly (e.g., supine wall slide to gain knee flexion should be avoided), and passive knee extension utilizing a heel prop. 8. The role of open-chain exercises in ACL reconstructions is controversial with some arguing that these exercises place excessive strain through the ACL graft. However, others report this is a safe exercise for patients to perform through a modified arc of motion. Ultimately, the orthopaedic surgeon's preference should be adhered to with this exercise. Most ACL protocols suggest knee active ROM from 90 to 45 degrees of knee extension with open-chain exercises to decrease anterior translation of the tibia.
Apply	9. In the early rehabilitation stages, the progression of quadriceps activation and strengthening postoperatively usually advances from isometric contractions to open-chain AROM in a limited arc (90–45 degrees), open-chain resisted AROM in a limited arc (90–45 degrees), and closed-chain strengthening in pain-free range and with a limited arc (0–45 degrees). For this patient with both an ACL and PCL reconstruction, knee open-chain AROM is restricted from 90 to 45 degrees. Strengthening of the quadriceps will likely begin with isometrics such as quadriceps setting and straight leg raises, in addition to the inclusion of neuromuscular electrical stimulation (NMES) to the quadriceps (▶ Fig. 1.3). It is recommended that patients progress away from crutches once an individual can complete 20 consecutive straight leg raises without a knee extension lag. 10. Due to the use of the patient's hamstring tendon for the ACL reconstruction, hamstring resistance training is contraindicated for 12 weeks. After 12 weeks, the hamstring tendon can begin to handle resistance training loads, but the PCL protocol becomes more restrictive and requires 16 weeks prior to progressive resistance training for knee flexion. At a minimum of 6 weeks, he is allowed to complete 0–90 degrees of active ROM knee flexion against gravity.
Understand	11. The largest precaution to the patient's weight-bearing status at 1-week postoperative is the lack of full knee extension passive ROM. Once full passive knee extension is restored, the patient should be cleared for partial weight-bearing with his orthosis locked at 0 degrees of knee extension per most PCL postoperative guidelines. The patient can be weaned out of his orthosis once quadriceps maximal voluntary isometric contraction (MVIC) reaches >60% based on strength testing. Crutches can be discharged if the patient is >6 weeks postoperative and gait is normalized and relatively pain free.
Remember	12. The ability to complete 20 straight leg raises without observing a quadriceps lag, >60% quad MVIC strength ratio, knee ROM at least 0–110 degrees, trace effusion in joint, and demonstration of normal gait mechanics with crutches.

Key points

1. The utilization of a variety of physical therapy interventions is required to address pain, ROM, strength, and function of this patient's case.
   - Ice and transcutaneous electrical nerve stimulation (TENS) have demonstrated positive effects on decreasing arthrogenic muscle inhibition secondary to effusion while controlling pain.
   - Appropriate joint mobility and ROM are required for normal arthrokinematics of the tibiofemoral and patellofemoral joints.
   - Adequate progression of strengthening is important for quadriceps hypertrophy, but physical therapists need to consider the potential stress on the reconstructed structures with different exercises. Additionally, the inclusion of NMES has been shown to maximize quadriceps strength and provide for a more optimal outcome in postsurgical knee patients.

2. For the early phases of this case, primary physical therapy goals include the protection of reconstructed structures, minimizing pain, decreasing knee joint effusion, restoring knee joint and soft-tissue mobility, and facilitating quadriceps activation. To best achieve these goals and to restore the patient's functional mobility with ADLs, it is important to consider the following key concepts related to this procedure:
   - How quickly and safely can knee ROM progress, while minimizing stress on the PCL graft with knee ROM exercises?
   - Limiting knee open-chain ROM to prevent anterior shear of tibia due to the third-class lever biomechanics.
   - Knee loading progression through the harvested patella and hamstring tendons.

3. When working with patients with complex surgical procedures, physical therapists should have a strong working knowledge of the relevant anatomy and biomechanics to best understand how to protect the involved structures. Progression of knee joint motion, strength, and weight-bearing in a safe, controlled manner will allow for a smooth transition from a protection and early motion/loading stage to early functional recovery and progression of sport-specific activities in the later stages of physical therapy.

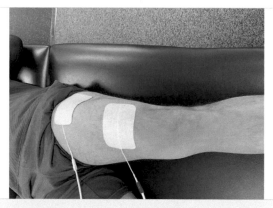

Fig. 1.3 Setup for neuromuscular electrical stimulation (NMES) of the quadriceps with the knee in full extension.

General Information	
Case no.	1.C
Authors	Christopher Tumminello, PT, DPT, EP-C Brian Eckenrode, PT, DPT, Board Certified Clinical Specialist in Orthopaedic Physical Therapy Ari Kaplan, PT, DPT, CSCS, COMT, Cert MDT, Board Certified Clinical Specialist in Sports Physical Therapy
Diagnosis	Knee dislocation with multiligamentous knee injury (KD III-MC)
Setting	Outpatient orthopaedic/sports medicine clinic: return-to-sport phase
Learner expectations	☐ Initial evaluation ☑ Re-evaluation ☑ Treatment session
Learner objectives	1. Identify the objective values for appropriate progression of a postoperative patient with multiligamentous knee reconstruction for return to running and sports participation. 2. Describe the common functional deficits that occur after ligament reconstructive surgery and preventive measure to minimize future injuries. 3. Apply the principles of movement science to develop functional and sport-specific exercises for athletes returning from knee injury.

Medical	
Chief complaint	Unable to run and play sports; he has read that people can return to sports after 6 months of rehab after ACL injury and he is only 1 week away from that timeline.
History of present illness	The patient is 16-year-old male who is 23 weeks postoperative and wants to return to high school football and baseball.
Past medical history	Asthma
Past surgical history	ACL and PCL reconstruction with partial lateral meniscectomy—left knee (23 weeks ago) See below for further information.
Allergies	Peanuts
Medications	Albuterol inhaler as needed
Precautions/Orders	Begin return to sport FWB LLE

Medical management	
Surgical intervention (vascular surgery—27 weeks ago)	The patient underwent a thrombectomy via catheter with suturing of the intimal flap. To avoid restenosis, the repair utilized a saphenous vein patch from the contralateral leg.
Surgical intervention (orthopaedic surgery—23 weeks ago)	A review of the patient's postoperative report shows that he underwent a hamstring tendon autograft for reconstruction of the ACL and patella tendon autograft for reconstruction of the PCL arthroscopically.

Social history	
Home setup	Prior to accident: • Lives with his parents, younger sister, and dog in a two-story home. • Four steps to enter, with right handrail when ascending. • Bedroom is on second floor. • Half bathroom on first floor, full bathroom on second floor. • Indoor stairs have handrails on both sides. Upon hospital discharge: • Modified independent with bilateral axillary crutches for transfers, gait, and stair negotiation. • Modified independent for ADLs—sits to dress, uses a shower bench for bathing. Currently: • Independent with all functional mobility and ADLs.
Occupation	• Full-time high school student. • Busses tables at a local restaurant on the weekends.
Prior level of function	• Independent with all activities of daily living.
Recreational activities	• Starting high school quarterback in the fall. • Starting shortstop for baseball in the spring.

Physical Therapy Examination		
Subjective		
"My knee feels like it forgot everything it used to do."		
Objective		
General	Observation	• Well-nourished, fit, high school male. Presents with no sign of antalgic gait, and no effusion.
	Pain level (left knee)	0/10 at rest. 2/10 with running on the treadmill for 5 minutes.

(Continued)

(Continued)

	Physical Therapy Examination		
	Effusion (sweep test) ▶ Fig. 1.2	Right knee: 0 Left knee: 0	
Cardiovascular and pulmonary	Blood pressure (mmHg)	115/76	
	Heart rate (beat/min)	68	
	Respiratory rate (breath/min)	14	
	Pulse oximetry on room air (SpO$_2$)	99%	
Integumentary	• Unremarkable, incisions well healed		
Musculoskeletal	Range of motion (knee flexion)	Right	Left
		4–0–136 degrees	4–0–134 degrees
	Strength (isometric MVIC[a] knee extension)	58 kg peak force	49 kg peak force
Neurological	Cognition	• Alert and oriented x four	
	Reflexes	• Patellar: 2 + bilaterally • Achilles: 2 + bilaterally	
	Sensation	• Intact bilaterally	
	Functional status		
Ambulation	• Ambulated more than 250 feet independently. • Gait deviations are unremarkable; none observed.		
Running on treadmill	• RLE: unremarkable • LLE: the patient exhibits a mild pelvic drop at midstance. He presents with excessive left hip internal rotation in terminal stance, decreased left knee flexion motion during swing, and decreased left knee flexion during midstance.		
Sport specific	Single leg hop tests: Single hop Triple hop	Right 137 cm 433 cm	Left 121 cm 363 cm
Functional outcomes	LESS[b] score = 8 IKDC[c] score = 82.8		

[a]Maximum volitional isometric contraction (MVIC) measured at 60 degrees of knee flexion.
[b]Landing error scoring system.
[c]International Knee Documentation Committee Subjective Knee Form.

Pause points
Based on the above information: • Review any tests and measures that are unfamiliar. • What factors can be contributing to his gait abnormalities with running? • What additional tests and measures does the physical therapist want to assess in this patient? • Will the patient be ready for his upcoming baseball season in 2 weeks?

	Assessment
☑ Physical therapist's	*Assessment left blank for learner to develop*
	Goals
Patient's	"I want to run so I can get back to football."
Short term	1.
	Goals left blank for learner to develop.
	2.

(Continued)

(Continued)

Assessment	
Long term	1.
	Goals left blank for learner to develop.
	2.

Plan	
☐ Physician's ☑ Physical therapist's ☐ Other's	Develop a treatment plan to meet the minimum acceptable criteria for return to sport (> 90% knee extension peak isometric strength ratio, IKDC > 90, LESS score < 5, hop testing ratio > 90%, and symmetrical running mechanics via video analysis of treadmill running.

Bloom's Taxonomy Level	Case 1.C Questions
Create	1. Synthesizing the medical data and physical examination findings, develop an appropriate physical therapy assessment of the patient. 2. Develop two short-term physical therapy goals, including an appropriate timeframe. 3. Develop two long-term physical therapy goals, including an appropriate timeframe.
Evaluate	4. How would the physical therapist explain to the patient and his parents, although he feels like he is ready to return to sport, current evidence suggests he is not ready?
Analyze	5. Compare the differences for each goal for return to sport minimum criteria in the physical therapy plan. Why is there a need for a battery of different tests for return to sport?
Apply	6. Identify two strength-related factors and one range of motion–related factor that can contribute to dynamic knee valgus with LESS testing and describe interventions to address these factors.
Understand	7. The physical therapist notices excessive hip internal rotation and increased pelvic drop with the patient's running mechanics. What should be assessed and addressed to improve these mechanical inefficiencies that were not assessed previously?
Remember	8. What is the risk for ACL reconstructions who return to competitive sport prior to 7 months? 9. What is the re-tear rate in individuals returning to sport following an ACL reconstruction? 10. How can ACL injury prevention programs reduce the rate of initial injuries?

Bloom's Taxonomy Level	Case 1.C Answers

Create	1. The patient is 23 weeks postoperative for an ACL and PCL reconstruction. He is able to perform all ADLs without any difficulty, but he is unable to complete age-appropriate activities such as running, jumping, and quickly changing direction. Upon the physical therapy assessment, knee flexion ROM is shy 2 degrees compared to the contralateral limb, quadriceps MVIC ratio is 84.4%, single leg single hop test scored is 88%, single leg triple hop test scored is 84%, and the IKDC is 82.8 points. At this time, the patient is not cleared for return to sport, as he is at a significantly higher risk of re-injury in his left knee based on the values noted earlier. The patient would benefit from additional physical therapy to improve lower extremity strength and neuromuscular control to maximize recovery to his prior level of function.
	2. Short-term goals:
	  • The patient will demonstrate single leg single hop test equal to his uninvolved lower extremity in 2 weeks.
	  • The patient will improve his IKDC score to > 90 in 2 weeks.
	3. Long-term goals:
	  • The patient will demonstrate > 90% quadriceps MVIC strength ratio compared to the uninvolved leg in 8 weeks to allow for full running, and beginning of a progressive return to on-field program.
	  • The patient will demonstrate a LESS score of < 5 in 8 weeks to allow for optimal lower extremity mechanics during age-appropriate functional activities.

(Continued)

(Continued)

Bloom's Taxonomy Level	Case 1.C Answers
Evaluate	4. While there is limited to no research at this time on return to sport criteria after a traumatic knee dislocation as in this current case, there is a growing body of evidence regarding return to sport time after an ACL reconstruction. Current research suggests that returning to sports after 6 months from surgery is possible but results in an approximately sevenfold increased rate of sustaining a second ACL injury compared to those that wait 9 months. Moreover, this does not account for the additional ligamentous involvement and initial vascular injury in this specific patient case. It is important that the patient and his parents understand that he has not met the minimum requirements in his physical therapy plan. With additional months of continued physical therapy, this will improve the odds for preventing a future knee injury.
Analyze	5. Strength, power, movement quality, and balance are all trained and assessed differently. Simply because a quadriceps MVIC ratio of 100% does not mean they will also successfully pass the hop test battery. Moreover, if the patient exhibits weak hip abductors or poor motor control patterns, the patient will likely not meet the minimum criteria on the LESS test. Due to the reduction in strength, power, and proprioception of the involved lower extremity after reconstructive surgery, each test needs to be considered individually for the full picture of the athlete prior to clearing them for returning to sport.
Apply	6. Dynamic knee valgus has many contributing factors including quadriceps strength, hamstring strength, ankle pronation, and others that increase the risk of ACL injuries when uncontrolled. The primary strength factors which should be assessed include quadriceps strength and gluteal strength, although knee flexion strength has been shown to be relevant. From a mobility perspective, decreased ankle dorsiflexion motion can cause excessive foot pronation with running and jumping, or contribute to excessive tibial internal rotation and dynamic knee valgus.
Understand	7. A wide variety of limitations can be contributing to the patient's movement pattern asymmetries with running. Suggested musculoskeletal objective measures for these asymmetries should include ankle dorsiflexion mobility and strength of the soleus or gastrocnemius, as deficits in these areas can cause biomechanical alterations through the principal of regional interdependence. Weakness of the hip abductors or extensors can lead to compensation of excessive hip internal rotation and is likely to contribute to the pelvic drop noted in midstance. Additionally, weakness of the hamstrings on the involved lower extremity could be contributing to his decreased knee flexion in swing phase of running.
Remember	8. Athletes returning prior to 7 months are nearly three times more likely to sustain a second ACL injury than those who return after 7 months. Furthermore, for each month of a delayed return to competitive sport, injury risk is reduced by 51% up to 9 months postoperative. 9. Research has shown a 21% re-injury rate to the involved knee, with additional 38% contralateral limb injury. 10. ACL injury prevention programs have shown a risk reduction of 52 and 85% in female and male soccer players, respectively.

Key points
1. Knee ROM, quadriceps MVIC, LESS scores, IKDC scores, and hop testing should all be utilized as objective measures prior to determining when a patient is able to return to sport. Increasing research is suggesting return to sport times increase to 9 months after surgery, as meeting minimum objective criteria is challenging to complete in 6 months or less.
2. Functional deficits after ACL and multiligament knee reconstruction mostly develop around the concept of preventing dynamic knee valgus. This movement can be altered by several factors including range of motion of the ankle, knee, and hip; strength of hamstrings, quadriceps, and gluteal muscles; functional power with hop testing; and neuromuscular control of landing mechanics.
3. Prior to initiating sport-specific training, the patient should demonstrate symmetrical strength and good neuromuscular control of the involved lower extremity. Progressive speed, agility, and change of direction should be added as necessary to help return this patient for football as a quarterback. If he was a volleyball player, additional time should be spent on jump landing mechanics and hopping progressions. While all athletes should have a foundational strength in each objective measure, additional challenges may be needed prior to returning to all unrestricted sport activities.

Suggested Readings

Adams D, Logerstedt DS, Hunter-Giordano A, Axe MJ, Snyder-Mackler L. Current concepts for anterior cruciate ligament reconstruction: a criterion-based rehabilitation progression. J Orthop Sports Phys Ther. 2012; 42(7):601–614

Beischer S, Gustavsson L, Senorski EH, et al. Young athletes who return to sport before 9 months after anterior cruciate ligament reconstruction have a rate of new injury 7 times that of those who delay return. J Orthop Sports Phys Ther. 2020; 50(2):83–90

Claiborne TL, Armstrong CW, Gandhi V, Pincivero DM. Relationship between hip and knee strength and knee valgus during a single leg squat. J Appl Biomech. 2006; 22(1):41–50

Gray JL. Management of arterial and venous injuries in the dislocated knee. Oper Tech Sports Med. 2015; 23(4):362–371

Green NE, Allen BL. Vascular injuries associated with dislocation of the knee. J Bone Joint Surg Am. 1977; 59(2):236–239

Grindem H, Snyder-Mackler L, Moksnes H, Engebretsen L, Risberg MA. Simple decision rules can reduce reinjury risk by 84% after ACL reconstruction: the Delaware-Oslo ACL cohort study. Br J Sports Med. 2016; 50(13):804–808

Henrichs A. A review of knee dislocations. J Athl Train. 2004; 39(4):365–369

Hewett TE, Myer GD, Ford KR, et al. Biomechanical measures of neuromuscular control and valgus loading of the knee predict anterior cruciate ligament injury risk in female athletes: a prospective study. Am J Sports Med. 2005; 33(4):492–501

Holm I, Oiestad BE, Risberg MA, Gunderson R, Aune AK. No differences in prevalence of osteoarthritis or function after open versus endoscopic technique for anterior cruciate ligament reconstruction: 12-year follow-up of a randomized controlled trial. Am J Sports Med. 2012; 40(11):2492–2498

Honsik K, Boyd A, Rubin AL. Sideline splinting, bracing, and casting of extremity injuries. Curr Sports Med Rep. 2003; 2(3):147–154

Hopkins JT, Ingersoll CD. Arthrogenic muscle inhibition: a limiting factor in joint rehabilitation. J Sport Rehabil. 2000; 9(2):135–159

Irrgang JJ, Anderson AF, Boland AL, et al. Development and validation of the international knee documentation committee subjective knee form. Am J Sports Med. 2001; 29(5):600–613

Irrgang JJ, Anderson AF. Development and validation of health-related quality of life measures for the knee. Clin Orthop Relat Res. 2002(402):95–109

Karkos CD, Koudounas G, Giagtzidis IT, Mitka MA, Pliatsios I, Papazoglou KO. Traumatic knee dislocation and popliteal artery injury: a case series. Ann Vasc Surg. 2018; 50:298.e13–298.e16

Laboute E, Savalli L, Puig P, et al. Analysis of return to competition and repeat rupture for 298 anterior cruciate ligament reconstructions with patellar or hamstring tendon autograft in sportspeople. Ann Phys Rehabil Med. 2010; 53(10):598–614

Lima YL, Ferreira VMLM, de Paula Lima PO, Bezerra MA, de Oliveira RR, Almeida GPL. The association of ankle dorsiflexion and dynamic knee valgus: a systematic review and meta-analysis. Phys Ther Sport. 2018; 29:61–69

Medina O, Arom GA, Yeranosian MG, Petrigliano FA, McAllister DR. Vascular and nerve injury after knee dislocation: a systematic review. Clin Orthop Relat Res. 2014; 472(9):2621–2629

Nessler T, Denney L, Sampley J. ACL injury prevention: what does research tell us? Curr Rev Musculoskelet Med. 2017; 10(3):281–288

Pardiwala DN, Rao NN, Anand K, Raut A. Knee dislocations in sports injuries. Indian J Orthop. 2017; 51(5):552–562

Palmieri-Smith RM, Thomas AC, Wojtys EM. Maximizing quadriceps strength after ACL reconstruction. Clin Sports Med. 2008; 27(3):405–424, vii–ix

Padua DA, DiStefano LJ, Beutler AI, de la Motte SJ, DiStefano MJ, Marshall SW. The landing error scoring system as a screening tool for an anterior cruciate ligament injury-prevention program in elite-youth soccer athletes. J Athl Train. 2015; 50(6):589–595

Robertson A, Nutton RW, Keating JF. Dislocation of the knee. J Bone Joint Surg Br. 2006; 88(6):706–711

Schenck RC, Jr. The dislocated knee. Instr Course Lect. 1994; 43:127–136

Sekiya JK, Whiddon DR, Zehms CT, Miller MD. A clinically relevant assessment of posterior cruciate ligament and posterolateral corner injuries. Evaluation of isolated and combined deficiency. J Bone Joint Surg Am. 2008; 90(8):1621–1627

Senese M, Greenberg E, Todd Lawrence J, Ganley T. Rehabilitation following isolated posterior cruciate ligament reconstruction: a literature review of published literature. Int J Sports Phys Ther. 2018; 13(4):737–751

Seroyer ST, Musahl V, Harner CD. Management of the acute knee dislocation: the Pittsburgh experience. Injury. 2008; 39(7):710–718

Smith D. Are all physical therapists qualified to provide sideline coverage of athletic events? Int J Sports Phys Ther. 2012; 7(1):120–123

Stannard JP, Sheils TM, Lopez-Ben RR, McGwin G, Jr, Robinson JT, Volgas DA. Vascular injuries in knee dislocations: the role of physical examination in determining the need for arteriography. J Bone Joint Surg Am. 2004; 86(5):910–915

Sturgill LP, Snyder-Mackler L, Manal TJ, Axe MJ. Interrater reliability of a clinical scale to assess knee joint effusion. J Orthop Sports Phys Ther. 2009; 39(12):845–849

Swartz EE, Boden BP, Courson RW, et al. National athletic trainers' association position statement: acute management of the cervical spine-injured athlete. J Athl Train. 2009; 44(3):306–331

Waschar DC, Bulthuis L. Extremity trauma: field management of sports injuries. Curr Rev Musculoskelet Med. 2014; 7(4):387–393

Wright RW, Haas AK, Anderson J, et al. MOON Group. Anterior cruciate ligament reconstruction rehabilitation: MOON guidelines. Sports Health. 2015; 7(3):239–243

Wellsandt E, Failla MJ, Snyder-Mackler L. Limb symmetry indexes can overestimate knee function after anterior cruciate ligament injury. J Orthop Sports Phys Ther. 2017; 47(5):334–338

2 Breast Cancer

General Information	
Case no.	2.A Breast Cancer
Authors	Aubree Colorito, PT, DPT, COS-C, Board-Certified Clinical Specialist in Oncologic Physical Therapy Kathleen L. Ehrhardt, MMS, PA-C, DFAAPA Judith Schaad, PT, DPT, CWS, CLT-LANA, Board Certified Clinical Specialist in Oncology Physical Therapy
Diagnosis	Right breast cancer
Setting	Outpatient clinic
Learner expectations	☑ Initial evaluation ☐ Re-evaluation ☐ Treatment session
Learner objectives	1. Understand rationale for the prospective surveillance model for detection of early lymphedema. 2. Understand significance of gathering key baseline data prior to cancer therapy. 3. Know risk reduction strategies for patients undergoing lymph node dissection.

Medical	
Chief complaint	Pre-op evaluation prior to mastectomy.
History of present illness	Patient is a 39-year-old female who presents for evaluation prior to right breast mastectomy and sentinel node biopsy for early breast cancer. Stage 2A cT2 cN0 cM0. Surgical procedure is scheduled in 1 week.
Past medical history	Infiltrating ductal carcinoma of the right breast, BRCA 1/2 negative, hypothyroidism, two uncomplicated pregnancies with vaginal deliveries.
Past surgical history	Breast biopsy right breast, appendectomy age 18
Family history	Mother: breast cancer diagnosed at age 49, no residual disease, hypothyroidism. Father: hypertension, hypercholesterolemia, myocardial infarction at age 62. Brother: alive and well.
Allergies	No known drug allergies.
Medications	Levothyroxine, Multivitamin
Precautions/Orders	Activity as tolerated.

Social history	
Home setup	• Resides in a multilevel home with husband and children. • Three steps + two handrails to enter. • Half bathroom is on the first floor. • Master bedroom and bathroom are located on the first floor. • Children's bedrooms located on the second floor. • Flight of stairs + two handrails to second floor.
Occupation	• College professor, currently off for summer.
Prior level of function	• Independent with functional mobility and activities of daily living. • Right handed • (+) Driver
Recreational activities	• Swims daily at local health club. • Enjoys cooking and spending time with husband and two children aged 12 and 15.

Imaging/Diagnostic tests	
Bilateral screening mammography	Right breast revealing suspicious microcalcifications. BIRADS 4—biopsy should be considered. Left breast without abnormalities.
Diagnostic mammography	Confirms screening mammography results.
Breast biopsy	Infiltrating ductal carcinoma, stage 2A cT2 cN0 cM0.
Hormone receptor tests, HER2 neu test	ER–/PR–/HER2 neu– Triple negative breast cancer
BRCA testing	BRCA negative
Transvaginal ultrasound	Normal appearance of uterus, tubes, and ovaries.

Medical management	
Right breast cancer, BRCA negative, triple negative tumor	Plan for right mastectomy and right sentinel lymph node biopsy in 1 week. Will perform lymph node dissection if sentinel lymph node biopsy positive.

Pause points
Based on the above information, what are the priority • Diagnostic tests and measures? • Outcome measures? • Treatment interventions?

Physical Therapy Examination		
Subjective		
"I am nervous about getting lymphedema."		
Objective		
Vital signs	Pre-treatment	Post-treatment
Blood pressure (mmHg)	112/70	113/72
Heart rate (beats/min)	87	75
Respiratory rate (breaths/min)	19	15
Pulse oximetry on room air (SpO$_2$)	98%	97
Pain	0/10	0/10
General	• Patient sitting in examination room, appears anxious. • Husband accompanies patient to visit.	
Head, ears, eyes, nose, and throat (HEENT)	• NCAT, neck FROM without lymphadenopathy.	
Cardiovascular and pulmonary	• Normal rate and rhythm • Auscultation: clear to adventitious sounds	
Musculoskeletal	Range of motion	• Bilateral upper extremities (BUE): within functional limit (WFL). • Bilateral lower extremities (BLE): WFL. • All ROM is pain free.
	Strength	• BUE: Grossly 5/5 • BLE: Grossly 5/5 • Five Times Sit-to-Stand Test = 11 seconds
	Aerobic	• Able to walk > 250 feet with an RPE 2/10

(Continued)

(Continued)

Physical Therapy Examination		
	Flexibility	• Good appropriate hamstring length as shown by long sit to get out of bed.
	Other	• N/A
Neurological	Balance	• SLS = 15 seconds on left lower extremity, 20 seconds on RLE. • Tandem stance: 25 seconds, mild postural sway, self corrects.
	Cognition	• Alert and oriented x 4 • Follows 100% of multistep commands.
	Coordination	• Finger-to-nose: intact BUE • Heel-to-shin: intact BLE
	Cranial nerves	• II–XII: intact
	Reflexes	• Biceps: 2 + bilaterally • Patellar: 2 + bilaterally
	Sensation	• Vibration testing with 128 Hz tuning fork: normal at ulnar styloid and MTP bilaterally.
	Tone	• Normal throughout BUEs and BLEs
	Other	• N/A
Integumentary	Skin integrity	• BUE and chest wall: intact; negative for irritation, drainage, erythema, and scars
	Limb volumes	• Left upper extremity (LUE): 2.38 L • Right upper extremity (RUE): 2.45 L • RUE > LUE by 2.9% ▶ Fig. 2.1
Functional status		
Bed mobility		• Supine to/from sit: independent
Transfers		• Sit to/from stand: independent
Ambulation		• Ambulated 250 feet independently. • Demonstrated normal gait pattern.
Stairs		• Ascend/descend 12 steps independently with no railing. • Demonstrated step-over-step pattern.
Other		• Health-related quality-of-life outcome measure: FACT B + 4: Score = 111/148 = 75%

Assessment	
☑ Physical therapist's	*Assessment left blank for learner to develop.*
Goals	
Patient's	"I want to do anything I can to prevent getting lymphedema."
Short term	1. *Goals left blank for learner to develop.* 2.
Long term	1. *Goals left blank for learner to develop.* 2.

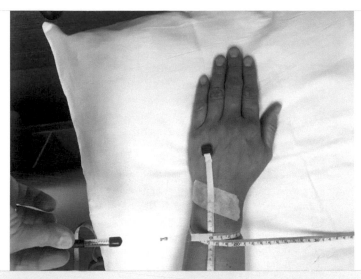

Fig. 2.1 Standardized evidence-based protocol for facility/health system is to mark off limb at 4-cm intervals. One should start at the wrist and progress along the length of the arm, using a tape measure. Measurements are then recorded using a calibrated tape measure to standardize results. Once circumferential measurements are recorded, they are entered into a formula that calculates the volume of a truncated cone. The result is an approximation of the limb volume. One can then compare the difference between the involved arm volume and the uninvolved as a percentage.

Plan	
☐ Physician's ☑ Physical therapist's ☐ Other's	Physical therapist provided home exercise program (HEP) ▸ Fig. 2.2 Physical therapist provided post-op education re: ROM precautions, limiting shoulder flexion to 90 degrees on surgical side until drains removed. Physical therapist provided education re: rationale and protocol for prospective surveillance for early lymphedema and lymphedema risk reduction practices.

Bloom's Taxonomy Level	Case 2.A Questions
Create	1. Synthesizing the medical data and physical examination findings, develop an appropriate physical therapy assessment of the patient. 2. Develop 2 short-term physical therapy goals, including an appropriate timeframe for home care. 3. Develop 2 long-term physical therapy goals, including an appropriate timeframe for home care.
Evaluate	4. Explain the physical therapy findings and plan of care to the medical team.
Analyze	5. Compare and contrast lymphedema incidence after sentinel node biopsy versus axillary lymph node dissection. 6. Compare and contrast interventions for breast cancer–related lymphedema when detected early (subclinical or < 5% change) to when detected visibly or 10% or more change.
Apply	7. Explain the different types of breast cancer receptor testing that should be done on patient's breast cancer and why testing is beneficial.
Understand	8. Discuss the indications for mastectomy in a patient with early breast cancer 9. Explain the significance of triple negative breast cancer. 10. Explain what it is and the general application of the American Joint Committee on Cancer staging system. Interpret the TMN nomenclature.
Remember	11. What is the most common diagnosed cancer in women and the second most common cause of cancer death in women? 12. Recall the most common histologic type of invasive breast cancer. 13. What is BRCA testing? What are the indications for BRCA testing in men and women?

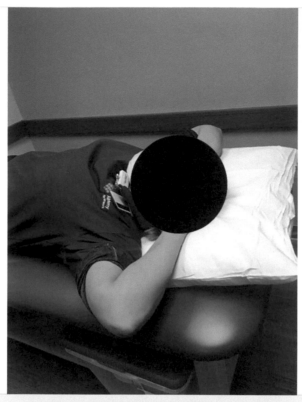

Fig. 2.2 Example of a pectoralis stretch, which can be provided as part of the home exercise program.

Bloom's Taxonomy Level	Case 2.A Answers

Create	1. Patient is a 39-year-old female who presents for evaluation prior to right breast mastectomy and sentinel node biopsy for early breast cancer—stage 2A cT2 cN0 cM0. The patient demonstrates normal AROM and strength of BUE and BLEs, normal vibration sense of BUEs and BLEs, normal postural stability, and normal functional mobility on even and uneven levels. Baseline UE limb volume difference is 2.9%, involved dominant RUE is greater than nondominant LUE. This difference is likely due to typical increased in size of dominant UE. At this time, patient was provided with HEP, of which she verbalized and demonstrated understanding. Patient will be seen 1-month post-op to reassess her functional status and modify program accordingly. Will continue to follow per Prospective Surveillance Model.
	2. Short-term goals:
	  • Patient will independently verbalize understanding of rationale for prospective monitoring for early lymphedema and ways to decrease risk of developing lymphedema within one visit.
	  • Patient will independently demonstrate post-op HEP within one visit to maintain ROM and strength in BUEs and BLEs.
	3. Long-term goals:
	  • Patient will follow up with outpatient physical therapist within 4–6 weeks post-op.

Evaluate	4. Patient exhibited baseline arm volume differences with normal functional levels. The baseline arm volume difference is expected in the pre-op setting. Typically, the volume of the dominant arm is 3–5% greater than the nondominant side, due to greater use and muscle hypertrophy. Certain athletes, such as tennis players, may have as much as 10% volume difference at baseline. Baseline information is critical to gather in cancer patients prior to beginning any medical treatments, as they can be used for later comparisons. These data points may be critical to compare later. This is especially true if the patient

(Continued)

(Continued)

Bloom's Taxonomy Level	Case 2.A Answers
	should receive chemotherapy, as it can cause peripheral neuropathy or breast cancer–related lymphedema. The patient is aware of the risk for lymphedema after lymph node dissection, recommendations to follow that may help reduce her risk, and how to restart upper body activity after breast cancer surgery. The Prospective Surveillance Model of care for breast cancer survivors is the current standard for accredited breast centers. Risk reduction strategies should they arise include: • A gradual return to normal activities: avoid overuse and lymph congestion in the early weeks after surgery. • Pay close attention to any break in the skin: wash with soap and water, apply antibiotic ointment and cover until healed, inspecting for any signs of infection. • Call a physician immediately if any signs of infection are noted in the lymphatic drainage quadrant (arm, chest, lateral and posterior trunk): warmth, redness, pain, swelling, tenderness. • Avoid blood pressures and injections/blood draws on the affected arm, and consider a prophylactic compression sleeve and gauntlet for long air flights.
Analyze	5. The risk of developing lymphedema after a sentinel node biopsy is 3–6%. The risk of developing lymphedema after an axillary lymph node dissection is 15–25%. 6. When lymphedema is detected at the subclinical stage (5% relative limb volume change), patients should be fitted with a light (20–30 mmHg) compression sleeve and gauntlet (handpiece) and wear it from wakeup until bedtime, 10–12 hours per day for 4–5 weeks. When relative limb volume differences return to baseline, the patient can reduce wear time of the compressive sleeve and gauntlet to strenuous activities. In contrast, when lymphedema is detected later (> 10% relative limb volume change), complex decongestive therapy (CDT) is required to reduce swelling. This intervention includes the following components: • Phase 1: lymph drainage massage, multilayer compression bandaging 24/7, decongestive exercises, and skin care education. In-person treatments are required three to five times per week. • After 4–6 weeks of Phase 1, when the limb volume is decreased and stabilized (often not to baseline level), patient must wear substantial day and night compression garments for the rest of their lives. This is Phase 2, or the maintenance phase.
Apply	7. Breast pathology specimens are tested for estrogen receptor (ER) and progesterone receptors (PR). Patients who are positive for ER, PR, or both are candidates for endocrine therapy in the treatment of their breast cancer. If human epidermal growth factor receptor 2 (HFR2) is positive, patients are given HER2-directed therapy.
Understand	8. Mastectomy is recommended for women with early breast cancer when (a) the tumor is large in size compared to the breast; (b) there are diffuse malignant-appearing calcifications on imaging; (c) the patient has a prior history of chest radiation, pregnancy, multicentric disease; or (d) the patient has persistently positive margins. Mastectomy is also a patient-preferred choice in some instances. 9. The significance of triple negative breast cancer is that these tumors do not express ER, PR, and HER2. These types of tumors tend to be more aggressive. There is no targeted therapy available for these patients. Unfortunately, these tumors tend to occur in women younger than 40. 10. The American Joint Commission on Cancer (AJCC) created a rating system to determine the extent of cancer, the location, and subtype. It includes a number and letter and TMN indicators. Number stages range from stage 1 to stage 4, with 4 being the most advanced. Letters (A–C) add more information to the stage. Determining the letter assignment is beyond the scope of this discussion. Invasive breast cancer is indicated by stages 2–4 and is a cancer that has spread from the ducts or lobules into surrounding breast tissue or nearby lymph nodes. TMN nomenclature provides more details about the cancer. T: stands for the size of the tumor and extent of spread to nearby tissues. N: stands for nodes, indicates if the cancer has spread to the nearby lymph nodes and how many nodes are involved.

(Continued)

(Continued)

Bloom's Taxonomy Level	Case 2.A Answers
	M: stands for metastasis and indicated Yes (1) or No (0), whether metastasis has been detected elsewhere in the body.
	Clinical stage (c) is the rating before any treatment. It is based on the physical exam, biopsy, and imaging results. Pathologic stage (p) or surgical stage is determined by the evaluation of tissue removed at the time of surgery. If drug therapy is given before surgery, then the stage nomenclature will indicate by adding (y) to the TMN stage. For this patient at the presurgery visit, her stage is 2A: cT2 cN0 cM0. If drug therapy has been administered prior to surgery with the same clinical findings, TNM stage would be 2A: yT2 yN0 yM0.
Remember	11. Breast cancer is the most diagnosed cancer in women as well as the second most common cause of cancer death in women. The most common cause of cancer death in women is lung cancer.
	12. Infiltrating ductal carcinoma is the most common histologic type of invasive breast cancer occurring in 76% of patients.
	13. Indications for BRCA testing in females include: • A personal history of breast cancer diagnosed at younger than 50 years and a second primary breast cancer, one or more relatives with breast cancer, or an unknown or limited family medical history. • A personal history of triple-negative breast cancer diagnosed at younger than 60 years. • A personal history of ovarian cancer. • Two or more of the following: breast cancer; ovarian, fallopian, or primary peritoneal cancer; male breast cancer; or metastatic prostate cancer. Indications for BRCA testing in males include: • A personal history of male breast cancer. • A personal history of prostate or pancreatic cancer with two or more relatives with BRCA-associated cancers. Indications for BRCA testing in females and males include: • A personal history of two or more types of cancer. • A personal history of breast cancer and Ashkenazi Jewish ancestry. • A history of breast cancer at a young age in two or more blood relatives. • A relative with a known BRCA1 or BRCA2 mutation.

Key points
1. It is important to measure and document pre-op circumferences and volumes of both arms. This can help detect breast cancer–related lymphedema at a subclinical, early stage and treat timely. This model of care can effectively prevent the onset of clinical lymphedema, which requires lifelong and costly care that impacts quality of life.
2. Patients seen for a pre-op visit should have baseline multisystem screening of all relevant tests and measures that could be impacted by later treatments, including surgery, radiation, and/or chemotherapy. Examples of side effects of these treatments can include soft-tissue restrictions, weakness, peripheral neuropathy, balance impairments, functional deficits, and pain.
3. It is important to educate patients early and often regarding lifelong risk reduction strategies, which can help avoid the onset of lymphedema, when possible.

General Information	
Case no.	2.B
Authors	Aubree Colorito, PT, DPT, COS-C, Board-Certified Clinical Specialist in Oncologic Physical Therapy Kathleen L. Ehrhardt, MMS, PA-C, DFAAPA Judith Schaad, PT, DPT, CWS, CLT-LANA, Board Certified Clinical Specialist in Oncology Physical Therapy
Diagnosis	Right breast cancer, positive sentinel node biopsy s/p right modified radical mastectomy, and lymph node dissection
Setting	Acute care hospital

(Continued)

(Continued)

General Information	
Learner expectations	☑ Initial evaluation ☐ Re-evaluation ☐ Treatment session
Learner objectives	1. Understand the differences in surgical procedures and their associated side effects. 2. Understand the importance of maintaining postoperative protocols during physical therapy assessment and intervention to minimize side effects while maximizing outcomes. 3. Understand the importance of patient education to improve compliance with a HEP.

Medical	
Chief complaint	s/p right mastectomy and full lymph node dissection yesterday.
History of present illness	Patient is a 39-year-old female who is hospital day 1, post-op day 1 s/p right modified radical mastectomy and lymph node dissection. Triple negative tumor. No reconstruction done due to patient wishes. Patient had sentinel node biopsy during procedure and frozen section was positive for tumor. Patient has been out of bed to bathroom and has ambulated once in the hall with nursing.
Past medical history	Infiltrating ductal carcinoma of the right breast, s/p right mastectomy and lymph node dissection, BRCA 1/2 negative, hypothyroidism, two uncomplicated pregnancies with vaginal deliveries.
Past surgical history	Right mastectomy, lymph node dissection, breast biopsy of right breast, appendectomy at age 18.
Family history	Mother: breast cancer diagnosed at age 49, no residual disease, hypothyroidism Father: hypertension, hypercholesterolemia, myocardial infarction at age 62 Brother: alive and well.
Allergies	No known drug allergies.
Medications	Levothyroxine, Hydrocodone, Ibuprofen, Docusate sodium, Zolpidem tartrate.
Precautions/Orders	Activity as tolerated, right arm in sling, right axillary drain. Right upper extremity (RUE) post-op precautions: non–weight-bearing, no flexion > 90 degrees until right axillary drain removed and no lifting.

Social history	
Home setup	• Resides in a multilevel home with husband and children. • Three steps plus two handrails to enter. • Half bathroom is on the first floor. • Master bedroom and bathroom are located on the first floor. • Children's bedrooms are located on the second floor. • Flight of stairs plus two handrails to second floor.
Occupation	• College professor, currently off for summer.
Prior level of function	• Independent with functional mobility and activities of daily living. • Right handed • (+) driver
Recreational activities	• Swims daily at local health club. • Enjoys cooking and spending time with husband and two children aged 12 and 15.

Vital signs	Hospital day 1: postoperative day 1, ward
Blood pressure (mmHg)	130/82
Heart rate (beats/min)	83

(Continued)

Vital signs	Hospital day 1: postoperative day 1, ward
Respiratory rate (breaths/min)	16
Pulse oximetry on room air (SpO$_2$)	94%
Temperature (°F)	98.8

Lab		Reference range	Hospital day 0: pre-op	Hospital day 1: ward
Complete blood cell count	White blood cell	5.0–10.0 × 10^9/L	9.8	9.2
	Red blood cell	4.1–5.3 million/mcL	4.0	5.24
	Hemoglobin	12–16 g/dL	14	11.6
	Hematocrit	37–47%	42%	35.5%
	Platelets	140–400 K/µL	260	178

Medical management	Hospital day 1: postoperative day 1, ward
Medications	1. Acetaminophen PRN pain 2. Ibuprofen PRN pain 3. Oxycodone PRN pain
Surgical oncology team.	1. Infiltrating ductal carcinoma with positive sentinel node, final pathology report pending. 2. Maintain sling, drain, and dressing for 2 weeks post-op. 3. Education on axillary drain to be provided upon hospital discharge.
Oncology team	1. Expected hospitalization is 3–5 days.
Precautions	• Activity as tolerated • Fall risk • No blood pressure in RUE • RUE in sling • Post-op precautions for RUE: non–weight-bearing, no flexion > 90 degrees until right axillary drain removed, no lifting.

Pause points
Based on the above information, what are the priority • Diagnostic tests and measures? • Outcome measures? • Treatment interventions?

Hospital Day 1, Postoperative Day 1, Ward: Physical Therapy Examination		
Subjective		
"I feel a little tired today"		
Objective		
Vital signs	Pre-treatment	Post-treatment
Blood pressure (mmHg)	126/82	128/84
Heart rate (beats/min)	78	87
Respiratory rate (breaths/min)	16	16

(Continued)

(Continued)

Hospital Day 1, Postoperative Day 1, Ward: Physical Therapy Examination		
Pulse oximetry on room air (SpO₂)	94%	96%
BORG scale	6	7
Pain	5/10 incisional	7/10 incisional
	• Patient with 5/10 pain at rest that increases with RUE in dependent position and during HEP. • Patient describes that pain as a stretching/pulling sensation in the front of her shoulder and around the incision.	
General	• Patient resting in hospital bed, holding pillow over right side of chest. Occasionally winces with movement. • Dressing clean, dry, and intact • Lines notable for peripheral IV access and 2 Jackson-Pratt drains with 20 mL serosanguinous fluid, peripheral IV access (▶ Fig. 2.3).	
Cardiovascular and pulmonary	• Normal rate and rhythm • Auscultation: mild decrease in breath sounds in right lower lobe. • Radial pulse: 2 + bilaterally	
Gastrointestinal	• Bowel sounds present × 4 quadrants • Soft, nontender, no organomegaly	
Musculoskeletal	Range of motion	• R scapular movements: poor coupling, increased scapular elevation noted • R shoulder flexion: 0–90 degrees • R shoulder abduction: 0–90 degrees *limited due to post-op precautions* • R elbow: 0–120 degrees • Left upper extremity (LUE): within functional limit (WFL) • Bilateral lower extremities (BLE): WFL
	Strength	• R shoulder flexion: 3/5 • R shoulder abduction: 3/5 • R elbow flexion: 3/5 • R elbow extension: 3/5 • R hand grip: good *resistance not applied due to post-op precautions* • LUE: grossly 5/5 • BLE: grossly 5/5
	Aerobic	• Did not perform formal assessment at this time.
	Flexibility	• Patient seated in a forward flexed posture guarding right shoulder with noted increase in pain to neutral position.
	Other	• N/A
Neurological	Balance	• Static sitting: normal • Dynamic sitting: normal • Static standing: good • Dynamic standing: fair
	Cognition	• Alert and oriented × 4
	Coordination	• Finger-to-nose: intact bilaterally • Heel-to-shin: intact bilaterally
	Cranial nerves	• II–XII: intact
	Reflexes	• Patellar: 2 + bilaterally

(Continued)

(Continued)

Hospital Day 1, Postoperative Day 1, Ward: Physical Therapy Examination		
	Sensation	• BUE: intact to light touch bilaterally
	Tone	• BUE: within normal limit (WNL) • BLE: WNL
	Other	• N/A
Integumentary	Skin integrity	Incisions R anterior-lateral chest wall and R axilla: both closed with surgical glue. Minimal erythema surrounding each wound with local post-op edema R anterior chest wall. Noted mild visible post-op edema of RUE at proximal arm to medial elbow.
Functional status		
Bed mobility		• Scooting up in bed: independent • Bridging: independent • Supine to/from sit: supervision, prefers getting out of bed on the left side
Transfers		• Sit to/from stand: supervision without an AD
Ambulation		• Ambulated 150 feet×2 with contact guard assist and no AD. • Gait deviations notable for wide base of support, decreased trunk rotation, minimal to no arm swing bilaterally, forward flexed and guarded posture of right shoulder.
Stairs		• Ascend 12 steps with supervision and left handrail. • Descend 12 steps with contact guard assistance and right handrail. • Demonstrated step-to pattern.
Other		Health-Related Quality-of-Life Outcome Measure: FACT B + 4: score = 75.8/148 = 51%

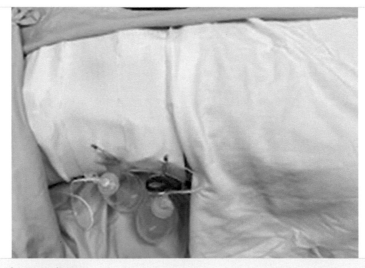

Fig. 2.3 Example of post-op dressing.

Assessment	
☑ Physical therapist's	*Assessment left blank for learner to develop.*

Goals	
Patient's	"To regain full motion in right arm and return to swimming"
Short term	1. *Goals left blank for learner to develop.* 2.
Long term	1. *Goals left blank for learner to develop.* 2.

Plan	
☐ Physician's ☑ Physical therapist's ☐ Other's	Will continue to provide therapy services once a day for 2 days to continue to assess ROM, strength, balance, edema, pain, and functional mobility to maximize functional mobility and safety in preparation for safe discharge home. Physical therapy to provide interventions and education on: • Post-op ROM precautions, limiting shoulder flexion to 90 degrees and non–weight-bearing on surgical side until drains removed. • HEP program. • Edema management and signs and symptoms (s/s) of lymphedema due to axillary lymph node dissection.

Bloom's Taxonomy Level	Case 2.B Questions
Create	1. Synthesizing the medical data and physical examination findings, develop an appropriate physical therapy assessment of the patient. 2. Develop two short-term physical therapy goals, including an appropriate timeframe for discharge. 3. Develop two long-term physical therapy goals, including an appropriate timeframe for discharge.
Evaluate	4. Explain the physical therapy findings and expected discharge disposition to the resident physician.
Analyze	5. Compare and contrast a radical mastectomy from a modified radical mastectomy. Discuss the indications for each. 6. Compare and contrast an axillary lymph node dissection from a sentinel lymph node biopsy.
Apply	7. Design and implement a HEP to improve the patient's RUE ROM and strength, while still ensuring maintenance of post-op precautions. 8. Design patient education for proper completion of steps with railing on left side during ascent. Ensure the patient maintains non–weight-bearing in RUE throughout.
Understand	9. Explain what education regarding axillary lymph node dissection needs to be conveyed to the patient prior to hospital discharge. 10. Identify the impact lab values could have on an acute care therapy session.
Remember	11. List the motor nerves that may be injured with an axillary dissection and discuss what type of finding would be associated with each injury. 12. What are the signs/symptoms of lymphedema?

Bloom's Taxonomy Level	Case 2.B Answers
Create	1. Patient is a 39-year-old female who is hospital day 1, post-op day 1 s/p right modified radical mastectomy and lymph node dissection. Triple negative tumor. The patient presents with the following findings post-op—a modified radical mastectomy and axillary dissection: • Limitations in RUE ROM and strength are due to post-op precautions and not directly related to musculoskeletal and neurological deficits.

(Continued)

(Continued)

Bloom's Taxonomy Level	Case 2.B Answers
	• The patient's forward flexed posture and poor scapular mechanics are due to pain and fear of injury to surgical site.
	The above are findings consistent in patient's s/p right modified radical mastectomy and axillary dissection. Patient would benefit from continued physical therapy to improve above deficits and to maximize functional mobility and safety within confines of precautions.
	2. Short-term goals:
	• Patient will ambulate 150 feet twice with supervision and no AD within 4 days to ensure safe discharge home with spouse.
	• Patient will be independent with all bed mobility within 4 days to promote independence upon hospital discharge.
	• Patient will independently verbalize and implement post-op precautions within 4 days to promote safety and decrease adverse reactions.
	3. Long-term goals:
	• Patient will ascend/descend three steps with one rail with supervision and non–weight-bearing RUE within 7 days to safely enter/exit home.
	• Patient will independently demonstrate teach-back of HEP instruction within 7 days to ensure independence and compliance upon hospital discharge.
	• Patient will independently demonstrate teach-back of lymphedema signs and symptoms within 7 days to ensure independence and compliance with self-monitoring for symptoms.
Evaluate	4. Patient is a 39-year-old female who is hospital day 1, post-op day 1 s/p right modified radical mastectomy and lymph node dissection. Post-op precautions verbalized and implemented during session. Pain levels, ROM, and strength are within normal limits for acute care setting. Patient currently performs all functional mobility with independence—contact guard assistance. Assistance and increased time are warranted during specific activities—such as ambulation and stair negotiation—due to newly implemented post-op precautions. Patient has been educated on HEP to improve strength and ROM, while maintaining postoperative precautions. Patient has also been educated on risk of lymphedema following an axillary lymph node dissection and signs and symptoms to monitor for. Patient is safe for discharge to home with husband without an assistive device (AD).
Analyze	5. A radical mastectomy removes the breast, overlying skin, pectoralis major and minor muscles, and the contents of the axilla. This type of mastectomy is rarely done today because of significant morbidity and lack of improvement in survival. A modified radical mastectomy is the removal of the breast and fascia underneath the pectoralis major muscle and removal of level I and II lymph nodes.
	6. The sentinel lymph node biopsy procedure is done in patients with early-onset breast cancer instead of a full lymph node dissection. During the procedure, the surgeon injects blue dye into the area around the breast tumor. The breast is then massaged for several minutes to help spread the blue dye into lymphatic channels. An axillary incision is made, and the surgeon follows the path of the blue dye to a lymph node or nodes. This node is surgically removed and evaluated for the presence of metastatic disease. If this node is positive for tumor, a lymph node dissection will be done for further evaluation for metastatic disease. Sentinel lymph node biopsy has reduced the need for axillary lymph node dissection and resultant morbidity such as lymphedema.
	An axillary lymph node dissection involves removal of axillary lymph nodes from zones 1, 2, and/or 3 significantly impacting the lymphatic flow within the surgical region.
Apply	7. A HEP post-op should focus on pain management and BUE ROM and strengthening to improve posture and shoulder mobility, all while maintaining postoperative precautions. Examples of interventions to include in the HEP include:
	Upon hospital discharge:
	• Neck: Cervical ROM and mild stretching demonstrated with side bending and rotation bilaterally. Chin tucks performed to improve strength and ROM for posturing. Chin tucks should be performed seated without resistance.
	• Shoulder: Postural strengthening and stretching performed bilaterally through seated scapular retractions with isometric hold and shoulder circles with arms resting at side.
	1-week post-op:
	• RUE strengthening and ROM achieved through active assisted ROM only working up to 90 degrees until drains removed (▶ Fig. 2.4). Delaying shoulder ROM by 1 week has

(Continued)

Bloom's Taxonomy Level	Case 2.B Answers
	been shown to decrease postoperative drainage, allowing for drains to be removed earlier than if shoulder ROM exercises were initiated and also decreasing the risk of seroma formation postoperatively. Postoperative protocol maintained until drain removed at surgical follow-up appointment after discharge. HEP can be progressed after initial follow-up appointment. 8. To help the patient negotiate stairs, the patient should be educated to use the step-to technique to decrease the risk of falling. During ascent, the railing on the left side can be utilized by the LUE. During descent, the patient can face the railing and perform a side-stepping technique with the LUE on railing. In both directions, cues should be provided for minimal pushing and pulling. The RUE should not be used on the railing as pushing/pulling would break the patient's RUE non–weight-bearing precautions.

Understand	9. The physical therapist needs to provide education related to the risk of lymphedema and how to decrease that risk to the patient. Risk reduction can occur through limiting unnecessary stress to the surgical side, including, but not limited to:
	• No blood pressure or needle sticks
	• Maintaining skin and nail care
	• Avoiding submerging of the limb in hot water, such as hot tubs.
	• Maintaining acute precautions including maintaining non–weight-bearing status (no pushing, pulling, lifting until cleared by medical team). This may be applicable to day-to-day life in carrying heavy purses on the surgical side and lifting children.
	10. As an acute care physical therapist, especially one who is working with patients who have an oncology diagnosis, it is imperative to review lab values as part of the medical record review prior to treatment at every therapy session. When reviewing, it is important to determine if the lab values are normal, elevated, or decreased. From there, consider therapeutic implications. Specific to this case, consider the following:
	• White blood cells (WBCs):
	  ○ If a patient has WBC > 11.0×10^9/L (leukocytosis), monitor for fever, malaise, lethargy, dizziness, bleeding, bruising, weight loss, lymphadenopathy, and painful inflamed joints.
	  ○ If a patient has WBC < 4.0×10^9/L (leukopenia), monitor for anemia, weakness, fatigue, fever, headache, and shortness of breath.
	  ○ If a patient has a WBC < 1.5×10^9/L (neutropenia), follow neutropenic precautions as outlined by the facility.
	  ○ Follow appropriate infection control to reduce the patient's risk for developing infections.
	• Hemoglobin:
	  ○ If a patient has Hgb < 11 g/dL (anemia), be sure to monitor symptoms. Patient may be tachycardic or present with signs or symptoms of orthostatic hypotension.
	  ○ If a patient has a Hgb < 8 g/dL, interventions should be symptom based, and it is important to have a discussion with the interprofessional team.
	• Platelets:
	  ○ If a patient has platelets > 450 k/µL (thrombocytosis), be sure to monitor for weakness, headache, dizziness, chest pain, and tingling in hands/feet; thromcytosis can also occur from malignancy.
	  ○ If a patient has platelets < 150 k/µL (thrombocytopenia), be sure to monitor for petechiae, ecchymosis, fatigue, jaundice, and splenomegaly. Also realize that with low platelets, the risk of bleeding is increased, and therefore, interventions should be modified accordingly to further reduce fall risk.

Remember	11. The motor nerves that are at risk for injury during axillary dissection are the long thoracic nerve, the thoracodorsal nerve, and the medial and lateral pectoral nerve. Injury to the long thoracic nerve will cause a winged scapula ipsilateral to the injury. Injury to the thoracodorsal nerve may cause mild weakness of internal rotation and adduction of the ipsilateral shoulder. Injury to the medial and lateral pectoral nerves will cause atrophy of pectoral muscles causing decrease movement of the shoulder. 12. Signs and symptoms related to lymphedema include swelling in the hand, which can lead to a sensation of heaviness, aching, or pain in the arm. Ways to identify this using rings become tighter, decreasing range of motion, or hardening and thickening of the skin. Education on such should be provided to the patient.

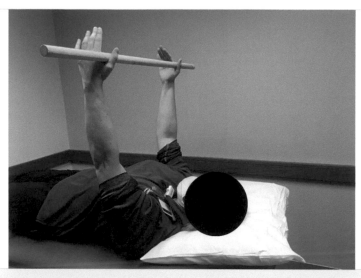

Fig. 2.4 An example of post-op active assisted range of motion shoulder flexion to 90 degrees.

Key points
1. The sentinel lymph node biopsy is a less invasive procedure compared to the axillary lymph node dissection. When possible, the sentinel lymph node biopsy is the favored procedure to reduce the risk of side effects, including lymphedema.
2. Post–mastectomy protocols typically involve weight-bearing and ROM restrictions during the acute phase. Although ROM is limited for a period of time postoperatively, if ROM exercises within restrictions are started early, patient will not experience long-term ROM limitations, but will see a reduction in post-op complications. It is imperative that physical therapy assessments and interventions are tailored to maintain postoperative protocols, including no overpressure during MMT, limitations in ROM assessments, modifications to functional activities to maintain weight-bearing status, and limitations in the selection of balance assessments to decrease unnecessary risk for falls.
3. In the acute care hospital, clinicians have minimal interactions with patients as discharges can be anywhere from same day to 5 days post-op. It is imperative during this time that the patient understands all safety education, postoperative protocols, red flags that would warrant communication with the medical team, HEP expectations and expected progression of therapy, and the recovery process.

General Information	
Case no.	2.C
Authors	Aubree Colorito, PT, DPT, COS-C, Board-Certified Clinical Specialist in Oncologic Physical Therapy Kathleen L. Ehrhardt, MMS, PA-C, DFAAPA Judith Schaad, PT, DPT, CWS, CLT-LANA, Board Certified Clinical Specialist in Oncology Physical Therapy
Diagnosis	Generalized weakness and new-onset swelling in right upper extremity
Setting	Home
Learner expectations	☑ Initial evaluation ☐ Re-evaluation ☐ Treatment session
Learner objectives	1. To understand advanced disease progression of breast cancer, including location of metastases. 2. To understand side effects of cancer treatments, including chemotherapy-induced peripheral neuropathy, vestibular dysfunction, cardiac dysfunction, and lymphedema. 3. To understand the escalation process for red flags and how to develop a plan of care when red flags exist

Medical	
Chief complaint	Swelling in right upper extremity (RUE)
History of present illness	Patient is a 43-year-old female with a history of T2N2 M0 triple negative breast cancer diagnosed 4 years ago who presented to primary care office for evaluation of fatigue. Patient was evaluated in office and found to have significant lymphedema in right arm and referred to physical therapy for further evaluation and treatment. Due to functional limitations leaving the home, primary team ordered home physical therapy. Patient complains of heaviness in right arm and mentions that her arm aches after physical activity. Lastly, the patient also reports numbness and tingling of bilateral feet and legs since chemotherapy. She reports a history of loss of balance when turning too quickly and expresses a feeling of "never feeling grounded" and feeling like she is "on a boat."
Past medical history	Infiltrating ductal carcinoma of the right breast, BRCA 1/2 negative, triple negative tumor, received adjuvant chemotherapy for six cycles with doxorubicin (Adriamycin) and cyclophosphamide followed by paclitaxel (Taxol) AC-T; chemotherapy-induced peripheral neuropathy bilateral lower extremities; hypothyroidism; two uncomplicated pregnancies with vaginal deliveries.
Past surgical history	Right modified radical mastectomy with lymph node dissection—4 years ago, breast biopsy right breast—4 years ago, appendectomy at age 18.
Family history	Mother: breast cancer diagnosed at age 49, no residual disease, hypothyroidism Father: hypertension, hypercholesterolemia, myocardial infarction at age 62 Brother: alive and well.
Allergies	No known drug allergies.
Medications	Levothyroxine, Gabapentin, Ibuprofen PRN occasional upper back discomfort
Precautions/Orders	Activity as tolerated

Social history	
Home setup	• Resides in a multilevel home with husband and children. • Three steps plus two handrails to enter. • Half bathroom is on the first floor. • Master bedroom and bathroom are located on the first floor. • Children's bedrooms are located on the second floor. • Flight of stairs plus two handrails to second floor.
Occupation	• College professor, currently off for summer.
Prior level of function	• Independent with functional mobility and activities of daily living • Right handed • (+) Driver
Recreational activities	• Swims daily at local health club. • Enjoys cooking and spending time with husband and two children aged 12 and 15.

Vital signs	PCP office, 2 days ago
Blood pressure (mmHg)	126/84
Heart rate (beats/min)	86
Respiratory rate (breaths/min)	17
Pulse oximetry on room air (SpO$_2$)	96%
Temperature (°F)	98.5

Imaging/diagnostic test	PCP office, 2 days ago
Doppler of right extremity	1. Negative for deep vein thrombosis.
3D echocardiography	1. Normal LV size and wall thickness with normal ejection function of 69%. No regional wall motion abnormalities. No clots or effusions.

Lab		Reference range	PCP office, 2 days ago
CBC	WBC	5.0–10.0 × 10^9/L	5.7
	RBC	4.1–5.3 million/mcL	5.27
	Hemoglobin	12–16 g/dL	15.4
	Hematocrit	37–47%	44.1%
	Platelets	140–400 k/µL	168
Other	Thyroid-stimulating hormone	0.3–3.0 U/mL	2.8 mU/L
Comprehensive metabolic profile	Glucose	65–99 mg/dL	83 mg/dL
	Calcium	8.7–10.3 mg/dL	12.5 mg/dL
	Chloride	96–106 mmo/L	101 mmo/L
	Carbon dioxide	20–29 mmo/L	24 mmo/L
	Potassium	3.7–5.2 mEq/L	4.5 mEq/L
	Sodium	136–144 mEq/L	140 mEq/L
	BUN	8–27 mg/dL	9 mg/dL
	Creatinine	0.8–1.4 mg/dL	0.9 mg/dL
	BUN/Creatinine ratio	10:1–20:1	10.1
	Estimated glomerular filtration rate	90–120 mL/min	102 mL/min
	Total bilirubin	0.3–1.9 mg/dL	0.1 mg/dL
	Aspartate aminotransferase	10–34 IU/L	20 IU/L
	Alanine aminotransferase	8–37 IU/L	10 IU/L
	Alkaline phosphatase	44–147 IU/L	250 IU/L
	Total protein	6.3–7.9 g/dL	7.1 g/dL
	Albumin	3.9–5.0 g/dL	4.5 g/dL

Medical management	PCP office, 1 week ago
Follow-up	Patient to return to primary care office in 2 weeks to review laboratory test results and discuss progression in physical therapy.

Pause points
Based on the aforementioned information, what are the priority • Diagnostic tests and measures? • Outcome measures? • Treatment interventions?

Physical Therapy Examination		
Subjective		
"During movement, I have some pain in my upper back between scapulae. It gets worse at night. My right arm also feels really heavy."		
Objective		
Vital signs	Pre-treatment	Post-treatment
	Sitting	Sitting
Blood pressure (mmHg), LUE	120/78	134/82
Heart rate (beats/min)	88	92
Respiratory rate (breaths/min)	16	18
Pulse oximetry on room air (SpO_2)	100%	98%
BORG scale	6	11
Pain	4/10	5
	• Reports pain, described as aching, 4/10 at rest in RUE. • Notes 2/10 pain back between shoulder blades but notes increased pain 7–8/10 at nighttime that is nagging. She feels that no matter what position she sleeps in, she cannot get comfortable enough to sleep.	
General	• Appears uncomfortable and older than stated age. • Right arm visibly enlarged.	
Head, ears, eyes, nose, and throat (HEENT)	• NCAT, PERRL, no scleral icterus, no palpable lymphadenopathy	
Cardiovascular and pulmonary	• Normal rate and rhythm. • Auscultation: mild decreased in breath sounds in bilateral lower lobes, mild accessory muscle use with increased exertion.	
Gastrointestinal	• Soft, NT, no masses, no organomegaly.	
Musculoskeletal	Range of motion	LUE: within functional range. RUE: • R shoulder flexion: 0–110 degrees with firm end feel. No increase in pain with ROM. • R shoulder abduction: 0–100 degrees with firm end feel. No increase in pain with ROM. • R shoulder external rotation: 0–65 degrees with soft-tissue restriction/tight heavy cording in axilla/anterior-lateral chest. • R shoulder internal rotation: 0–70 degrees. • R elbow: 0–120 degrees. • R wrist flexion: 0–78 degrees. • R wrist extension: 0–60 degrees. • LUE: WFL • BLE: WFL
	Strength	• LUE: 4/5 • RUE: 4-/5 • Left lower extremity: 4/5 • RLE: 4/5
	Aerobic	• Formal assessment deferred at this time. Will assess at future session when cleared by medical team for continued care.
	Flexibility	• Able to assume long sitting to get in/out of bed.
	Other	• Proprioception: decreased in bilateral ankles and great toes. (▶ Fig. 2.5)

(Continued)

(Continued)

Physical Therapy Examination		
Neurological	Balance	• Static seated: normal • Dynamic seated: normal • Static standing: good • Dynamic standing: fair
	Cognition	• Alert and oriented x 4
	Coordination	• Finger-to-nose: intact bilaterally • Heel-to-shin: intact bilaterally
	Cranial nerves	• II–XII: intact • VOR (−)
	Reflexes	• Patellar: 2 + bilaterally
	Sensation	• Light touch: decreased from mid-calf and distal in bilateral lower extremities. • Vibration testing with 128 Hz tuning fork: Absent at bilateral medial malleoli and great toes (▶ Fig. 2.6).
	Tone	• Normal throughout BUEs and BLEs
	Other	• N/A
Integumentary	Skin condition	• Right axillary and chest wall scars well healed, though scar tightness and adhesions are observed. • R arm tissues exhibit moderate fibrosis with 2 + pitting edema, particularly at the dorsal forearm and lateral elbow.
	Limb volumes	• RUE: 2.69 L • LUE: 2.41 L
Functional status		
Bed mobility		• Rolling either direction: independent on flat surface. • Supine to/from sit: supervision with increased time to complete.
Transfers		• Sit to/from stand: supervision
Ambulation		Level surfaces: • Ambulated 100 feet with contact guard assistance and no AD. • Occasionally uses external support (i.e., wall) to help stabilize. • Gait deviations notable for wide base of support, external rotation of bilateral lower extremities, increased hip flexion during swing phase, decreased bilateral dorsiflexion but no presentation of foot drop. Uneven surfaces: • Ambulated 30 feet with minimal assistance and no AD. • Reports only leaving home with family/friends present due to fear of falling on gravel driveway.
Stairs		• Ascend 12 steps with supervision and left handrail, demonstrates step-over-step pattern. • Descend 12 steps with contact guard assistance and right handrail, demonstrates step-to pattern. • Reports not trusting her foot placement during descent resulting in increased time to complete.
Other		Health-Related Quality-of-Life Outcome Measure: FACT B + 4: score =76.6/148 = 51.7%

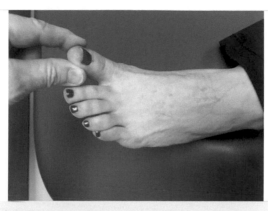

Fig. 2.5 Assessment of proprioception at great toe.

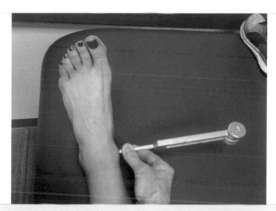

Fig. 2.6 Vibration testing over medial malleolus.

Assessment	
☑ Physical therapist's	*Assessment left blank for learner to develop.*
Goals	
Patient's	"To feel confident leaving the house alone again." "To improve my balance and motion in right arm to safely drive short distances." "To decrease swelling in right arm to be able to wear her mother's wedding band again."
Short term	1. 　　　*Goals left blank for learner to develop.* 2.
Long term	1. 　　　*Goals left blank for learner to develop.* 2.

Plan	
☐ Physician's ☑ Physical therapist's ☐ Other's	Physical therapist to develop a treatment plan for: • Lymphedema, which is to include complete decongestive therapy (CDT). • Chemotherapy-induced peripheral neuropathy to address balance deficits. Aerobic deficits from possible cardiotoxicity (to be evaluated further at follow-up visit) with the goal of improving overall function and quality of life. Plan to see patient twice a week for 4 weeks followed by once a week for 2–4 weeks once cleared by medical team to resume care.

(Continued)

Bloom's Taxonomy Level	Case 2.C Questions
Create	1. Synthesizing the medical data and physical examination findings, develop an appropriate physical therapy assessment of the patient.
	2. Develop one short-term goal specific to lymphedema and two short-term functional therapy goals, including an appropriate timeframe.
	3. Develop one long-term goal specific to lymphedema and two long-term functional therapy goals, including an appropriate timeframe.
Evaluate	4. Explain the physical therapy findings and recommendations to the medical team.
Analyze	5. Link the patient's symptomology with concerns for bone metastases and explain why therapy would be held until MD clearance.
Apply	6. Explain characteristics of the four stages of lymphedema and determine which stage would apply to this patient's swelling.
Understand	7. Discuss what laboratory evaluation should be done to evaluate for bony metastasis from malignancies.
	8. Summarize the classic presentation of chemotherapy-induced peripheral neuropathy (CIPN) and how to complete a thorough assessment of CIPN.
Remember	9. Recall the malignancies that most commonly metastasize to bone.
	10. Recall four areas where systemic metastases are more prone to occur in patients with metastatic breast cancer.
	11. Recognize common side effects of AC-T treatment.

Bloom's Taxonomy Level	Case 2.C Answers
Create	1. Patient is a 43-year-old female who was referred to home physical therapy due to fatigue, weakness, and increased right upper extremity swelling. Past medical history is notable for T2N2MO triple negative breast cancer diagnosed 4 years ago. Medical management included right modified radical mastectomy, lymph node dissection, breast biopsy, and chemotherapy. Subjective and objective findings are consistent with chemo-induced peripheral neuropathy. As a result, the patient presents with decreased balance, noted during ambulation on level and uneven surfaces, and exacerbated with turns. Patient would benefit from balance training to address deficits, teach compensatory strategies, and decrease risk for falls.
	From a lymphedema perspective, this patient has a significant increase in her RUE limb volume compared to the left. Pre-op limb volume difference showed that her involved, dominant RUE was 2.9% greater than LUE. This was a normal, expected difference in a dominant arm. However, at this visit, her involved, dominant RUE is 11.6% greater than LUE, a change of 8.7%. In addition, the swelling does not resolve with elevation (considered "non-reversible") and moderate tissue fibrosis is present, indicating at least a stage 2 lymphedema. She does not exhibit nonpitting edema and hyperkeratosis, which would indicate stage 3 lymphedema. Therefore, the patient's swelling presents as stage 2 lymphedema.
	It is important to note that the patient was negative for deep vein thrombosis prior to beginning physical therapy.
	In addition, her axillary and chest wall scars have caused adhesions and restricted shoulder mobility that has reduced use of RUE for functional activities and reduced lymphatic decongestion.
	Pain assessment consistent with red flags for possible bony metastases due to location of pain, description of pain, and time of day that pain increases. Medical team to be notified of findings and therapy will be held until cleared by medical team for functional training and lymphedema management.
	2. For STGs and LTGs, it is important to recognize that goals would be created to build the POC, but the physician would be notified immediately of the red flags found during the session related to possible bone metastases and care would be held until cleared by the MD.
	Short-term goals for lymphedema:
	• Within 4 weeks of start of treatment, there will be reduced limb volume difference to < 6% between BUE, reduced tissue fibrosis R forearm, and elbow to slight/mild.

(Continued)

(Continued)

Bloom's Taxonomy Level	Case 2.C Answers
	Short-term goals for function: • Patient will be modified independent to ascend/descend 12 steps, while demonstrating step-over-step pattern, with 1 HR within 4 weeks to improve functional mobility. • Patient will demonstrate Romberg EO: 1 minute and Romberg EC: 30 seconds with supervision within 4 weeks to improve balance. 3. Long-term goal for lymphedema: • Within 8 weeks of start of treatment, patient will be successfully fitted into a custom, flat knit compression sleeve and glove for daytime and an inelastic night compression garment that covers her fingers and arm. Success is defined as comfortable, tolerable, and effective in controlling her swelling. Long-term goal for function: • Patient will ambulate 300 feet without AD on level and uneven surface independently in 8 weeks to improve functional mobility and balance. • Patient will score 45/56 on the Berg Balance Scale to decrease risk of falling in 8 weeks: a) *Note*: Berg held at the start of care due to conservative assessment in relation to "red flag" for bony metastases. Once patient is cleared for return to activity with therapy, it would be beneficial to incorporate the Berg Balance Scale and set a long-term goal to show functional gains specific to balance and reduced risk for falling.
Evaluate	4. Treatment of stage 2 lymphedema: The "gold standard" treatment for stage 2 lymphedema is complete (or complex) decongestive therapy or CDT. It is also known as DLT (decongestive lymphatic therapy). This treatment includes multilayer bandaging worn 24/7, changed three to five times per week for 2–4 weeks, manual lymphatic drainage applied at the time of bandage changes, decongestive exercise to promote muscle pump and improve lymphatic drainage, and education regarding meticulous skin care to prevent infection. After this initial active phase of treatment, "Phase 1," the patient would be fitted with a compression sleeve and glove for day and an inelastic night compression garment. For a patient without the complaint of back pain, management would include manual therapy techniques to her right shoulder, such as joint mobilizations and myofascial trigger point releases. However, these techniques would need to be held, until her new mid back pain is evaluated, and she is cleared of bony metastases.
Analyze	5. Red flags for bony metastases include increased pain at night, loss of function, and functional pain, defined as increasing pain with movement. Symptoms of functional back pain and/or neurologic pain should be evaluated immediately for possible nerve root compression, vertebral fracture, or spinal instability in those with a history of cancer. This patient exhibits the red flags of increased pain at night and loss of function. It is also important to understand that in many cases, metastatic spread follows hematologic and lymphatic drainage. In this patient's case, breast cancer has a preference to metastasize to the thoracic spine—where her scapular pain is—due to venous drainage. Lastly, physical therapy would need to be held until cleared by the medical team due to the concerns for possible bony metastases. Dr Stubblefield, author of Cancer Rehabilitation: Principles and Practice, explains in simple terms that "Bone pain in a patient with a history of cancer should be considered secondary to metastasis until proven otherwise." When physical therapists see signs/symptoms of red flags, regardless of how minimal they seem, always notify the medical team and seek clearance for care before continuing with the plan of care, especially in patients with a history of cancer.
Apply	6. There are four stages of lymphedema, defined as a chronic progressive high protein swelling: • Stage 0: Abnormal flow in the lymphatic system due to surgery, radiation, trauma, infection, obesity, other medical conditions, or congenital abnormality of lymphatic anatomy. At Stage 0, no signs or symptoms are observed of felt by the patient. At this stage, close observation and education is required. • Stage 1: Spontaneously reversible. A progression from Stage 0, where mild swelling completely (or nearly) resolves overnight. At this stage, education and a circular knit compression garment is recommended in the daytime to support lymphatic drainage and avoid progression.

(Continued)

(Continued)

Bloom's Taxonomy Level	Case 2.C Answers
	• Stage 2: Spontaneously irreversible: the swelling increases, and early fibrosis is noted in the tissues with pitting edema. It does not resolve or change overnight very slightly. At this stage, CDT is required to treat and control the swelling. • Stage 3: Edema is more extreme and causes tissue deformities, the swelling is nonpitting (hard), and skin becomes thickened with hyperkeratosis and wart-like growths or papillomas are seen on exam. These patients require CDT and lifelong diligence to contain the swelling and skin condition. In Stage 3, treatment will not completely resolve the swelling, though can significantly improve it and provide for an improved quality of life. This patient has stage 2 lymphedema.
Understand	7. The laboratory tests that should be ordered to evaluate for the presentation of bony metastasis from malignancy include a CBC, calcium level, and alkaline phosphatase level. Patients with bony metastases may have anemia due to the bone marrow being affected by disease. Additionally, patients with metastatic disease to the bone will have high levels of calcium and alkaline phosphatase due to the bone being disintegrated by tumor. 8. Patients with chemotherapy-induced peripheral neuropathy present with a symmetric distal "stocking glove" distribution of their symptoms. Symptoms most commonly are sensory not motor. To ensure thorough assessment of CIPN, physical therapists will need to complete a thorough sensory assessment including light touch, pain, proprioception, and vibration assessments. Clinicians may also find benefit in incorporating self-reported assessments, such as the FACT/GOG-Ntx to screen patients for self-reported symptoms of CIPN. The Oncology EDGE Taskforce has created recommendations of oncology-specific outcomes assessments based on what the tools are measuring for and diagnoses. FACT/GOG-Ntx has been identified as "Highly Recommended" for breast cancer patients with CIPN.
Remember	9. The malignancies that most commonly metastasize to bone are prostate, thyroid, breast, lung, and kidney. This can be remembered by the pneumonic physical therapy Barnum Loves Kids. 10. Systemic metastasizes are likely to affect the brain, bones, lungs, and liver for patients with a diagnosis of metastatic breast cancer. 11. The cell cycle includes the G1, S, G2, and M phases. It is important to understand that chemotherapy treatments kill cells at different points within the cell cycle. Therefore, in order to increase the chances of killing cancer cells at different phases within their cell cycle, combination chemotherapy regimens are used. In this patient's case, the patient is receiving the AC-T regimen, including doxorubicin (Adriamycin) and cyclophosphamide followed by paclitaxel (Taxol). Adriamycin is an anthracycline, Cyclophosphamide is an alkylating agent, and Taxol is a taxane/antimicrotubule agent, impacting the cells at different points within their cell cycle. Another important concept to understand is chemotherapy kills all rapidly dividing cells, healthy and unhealthy. The damage to healthy cells results in chemotherapy-specific side effects: Doxorubicin (Adriamycin) patients are at an increased risk for cardiotoxicity, which can lead to early-onset heart failure. Cyclophosphamide—patients may experience an acute drop in WBCs during treatment and risk for inflammation to the kidneys. Taxanes are known to increase the risk for peripheral neuropathy. One way to remember this is Taxanes "Tax the nervous system." Taxol specifically is known to cause a sensory chemo-induced peripheral neuropathy. Patients may experience increased burning/tingling and loss of proprioception and vibration distally. Chemo-induced peripheral neuropathy symptoms will be present bilaterally. Lastly, it is important to remember cranial nerves are peripheral nerves. Patients who have received chemotherapy in the past should always receive a cranial nerve assessment at their first visit, with an increased emphasis assessing the vestibular nerve for dysfunction.

Key points

1. The homecare setting offers many challenges that are not commonly seen in other settings, including the need to provide a thorough medical screening for patients at any point within their clinical continuum. The home health clinicians may be the first to identify a new onset of symptoms that the patient has not been forthcoming in sharing with the medical team at office visits. The home health setting also offers challenges in selection of objective tests and measures and interventions that can be used within available space and resources.

2. Patients with a history of cancer should always be evaluated for the potential of recurrent or metastatic disease. In this patient's case, the patient has new-onset pain that has not been evaluated by a physician. The physical therapy evaluation will need to be modified to a more conservative assessment and the patient must be evaluated and cleared by the medical team before interventions can begin.

3. Patients with a history of cancer experience impairments secondary to the cancer itself and the treatments for cancer. In this patient's case, she is experiencing long-term treatment side effects including lymphedema, chemo-induced peripheral neuropathy, and possible cardiotoxicity. Physical therapists can develop a plan of care to address all three deficits, which will result in improved function and quality of life for the patient.

4. After surgery or radiation for breast cancer, lymph nodes and vessels are dissected or damaged. The result is impaired lymphatic drainage. The patient is at lifelong risk of developing lymphedema. Lymphedema can develop in the extremity or territory of the body impacted by the reduced lymphatic drainage. After breast cancer, it may be seen in the UE, the posterior-lateral trunk, or the breast. Without treatment, it tends to progress over time and must be properly managed. Risk reduction practices must be followed for the remainder of the patient's life.

Suggested Readings

American Joint Committee on Cancer. AJCC Cancer Staging Manual. 8th ed. Chicago, IL: Springer International Publishing; 2018

Dent R, Trudeau M, Pritchard KI, et al. Triple-negative breast cancer: clinical features and patterns of recurrence. Clin Cancer Res. 2007; 13(15, Pt 1):4429–4434

Feigelson HS, James TA, Single RM, et al. Factors associated with the frequency of initial total mastectomy: results of a multi-institutional study. J Am Coll Surg. 2013; 216(5):966–975

Halsted WS. I. The results of radical operations for the cure of carcinoma of the breast. Ann Surg. 1907; 46(1):1–19

Hammond MEH, Hayes DF, Dowsett M, et al. American Society of Clinical Oncology/College Of American Pathologists guideline recommendations for immunohistochemical testing of estrogen and progesterone receptors in breast cancer. J Clin Oncol. 2010; 28(16):2784–2795

Harrington S, Miale S, Ebaugh D. Breast Cancer EDGE Task Force Outcomes: clinical measures of health-related quality of life. Rehabil Oncol. 2015; 33(1):5–17

Knight CD, Jr, Griffen FD, Knight CD, Sr. Prevention of seromas in mastectomy wounds. The effect of shoulder immobilization. Arch Surg. 1995; 130(1):99–101

Li CI, Uribe DJ, Daling JR. Clinical characteristics of different histologic types of breast cancer. Br J Cancer. 2005; 93(9):1046–1052

Lin NU, Vanderplas A, Hughes ME, et al. Clinicopathologic features, patterns of recurrence, and survival among women with triple-negative breast cancer in the National Comprehensive Cancer Network. Cancer. 2012; 118(22):5463–5472

Maltser S, Cristian A, Silver JK, Morris GS, Stout NL. A focused review of safety considerations in cancer rehabilitation. PM R. 2017; 9 9S2:S415–S428

McNeely ML, Campbell K, Ospina M, et al. Exercise interventions for upper-limb dysfunction due to breast cancer treatment. (Review). Cochrane Database Syst Rev. 2010(6):CD005211

Moore KL, Dalley AF, Agur AMR. Clinically Oriented Anatomy. 8th ed. New York, NY: LWW; 2017

Mundy GR. Metastasis to bone: causes, consequences and therapeutic opportunities. Nat Rev Cancer. 2002; 2(8):584–593

National Comprehensive Cancer Network. NCCN Clinical Practice Guidelines in Oncology. Genetic/Familial High-Risk Assessment:

Breast and Ovarian. Version 1.2020. Available at: www.nccn.org/professionals/physician_gls/pdf/genetics_screening.pdf. Accessed June 1, 2020

National Comprehensive Cancer Network. NCCN Guidelines for Patients, Invasive Breast Cancer. 2020. Available at: www.nccn.org/patients/guidelines/content/PDF/breast-invasive-patient.pdf. Accessed June 1, 2020

O'Sullivan SB, Schmitz TJ. Physical Rehabilitation. 5th ed. Philadelphia, PA: F.A. Davis Company; 2007

Peto R, Davies C, Godwin J, et al. Early Breast Cancer Trialists' Collaborative Group (EBCTCG). Comparisons between different polychemotherapy regimens for early breast cancer: meta-analyses of long-term outcome among 100,000 women in 123 randomised trials. Lancet. 2012; 379(9814):432–444

Rao R, Euhus D, Mayo HG, Balch C. Axillary node interventions in breast cancer: a systematic review. JAMA. 2013; 310(13):1385–1394

Schultz I, Barholm M, Gröndal S. Delayed shoulder exercises in reducing seroma frequency after modified radical mastectomy: a prospective randomized study. Ann Surg Oncol. 1997; 4(4):293–297

Siegel RL, Miller KD, Jemal A. Cancer statistics, 2020. CA Cancer J Clin. 2020; 70(1):7–30

Stout Gergich NL, Pfalzer LA, McGarvey C, Springer B, Gerber LH, Soballe P. Preoperative assessment enables the early diagnosis and successful treatment of lymphedema. Cancer. 2008; 112(12):2809–2819

Stout NL, Binkley JM, Schmitz KH, et al. A prospective surveillance model for rehabilitation for women with breast cancer. Cancer. 2012; 118(8) Suppl:2191–2200

Stubblefield MD. Cancer Rehabilitation: Principles and Practice. 2nd ed. Springer Publishing Company; 2018

Turner L, Swindell R, Bell WG, et al. Radical versus modified radical mastectomy for breast cancer. Ann R Coll Surg Engl. 1981; 63(4):239–243

Wolff AC, Hammond ME, Hicks DG, et al. American Society of Clinical Oncology, College of American Pathologists. Recommendations for human epidermal growth factor receptor 2 testing in breast cancer: American Society of Clinical Oncology/College of American Pathologists clinical practice guideline update. J Clin Oncol. 2013; 31(31):3997–4013

3 Burn

General Information	
Case no.	3.A Burn
Authors	Brian Stagno, PT
Diagnosis	Thermal burns to 14% total body surface area (TBSA)
Setting	Burn trauma unit in an acute care hospital
Learner expectations	☑ Initial evaluation ☐ Re-evaluation ☐ Treatment session
Learner objectives	1. Explain the pathophysiology of the patient's diagnosis and the multisystem effects of the injury. 2. Understand medical and surgical management of a patient with partial- and full-thickness burns. 3. Achieve a general understanding of the timeframe for the introduction and progression of physical therapy interventions with this patient population.

Medical	
Chief complaint	14% TBSA
History of present illness	A 66-year-old male presents to the hospital status post a fall from a stool while using a welding torch overhead. Per patient, once on the ground, his clothes caught on fire. Due to hip pain from the fall, the patient was unable to get up quickly. He did, however, put the flames out by patting them with his gloved hands and rolling his body.
Past medical history	Hypertension, chronic lower extremity edema, dyspnea on exertion
Past surgical history	None
Allergies	Morphine (depresses respiration) Lisinopril (cough)
Medications	Aspirin, Furosemide, Losartan
Precautions/Orders	Activity as tolerated Evaluate and treat

Social history	
Home setup	• Resides in a ranch style home with wife • One step to enter • Flight of stairs plus one handrail to basement, where work area/garage is located
Occupation	• Auto mechanic, part time, self-employed
Prior level of function	• Independent with functional mobility and activities of daily living; however, mildly limited by occasional shortness of breath
Recreational activities	• Projects around the house and in garage: "I'm always working on something."

Vital signs	Hospital day 0: direct admit to burn unit	Hospital day 1: burn unit
Blood pressure (mmHg)	190/96	162/88
Heart rate (beats/min)	140	115
Respiratory rate (breaths/min)	26	22
Pulse oximetry on room air (SpO$_2$)	96	96
Temperature (°F)	98.9 (tympanic)	99.0 (tympanic)

Imaging/Diagnostic test	Hospital day 0: direct admit to burn unit	Hospital day 1: burn unit
Lund and Browder chart	1. Partial-thickness burns: • 1% Right thigh • 4% Anterior torso 2. Full-thickness burns: • 1% left hand • 1% right hand • 2% left forearm • 5% left thigh	1. Unchanged
Right hip X-ray	1. Negative for acute fracture	N/A
CT right hip	1. Hyperdense foci in medial thigh consistent with large hematoma	N/A
CT head without contrast	1. No acute Intracranial trauma	N/A
CT cervical spine without contrast	1. Degenerative changes, no acute fractures	N/A
CT of the chest/abdomen/pelvis with contrast	1. No visceral thoracic or abdominal posttraumatic findings 2. Notable cardiomegaly with pulmonary hypertension	N/A

Medical management	Hospital day 0: direct admit to burn unit	Hospital day 1: burn unit	Hospital day 2: burn unit	Hospital day 5: burn unit
Medications	1. Fluid bolus: lactated ringer 2. Fentanyl 3. Gabapentin capsule 4. Ibuprofen 5. Cefazolin 6. Tdap vaccine for adult injection 7. Zinc sulfate capsule 8. Ascorbic acid tab 9. Vitamin A	1. Lactated ringer, continued with titration contingent on urine output 2. Continued 3. Continued 4. Continued 5. Continued 6. One time 7. Continued 8. Continued 9. Continued	1. Lactated ringer, continued with titration contingent on urine output 2. Continued 3. Continued 4. Continued 5. Continued 6. N/A 7. Continued 8. Continued 9. Continued	1. Titrate to PRN 2. Continued 3. Continued 4. Continued 5. Continued 6. N/A 7. Continued 8. Continued 9. Continued
Procedures	1. Sharp debridement and deep cleansing of burn injuries; Covered in silver sulfadiazine cream.		1. Operative procedure: excisional debridement of anterior torso, left forearm, bilateral hands, and bilateral lower extremities, with application of split-thickness skin autograft to bilateral hands (▶ Fig. 3.1) and left lower extremity, with donor skin from bilateral thighs (▶ Fig. 3.2).	1. Dressing change and staple removal at skin grafting sites completed under anesthesia with near 100% graft take noted. Graft sites covered with Bacitracin/Cuticerin/gauze/Kerlix web roll; donor sites covered with Mepilex Ag sheet, Kerlix web roll, compression wrap.

(Continued)

(Continued)

Medical management	Hospital day 0: direct admit to burn unit	Hospital day 1: burn unit	Hospital day 2: burn unit	Hospital day 5: burn unit
Consultations	1. Orthopaedic surgery: no surgical intervention to right hip necessary; will treat conservatively, weight-bearing as tolerated.	1. Cardiology: TTE performed with moderated left ventricle hypertrophy, preserved ejection fraction of 60–64%; given clearance for surgery.	N/A	N/A

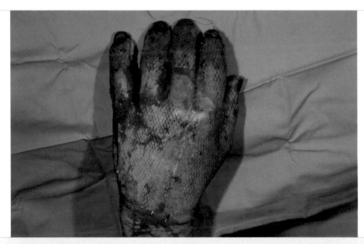

Fig. 3.1 Example of newly placed split thickness skin autograft.

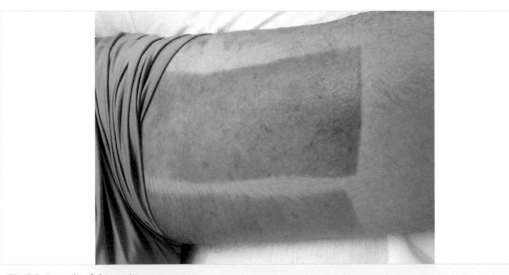

Fig. 3.2 Example of donor site appearance.

Lab values		Reference range	Hospital day 0: direct admit to burn unit	Hospital day 1: burn unit	Hospital day 5: burn unit
Complete blood count	WBC	$5.0–10.0 \times 10^9$/L	12.19	14.4	14.8
	Hemoglobin	14.0–17.4 d/dL	15	11.1	9.1
	Hematocrit	42–52%	45.8	34.8	28.8
	Platelets	140–400 k/μL	390	355	299
Other select labs	Albumin	3.5–5.2 g/dL	3.0	2.7	2.4
	BUN	7–20 mg/dL	6	8	8
	Creatinine	0.7–1.3 mg/dL	0.7	0.4	0.4
	Protein	6–8.3 g/dL	5.5	5.1	4.5

Pause points

Based on the above information, what are the priority
• Diagnostic tests and measures?
• Outcome measures?
• Treatment interventions?

Hospital Day 5:
Post-Op Day 3 from Excisional Debridement and Split-Thickness Skin Grafting
Post-Op Day 0 from Dressing Change Under Anesthesia:
Physical Therapy Examination

Subjective

"Everything is tight, and it feels like my (left) leg is going to explode when I move it."

Objective

Vital signs	Pre-treatment			Post-treatment
	Supine	Sitting	Standing	
Blood pressure (mmHg)	126/74	106/57	N/A	115/67
Heart rate (beats/min)	72	83	93	88
Respiratory rate (breaths/min)	16	18	24	20
Pulse oximetry on 2 L NC (SpO_2)	99	98	98	99
Pain	7/10 at bilateral thighs 9/10 at bilateral hands	8/10 at bilateral thighs 9/10 at bilateral hands	10/10 at bilateral thighs 10/10 at bilateral hands	9/10 at bilateral thighs and bilateral hands

General	• Patient presents supine in bed with dressings to bilateral hands, trunk, and bilateral lower extremities intact. • Lines notable for peripheral IV in right antecubital space, telemetry, nasal cannula, pulse ox, and urinary catheter.
Cardiovascular and pulmonary	• Auscultation: no adventitious breath sounds • Normal sinus rhythm and rate • Peripheral pulses: Bilateral upper extremities (BUE): 2 + radial (however, difficult to find due to bandages) BLE: 2 + pedal
Gastrointestinal	• Soft, nontender, nondistended • No hepatosplenomegaly
Genitourinary	• Urinary catheter in place
Musculoskeletal	Range of motion • L shoulder, active range of motion (AROM): within normal limit (WNL) • R shoulder, AROM: WNL

(Continued)

(Continued)

	Hospital Day 5:
	Post-Op Day 3 from Excisional Debridement and Split-Thickness Skin Grafting
	Post-Op Day 0 from Dressing Change Under Anesthesia:
	Physical Therapy Examination

		• Left elbow, AROM: WNL
		• R elbow, AROM: WNL
		• L wrist flexion, active assisted range of motion (AAROM): 0–20 degrees
		• R wrist flexion, AAROM: 0–15 degrees
		• L wrist extension, AAROM: 0–10 degrees
		• R wrist extension, AAROM: 0–15 degrees
		• B metacarpopphalangeal joint/proximal interphalangeal joint/ distal interphalangeal joint (MCP/PIP/DIP) flexion/extension: limited and painful
		• L hip flexion, AROM: 0–60 degrees
		• L hip flexion, AAROM: 0–75 degrees
		• R hip flexion, AROM: 0–65 degrees
		• R hip flexion, AAROM: 0–80 degrees
		• L knee, AROM: 0–40 degrees
		• L knee, AAROM: 0–50 degrees
		• R knee, AROM: 0–90 degrees
		• B ankle DF, AROM: WNL
		• B ankle PF, AROM: WNL
	Strength	• B shoulder flexion: 5/5
		• B shoulder abduction: 5/5
		• L elbow flexion: 3/5 (resistance not applied due to forearm burn)
		• R elbow flexion: 5/5
		• L wrist flexion: not formally assessed
		• R wrist flexion: 2/5
		• L hip flexion: not formally assessed
		• R hip flexion: 2/5
		• L knee extension: 2/5
		• R knee extension: 4/5
		• B ankle DF: 4/5
		• B ankle PF: 4/5
	Aerobic	• Not formally assessed at this time
	Flexibility	• Not formally assessed at this time
	Other	• Muscle guarding with LLE > RLE ROM assessment
Neurological	Balance	• Static sitting, unsupported: supervision × 10 minutes
		• Dynamic sitting, unsupported: minimal assistance for weight shifting, limited UE reach activity
		• Static standing: moderate assistance twice to maintain upright posture with rolling walker × 20–30 seconds
	Cognition	• Alert and oriented x 4
	Coordination	• Finger-to-nose: grossly intact bilaterally
	Cranial nerves	• II–XII: intact
	Sensation	• Hypersensitive to light touch at bilateral C6, C7, C8, and left L1, L2, L3, L4, L5
	Functional status	
Bed mobility		• Rolling either direction: moderate assistance once
		• Supine to sit: maximal assistance once
		Upon sitting, patient-reported dizziness, which resolved within ~1 minute.
		• Sit to supine: maximal assistance once
Transfers		• Sit to/from stand: moderate assistance twice with rolling walker
		• Posture notable for flexed posture.
Ambulation		• Not assessed at this time

Assessment	
☑ Physical therapist's	*Assessment left blank for learner to develop.*

Goals	
Patient's	"Get out of this bed." "Use my hands again."
Short term	1. *Goals left blank for learner to develop.* 2.
Long term	1. *Goals left blank for learner to develop.* 2.

Plan	
☐ Physician's ☑ Physical therapist's ☐ Other's	Will follow up patient five to seven times per week to address deficits in range of motion, strength, balance, endurance, and functional mobility through interventions including but not limited to stretching, strengthening exercises, mobility training with assistive device, and general conditioning activities.

Bloom's Taxonomy Level	Case 3.A Questions
Create	1. Synthesizing the medical data and physical examination findings, develop an appropriate physical therapy assessment of the patient. 2. Develop two short-term physical therapy goals, including an appropriate timeframe. 3. Develop two long-term physical therapy goals, including an appropriate timeframe.
Evaluate	4. What impact does the TBSA percentage have in medical management of the patient? 5. What steps are medically taken to prevent infection in this patient given the extensive damage to his skin organ? 6. Why was skin grafting surgery delayed until hospital day 2? Why was a full physical therapy assessment not completed until day 5? 7. What specific intermediate steps should be trialed in subsequent physical therapy sessions to determine best discharge disposition?
Analyze	8. What factors may contribute to the patient's decreased range of motion at the involved joints? 9. What other obstacles may be limiting the patient's activity tolerance at the time of initial evaluation?
Apply	10. What specific functional mobility tasks may be impaired by the injuries to the patient's hands? 11. How can the physical therapist address orthostatic hypotension and lower extremity pain as mobility is reintroduced after prolonged bed rest?
Understand	12. What does the surgical application of an autologous split-thickness skin graft entail?
Remember	13. What are the different classifications of burn injury with regard to depth, and what are their characteristics? 14. What topical agents are used in wound care for this patient, and what are distinctions between their classifications?

Bloom's Taxonomy Level	Case 3.A Answers
Create	1. The patient is a 66-year-old male who presents with partial-thickness burns to his right thigh and anterior torso and full-thickness burns to his left hand, right hand, left forearm, and left thigh. On hospital day 2, the patient underwent excisional debridement of left forearm, bilateral hands, bilateral lower extremities, and anterior torso, and application of split-thickness skin autograft to bilateral hands and left lower extremity. On hospital day 5, dressing changes and staple removal at skin grafting

(Continued)

Bloom's Taxonomy Level	Case 3.A Answers
	sites were performed under anesthesia, with near 100% graft take noted. The patient now presents with significant pain; decreased range of motion of multiple joints from the burn injury, skin grafting, and prolonged immobility; decreased endurance from his injuries and bedrest; and decreased functional mobility. The patient will benefit from continued physical therapy interventions, including but not limited to range of motion and strength training, functional mobility training, and integration of adaptive equipment, to improve the aforementioned deficits. The patient and family will also need extensive education on long-term management of current deficits and self-care strategies to minimize risk of long-term impairments involving areas of skin grafting. Will continue to follow.
	2. Short-term goals:
	• Patient will perform a bed to/from chair transfer with moderate assistance × 1 and rolling walker within 1 week to decrease caregiver burden.
	• Patient will achieve AROM of bilateral hip and knees to ≥ 90 degrees of flexion within 1 week to improve comfort and independence with functional mobility tasks.
	• Patient will independently ensure that dressings over donor sites are clean, dry, and intact 100% of the time within 1 week to improve healing.
	3. Long-term goals:
	• Patient will perform all functional transfers with supervision and least restrictive assistive device within 3 weeks to improve functional independence.
	• Patient will ambulate 50 feet with minimal assistance and rolling walker within 3 weeks to improve household mobility.
	• Patient will independently verbalize his dressing change process, including order of application and dressing materials, within 3 weeks.
Evaluate	4. The TBSA and depth of injury are first and foremost an indication of the severity of the injury. The systemic effects of a burn injury are proportionally related to the TBSA. The breakdown of the extracellular matrix of the skin organ causes fluid shift and places a large burden on the kidneys and cardiovascular and pulmonary systems. Therefore, the fluid resuscitation that is necessary to keep these systems in balance is guided by the TBSA. The hypermetabolic effects are also proportional to TBSA, which means that calorie and protein needs of wound healing are correlated to the TBSA number.
	5. The loss of the protective function of the skin leads to a high risk of infection. The patient's wounds were immediately debrided to remove necrotic tissue from the wound bed. The application of Silvadene, a topical broad-spectrum antimicrobial cream, further helps prevent infection. Skin grafting of the full-thickness burns provides the necessary coverage over a healthy wound bed to further protect from infection. Prophylactic use of an antibiotic, such as cefazolin (Ancef), as well as immune boosting oral agents, like vitamin A, ascorbic acid (vitamin C), and zinc sulfate, can also be used. Surgical skin donor sites are covered with Mepilex Ag to minimize exposure of these sites to infection. WBC count and temperatures are taken to monitor for signs of infection.
	6. Skin grafting was done on hospital day 2 because additional consultation services were warranted to medically clear the patient for surgery. First, orthopaedic surgeon needed to be sure that the trauma to the right hip did not require emergent surgery. Second, cardiologist had to assess the patient and determine any risks given the patient's chest CT findings. While physical therapist was consulted upon admission for positioning, splinting, and skin integrity management, a full physical therapy evaluation was deferred until after the first dressing change and staple removal at the skin graft site.
	The physical therapy evaluation occurred on day 5, as this allowed the skin graft to have sufficient time to adhere to the wound bed. This is especially necessary for a graft that crosses an anatomic joint and will be taught or stretched with functional mobility. For this reason, grafts that do cross a joint are commonly immobilized with splinting or bracing for a 2–3-day period until the dressings are first changed and the surgeons confirm the integrity of the graft. Functional mobility may be assessed in a patient with grafting to an area that is not strained or appropriately immobilized, as the patient's tolerance allows.

(Continued)

(Continued)

Bloom's Taxonomy Level	Case 3.A Answers
	7. It is important to gauge the patient's response to physical therapy interventions with regard to pain management and activity tolerance (i.e., monitoring of vital signs) to determine discharge disposition. Specifically, time spent out of bed in a seated position and tolerance to stretching, strength, and mobility training will help determine the appropriate level of rehabilitation at discharge.
Analyze	8. The patient's burn injury, skin grafts, period of immobility, and bulky dressings all limit the available motion at the wrists and hands. The pain related to the orthopaedic injury as well as the skin donor site at the right thigh limit comfort with right hip and knee motion. The burn injury, skin graft, and skin donor site of the left thigh and period of immobility limit comfort with the left hip and knee motion.
	9. Acute pain and sedative side effects of pain medications, recent anesthesia administration, orthostatic hypotension, and generalized weakness from prolonged immobility may all be contributing to the patient's poor activity tolerance on initial assessment.
Apply	10. On the initial evaluation, the patient's hands are painful, edematous, and wrapped in bulky dressings, all limiting functional grip and weight-bearing tolerance. Specifically, the patient has great difficulty gripping the bedrail and the physical therapist's hand to achieve rolling and the supine to/from sit task. The patient also has difficulty pushing down with the hands at the edge of the bed to initiate forward weight shift for maintaining sitting balance and for the sit-to-stand task. Lastly, the patient's poor grip limits the use of the walker to support weight, as the patient does have bilateral lower extremity injuries.
	11. To address orthostatic hypotension, the physical therapist can have the patient complete range-of-motion exercises, such as long arc quads and/or ankle pumps, prior to attempting bed mobility. These exercises can again be completed once sitting on edge of bed. Additionally, applying compression (i.e., ace wraps) to the legs over top of the wound care dressings can help mitigate pain and the pooling effect that come with introducing a gravity-dependent position in this patient.
Understand	12. The autologous split-thickness skin graft is the standard of care for full-thickness and deep partial-thickness burns. Surgeons look for healthy donor skin on the patient; preferably a large, flat part of the body such as the thigh, flank, or back. Using a tool called dermatome, they remove the epidermal layer and papillary dermis of the skin. Surgeons then place the donor skin through a meshing machine, which increases the size of the donor skin graft, thus allowing less skin to be taken to cover a larger burn area. The graft is then placed over the borders of the burn injury, and attached at the periphery usually with staples, fibrin glue, or sutures. The meshed appearance of the graft allows for the newly generated epithelial cells to fill in the space at the junction of the wound and graft. The graft is typically left immobilized and in surgical dressings for 48–72 hours. After that period, the dressings are removed, the surgeons examine the attachment of the graft to the wound bed, and staples or sutures are removed as appropriate.
Remember	13. The different classifications of burn injury with regard to depth and their descriptions are as follows: *Superficial (formerly first degree):* • Damage is to the epidermis. • Skin presents as red or erythematous, dry surface, and without blisters. • Pain is moderate. • Healing occurs within 5–10 days with no scar formation. *Superficial partial thickness (formerly second degree):* • Damage is to the entire epidermis and superficial (papillary) dermis, with preservation of underlying vasculature. • Skin presents as red and blanchable and weeping, with blisters. • Pain is severe. • Healing occurs within 3 weeks with minimal scarring.

(Continued)

(Continued)

Bloom's Taxonomy Level	Case 3.A Answers
	Deep partial thickness (formerly second degree): • Damage is to the entire epidermis and superficial (papillary) and deeper (reticular) dermis, with involvement of underlying vasculature. • Skin presents as yellow or white (leathery in appearance), dry, and minimal to no blanching. • Pain is minimal due to decreased sensation. • Healing occurs within 3–8 weeks with scarring present. *Full thickness (formerly third degree):* • Damage is through the entire skin and subcutaneous structures. • Skin presents as white or black/brown (leathery in appearance) and dry with no blanching. • Pain is minimal to absent due to decreased sensation. • Healing takes greater than 8 weeks and requires skin grafting. 14. The topic agents used in wound care for this patient are enzymatic debriders and antimicrobials. Distinctions between the two are as follows: • Enzymatic debriders: Clean the wound bed of necrotic tissue • Antimicrobials: preserve the healthy environment of an already clean wound bed

Key points

1. Burn injuries are painful injuries that damage the skin organ and impair healthy movement as well as limit the patient's ability to fight infection. This damage has profound effects on the renal, cardiovascular and pulmonary, and vascular systems and places a high demand on the patient's metabolic system with increased calories and proteins needed for healing.

2. Superficial and superficial partial-thickness burns should heal spontaneously through the process of reepithelialization. The management is to create and maintain a healthy wound bed and prevent infection. Most deep partial and all full-thickness burn injuries will require skin grafting surgery once a wound bed is prepared and the patient's medical and nutritional status have been optimized.

3. Basic physical therapy interventions can be introduced immediately to prevent the secondary effects of immobilization, maximizing preserved motion and strength. Skin grafts require a period of immobility to fully adhere to wound bed before introducing range of motion or shearing force to the affected area.

General Information

Case no.	3.B
Authors	Brian Stagno, PT
Diagnosis	Thermal burns to 14% total body surface area (TBSA)
Setting	Acute inpatient rehabilitation
Learner expectations	☑ Initial evaluation ☐ Re-evaluation ☐ Treatment session
Learner objectives	1. Gain a greater understanding of the subacute medical management and physiologic healing process of a burn injury. 2. Construct a plan of care that prioritizes deficits, addresses barriers to discharge from a rehabilitation unit, and achieves requirements for discharge to community. 3. List topics of patient education to prepare patient for long-term self-management of burn injuries.

Medical

Chief complaint	"I can't go home like this. I can't take care of myself at all."
History of present illness	A 66-year-old male presents to the hospital status post a fall from a stool while using a welding torch overhead. Per patient, once on the ground, his clothes caught on fire. Due to hip pain from the fall, the patient was unable to get up quickly. However, he did put out the flame by patting with his gloved hands and rolling his body over the flames.

(Continued)

(Continued)

Medical	
	During his acute hospitalization, the patient underwent sharp debridement and deep cleansing of burn injuries on hospital day 0, excisional debridement of all burns, and split-thickness skin grafting surgery to bilateral hands and left lower extremity using donor skin from bilateral thighs on hospital day 2, and operative dressing change and removal of staples on hospital day 5. The patient continued with daily dressing changes and daily physical therapy until transfer to acute inpatient rehabilitation on hospital day 9.
Past medical history	Hypertension, chronic lower extremity edema, dyspnea on exertion
Past surgical history	See HPI
Allergies	Morphine (depresses respiration) Lisinopril (cough)
Medications	Prehospitalization: Aspirin, Furosemide, Losartan Currently: Gabapentin, Ibuprofen, Acetaminophen, Iron supplement, Zinc sulfate, Ascorbic acid, Vitamin A PRN medication: Roxicodone, Anti-anxiety medication
Precautions/Orders	Activity as tolerated

Social history	
Home setup	• Resides in a ranch style home with wife • One step to enter • Flight of stairs plus one handrail to basement, where work area/garage is located
Occupation	• Automechanic, part time, self-employed
Prior level of function	• Independent with functional mobility and activities of daily living; however, mildly limited by occasional shortness of breath.
Recreational activities	• Projects around the house and in garage: "I'm always working on something."

Vital signs	Day 1: acute inpatient rehabilitation
Blood pressure (mmHg)	148/92
Heart rate (beats/min)	105
Respiratory rate (breaths/min)	22
Pulse oximetry on room air (SpO_2)	97
Temperature (°F)	99.0 (tympanic)

Medical management	Day 1: acute inpatient rehabilitation
Wound care	1. Daily dressing changes to be completed as follows: • Wash all areas with gentle antibacterial soap, dry completely. • Cover areas of injury with bacitracin/Cuticerin/gauze web roll and stockinette. • Mepilex to remain in place covering donor sites until post-op day 7.
Nutrition	1. Added nutritional supplement drinks: ensure with 1–2 meals/day, as well as high protein snack once a day.

Pause points
Based on the above information, what are the priority • Diagnostic tests and measures? • Outcome measures? • Treatment interventions?

Day 1, Acute Inpatient Rehabilitation: Physical Therapy Examination		
Subjective		
"This is really hard, but I know I have to get moving."		
Objective		
Vital signs	Pre-treatment	Post-treatment
Blood pressure (mmHg)	116/67	111/72
Heart rate (beats/min)	84	101
Respiratory rate (breaths/min)	18	24
Pulse oximetry on room air (SpO_2)	98	96
Pain	6 /10 at bilateral thighs 7/10 at bilateral hands	8/10 at bilateral thighs and bilateral hands
General	• Patient presents in bed, anxious appearing. • Dressings are intact to bilateral hands and left lower extremity, with moderate exudate noted. Bilateral thighs are covered with Mepilex Ag sheets, reinforced with gauze wrap. • Per chart notes and patient report, dressings changed last evening • Lines notable for peripheral IV access	
Cardiovascular and pulmonary	• Normal sinus rhythm and rate • No adventitious breath sounds	
Musculoskeletal	Range of motion	• L shoulder: WNL • R shoulder: WNL • L elbow: WNL • R elbow: WNL • L wrist flexion: 0–25 degrees • R wrist flexion: 0–25 degrees • L wrist extension: 0–15 degrees • R wrist extension: 0–20 degrees • B MCP/PIP/DIP flexion/extension: limited and painful • L hip flexion, AROM: 0–65 degrees • L hip flexion, AAROM: 0–80 degrees • R hip flexion, AROM: 0–70 degrees • R hip flexion, AAROM: 0–90 degrees • L knee, AROM: 0–60 degrees • R knee, AROM: 0–95 degrees • B ankle DF, AROM: WNL • B ankle PF, AROM: WNL
	Strength	• B shoulder flexion: 5/5 • B elbow flexion: 5/5 • B elbow extension: 5/5 • B wrist flexion: 2/5 • B wrist extension: 2/5 • B grip strength: 1/5 • L hip flexion: 2/5 • R hip flexion: 3 + /5 • L knee extension: 2/5 • R knee extension: 4/5 • B ankle dorsiflexion: 4/5 • B ankle plantarflexion: 4/5
	Aerobic	• Notable dyspnea on exertion, increased accessory muscle breathing, verbal cues required for deep breathing techniques.
Neurological	Balance	• Static sitting, unsupported: independent • Dynamic sitting, unsupported: supervision

(Continued)

(Continued)

		Day 1, Acute Inpatient Rehabilitation: Physical Therapy Examination
		• Static standing, unsupported: deferred due to safety concerns • Static standing, supported: minimal assistance with platform rolling walker, (+) retropulsion and significant UE support needed • Dynamic standing, unsupported: deferred due to safety concerns • Dynamic standing, supported: minimal assistance × 2 with platform rolling walker
	Cognition	• Alert and oriented × 4 • Anxious • Easily distracted, requires cuing to attend to task. • Encouragement and positive reinforcement needed for most tasks.
	Coordination	• Finger-to-nose: grossly intact bilaterally, though limited by hand dressings and pain with movement.
	Cranial nerves	• II–XII: intact
	Sensation	• Intact to light touch throughout BUE and BLE, though diminished at areas of dressings.
	Tone	• Muscle guarding at hip and knee groups, noted with initial introduction of ROM.
Integumentary	Partial-thickness burns	• 100% reepithelization • Appears erythematous with scant bleeding, particularly with range of motion and functional mobility. • Open to air, with daily application of antimicrobial lotion.
	Split-thickness skin grafts	• Left forearm and bilateral hands: partial epithelialization, retaining cyclone, meshed appearance. • Left thigh: healthy pink, with scattered raised areas indicating scar formation.
	Donor sites	• Neat borders, slight erythema
		Functional status
Bed mobility		• Rolling to left: minimal assistance • Rolling to right: moderate assistance • Supine to sit: moderate assistance at leading LE and trunk; patient initiates well with trunk • Sit to supine: maximal assistance for trunk control and BLEs into bed
Transfers		• Sit to stand: moderate assistance × 2 people with platform rolling walker. Patient demonstrates fair initiation and BLE stability; initial retropulsion, verbal and tactile cuing for anterior weight shift and UE grip on bariatric walker. • Stand pivot transfer: minimal assistance × 2 with platform rolling walker. Patient demonstrates postural instability, difficulty with weight shifting. Patient achieved pivot with physical therapists' assistance to initiate weight shifts.
Ambulation		• Ambulated 15 feet with minimal assistance × 2 with platform rolling walker (▶ Fig. 3.3). • Gait deviations notable for rigidness, with increased time in double stance between steps, absent heel strike bilaterally, and flexed trunk posture.
Stairs		• N/A due to safety concerns

Task specific		• Modified functional reach test while sitting unsupported:
		  ○ Forward reach: 18 cm
		  ○ Right lateral reach: 10 cm
		  ○ Left lateral reach: 9 cm

Assessment	
☑ Physical therapist's	*Assessment left blank for learner to develop.*

Goals	
Patient's	"I want to be able to walk better."
Short term	1. *Goals left blank for learner to develop.* 2.
Long term	1. *Goals left blank for learner to develop.* 2.

Plan	
☐ Physician's ☑ Physical therapist's ☐ Other's	Will benefit from intensive physical therapy for stretching, strengthening exercises, functional mobility with assistive device use, and general conditioning. Overall goal is to return home with spouse's assistance.

Bloom's Taxonomy Level	Case 3.B Questions
Create	1. Synthesizing the medical data and physical examination findings, develop an appropriate physical therapy assessment of the patient. 2. Develop two short-term physical therapy goals, including an appropriate timeframe. 3. Develop two long-term physical therapy goals, including an appropriate timeframe.
Evaluate	4. What durable medical equipment may be used to improve patient's independence with bed mobility, transfers, and gait training? How would the physical therapist expect to progress the patient away from such devices? 5. What impact may the patient's anxiety play in his rehabilitation course? What compensatory strategies may be used to overcome this limitation?
Analyze	6. What should the physical therapist instruct the patient to do in between therapy sessions and overnight to maintain the motion gains being made?
Apply	7. How can the physical therapist best use the modified functional reach test scores?
Understand	8. How do topical agents and dressings progress over the course of healing for areas of partial-thickness burns, skin grafted sites, and donor sites?
Remember	9. What topics should be included in patient education and discharge planning?

Bloom's Taxonomy Level	Case 3.B Answers

Create	1. The patient is a 66-year-old male who presents with partial-thickness burns to his right thigh and anterior torso and full-thickness burns to his left hand, right hand, left forearm, and left thigh. His acute care hospital course was notable for sharp debridement on hospital day 0, excisional debridement of all burns, and split-thickness skin grafting surgery to bilateral hands and left lower extremity using donor skin from bilateral thighs on hospital day 2, and operative dressing change and removal of staples of hospital day 5. As a result, the patient has had a functional decline and presents to acute inpatient rehabilitation. During today's physical therapy examination, the patient demonstrates a significant increase in pain, decreased range of motion, decreased strength, postural instability and impaired balance, and decreased activity tolerance, all limiting safe and independent functional mobility. Patient would benefit from continued physical therapy to improve the aforementioned deficits. Will continue to follow.
	2. Short-term goals:
	  • Patient will complete supine to/from sit with minimal assistance within 10 days to improve independence.
	  • Patient will complete sit to/from stand transfers with minimal assistance and least restrictive assistive device within 10 days to improve independence.
	  • Patient will independently remove > 50% of wound dressings within 10 days to decrease caregiver burden and promote independence.
	3. Long-term goals:
	  • Patient will ambulate 100 feet with modified independence and rolling walker within 3 weeks to allow safe access through home environment.

(Continued)

(Continued)

Bloom's Taxonomy Level	Case 3.B Answers
	• Patient will independently demonstrate home exercise program within 3 weeks to maximize BUE and BLE ROM and strength. • Patient's spouse will demonstrate proper body mechanics 100% of the time when assisting patient within 3 weeks to reduce her risk of injury. • Patient and caregiver will demonstrate independence and effectiveness with scar management techniques to left lower extremity within 3 weeks to decrease risk of adverse reactions.
Evaluate	4. For bed mobility, a hospital bed with a trapeze attachment may allow the patient more independence with mobility while his leg motion is limited. However, pain and dressings at the hand injuries may limit grip strength and comfort using the trapeze, as well when using a walker. For more comfort while using the trapeze during bed mobility and walker during transfers and gait, increasing the size and softness of the grips with towel rolls or wash cloths may help. The cushioned platform walker may be helpful for initial gait training to provide more upper extremity support and allow focus on gait mechanics at the legs. As the left leg and bilateral hands become more flexible and comfortable bearing weight, the patient may progress to a more traditional rolling walker. 5. Any patient experiencing the trauma of a burn injury may require increased time, as well as patience and encouragement from the physical therapist to achieve the therapeutic goals. Monitoring pain levels and ensuring that medications for pain and/or anxiety are scheduled in advance of physical therapy will help maximize outcomes of each session. Allowing the patient to play a greater role in selecting from choices of interventions or the sequence of those interventions may help him feel more in control of his rehabilitation course. Giving clear explanations of benefits of each intervention, as well as expectations with regard to repetitions or duration of an intervention, may help the patient focus on the task and have a sense of achievement after completing the activity.
Analyze	6. The physical therapist should encourage the patient to complete. • Stretching. An example of this is having the patient lay flat and/or prone to stretch the hip flexors, since he is likely in a wheelchair the majority of the day. • Therapeutic exercise. An example of this is heel slides, which can not only strengthen the muscle but also improve range of motion. After encouraging motion all day, nighttime may be a good time to use resting hand splints or a knee immobilizer to prevent the patient from inadvertently reverting to positions of comfort. Additionally, the patient can be encouraged to perform dressing changes at night to ensure that they are in place during a long, period of inactivity (overnight). This also minimizes the impact therapy interventions may have on displacing the bandages. Because burn dressing changes may be painful, it's also beneficial to let the patient rest after the dressing change.
Apply	7. Though there is limited normative data for seated functional reach measurements, especially with regard to this patient population, it can be inferred that this patient has a significant impairment in dynamic sitting balance. Interventions may address seated balance and flexibility exercises, which can eventually simulate his occupation. Ultimately, a repeated measure of the seated functional reach test should be performed to assess patient's progression or regression.
Understand	8. Enzymatic debriders (Santyl) may be used after injury to ensure that any necrotic tissue is cleared from the wound bed. They are also chosen if there is any evidence of infection at the wound site. Once a partial-thickness burn injury wound has been sufficiently cleaned, antimicrobial agents (e.g., Silvadene, Bacitracin) may be used to maintain a clean, healthy, moist environment for reepithelialization. Following grafting for a full-thickness burn, Bacitracin may be used to maintain a moist wound environment. Donor sites are treated similarly to a superficial partial thickness burn and topically receive antimicrobial treatments as long as they remain free of infection. The neat borders of donor sites are managed well with silver sulfate sheets (Mepilex Ag) that provide coverage for up to 7 days without the need to remove or change dressings.

(Continued)

(Continued)

Bloom's Taxonomy Level	Case 3.B Answers
	Characteristically, superficial burns heal in 5–10 days and superficial partial-thickness burns heal within 3 weeks. Once epidermal coverage is consistent across the wound, dressings can be eliminated. However, it is advised that topical application of moisturizers, such as vitamin E cream or coconut oil, is important for an extended period of weeks to months.
	Deep partial- or full-thickness burns that receive surgical skin grafting will require antimicrobials and dressing coverage until epidermal coverage is consistent across the wound, at which time dressings can be eliminated and topical agents switched to moisturizers.
Remember	9. Education during the patient's acute inpatient rehabilitation stay should promote independent management of his injuries. The patient should be informed of the normal course of wound healing and the scar formation process, which can last for up to a year. For this reason, emphasis must be placed on preparing the patient to self-manage his deficits and preventing long-term complications postinjury. Examples of self-management include educating the patient on: • Stretching exercises with low reps and long holds are important to restore and maintain flexibility at affected areas. • Adding deep pressure or scar massage techniques with moisturizer application, particularly in areas of superficial tendons to prevent hypertrophic scarring. Emphasizing that scar formation can be severely limiting and lead to further repeat surgeries is a necessary element of educating a patient with a full-thickness burn. • Future use of compression garments may also be appropriate.

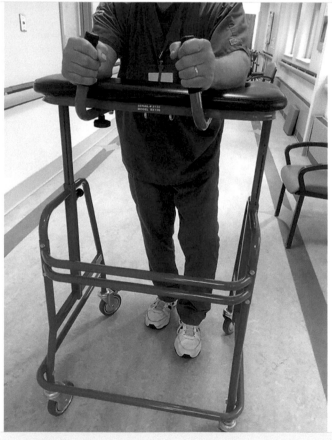

Fig. 3.3 Gait training with a platform rolling walker.

Key points

1. One of the essential characteristics of the skin is elasticity. Introducing range of motion to areas of a burn injury should be done as soon as pain allows for partial-thickness burns, or after the placement of a skin graft, as long as graft adherence is acceptable to the surgeons and surgical staples/sutures are removed.

2. Stretching, strengthening, and functional mobility outcomes will be maximized if consideration is given to the patient's pain, anxiety, medical, and nutritional status.

3. Patient and caregiver education should begin immediately and repeated often. Topics to include are wound and dressing care, the importance of stretching/range of motion exercises, functional use of injured extremities, and the signs and symptoms of possible infection and scar formation.

General Information

Case no.	3.C
Authors	Mike Fletcher, PT, DPT Brian Stagno, PT
Diagnosis	Thermal burns to 14% total body surface area (TBSA)
Setting	Outpatient clinic
Learner expectations	☑ Initial evaluation ☐ Re-evaluation ☐ Treatment session
Learner objectives	1. Relate multisystem impairment to initial injury and overall functional mobility. 2. Construct a plan of care that prioritizes deficits, as well as impairments that have developed secondary to the initial injury. Develop appropriate interventions and goals. 3. List topics of patient education to prepare patient for long-term self-management of burn injuries and overall secondary impairments.

Medical

Chief complaint	"I just am not getting around as well as I want to. I also feel weak and cannot tolerate a lot of activity. My hips just feel so limited."
History of present illness	A 66-year-old male presents to outpatient physical therapy status post multisite burns 6 weeks ago. Per the patient, he was standing on a stool using a welding torch overhead. He unfortunately fell and his clothes caught on fire. He was unable to quickly move secondary to instant right hip discomfort. Therefore, he put the burn out by rolling his body and utilizing his gloved hands to pat the flames. He sustained partial-thickness burns to his right thigh (1%) and anterior torso (4%), and full-thickness burns to his left hand (1%), right hand (1%), left forearm (2%), and left lower extremity (5%). He underwent skin excision and debridement with autografting to all full-thickness areas via split-thickness skin grafting. His right hip was negative for acute fracture. Following his acute care stay, he was admitted to acute inpatient rehabilitation for a 12-day stay. Per patient, upon discharge from rehabilitation, he follows up with the burn surgeons as an outpatient for wound care twice a month; however, they recently decreased to once a month because wounds are all closed and healing well. He presents today with chief complaint of mobility deficits, generalized tightness and weakness in bilateral hips, and decreased endurance.
Past medical history	Hypertension, chronic lower extremity edema, dyspnea on exertion
Past surgical history	None except for above mentioned procedures post burn
Allergies	Morphine (depresses respiration) Lisinopril (cough)
Medications	Aspirin, Furosemide, Losartan, Gabapentin, Ibuprofen, Acetaminophen, Iron supplement, Zinc sulfate, Ascorbic acid tab, Vitamin A, Sertraline (Zoloft)
Precautions/Orders	Activity as tolerated

Social history	
Home setup	• Resides in a ranch style home with wife • One step to enter • Flight of stairs plus one handrail to basement, where work area/garage is located
Occupation	• Automechanic, part time, self-employed
Prior level of function	• Independent with functional mobility and activities of daily living; however, mildly limited by occasional shortness of breath.
Recreational activities	• Projects around the house and in garage: "I'm always working on something."

Medical management	
Wound care	• All wounds have closed. • Epithelialization is occurring at all grafting sites. • Nongrafted sites have healed well. • Eschar noted mid left thigh at top of graft site which is the only site that has not fully epithelialized. • Increased raised scarring at donor sites (▶ Fig. 3.4), left wrist, and left anterolateral hip.
Nutrition	• Physician has patient on regimen to maintain 1–2 g of protein per kilogram body weight per day. • Patient taking two protein shakes throughout day and protein bar snack mid-day.

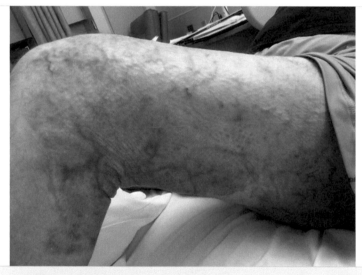

Fig. 3.4 Raised scarring at donor site of left anterolateral hip.

Pause points
Based on the above information, what are the priority • Diagnostic tests and measures? • Outcome measures? • Treatment interventions?

Physical Therapy Examination		
Subjective		
"I am feeling okay; but I am so stiff when I wake up and it feels like my hips pull me forward"		
Objective		
Vital signs	Pre-treatment	Post-treatment
Blood pressure (mmHg)	118/68	120/68
Heart rate (beats/min)	86	104
Respiratory rate (breaths/min)	16	20
Pulse oximetry on room air (SpO$_2$)	98	97
Pain	5/10 at low back and bilateral hips	6/10 at low back and bilateral hips
General	• Patient is sitting on plinth, appears anxious. • There are no dressings to any burn sites. • Observations notable for guarding of right hand and guarding of bilateral lower extremities. As a result, patient demonstrates rigid gait and is using a single point cane in left hand.	
Cardiovascular and pulmonary	• Normal increase in HR and RR with activity is noted.	
Musculoskeletal	Range of motion	*All UE ROM measurements were taken from AROM. BLE ROM measurements as indicated below.* • L shoulder flexion: 0–166 degrees • R shoulder flexion: 0–170 degrees • L shoulder abduction: 0–164 degrees • R shoulder abduction: 0–166 degrees • B shoulder extension, ER, IR: WFL • B elbow: 0–102 degrees • L wrist flexion: 0–50 degrees • R wrist flexion: 0–48 degrees • L wrist extension: 0–25 degrees • R wrist extension: 0–22 degrees • R MCP, digits 1–4, flexion: 0–75 • R MCP, digits 1–4, extension: 0–3 degrees • B MIP, digits 1–5, flexion: 0–82 degrees • B MIP, digits 1–5, extension: 0–5 degrees • B DIP, digits 1–5, flexion: 0–80 degrees • B DIP, digits 1–5, extension: 0–6 degrees • L hip flexion, AROM: 0–93 degrees • L hip flexion, PROM: 0–99 degrees • R hip flexion, AROM: 0–86 degrees • R hip flexion, PROM: 0–95 degrees • L hip abduction, AROM: 0–36 degrees • L hip abduction, AAROM: 0–44 degrees • R hip abduction, AROM: 0–32 degrees • R hip abduction, AAROM: 0–41 degrees • B ER/IR deferred due to discomfort • L knee, AROM: 0–109 degrees • R knee, AROM: 0–118 degrees • B knee, PROM: increased tightness at end range of extension • B ankle DF, AROM: WFL • B ankle PF, AROM: WFL
	Strength	• B shoulder flexion: 5/5 • B shoulder abduction: 5/5 • B elbow flexion: 5/5 • B elbow extension: 5/5 • B wrist extension: 3/5

(Continued)

(Continued)

Physical Therapy Examination		
		• B wrist flexion: 4–/5 • B hip flexion: 4–/5 • B hip abduction: 3+/5 • B hip extension: 4–/5 • B hip internal rotation: 3+/5 • B hip external rotation: 4–/5 • B knee flexion: 4+/5 • B knee extension: 3+/5 • B ankle dorsiflexion: 4/5 • B ankle plantar flexion: 3/5 • B ankle inversion: 4–/5 • B ankle eversion: 4–/5 *Through hip flexors and knee extensors, patient with decreased muscular endurance and decreased VMO recruitment.*
	Aerobic	• With transfers and initial ambulation, patient utilizes Valsalva maneuver. This creates reported shortness of breath, which was corrected with verbal cuing. • 6-Minute Walk Test: 507 m
	Special tests	• Ober Test: (+) bilaterally • Thomas Test: (+) bilaterally • FADIR: (–) bilaterally • FABER: (–) bilaterally
Integumentary	Joint integrity	• Hypomobility noted with B wrist extension, MIP extension, and DIP extension glides • Bilateral inferior, posterior, and lateral hip glide mobility deficits
	Soft tissue	• Increased tension B wrist and hand extensor musculature limiting ROM and extensibility • Increased quad tightness and TTP B; ITB TTP B; hip flexor tenderness, restriction, and slight contracture B • Hip adductor tightness and discomfort bilaterally
Neurological	Balance	• Static sitting, unsupported: independent, increased forward flexed positioning • Static standing, unsupported: independent • Dynamic standing, unsupported: contact guard assistance • Romberg, eyes open: 30 seconds with increased sway • Romberg, eyes closed: 15 seconds before needing to open eyes for visual input and stability • Tandem stance: minimal assistance Right in front of left: 8 seconds Left in front of right: 7 seconds • Mini-BESTest: 19/28
	Cognition	• Alert and oriented x 4 • Anxious • Slight impulsivity • Follows simple commands, difficulty sequencing multistep commands
	Coordination	• Finger-to-nose: grossly intact bilaterally, though limited by hand dressings and pain with movement
	Cranial nerves	• II–XII: intact
	Reflexes	• Patellar: 2+ bilaterally
	Sensation	• Intact to light touch throughout BUE and BLE • Slightly diminished at L L2, L3, L4

(Continued)

(Continued)

Physical Therapy Examination		
	Tone	• Muscle guarding hip and knee groups noted with initial introduction of ROM bilaterally • Hypertonic throughout bilateral anterior hip compartments
	Other	
Functional status		
Bed mobility	• Supine to/from sit: independent	
Transfers	• Sit to/from stand: independent, frequently uses arms for assistance	
Ambulation	• Ambulated for 100 feet with modified independence and single point cane. • Gait deviations notable for antalgic gait, increased left lateral lean, decreased bilateral heel strike with increased mid-foot landing creating increased waddle sequencing and Trendelenburg sequence, and decreased toe off.	
Stairs	• Ascend/descend curb step with supervision and single point cane	
Functional movement	• Increased genu valgus with squatting; increased L lateral lean	

Assessment	
☑ Physical therapist's	*Assessment left blank for learner to develop.*
Goals	
Patient's	"I want to get back to work."
Short term	1. *Goals left blank for learner to develop.* 2.
Long term	1. *Goals left blank for learner to develop.* 2.

Plan	
☐ Physician's ☑ Physical therapist's ☐ Other's	Patient will benefit from skilled physical therapy two to three times per week for 6 weeks to address the aforementioned impairments. Treatment will consist of soft-tissue and joint mobilization, flexibility, progressive resistive therapeutic exercise, gait training, neuromuscular reeducation, body mechanics, and instruction on a comprehensive home exercise program.

Bloom's Taxonomy Level	Case 3.C Questions
Create	1. Synthesizing the medical data and physical examination findings, develop an appropriate physical therapy assessment of the patient. 2. Develop two short-term physical therapy goals, including an appropriate timeframe. 3. Develop two long-term physical therapy goals, including an appropriate timeframe. 4. Construct simulation activities to coincide with patient's return to work, which is scheduled for 2 weeks from the date of physical therapy initial evaluation.
Evaluate	5. Determine the patient's psychosocial concerns/status and correlate this to patient's overall presentation. How may this affect his course of therapy? 6. Assess the need for multidisciplinary approach and determine appropriate referral(s) if applicable.
Analyze	7. Analyze relationship of proximal musculature recruitment and locations of burn sites and grafts, and then correlate to balance impairments.
Apply	8. Based on the patient's gait deviations, what physical therapy interventions can be implemented to help correct?

(Continued)

(Continued)

Bloom's Taxonomy Level	Case 3.C Questions
	9. What are appropriate manual therapy interventions that can be implemented to promote tissue healing and joint integrity?
	10. What are three interventions that can be implemented to improve patient's postural awareness/balance?
Understand	11. Interpret the patient's 6-Minute Walk Test (6MWT) score.
	12. Based on healing graft sites, describe how the healing process will affect progressing the rehabilitation program in terms of weight-bearing, repetitions, and resistance levels.
	13. Interpret the patient's Mini-BESTest scores and locate areas needed for improvement. What is the MCDI of the Mini-BESTest?
Remember	14. What are the properties of the dermis and how does this affect the outpatient rehabilitation process?
	15. List the most appropriate outpatient rehabilitative planning for individuals who have sustained burns.

Bloom's Taxonomy Level	Case 3.C Answers
Create	1. The patient is a 66-year-old male status post multisite burns who presents with multisystem involvement. The patient demonstrates generalized weakness, decreased balance, decreased endurance, integumentary deficits including but not limited to decreased skin extensibility and multi-joint tension restrictions, and impaired functional mobility. Patient will benefit from continued skilled physical therapy to address these impairments and to maximize functional mobility and safety. Will continue to follow.
	2. Short-term goals:
	• Patient will increase bilateral hip flexion active range of motion to 100 degrees within 3 weeks to improve his ability to negotiate stairs.
	• Patient will increase proximal hip muscle strength (of all major muscle groups) by grade 1/2 to improve pelvic stability, weight-bearing tolerance, and muscular endurance.
	3. Long-term goals:
	• Patient will increase his Mini-BESTest score to 24/28 within 6 weeks to improve dynamic functional balance and maximize safety.
	• Patient will increase his 6MWT distance to 575 m within 6 weeks to improve his cardiovascular endurance.
	4. The patient is an automechanic. This job requires frequent positional changes, reaching outside of base of support, static and dynamic balance, and fine motor tasks. Therefore, as his return to work nears, many factors must be considered for simulation activities. Examples of simulation activities that can be performed to help prepare the patient to return to work include:
	• Positional changes on various surfaces. Positions that should be trialed may include supine, prone, half kneeling, kneeling, sitting, and standing.
	• Balance activities such as reaching for various weighted objects, located at various heights, outside of base of support; obstacle course to simulate a garage; activities with narrow base of support (including single limb stance), etc.
	• Fine motor activities such as sifting through hardware (bolts, straps, etc.), extending fingers through resistance, and completing A/AAROM from wrist through distal finger joints.
	Education on body mechanics should also be provided.
Evaluate	5. As noted from the acute care and acute inpatient rehabilitation settings, it is imperative to examine how the patient is coping during the rehabilitation process. It is important to remember that this patient may have an altered body image/appearance. This can impact motivation and/or potentially lead to fear, anxiety, and/or depression. If the individual is struggling with any of these emotions, this can

(Continued)

(Continued)

Bloom's Taxonomy Level	Case 3.C Answers
	negatively affect his physical performance, activity engagement, and progression. In general, individuals with burns tend to have an altered outlook on progress secondary to months of altered daily routines which have all strayed from their sense of normalcy. If these are noticed during physical therapy sessions, it is appropriate to have the discussion with the patient and complete appropriate referrals to mental health professionals. If a patient is in need of anxiety/depression medication, the earlier in the rehabilitation process the better; therefore, some clients may present to the clinic already on a particular dosage. For this patient, he has been prescribed Zoloft. 6. Multidisciplinary approaches for treatment of individuals post–burn injury are typically utilized. As noted earlier, referral for psychosocial issues has high significance. Beyond that, referrals to other medical professionals are commonly made. Depending on severity of burn, occupational therapy, speech therapy, and recreational therapy may also be involved in the patient's care.
Analyze	7. Proximal musculature recruitment in relation to posture and burn site areas is significant for this patient. Injuries that crossover the hip joint, from abdomen to thigh, tend to force an individual into a forward flexed posture. There is also a decrease in back extensors activation and increased tightness through the anterior hip compartment. With deficits in muscle recruitment and abnormal muscle coupling (hip flexors and back extensors, hip extensors, and core), the patient is more likely to develop contractures secondary to such compensations. Therefore, proper alignment with upright positions and gait is varied, providing altered center of mass and abnormal gait sequencing at more distal joints.
Apply	8. The patient's gait deviations are notable for antalgic gait, increased left lateral lean, decreased bilateral heel strike with increased mid-foot landing creating increased waddle sequencing and Trendelenburg sequence, and decreased toe off. The gait sequence with decreased bilateral heel strike and toe off along with decreased right weight-bearing indicate the need for increased weight-bearing activity on the right lower extremity. Treatment ideas may include weight shifts, single leg activity as tolerated, high kneeling positions to RLE, left lunges, and increasing isolated resistive exercises to weak musculature (single leg raises, side lying hip abductions, etc.). Promoting multiple joint involvement is typically successful at increased weight loading such as squats and progressing activity to uneven terrain/surfaces. For increased core involvement and posture, prone exercise program should be initiated early to promote extensibility of the anterior compartment musculature in the core and hips. However, it is important to remember those both lower extremities have involvement and symmetry should also be emphasized. 9. Appropriate manual therapy interventions that can be implemented to promote tissue healing and joint integrity include: • Passive range of motion to (a) proximal hip musculature (hip flexors, hip adductors, and gluteals) (b) wrist/hand/finger extension stretches especially at MCP, MIP, and DIP joints to avoid static flexion. • Increased transverse friction scar massage for to decrease risk of scar tissue formation and hypertrophic scarring. Emphasis should be placed on areas that cross joint lines or that cover superficial tendons. 10. Three interventions that can be implemented to improve this patient's postural awareness/balance include: • Prone lying to improve extensibility of tissues throughout abdominal wall and anterior hip regions. • Weight bearing exercises such as bridging, squatting, steamboats and lunging to increase weight bearing, strengthening, and stability through BLEs. • Upper extremity exercises such as scapular retraction, pectoralis stretches, and cervical retraction to promote posture and assist with upright positioning during gait/balance.

(Continued)

(Continued)

Bloom's Taxonomy Level	Case 3.C Answers
Understand	11. During the 6MWT, the patient was able to ambulate 507 m. This is indicative of an endurance deficit, as the norm for a male between the ages of 60 and 69 years old is > 572 m. As the patient begins endurance training, retesting the 6MWT is a good comparative measure and a change of 50 m is considered significant according to the MCID for community dwelling individuals.
	12. Healing graft areas will affect overall extensibility of the skin and soft tissue structures in the surrounding areas such as muscles and tendons. This will affect progression of exercises because through the healing process there will be limitations of ROM and stretching due to this extensibility and it is a gradual healing process to assist promotion of extensibility to the above-mentioned tissues to increase activity level to the graft regions. When performing interventions, it is imperative to screen for scar blanching to decrease the risk of skin tears.
	13. The Mini-BESTest (Balance Evaluation Systems Test) is a clinical assessment tool that assesses 6 different balance control systems through 14 items. This allows optimal interventions to be implemented. The test's MCID is a 4-point change. The normative value for ages 60–69 is 24.7/28. This patient scored a 19/28 at physical therapy initial evaluation, and, therefore, is below the norm for his age. A goal can be set based on a 4-point increment utilizing the MCID.
Remember	14. Collagen and elastin fibers develop networks that create properties in the dermis which are elasticity, strength, extensibility. Due to trauma, in this case a burn, the patient is susceptible to increased stiffness, roughness, and hardness through the dermal level secondary to such fibers being traumatized which limits all the dermal qualities which reinforces why treatment to improve conditions and to prevent further damage is indicated.
	15. The most appropriate outpatient rehabilitation planning for this individual is to limit the loss of and promote ROM, reduce edema, prevent contractures and promote flexibility, assist with scar management, increase strength, and encourage higher balance and functional activities. It is important to create and maintain an open conversation throughout the treatment plan. Lastly, education must be provided at the patient's level of understanding.

Key points
1. Contractures are defined as a joint's inability to complete full range of motion. This can be caused by a multitude of reasons including surrounding soft tissue as well as bones that make up the joint. With burns, these areas are susceptible to damage and subsequently the body produces a physiological response creating increased fibroblast and myofibroblast activity which can result in increased scarring as well as damaged soft tissue which loses extensibility creating scar contractures as well as joint contractures. These contractures can lead to functional inhibitions of ambulation, activities of daily living, transfers, and fine motor skills. This is why addressing soft tissue, joint, and scar mobilization early is crucial for the patient's function.
2. Relating physical impairments to the whole body is imperative. Relating functional mobility to job tasks as well as relating mind set and motivation to rehabilitation goals helps create a plan of care that is encompassing the entire patient. Setting up a broader whole-patient spectrum is likely to have better goal attainment.
3. In the outpatient phase of rehabilitation for individuals post burn, the deficits addressed are the subsequent impairments that have accumulated after the injury itself. As the wound sites are mostly healed focusing on compensations, muscular restrictions, gait deficits, and balance are crucial at this stage. Impairments manifest due to our body's responses to a trauma. This can lead to compensations. Therefore, rehabilitation at the outpatient setting is pulling together multisystem involvement to promote overall function.

Suggested Readings

6 Minute Walk Test. Available at: https://www.sralab.org/rehabilitation-measures/6-minute-walk-test. Accessed June 1, 2020

Dodd H, Fletchall S, Starnes C, Jacobson K. Current concepts burn rehabilitation, Part II: Long-term recovery. Clin Plast Surg. 2017; 44(4):713–728

Finnerty CC, Jeschke MG, Branski LK, Barret JP, Dziewulski P, Herndon DN. Hypertrophic scarring: the greatest unmet challenge after burn injury. Lancet. 2016; 388(10052):1427–1436

Goodman CC, Fuller KS. Pathology: Implications for the Physical Therapist. 4th ed. St. Louis, MO: Saunders Elsevier; 2015

Goverman J, Mathews K, Goldstein R, et al. Adult contractures in burn injury: a burn model system national database study. J Burn Care Res. 2017; 38(1):e328–e336

Hundeshagen G, Suman OE, Branski LK. Rehabilitation the acute versus outpatient setting. Clin Plast Surg. 2017; 44(4):729–735

Jacobson K, Fletchall S, Dodd H, Starnes C. Current concepts burn rehabilitation, Part I: Care during hospitalization. Clin Plast Surg. 2017; 44(4):703–712

Kwan PO, Tredget EE. Biological principles of scar and contracture. Hand Clin. 2017; 33(2):277–292

Mini Balance Evaluation Systems Test. Available at: https://www.sralab.org/rehabilitation-measures/mini-balance-evaluation-systems-test. Accessed June 1, 2020

O'Sullivan SB, Schmitz TJ, Fulk G. Physical Rehabilitation. 7th ed. Philadelphia, PA: FA Davis; 2019

Porter C, Hardee JP, Herndon DN, Suman OE. The role of exercise in the rehabilitation of patients with severe burns. Exerc Sport Sci Rev. 2015; 43(1):34–40

Sevgi D, Sevban A. Pain and anxiety in burn patients. Int J Caring Sci. 2017; 10(5):1723

Snell JA, Loh NH, Mahambrey T, Shokrollahi K. Clinical review: the critical care management of the burn patient. Crit Care. 2013; 17(5):241

Warby R, Maani CV. Burns Classification. Available at: https://www.ncbi.nlm.nih.gov/books/NBK539773/. Accessed June 1, 2020

Williams FN, Branski LK, Jeschke MG, Herndon DN. What, how, and how much should patients with burns be fed? Surg Clin North Am. 2011; 91(3):609–629

4 Cerebral Palsy

General Information	
Case no.	4.A Cerebral Palsy
Authors	Suzanne F. Migliore, PT, DPT, MS, Board Certified Specialist in Pediatric Physical Therapy Karen Warenius, PT, DPT, C/NDT
Diagnosis	Spastic diplegic cerebral palsy, impaired functional mobility, balance gait, and endurance
Setting	Acute care hospital
Learner expectations	☑ Initial evaluation ☐ Re-evaluation ☐ Treatment session
Learner objectives	1. Explain the pathophysiology of cerebral palsy. 2. Recognize the different surgical interventions utilized for patients with muscle imbalance/shortening due to spasticity. 3. Select, implement, and interpret physical therapy interventions based on initial examination findings.

Medical	
Chief complaint	Worsening of gait pattern
History of present illness	Patient is a 16-year-old male with a history of spastic diplegic cerebral palsy Gross Motor Function Classification System (GMFCS) level II who presented to orthopaedics with complaints of worsening in-toeing and scissoring with his gait pattern in addition to hammertoes on both feet. He and his family had considered surgical intervention in the past 2 years, but now, with his worsening gait pattern, the decision was made to move forward with surgery.
Past medical history	Attention-deficit hyperactivity disorder (ADHD); bladder incontinence; global developmental delay; learning disability; platelet dense granule deficiency; mild persistent asthma; Botox injections at ages 9, 10, and 11; serial casting for bilateral gastrocnemius/soleus.
Past surgical history	Adenoidectomy
Allergies	Ibuprofen (due to platelet dense granule deficiency)
Medications	Acetaminophen, Albuterol, Baclofen, Fexofenadine, Fluticasone HFA, Miralax
Precautions/Orders	Non–weight-bearing (NWB) bilateral lower extremities (LEs) Hip abduction pillow in place at all times

Social history	
Home setup	• Lives with his mom, stepdad, and three siblings in a two-story home with three steps to enter. Mom has lifting restrictions and is unable to assist. • Bedroom is on the second floor. • Shower/tub combination as well as a shower stall with a small lip to step over/into the shower are on the second floor.
Occupation	• High school student
Prior level of function	• Independent with bed mobility • Modified independent for transfers, community ambulation, and activities of daily living with bilateral Lofstrand /forearm crutches and bilateral Molded ankle-foot orthosis (MAFOs) • Occasional use of a wheelchair for extended community distances • GMFCS level III
Recreational activities	• Participates in modified track and field events

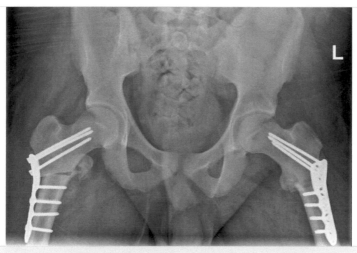

Fig. 4.1 Hip X-ray showing post-operative internal fixation

Imaging/Diagnostic test	Hospital day 1: pediatric ward
Hip X-ray	► Fig. 4.1

Medical management	Hospital day 2, post-op day 1: pediatric ward
Surgical intervention	• Status post bilateral femoral derotational osteotomies, bilateral adductor tenotomies, bilateral gastrocnemius recessions, left split tibialis anterior tendon transfer (SPLATT), bilateral hammertoe corrections • Intraoperative bilateral femoral nerve blocks for postoperative pain management • Placed in bilateral short leg casts (SLCs) and a hip abduction wedge postoperatively
Pain management	1. Patient-controlled analgesia (PCA) pump hydromorphone (Dilaudid) 2. Tylenol/oxycodone
Medications	1. Lactated ringers' infusion 2. Morphine 3. Albuterol 4. Dextrose 5. Ondansetron 6. Baclofen 7. Docusate 8. Diazepam

Lab	Reference range	Hospital day 2, post-op day 1: pediatric ward
White blood cells	$5.0–10.0 \times 10^9$/L	14.7
Hemoglobin	14–17.4 g/dL	10.8
Hematocrit	42–52%	32.3
Red blood cells	4.1–5.3 million/mm³	3.61
Platelets	140–400 k/μL	261
Mean corpuscular volume	78.0–98.0 fL	89.5
Mean platelet volume	9.6–11.8 fL	9.1

Pause points
Based on the above information, what are the priority: • Diagnostic tests and measures? • Outcome measures? • Treatment interventions?

Hospital Day 2, Post-Op Day 1, Pediatric Ward: Physical Therapy Examination		
Subjective		
"My legs hurt and I'm scared to get out of bed"		
Objective		
Vital signs	**Pre-treatment**	**Post-treatment**
	Supine	Sitting
Blood pressure (mmHg)	120/55	129/60
Heart rate (beats/min)	96	100
Respiratory rate (breaths/min)	20	22
Pulse oximetry (SpO$_2$)	96	96
Pain	6/10 at bilateral LEs	8/10 at bilateral LEs
General	• Young male, sitting up in hospital bed, bilateral SLCs and hip abduction pillow in place. • Lines/equipment notable for left upper extremity (UE) peripheral intravenous catheter (PIV), patient-controlled analgesia (PCA).	
Integumentary	• Hip/thigh incisions under postoperative bandages which are clean/dry/intact. • Unable to visualize gastrocnemius/foot incisions due to bilateral SLCs.	
Cardiovascular and pulmonary	• Normal sinus rhythm • No adventitious lung sounds • Capillary refill: < 2 seconds bilateral toes	
Musculoskeletal	Range of motion	• Bilateral upper extremities (BUEs): within normal limit (WNL) • B hips/knees/ankles: unable to fully assess due to hip abduction wedge in place at all times, knee immobilizers, and bilateral SLCs
	Strength	• Bilateral UEs: WNL • Bilateral LEs: unable to fully assess due to hip abduction wedge in place at all times, knee immobilizers, and bilateral SLCs • B ankles/feet: active toe flexion/extension noted on both sides
Neurological	Balance	• Static unsupported sitting: moderate assistance x 2 therapists
	Cognition	• Alert and oriented x 4
	Sensation	• BLE: limited assessment due to orthopaedic devices • Bilateral toes: intact to light touch/deep pressure
	Tone	• Unable to assess due to precautions
	Other	• N/A
Functional status		
Bed mobility	• Rolling supine to side lying: maximal assistance x 3 therapists • Side lying to sitting: maximal assistance x 3 therapists attempted, unable to sit on the edge of the bed	
Transfers	• Bed to/from wheelchair: dependent transfer via mechanical lift	
Ambulation	• Unable to assess due to NWB bilateral LE precautions	
Stairs	• Unable to assess due to NWB bilateral LE precautions	
Other	Wheelchair mobility: propelled forward/backward for 5 feet within room with minimal assistance; oriented to having brakes on while sitting in the wheelchair	

Assessment	
☑ Physical therapist's	*Assessment left blank for learner to develop.*
Goals	
Patient's	"I want to go home."
Short term	1. *Goals left blank for learner to develop.* 2.
Long term	1. *Goals left blank for learner to develop.* 2.

Plan	
☐ Physician's ☑ Physical therapist's ☐ Other's	Continue treatment daily for transfer training, patient and caregiver education, and therapeutic activities. Encourage patient to be out of bed (OOB) to chair for all meals. Discharge planning for home equipment and services.

Bloom's Taxonomy Level	Case 4.A Questions
Create	1. Synthesizing the medical data and physical examination findings, develop an appropriate physical therapy assessment of the patient. 2. Develop two short-term physical therapy goals, including an appropriate timeframe for acute care. 3. Develop two long-term physical therapy goals, including an appropriate timeframe for post-acute care.
Evaluate	4. Explain the physical therapy examination findings and expected discharge recommendation to the acute care team.
Analyze	5. Compare the baseline mobility of a patient at GMFCS levels I and II and how they differ. 6. Analyze his postoperative CBC. What could be causing the low values listed? 7. How will the patient's low hemoglobin affect the treatment session?
Apply	8. Design and implement two in bed exercises to improve upper body strength to assist with bed mobility and transfers. 9. Design and implement bed mobility and transfers out of bed to wheelchair. 10. Design a bedside positioning program to protect the integumentary system and promote function.
Understand	11. What is a PCA? What are the physical therapy implications of hydromorphone? 12. What is the purpose of a derotational osteotomy?
Remember	13. What is spastic diplegia? What are the most common causes? 14. What are the patient's precautions for mobility? How long will they be in place?

Bloom's Taxonomy Level	Case 4.A Answers

Create	1. The patient is a 16-year-old male with a history of spastic diplegia who presents with worsening gait pattern. He was having difficulty ambulating at home, in the community and at school. His loss of quality of gait was interfering with his participation in adaptive sports. He underwent major orthopaedic surgery to correct the alignment of both lower extremities and improve flexibility at his ankles and hips. He presents with pain, limited strength, decreased balance, requiring significant assistance for transfers and will be NWB bilateral LEs for 6 weeks. He will benefit from continued skilled physical therapy to address these impairments, provide patient and caregiver education, and minimal assistance x 1 caregiver with discharge planning. Patient would be appropriate for intensive inpatient rehabilitation once cleared for weight-bearing.
	2. Short-term goals:
	   • Patient will perform rolling either direction in bed with minimal assistance x 1 to reposition self and assist in pressure relief within 5 days.
	   • Patient will independently perform incentive spirometer and deep breathing exercises twice per hour to aid in the prevention of atelectasis within 5 days.

(Continued)

(Continued)

Bloom's Taxonomy Level	Case 4.A Answers
	3. Long-term goals: • Patient will mobilize bed to/from wheelchair via slide board transfer, NWB bilateral LEs, with minimal assistance once to improve independence within 10 days. • Patient's caregiver will perform a wheelchair transfer up/down one threshold step independently in order to safely get the patient into/out of home within 10 days.
Evaluate	4. During the physical therapy examination, the patient demonstrates pain despite being on a PCA. He also had slightly elevated systolic blood pressure and heart rate at rest. He had significant difficulty with bed mobility due to pain, restriction of his LE bracing/casting, and his baseline cardiovascular endurance. He needed maximal assistance with three caregivers to roll in bed and was unable to assist much with bed-to-wheelchair transfers. Due to his size and inability to effectively assist with transfers, a mechanical lift was implemented. He had overall a low tolerance to mobility activities, becoming easily fatigue. Due to his anticipated length of time in non–weight-bearing, and needing increased level of support for transfers, a brief inpatient rehabilitation stay was recommended so that he could improve his bed mobility, his caregivers could learn to assist him with transfers (slide board or mechanical lift), and that his pain could be managed without intravenous medication.
Analyze	5. GMFCS level I: between the 12th and 18th birthday, those classified as level I are able to walk at home, school, outdoors, and in the community. The child is able to walk up/down stairs without using a railing. He can run and jump, but speed and coordination are limited. Participating in sports and physical activities is possible, depending on environmental factors and patient choice. GMFCS level II: The child is able to walk in most settings. Uneven surfaces (terrain/inclines/long distances) may influence whether or not he uses an assistive device or wheelchair. In school, he is able to use a handheld mobility device. In the community, he may choose to use wheel mobility. When ascending/descending stairs, he will use a railing or need physical assistance if there is no railing. Participation in physical activities and sports may need adaptations/accommodations. 6. The patient's hemoglobin and hematocrit levels are lower than the reference ranges for his gender and age. The total number of procedures included in this surgery are the likely causes of these levels due to blood loss. These levels will be monitored for the first few days postoperatively to ensure there is no active bleeding and that he can recover these counts on his own versus needing a blood transfusion. 7. Implications for physical therapy sessions with low hemoglobin include the potential for lightheadedness and fatigue with even minimal exertion. He may present with pallor and may have tachycardia. Monitoring his vitals during the session would be important, especially with mobility. Monitoring his hemoglobin if it were to trend further downwards (<8 g/dL) may indicate the need for transfusion.
Apply	8. In-bed exercises: a) Due to his recent surgery and limited in-bed mobility, maintaining active range of motion (ROM) of those joints not affected by surgery is important. He is fearful of moving, having LE pain, and will need his arms and core to help him start mobilizing. Start with UE active range of motion (AROM) via shoulder flexion and abduction. Keep it simple, selecting repetitions or even challenging him to keep moving for a set amount of time. The physical therapist can add in a functional component by having him reach for the bed rails to assist with rolling (pulling self to the side), or if he has an overhead trapeze, pulling himself up (modified biceps curls) to relieve pressure and assist with repositioning. b) He will also benefit from deep breathing exercises to assist after anesthesia, and to improve aeration while spending most of his time in bed. He is at risk for atelectasis or pneumonia if allowed to just rest supine in bed while recovering. Use of a bedside incentive spirometer may be beneficial. In addition to the incentive spirometer, consider putting the head of the bed up, work with him on diaphragmatic breathing with a 1:2 ratio. If he is able to combine the exercise, consider an UE D2 PNF pattern incorporated with deep breathing. 9. He will require assistance to roll for hygiene, repositioning to relieve pressure, and to start with bed mobility for transfers. Start with raising the head of the bed and monitoring his vital signs for orthostatic hypotension. Utilize the bed environment as an advantage, using the side rails or overhead trapeze to have him participate as much

(Continued)

(Continued)

Bloom's Taxonomy Level	Case 4.A Answers
	as possible. He needs assistance with rolling his lower body, especially since he must keep the hip abduction wedge on due to the pelvic surgery and is non–weight-bearing bilateral LEs, so he can't do a traditional bridge.
	Due to the amount of assistance he needs, he would be most appropriate for a mechanical lift OOB to reclining wheelchair. Many hospitals have specific policies and procedures regarding the amount a practitioner may lift, and when a patient needs to utilize a mechanical lift. These policies may be classified as "no lift" or "safe patient handling" and have the patient and caregivers' safety in the forefront. Incorporate a pressure reducing surface in the wheelchair to aid in pressure relief. Once up in the wheelchair, teach him pressure relief via lateral weight shifts and wheelchair/triceps pushups. Limit his time out of bed to less than an hour for the first trial, monitoring vitals, pain tolerance, and fatigue level. If he tolerates this well, have him up and OOB for all meals.
	10. Considerations for in-bed positioning include his level of mobility, his NWB status, the need for the ABD wedge to be in place at all times, and that he is in bilateral short leg casts. To determine the patient's overall risk for developing pressure injuries, a pressure injury risk assessment tool such as the Braden Q Scale may be appropriate to implement. Positioning programs could include raising the heels of his casts slightly off the bed surface so that he is not lying supine, with his heels bottoming out in the casts all day. He will be able to be in supine position, modified semi-side lying, and semi-Fowler and Fowler positions throughout the day. The physical therapist may want to consider using the clock method for position changes, for example, 8 a.m.: supine; 10 a.m.: semi-Fowler, 12 p.m.: modified side lying, 2 p.m.: Fowler, and continue to change his position every 2 hours. He should also be on a pressure reducing mattress (▶ Fig. 4.2).
Understand	11. A patient-controlled analgesia device is a machine that will deliver specific dosages of pain medicine, through an IV, accessed via a button which is controlled by the patient. The patient is able to self-dose with a PCA at specific locked-out intervals (to avoid overdosing) when they are having pain, rather than waiting for oral or IV pain medicine to be brought to them by nursing. The hydromorphone this patient is getting is an opioid used for pain management. This medication has side effects including nausea, vomiting, constipation, dry mouth, lightheadedness, dizziness, drowsiness, and sweating. While on this medication, the physical therapist would want to monitor his vitals, his pain levels, and his complaint of dizziness/lightheadedness while coming up to sitting. It would be appropriate to have the patient self-administer the PCA prior to starting LE ROM exercises or bed mobility to improve his comfort level during therapy sessions. Patients who are able to self-administer should continue to do so, and not have their parent/caregiver administer for them.
	12. The derotational osteotomy is a common reconstructive, orthopaedic surgery for a patient with spastic diplegic cerebral palsy. In this patient's case, it was utilized to correct his severe in-toeing, with the aim of surgery to correct excessive femoral neck anteversion. The surgical site is typically intertrochanteric, with the bone cut, rotated to the new position and held in place with screws or a blade/plate. Adverse effects of this surgery include infection, hardware failure, penetration of the hardware into the femoral neck, and delayed union (if NWB status is not maintained) for at least 6 weeks postoperatively.
Remember	13. Cerebral palsy occurs when there is abnormal development of the brain or damage to the developing brain. The damage can occur in utero, during the birthing process, or during the first month of birth (often following meningitis or a stroke). Triggers in utero may be bacterial or viral infections, or events that cause hypoxic events including placental abruption or a tight nuchal cord. Spastic diplegic CP is a diagnosis in patients whose lower extremities are affected, while their trunk and upper extremities are not. The most common cause of spastic diplegic CP is periventricular leukomalacia (PVL). PVL affects premature infants and presents with brain tissue death in the areas surrounding the ventricles. This area contains the long descending motor tracts as they travel from the motor cortex to the spinal cord. The motor tracts that control the lower extremities are closest to the ventricles and are more likely to be damaged and present as spastic diplegia. Patients with spastic diplegic cerebral palsy may have typical cognition, or a range of learning and cognitive deficits.
	14. The patient has NWB orders for bilateral LEs. This is due to the extensive orthopaedic surgery they had. While the osteotomies are healing, the patient will remain NWB for at least 6 weeks or until radiographic signs of acceptable union of the bones have occurred.

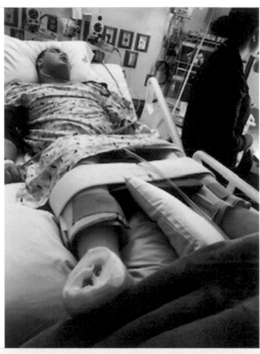

Fig. 4.2 In bed positioning with hip abduction brace and bilateral LE short leg casts

Key points
1. Patients with spastic diplegic cerebral palsy may have varied medical and surgical interventions to affect the quality of their gait.
2. Working with a patient postoperatively poses challenges including monitoring lab values, monitoring pain and vital signs, and selecting appropriate and safe mobility options.
3. Interventions for acute care patients must incorporate all the body systems. Being mindful of the patient's cardiovascular and pulmonary, integumentary, neuromuscular, and musculoskeletal needs will guide physical therapy interventions.

General Information	
Case no.	4.B
Authors	Suzanne F. Migliore, PT, DPT, MS, Board-Certified Specialist in Pediatric Physical Therapy Karen Warenius, PT, DPT, C/NDT
Diagnosis	Spastic diplegic cerebral palsy, impaired functional mobility, balance gait, and endurance
Setting	Acute inpatient rehabilitation
Learner expectations	☑ Initial evaluation ☐ Re-evaluation ☐ Treatment session
Learner objectives	1. Interpret initial examination findings from the inpatient rehabilitation setting. 2. Select appropriate physical therapy interventions based on initial examination findings. 3. Create a discharge plan for the next phase in the continuum of care.

Medical	
Chief complaint	"I need to get stronger and start walking."
History of present illness	Patient is now 6 weeks status post orthopaedic surgery and bilateral SLC placement. Patient was discharged home from the acute care hospital 10 days after surgery and received 16 hours a day of home health aide and home care nursing while NWB on

(Continued)

(Continued)

Medical	
	bilateral LEs. He had his SLC removed, had follow-up X-rays with orthopaedics, and referred to acute inpatient rehabilitation to start weight-bearing, gait training, and LE strengthening.
Past medical history	Attention-deficit hyperactivity disorder (ADHD); bladder incontinence; global developmental delay; learning disability; platelet dense granule deficiency; mild persistent asthma; Botox injections at ages 9, 10, and 11; and serial casting for bilateral gastrocnemius/soleus.
Past surgical history	Patient underwent bilateral femoral derotational osteotomies, bilateral adductor tenotomies, bilateral gastrocnemius recessions, left split tibialis anterior tendon transfer (SPLATT), and bilateral hammertoe corrections. Intraoperative bilateral femoral nerve blocks for postoperative pain management. He was placed on bilateral short leg casts (SLC) and a hip abduction wedge postoperatively.
Allergies	Ibuprofen (due to platelet dense granule deficiency)
Medications	Oxycodone, Acetaminophen, Diazepam, Baclofen, Fluticasone, Miralax, Dexmethylphenidate HCl
Precautions/Orders	Activity as tolerated WBAT BLEs

Social history	
Home setup	• Lives with his mom, stepdad, and three siblings in a two-story home with three steps to enter. Mom has lifting restrictions due to recent back surgery. • Bedroom is on the second floor. • Shower/tub combination as well as a shower stall with a small lip to step over/into the shower are on the second floor.
Occupation	• High school student
Prior level of function	• Independent with bed mobility • Modified Independent for transfers, community ambulation, and activities of daily living with bilateral Lofstrand/forearm crutches and bilateral MAFOs. • Occasional use of a wheelchair for extended community distances. GMFCS level III
Recreational activities	• Participates in modified track and field events

Imaging/Diagnostic test	Day 1: acute inpatient rehabilitation
Hip/Pelvis X-ray	• Signs of adequate healing and intact hardware • Both femoral heads were located

Medical management	Day 1: acute inpatient rehabilitation
Medications	1. Tylenol, valium, and oxycodone PRN for pain 2. Colace every 12 hours for bowel/bladder management
Diet	1. Regular
Vitals	1. Every 8 hours

Pause points
Based on the above information, what are the priority: • Diagnostic tests and measures? • Outcome measures? • Treatment interventions?

Day 1, Acute Inpatient Rehabilitation: Physical Therapy Examination		
Subjective		
"I'm scared to try and walk."		
Objective		
Vital signs	Pre-treatment Sitting	Post-treatment Standing
Blood pressure (mmHg)	127/54	130/60
Heart rate (beats/min)	102	110
Respiratory rate (breaths/min)	18	19
Pulse oximetry (SpO$_2$)	95	95
Pain	0/10	2/10 at bilateral ankles
General	• Young male, lying supine in bed, no apparent distress • Awake, alert, and conversing with caregivers	
Integumentary	• Healing incisions at bilateral lateral hips, inner groin, distal femur, calves, and dorsum of both feet	
Cardiovascular and pulmonary	• Normal heart rate and rhythm • Normal breath sounds • No cyanosis	
Gastrointestinal	• On Colace from home	
Genitourinary	• Able to void on his own	
Musculoskeletal	Range of motion	• Bilateral upper extremities (BUE): within functional limit (WFL) • L hip flexion: 80 degrees • R hip flexion: 80 degrees • L knee flexion: −5 to 75 degrees • R knee flexion: 0–70 degrees • L ankle dorsiflexion: 5 degrees • R ankle dorsiflexion: −3 degrees
	Strength	• BUE: WFL • B hip flexion: 2 + /5 • B hip extension: 3/5 • B hip abduction: 3 + /5 • B hip adduction: 3 + /5 • B knee flexion: 2 + /5 • B knee extension: 3–/5 • B ankle dorsiflexion: 2 + 5 • B ankle plantarflexion: 3–/5
Neurological	Balance	• Static unsupported sitting: minimal assistance
	Cognition	• Alert and oriented x 4
	Coordination	• Finger-to-nose: intact BUEs • Heel-to-shin: to be assessed at a later date
	Cranial nerves	• I–XII: intact
	Reflexes	• Biceps: 2 + • Patellar: not tested
	Sensation	• Intact to light touch/deep pressure throughout bilateral LEs
Functional status		
Bed mobility	• Rolling: minimal assistance x 1 caregiver • Supine to/from sit: maximal assistance x caregiver	
Transfers	• Mat to/from wheelchair: moderate assistance of 1 physical therapy once using sit pivot technique	

(Continued)

(Continued)

Day 1, Acute Inpatient Rehabilitation: Physical Therapy Examination	
Ambulation	• Unable to assess due to weakness and poor tolerance to bilateral MAFOs
Stairs	• N/A
Task specific	• Bed to commode/toilet transfers: moderate assistance
Other	WeeFIM: Transfers: chair/wheelchair: 1 Locomotion: walk, wheelchair, crawl: 6 Locomotion: stairs: 1 Eating: 7 Grooming: 7 Bathing: 1 Dressing upper body: 4 Dressing lower body: 2 Toileting: 2

Assessment	
☑ Physical therapist's	*Assessment left blank for learner to develop.*
Goals	
Patient's	"I want to walk better and get back to school."
Short term	1. *Goals left blank for learner to develop.* 2.
Long term	1. *Goals left blank for learner to develop.* 2.

Plan	
☐ Physician's ☑ Physical therapist's ☐ Other's	Patient will be seen 7 days per week for range of motion exercises, balance activities, gait training, endurance activities, patient/parent education, and discharge planning.

Bloom's Taxonomy Level	Case 4.B Questions
Create	1. Synthesizing the medical data and physical examination findings, develop an appropriate physical therapy assessment of the patient. 2. Develop two short-term physical therapy goals, including an appropriate timeframe. 3. Develop two long-term physical therapy goals, including an appropriate timeframe.
Evaluate	4. Explain the physical therapy examination findings and expected length of stay to the rehabilitation team. 5. From the initial examination findings, which other services the physical therapist conclude should be consulted during his rehabilitation stay? 6. Predict what the patient's needs are for a safe discharge to home.
Analyze	7. Analyze his WeeFIM scores and how his baseline mobility may influence his length of stay.
Apply	8. Design and implement three lower extremity exercises to improve strength in preparation for transfers and gait training. 9. Select and implement appropriate transfer training for bed to wheelchair mobility. 10. Select an appropriate therapeutic intervention for upright progressive mobility and gait training that can be used in future treatments.

(Continued)

(Continued)

Bloom's Taxonomy Level	Case 4.B Questions
Understand	11. Describe the different levels of the Modified Ashworth Scale (MAS). 12. What was the purpose of the SPLATT procedure and the effect on a patient's gait?
Remember	13. List the warning signs of a deep vein thrombosis (DVT) using the Wells criteria. 14. List three outcome measures that could be used for fall risk detection.

Bloom's Taxonomy Level	Case 4.B Answers
Create	1. Patient is a 16-year-old male, with GMFCS level III, spastic diplegic cerebral palsy, admitted to inpatient rehabilitation following 5 weeks at home to recover from bilateral femoral derotational osteotomies, bilateral adductor tenotomies, bilateral gastrocnemius recessions, left SPLATT, and left second toe hammertoe correction. He was NWB bilateral LEs for 6 weeks while his osteotomy sites healed. He had his short leg casts removed at his orthopaedic appointment, hip X-rays taken which showed good union at the osteotomy sites, and cleared for WBAT and admission for inpatient rehabilitation. He presents with impaired range of motion, decreased LE strength, decreased bed mobility, impaired sitting balance, decreased transfers, and currently unable to ambulate due to prolonged bedrest. He will benefit from skilled physical therapy as well as occupational therapy to address his body structures and functions, activity, and participation restrictions. 2. Short-term goals: • Patient will demonstrate supine-to-sit bed mobility with minimal assistance x 1 physical therapy once in 2 weeks to aid in functional mobility. • Patient will demonstrate sit-to-stand transfer up to parallel bars with minimum assistance x 1 once in 2 weeks in preparation for gait training. 3. Long-term goals: • Patient will be able to ambulate household distances with least restrictive device with close supervision in 6 weeks in preparation for discharge home. • Patient will be able to ascend/descend three steps with one handrail with minimal assist once in 6 weeks keep access his home safely.
Evaluate	4. The patient spent 5 weeks at home, with NWB bilateral lower extremity precautions as well as positioned with a hip abduction wedge and in bilateral short leg casts. Due to the postoperative precautions, he presents with limited lower extremity range of motion and strength which is anticipated at this point. He had been using a portable mechanical lift at home but was able to begin sit pivot transfers as his weight-bearing restrictions had been lifted. He requires assistance for many of his activities of daily living and was unable to start standing on day 1 due to poorly fitting ankle foot orthoses which must be worn while in an upright position to support his ankles and protect the gastrocnemius recession surgeries. Due to his size, his level of weakness, and current level of functional mobility, it is anticipated he will require at least 6–8 weeks of intensive inpatient physical therapy to meet his goals. 5. In addition to physical therapy, the patient will benefit from consultation from occupational therapy to address his activities of daily livings and instrumental activities of daily living. The patient would also benefit from some social activities as well as preparation for uncomfortable activities such as standing or walking for the first time. He will benefit from referrals to child life specialists and music therapists to complement his rehabilitation. In addition, as he is of school age and missing regular classes, referral to the school services the rehabilitation unit offers is important so that he can keep up with his classwork. 6. The patient will require intensive rehabilitation to regain lower extremity range of motion, lower extremity strength, gain independence with transfers, and gait. He will need to be able to walk household distances and safely go up/down three steps to get into and out of his home not only for appointments but also in the case of emergency. He will need to be able to get into/out of a shower and will likely benefit from a shower bench and handheld shower head to bathe in a seated position. He will benefit from referral to outpatient physical therapy to continue with his goals and progress his mobility from a rolling walker to a lesser device or no device at all. The outpatient physical therapist will need to address his ability to return to school and referral back to school-based physical therapy services to assess his safety in that environment.

(Continued)

(Continued)

Bloom's Taxonomy Level	Case 4.B Answers
Analyze	7. The WeeFIM was administered at admission and will be administered again at discharge to measure the change in the level of assistance needed during functional tasks. Transfers: chair/wheelchair: 1 (total assistance/performs less than 25% of the transferring task or requires two or more helpers). Locomotion: walk, wheelchair, crawl: 6 (walks or operates a wheelchair 150 feet without helper, increased time, or a safety concern). Locomotion: stairs: 1 (performs less than 25% or none of the effort required to climb stairs). Eating: 7 (complete independence). Grooming: 7 (complete independence). Bathing: 1 (total assistance). Dressing—upper body: 4 (minimal assistance). Dressing—lower body: 2 (maximal assistance). Toileting: 2 (maximal assistance). From these scores, the physical therapist and occupational therapist could base functional goals and be able to measure progress during the course of rehab.
Apply	8. There are many LE exercises that would be appropriate for the patient. Below are three suggestions: a) Bridges: in bed, getting the patient into a hook-lying position will aid in AROM for his hips, knees, and ankles. Now that he is able to weight bear, this activity is possible (in comparison to acute care or while he was at home). Bridging with symmetrical use of both LEs, holding for 3–5 seconds, and slow eccentric lowering to the support surface. Dosing may be dependent on his pain tolerance, fatigue level, or quality of his form. Not only an early strengthening activity but also functionality is important if he were to need to use a bedpan prior to improving his mobility OOB to a commode. b) Short arc quadriceps extension: in preparation for standing, activating his quads either in short arc (in bed) or long arc (sitting on edge of bed or in wheelchair) would be appropriate. Due to his hamstring spasticity, he may not be able to gain full extension when in an upright position. Dosing could start with 8–10 repetitions, likely with verbal cues for speed and quality for concentric and eccentric components. Rest for 1 minute, repeat for two to three total sets. c) Wheelchair pushups: in preparation for sit-to-stand transfers, improving his UE strength will aid in assisting him getting into an upright position. Due to his LE weakness, he will likely rely on his arms early on during transfers. In addition, for transfer training, helping him unweight his buttocks will be important as he spends time in his wheelchair between therapy sessions. Start with lifting/lowering self for 10. Progress to holding for 3 seconds once full elbow extension is achieved for 10 repetitions. Incorporate breathing techniques and cueing to not hold breath. 9. The patient was utilizing a mechanical lift at home, tolerating extended periods of time up in his wheelchair. He is able to sit at the edge of the bed with minimal assistance. He is able to utilize his arms to help reposition himself. The physical therapist would have two options for starting to do more functional transfers with him. The physical therapist could select a sliding board to aid in guiding his buttocks/lower body from bed to wheelchair. The sliding board would decrease friction/shear across his buttocks. The other option, and now that he can weight bear as tolerated, is to attempt squat pivot transfers. This will allow him to start doing some weight-bearing, utilize his upper body and core to aid in the transfer, and start a progression toward sit-to-stand transfers. 10. Due to his prolonged immobility after orthopaedic surgery, his premorbid gait status, and his current level of LE weakness, he may not be able to fully weight bear in an upright posture either in the parallel bars or up to an assistive device. He was also fearful of moving and standing. Due to his size, and these factors, he would be most appropriate for a partial weight-bearing harness system to aid in the initial stages of mobility. By unweighting his lower extremities, the therapist can slowly add more of his body weight as his leg strength improves. He can begin working on his gait pattern in a partially unweighted capacity, working on each phase of heel strike, loading response, midstance terminal stance, pre-swing, initial swing, mid-swing, and terminal swing. These harness

(Continued)

(Continued)

Bloom's Taxonomy Level	Case 4.B Answers
	systems not only unweight the patient but also provide a level of safety to avoid a fall during early mobilization. The other component of one of these systems is his energy conservation. Due to his prolonged immobility, his endurance level is decreased. It would be recommended to monitor vital signs as well as use an RPE Scale to gauge his tolerance to the activity. The partial weight-bearing harness system would be the bridge to traditional upright gait training in the parallel bars or with an assistive device. ▶ Fig. 4.3 ▶ Video 4.1
Understand	11. The Modified Ashworth Scale (MAS) is an objective measure of muscle spasticity. 0: No increase in muscle tone. 1: Slight increase in muscle tone, with a catch and release or minimal resistance at the end of the range of motion when an affected part(s) is moved in flexion or extension. 1 +: Slight increase in muscle tone, manifested as a catch, followed by minimal resistance through the remainder (less than half) of the range of motion. 2: A marked increase in muscle tone throughout most of the range of motion, but affected part(s) are still easily moved. 3: Considerable increase in muscle tone, passive movement difficult. 4: Affected part(s) are rigid in flexion or extension. 12. The SPLATT procedure is a surgical procedure to address a spastic varus foot deformity, common in children with cerebral palsy. The split tibialis anterior tendon transfer is one of the procedures to correct this deformity. During this surgery, the tendon is split longitudinally, with half of the tendon being detached from its medial border and reattached to the lateral side of the foot. This transfer is to provide the foot stability and retain flexibility. In addition, the patient underwent gastrocnemius recession due to spasticity and loss of ROM causing his equinovarus foot position. The surgery will also aid in balancing the foot which often shows weakness of the anterior tibialis muscle. The postoperative foot alignment is proposed to affect his gait pattern, allowing for more neutral alignment of the foot, avoid excessive plantarflexion, and the toe walking pattern he had preoperatively.
Remember	13. Physical therapists are responsible for screening for DVT. This patient had a prolonged period of immobility, decreased mobility/gait from preoperative status, and was immobilized in short leg casts. He demonstrated swelling in his right foot after the cast was removed. The Wells criterion is a screening tool that looks at the risk of DVT in a patient. Patients are given one point for each of the following criteria: • Active cancer (patient either receiving treatment for cancer within the previous 6 months or currently receiving palliative treatment): 1 • Paralysis, paresis, or recent cast immobilization of the lower extremities: 1 • Recently bedridden for ≥ 3 days, or major surgery within the previous 12 weeks requiring general or regional anesthesia: 1 • Localized tenderness along the distribution of the deep venous system: 1 • Entire leg swelling: 1 • Calf swelling at least 3 cm larger than that on the asymptomatic side (measured 10 cm below tibial tuberosity): 1 • Pitting edema confined to the symptomatic leg: 1 • Collateral superficial veins (non-varicose): 1 • Previously documented DVT: 1 • Alternative diagnosis at least as likely as DVT: −2 Total score: −2 to 0: low probability of DVT 1–2: moderate probability of DVT 3–8: high probability 14. Outcome measures that can address fall risk: a) TUG/TUG-c (cognitive)/TUG-m (motor) b) Pediatric Balance Scale/Berg Balance Scale c) Functional reach test d) Dynamic gait index (DGI) e) Functional gait assessment (FGA) f) 10 MWT (Meter Walk Test; gait speed)

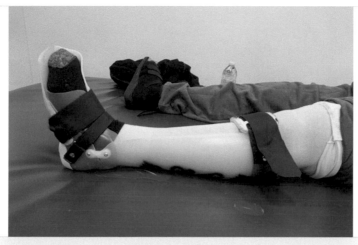

Fig. 4.3 Molded ankle-foot orthosis

Key points
1. Taking the information from the initial examination, the physical therapist is able to choose initial plan of care, make appropriate referrals, and recognize outcome measures that are appropriate for this case.
2. Interventions will start with the basics of improving ROM, strength, and mobility with the goal of improving his functional mobility in the preparation for discharge.
3. The patient will require additional outpatient physical therapy upon discharge to continue his progress with his gait pattern and to return him to his previous level of function.

General Information	
Case no.	4.C
Authors	Suzanne F. Migliore, PT, DPT, MS, Board-Certified Clinical Specialist in Pediatric Physical Therapy Karen S. Warenius, PT, DPT, C/NDT
Diagnosis	Cerebral palsy spastic diplegia; impaired functional mobility, gait, balance, and endurance
Setting	Outpatient clinic
Learner expectations	☑ Initial evaluation ☐ Re-evaluation ☐ Treatment session
Learner objectives	1. Identify impairments, activity limitations, and participation restrictions. 2. Identify relevant outcome measures and understand impact of results on function and participation. 3. Formulate relevant functional goals based on objective information provided. 4. Develop a treatment plan to maximize participation and quality of life. 5. Discuss recommendations for school participation and community-based activities

Medical	
Chief complaint	"It's hard to get up and down my stairs at home."
History of present illness	Patient is a 16-year-old male with past medical history (PMH) significant for spastic diplegia, cerebral palsy, delta granule storage pool deficiency, attention-deficit hyper-activity disorder (ADHD), and ODD who was seen by orthopaedics for difficulty walking

(Continued)

(Continued)

Medical	
	due to in-toeing and scissoring causing frequent tripping. Patient underwent bilateral femoral derotational osteotomies, bilateral adductor tenotomies, bilateral gastrocnemius recessions, left SPLATT (split anterior tibial tendon transfer), left second toe hammertoe correction, and right third toe hammertoe correction. He was placed in short leg casts bilaterally with knee immobilizers and an abduction pillow.
	Patient remained NWB for 6 weeks at which time his weight-bearing status was advanced to as tolerated. He was admitted to inpatient rehab to work on mobility and strengthening postsurgery to maximize potential. He completed 9 weeks of inpatient rehab that included physical therapy and OT 7 days a week. Upon discharge, he was referred to outpatient physical therapy 2 days a week.
Past medical history	ADHD, bladder incontinence, global developmental delay, learning disability, platelet dense granule deficiency, mild persistent asthma, Botox injections at ages 9, 10, and 11, serial casting for bilateral gastrocnemius/soleus.
Past surgical history	Adenoidectomy, bilateral femoral de-rotational osteotomies, bilateral adductor tenotomies, bilateral gastrocnemius recessions, SPLATT, bilateral hammertoe corrections 14 weeks ago.
Allergies	Ibuprofen—due to platelet insufficiency.
Medications	Baclofen, Albuterol, Fluticasone, Montelukast, Miralax, Sennosides, Melatonin
Precautions/Orders	Activity as tolerated WBAT BLE

Social history	
Home setup	• Lives with his mom, stepdad, and three siblings in a two-story home with three steps to enter. Mom has lifting restrictions due to recent back surgery. • Bedroom is on the second floor. • Shower/tub combination as well as a shower stall with a small lip to step over/into the shower are on the second floor.
Occupation	• 10th grade student at a large public high school attending a life skills program and taking culinary classes at a tech school.
Prior level of function	• Independent with bed mobility • Modified independent for transfers, community ambulation, and activities of daily living with bilateral Lofstrand/forearm crutches and bilateral MAFOs. • Occasional use of a wheelchair for extended community distances • GMFCS level III
Recreational activities	• Participates in modified track and field events—javelin and 100-m dash • Involved with school band
Other	Durable medical equipment (DME): manual wheelchair, anterior rolling walker, bilateral axillary crutches, bilateral custom-molded articulating ankle foot orthosis (AFO) with plantarflexion stop, gait belt

Medical management
• Follow up with orthopaedics, developmental pediatrics, and general pediatrician • Continue with current daily medications

Pause points
Based on the above information, what are the priority: • Diagnostic tests and measures? • Outcome measures? • Treatment interventions?

Day 1, Acute Inpatient Rehabilitation: Physical Therapy Examination			
Subjective			
"I can finally stand up straight since surgery"			
Objective			
Vital signs		**Pre-treatment**	**Post-treatment**
		Sitting	**Sitting**
Blood pressure (mmHg)		105/62	110/64
Heart rate (beats/min)		88	94
Respiratory rate (breaths/min)		18	22
Pulse oximetry on room air (SpO$_2$)		96	95
Pain		0/10	0/10
Musculoskeletal	Range of motion (ROM)	• Bilateral upper extremities (BUE): within functional limit • R hip flexion/extension: 0–114 degrees • L hip flexion/extension: 0–106 degrees • R knee flexion/extension: 0–125 degrees • L knee flexion/extension: 0–129 degrees • R popliteal angle: 36 degrees • L popliteal angle: 32 degrees • R ankle dorsiflexion/plantar flexion: 0–22 degrees • L ankle dorsiflexion/plantar flexion: 3–25 degrees	
	Strength	• BUE: within normal limit • B hip flexion: 2+/5 • B hip extension: 3/5 • B hip abduction: 4–/5 • R hip adduction: 3+/5 • B knee flexion: 2+/5 • B knee extension: 3–/5 • B dorsiflexion: 2+/5	
	Aerobic	• 6MWT: 112 m; –9.25 SD from the mean with anterior rolling walker and B AFOs	
	Flexibility	• Shortening of B hamstrings, gastrocnemius, and hip flexors	
	Other	• N/A	
Neurological	Balance	• BERG balance: 28 • TUG: 19.7 seconds	
	Cognition	• Alert and oriented ×4	
	Coordination	• Finger to nose: intact BUE	
	Cranial nerves	• I–XII: intact	
	Reflexes	• Biceps: 2+ bilaterally • Patellar: 2+ bilaterally	
	Sensation	• BLE: intact to light touch	
	Tone	Modified Ashworth Scale • Glutes: 0 bilaterally • Hip flexors: 0 bilaterally • Quadriceps: 0 bilaterally • Hamstrings: 1 bilaterally • Hip adductors: 1+ bilaterally • Gastroc-soleus: 1+ bilaterally • Clonus: absent bilaterally	

(Continued)

(Continued)

Day 1, Acute Inpatient Rehabilitation: Physical Therapy Examination		
	Other	• 10MWT: completed with anterior rolling walker and BLE bracing donned (B articulating AFOs) at preferred walking speed Trial 1 = 1.74 m/s Trial 2 = 1.81 m/s Average speed = 1.78 m/s
Functional status		
Bed mobility	• Rolling either direction: independent • Supine to/from sit: independent	
Transfers	• Sit to/from stand: supervision with BUE assist	
Ambulation	• Ambulates household ambulation and short community distances (max 500 feet) with anterior rolling walking and BLE articulating AFOs with close supervision. • ▶ Video 4.2 • Gait deviations notable for decreased hip and knee flexion bilaterally in swing phase of gait; foot flat at initial contact bilaterally; decreased R quadriceps activation, which impairs neutral knee extension in stance phase on right with resultant knee buckle; + Trendelenburg sign R > L; increased use of BUEs on RW for support.	
Stairs	• Ascend/descend full flight of stairs with support of single handrail and single Lofstrand/forearm crutch with contact guard assistance and verbal cues; necessary for caregiver to relocate walker to top/bottom of stairs.	
Task specific	• Activities of daily living—bathing, dressing, and toileting require minimal assistance	
Other	PROMIS: Parent Proxy Short Form—Physical Function Mobility Score = 20 Patient Entered Physical Function Mobility Score = 23	

Assessment	
☑ Physical therapist's	*Assessment left blank for learner to develop.*
Goals	
Patient's	"I want to do everything I could before surgery but do it better."
Short term	1. *Goals left blank for learner to develop.* 2.
Long term	1. *Goals left blank for learner to develop.* 2.

Plan	
☐ Physician's ☑ Physical therapist's ☐ Other's	Patient will be seen twice a week for 12 weeks followed by once a week for 12 weeks. Treatment will include: • Therapeutic exercise including strengthening and ROM of BLE and aerobic conditioning. • Gait training including even and uneven surfaces and stairs. • Balance training. • Transfer/transition training.

Bloom's Taxonomy Level	Case 4.C Questions
Create	1. Synthesizing the medical data and physical examination findings, develop an appropriate physical therapy assessment of the patient.

(Continued)

(Continued)

Bloom's Taxonomy Level	Case 4.C Questions
	2. Develop two short-term physical therapy goals, including an appropriate timeframe. 3. Develop two long-term physical therapy goals, including an appropriate timeframe.
Evaluate	4. Assess the patient's current durable medical equipment and bracing prescription and justify need for current equipment and any additional equipment recommendations. 5. Describe school accommodations and/or related services that may be indicated to maximize patient's participation in school. Based on ▶ **Video 4.3**, can the patient safely, effectively, and efficiently ascend/descend stairs or will he require elevator access? 6. In regard to ▶ **Video 4.2**, evaluate the patient's current gait speed and its impact on current mobility and participation.
Analyze	7. Analyze patient's ROM and strength values and discuss impact on gait. 8. Analyze results of the 6MWT and determine patient's ability to participate in a high school environment.
Apply	9. Choose four LE strengthening exercises that will be important given the patient's diagnosis and surgical intervention. 10. Design one gait-related activity to progress the patient to a less restrictive assistive device
Understand	11. Discuss how the patient's tone/spasticity may influence progress and functional improvements. 12. Identify two community-based activities that the physical therapist would refer the patient to upon discharge from outpatient physical therapy. State why each would be beneficial.
Remember	13. Describe the classic gait pattern of a patient with spastic diplegic cerebral palsy. 14. Define spasticity and recall spasticity management options. 15. List case-appropriate activity and participation outcome measures.

Bloom's Taxonomy Level	Case 4.C Answers

Create	1. Patient is a 16-year-old male, with past medical history significant for spastic diplegia cerebral palsy who underwent bilateral femoral derotational osteotomies, bilateral adductor tenotomies, bilateral gastrocnemius recessions, left SPLATT, left second toe hammertoe correction, and right third toe hammertoe correction on 10/4/19. He was recently discharged from inpatient rehab where he made significant progress in his gait. He has been referred to outpatient physical therapy to continue his progress in all areas to maximize his participation. On evaluation, patient presents with impaired ROM of BLE, impaired strength of BLE, impaired balance/fall risk as assessed via Berg Balance Scale, impaired transfers, decreased endurance as assessed via 6MWT, and impaired gait. The aforementioned impairments impact the patient's ability to fully access his home (bedroom) independently and participate in school and recreational activities as he did prior to surgery. Patient has good rehab potential and will benefit from outpatient physical therapy.
	2. Short-term goals:
	  • Patient will transfer sit to stand from a regular chair without UE assist independently 3/4 trials within 8 weeks to improve independence.
	  • Patient will walk 50 feet twice without assistive device with contact guard assistance in one session within 8 weeks to improve functional gait.
	3. Long-term goals:
	  • Patient will demonstrate 6MWT scoring less than 3 standard deviations below the mean for height and gender norms within 6 months as a demonstration of improved endurance to improve participation in school.
	  • Patient and parent proxy scores on the PROMIS Physical Function Mobility questionnaire will increase by at least 3 points, MCID, as a demonstration of meaningful improvement in physical health and mobility and a demonstration of improved participation.

Evaluate	4. The patient currently requires several pieces of durable medical equipment to maintain safety and optimize participation. He is currently using a manual wheelchair

(Continued)

(Continued)

Bloom's Taxonomy Level	Case 4.C Answers
	for long distance mobility due to impaired gait, speed, and endurance. The wheelchair is required for school and community mobility due to risk for falls. He also uses an anterior rolling walker. Due to poor balance and LE weakness, the patient requires an assistive device that offers a greater amount of stability to allow for safe mobility. In addition to the walker, he also has B axillary crutches for use when ascending and descending stairs. He is required to use the stairs in his home as the bathroom is on the second floor. In regard to bracing, the patient currently uses bilateral custom–molded articulating AFOs with a plantarflexion stop. The patient requires this type of bracing to provide stability during gait. The plantarflexion stop limits the influence of spasticity into plantarflexion, toe walking, and overuse and shortening of the gastrocnemius. The articulating component of the brace allows for free dorsiflexion which improves ability to function during transitions and when walking on stairs. It is necessary to monitor the patient's gait pattern and evidence of crouch allowed by the current brace due to LE weakness both pre- and postsurgery. For safety, the patient utilizes a gait belt during transfers and ambulation due to his continued impairment in balance, strength, and gait. Additional equipment considerations would include a shower chair. This will be recommended for safety during showering. The patient has limited standing endurance and impaired balance as well as a history of LE buckling. To maintain safety, it is recommended that the patient sit during showering tasks.
	5. Upon return to school, the patient will require accommodation to his learning environment to maximize his participation in a least restrictive environment as is outlined in Individuals with Disabilities Education Act (IDEA). The patient does not independently, safely, efficiently, and effectively ascend/descend stairs and, therefore, he is at a fall risk. Due to this, and that his primary mode of mobilization around the school is using his wheelchair, he will require elevator access. He will also require extra time between classes due to decreased gait speed, impaired balance, and risk for falls in a crowded high school hallway. In certain settings within the school environment, he may need modified seating or desk to accommodate the wheelchair when necessary. He will benefit from a one-to-one aide to assist with transfers, school mobility, and management of his school items (books, laptop, and backpack). The patient will also be eligible for several related services upon his return. Physical therapy will be necessary to promote independent access to and participation in the school environment including technical school (culinary classroom). Physical therapist will also make recommendations for use of assistive devices in regard to safety, speed, and endurance. He will benefit from occupational therapy to promote independence in the management of school items, toileting, and dressing. Specialized transportation will be another recommended related service. The patient continues to use a wheelchair and therefore, the bus must allow for wheelchair access/ lift with tie downs for safe transportation to and from school.
	6. Requirements for community gait speed vary greatly in the literature. Often, values are based on the ability to successfully cross a crosswalk in the time allotted by a traffic signal. In a systematic review by Salbach et al, they reported necessary community gait speed of 0.44–1.32 m/s. Currently, the patient's average gait speed is 1.78 m/s as was assessed via the 10MWT. This is significantly slower than the documented speed in the literature. This will impact the patient's ability to ambulate within his community and, more importantly, in his high school environment. High school students are typically given 3 to 5 minutes during class period changes to arrive at their next class. At the current gait speed, it is likely, depending on the distance needed to travel, that the patient will not arrive on schedule and wheelchair use at school must be considered. The patient will also require use of the elevator for safe transitions between floors of the building. This will also impact and slow down the time it will take him to mobilize between classes. Gait speed, quality of gait, and balance will all deteriorate with a less supportive assistive device. These must be taken into consideration when making recommendations for a device. Utilizing the patient's TUG score of 19.7 seconds indicates that his dynamic balance is impaired and not ready to advance to a less supportive device. Performing a 10MWT and a TUG when making recommendations for assistive devices would be beneficial. The patient needs to demonstrate safe, time-efficient gait to function in the community.
Analyze	7. Currently, the patient completes 112 meters in a 6-minute timeframe as was reported in the 6MWT placing him 9.25 standard deviations below the mean as compared to his

(Continued)

(Continued)

Bloom's Taxonomy Level	Case 4.C Answers

height-matched peers. In this case, it would be beneficial to compare the distance traveled to his healthy, age-matched peers to better understand how this will impact functional mobility in the school environment. In a study by Geiger et al, the mean distance traveled by healthy males 16 years old and older was 725.8 ± 61.2 meters. This represents a significant discrepancy when compared to the patient's distance. Based on the results of the 6MWT, the patient does not have the ability to walk the same distance in the same timeframe due to a deficit in endurance and gait speed. This will significantly impact his participation in regard to mobility within his school and keeping up with his peers.

Another consideration is the distance that the patient will be required to walk within his large high school environment. The current school environment is roughly 179,000 square feet. This size equates to a superstore (e.g., Target, Wal-Mart) which ranges from 130,000 to nearly 187,000 square feet. Andrews et al documented mean distances to traverse various community establishments. The mean distance to travel in a superstore was 606 meters, in a department store 346 meters, and at a pharmacy 206 meters. For the purpose of this case study, we are going to assume that the distance the patient is required to travel between classes is between 206 meters (0.13 miles) and 346 meters (0.21 miles). Currently, the patient is not demonstrating the endurance or gait speed to complete the distance necessary in the time allotted (3–5-minute school bell) to function in his school environment. It will be necessary for the patient to utilize his wheelchair for class changes upon returning to school. As his endurance and speed improve, he may be able to walk with his assistive device during shorter distance transitions and progress to a full school day.

8. The patient demonstrates impairments in LE ROM and strength that directly impact his gait. A decrease in popliteal angle measurements indicate shortening of bilateral hamstrings. This will impact the patient's step length and the ability to achieve heel strike at initial contact. The present decrease in bilateral dorsiflexion ROM and shortening of the gastrocnemius will limit heel strike at initial contact as well as toe clearance during swing phase of gait. Toe clearance will be more important when the patient is not wearing B AFOs such as in the home environment. Shortening of the gastrocnemius may also contribute to knee hyperextension in stance phase. A decrease in hip extension ROM leads to the inability to achieve terminal stance and therefore reduces the contralateral step length.

The patient demonstrates muscle weakness throughout his BLE. These impairments will also impact his gait pattern. His current hip abduction strength is 4–/5 B. This will create a decrease in hip stability in stance phase and resultant compensation of a Trendelenburg gait pattern. Hip extension MMT reveals 3/5 strength. This weakness will result in decreased step length contralaterally due to decreased propulsion which ultimately impacts gait speed. Bilateral quadriceps strength is 3–/5. This strength deficit will influence the ability to achieve terminal knee extension at late swing phase which will impact the achievement of heel strike. This may also create knee hyperextension from initial contact to midstance due to the inability of the quadriceps to control extension. The patient's dorsiflexion strength of 2 + /5 will be significant during swing phase of gait. The lack of dorsiflexion during this phase of gait will result in toe drag and an increased risk for falls. Compensatory strategies may include excessive hip and knee flexion or hip circumduction to assist in toe clearance.

Apply

9. Four LE strengthening exercises that will be beneficial for the patient include:

a) Hip abduction leg raise—This exercise targets the gluteus medius and gluteus minimus strength. Prior to surgery, the patient maintained a position of strong hip adduction and over lengthening of the hip abductor muscle group which leads to weakness. Due to bilateral adductor tenotomies, the patient now has improved passive and active ROM into hip abduction and requires strengthening of the hip abductor muscle group to improve hip alignment and stability in weight-bearing and ambulation.

b) Bridges—For strengthening of the gluteus maximus (primary) and hamstring (secondary), the patient would benefit from performing bridges. This is important to improve posture and alignment in standing. Presurgically, the patient utilized a crouched standing posture and gait pattern. Postsurgery, the patient demonstrates increased hip extension PROM and requires strengthening of hip extensors for improved standing posture and improved gait pattern with increased propulsion.

(Continued)

Bloom's Taxonomy Level	Case 4.C Answers
	c) Leg press—Performing a machine-based leg press will allow for quadriceps and gluteus maximus strengthening in modified weight-bearing. This will also allow for the progression of resistance as tolerated versus a wall slide exercise. Strengthening of these muscle groups is important to maintain upright posture in standing with hip and knee extension. Improved strength will also improve propulsion and the opportunity to achieve heel strike at initial contact. d) Terminal knee extension in weight-bearing—This exercise addresses activation and strengthening of the quadriceps in a weight-bearing position to promote strength and stability at the knee in stance phase of gait. Currently, the patient experiences buckling of R > L knee. 10. To promote improved sustaining of knee and hip extension in RLE stance, the patient will practice weight shifting over the RLE. The patient may require verbal cues, tactile cues, or hands-on facilitation of knee and hip extension initially. As the patient improves with sustaining weight-bearing and stance on the RLE, progression of single limb support can be performed with LLE stepping or kicking a ball, again providing assistance/facilitation as needed and reducing as the patient becomes stronger and more stable. ▶ Video 4.4 ▶ Video 4.5
Understand	11. The patient underwent multilevel orthopaedic surgery to improve ROM, posture, alignment, and overall function. While the surgery addressed the secondary musculoskeletal impairments of cerebral palsy, the patient's motor disorder influenced by spasticity remains unchanged. Spasticity is one of the underlying causes of muscle contractures and decreased ROM in children with CP. Some reduction of spasticity following muscle tendon lengthening surgeries has been documented. Damiano et al and Dreher et al attributed this decrease in tone and spasticity to an alteration in the muscle structure secondary to muscle tendon lengthening surgery and not a true reduction in tone from a neurophysiologic basis. As tension in the muscle returns, we can expect the influence of spasticity on movement patterns and alignment also to return, impacting the long-term progress and ability to sustain functional gains. It is important for the patient to continue with previous spasticity management, oral baclofen in this case. 12. Two community-based activities that the patient would benefit from include martial arts and swimming. Martial arts are able to offer the benefit of flexibility, strengthening, balance, and coordination, all of which the patient has impairments in. Another community-based activity is swimming or aquatic exercise. The buoyancy and resistance of the water will be beneficial to the patient in improving strength and aerobic endurance and allow the patient to work in an unweighted environment.
Remember	13. The typical gait pattern of spastic diplegic cerebral palsy is one of sustained hip flexion, adduction, and internal rotation and knee flexion throughout the gait cycle or a crouched gait pattern. In some cases, the knees may hyperextend during stance phase depending on the mobility of the pelvis and ankle musculature. The ankles may present with valgus alignment and subsequent foot pronation with an increased base of support or the ankle may sustain plantarflexion with the heels off the floor (toe walking) with a narrow base of support. In the case of ankle valgus and increased base of support, it is difficult to perform lateral weight shift during ambulation, and compensatory strategies of excessive head and upper trunk movements to unload their lower extremities for advancement are often used. 14. Spasticity is defined as velocity-dependent increase in muscle tone due to hyperexcitability of the stretch reflex secondary to an upper motor neuron lesion. Spasticity management options include oral medications such as diazepam, dantrolene, and baclofen. Another spasticity management option is neuromuscular blocks using botulinum toxin A and/or phenol. Lastly, neurosurgical interventions such as selective dorsal rhizotomy (SDR) and intrathecal baclofen pump are available as well. 15. The following outcome measures in the activity domain would be appropriate in this patient case: Dynamic Gait Index, Observational Gait Scale, Timed Up and Down Stairs, Timed Up and Go, Functional Independence Measure, Pediatric Evaluation of Disability Inventory-CAT, and Standardized Walking Obstacle Course. The following outcome measures in the participation domain would be appropriate in this patient case: Canadian Occupational Performance Measure, Children's Assessment of Participation and Enjoyment, School Function Assessment, PedsQL, Child Occupational Self-Assessment.

Key points
1. It is important to consider the patient's gait speed and ability to keep up with peers but keeping in mind safety and quality of gait when making recommendations for an assistive device for community ambulation.
2. Understand the demands of a high school environment and the activity and participation limitations of a student with a disability and how outpatient physical therapist will address these.
3. Emphasize the importance of participation and help the patient identify activities of interest to assist them in continued progress through fitness upon discharge.

Suggested Readings

Academy of Acute Care Physical Therapy. Laboratory Values Interpretation Resource. 2017. Available at: www.acutept.org. Accessed January 7, 2019

Alemdaroğlu E, Özbudak SD, Mandiroğlu S, Biçer SA, Özgirgin N, Uçan H. Predictive factors for inpatient falls among children with cerebral palsy. J Pediatr Nurs. 2017; 32:25–31

Andrews AW, Chinworth SA, Bourassa M, Garvin M, Benton D, Tanner S. Update on distance and velocity requirements for community ambulation. J Geriatr Phys Ther. 2010; 33(3):128–134

Bohannon RW, Smith MB. Interrater reliability of a modified Ashworth scale of muscle spasticity. Phys Ther. 1987; 67(2): 206–207

Bierman J, Franjoine M, Hazzard C, Howle J, Stamer M. Neuro-Developmental Treatment. Thieme Publishers; 2016:541

Child life, education and creative arts therapy. Available at: https://www.chop.edu/centers-programs/child-life-education-and-creative-arts-therapy. Accessed March 29, 2020

Corporate - US. 2020. Our Retail Divisions. [online]. Available at: https://corporate.walmart.com/newsroom/2005/01/06/our-retail-divisions. Accessed April 14, 2020

Damiano DL, Alter KE, Chambers H. New clinical and research trends in lower extremity management for ambulatory children with cerebral palsy. Phys Med Rehabil Clin N Am. 2009; 20(3): 469–491

Delmore B, Deppisch M, Sylvia C, et al. Pressure injuries in the pediatric population: a national pressure ulcer advisory panel white paper. Adv Skin Wound Care. 2019; 32(9):394–408

Department of Education. 2020. Frequently Asked Questions, Available at: https://www.education.pa.gov/Teachers%20-%20Administrators/School%20Construction%20and%20Facilities/Pages/Frequently-Asked-Questions.aspx. Accessed April 14, 2020

dos Santos PD, da Silva FC, Ferreira EG, da Rosa lop R, Bento GG, da Silva R. Instruments that evaluate functional independence in children with cerebral palsy: a systematic review of observational studies. Fisioter Pesqui. 2016; 23(3):318–328

Dreher T, Brunner R, Vegvari D, et al. The effects of muscle-tendon surgery on dynamic electromyographic patterns and muscle tone in children with cerebral palsy. Gait Posture. 2013; 38(2):215–220

Franki I, Desloovere K, De Cat J, et al. The evidence-base for basic physical therapy techniques targeting lower limb function in children with cerebral palsy: a systematic review using the International Classification of Functioning, Disability and Health as a conceptual framework. J Rehabil Med. 2012; 44(5):385–395

Geiger R, Strasak A, Treml B, et al. Six-minute walk test in children and adolescents. J Pediatr. 2007; 150(4):395–399, 399.e1–399.e2

Harmon LC, Grobbel C, Palleschi M. Reducing pressure injury incidence using a turn team assignment. J Wound Ostomy Continence Nurs. 2016; 43(5):477–482

Kratz AL, Slavin MD, Mulcahey MJ, Jette AM, Tulsky DS, Haley SM. An examination of the PROMIS(®) pediatric instruments to assess mobility in children with cerebral palsy. Qual Life Res. 2013; 22(10):2865–2876

Kutz MJ, Stuberg W, Dejong S, Arpin DJ. Overground body-weight-supported gait training for children and youth with neuromuscular impairments. Phys Occup Ther Pediatr. 2013; 33(3):353–365

Lee SJ, Lee JH, Gershon RRM. Musculoskeletal symptoms in nurses in the early implementation phase of California's safe patient handling legislation. Res Nurs Health. 2015; 38(3):183–193

Matthews DJ, Balaban B. Management of spasticity in children with cerebral palsy [in Turkish)]. Acta Orthop Traumatol Turc. 2009; 43(2):81–86

Mendes LPS, Teixeira LS, da Cruz LJ, Vieira DSR, Parreira VF. Sustained maximal inspiration has similar effects compared to incentive spirometers. Respir Physiol Neurobiol. 2019; 261:67–74

Modi S, Deisler R, Gozel K, et al. Wells criteria for DVT is a reliable clinical tool to assess the risk of deep venous thrombosis in trauma patients. World J Emerg Surg. 2016; 11(24):1–6

Nahm NJ, Graham HK, Gormley ME, Jr, Georgiadis AG. Management of hypertonia in cerebral palsy. Curr Opin Pediatr. 2018; 30(1): 57–64

Pediatricapta.org. Available at: https://pediatricapta.org/includes/fact-sheets/pdfs/13%20Assessment&screening%20tools.pdf. Published 2020. Accessed February 2020

Salbach NM, O'Brien K, Brooks D, et al. Speed and distance requirements for community ambulation: a systematic review. Arch Phys Med Rehabil. 2014; 95(1):117–128.e11

Shrader MW, Jones J, Falk MN, White GR, Burk DR, Segal LS. Hip reconstruction is more painful than spine fusion in children with cerebral palsy. J Child Orthop. 2015; 9(3):221–225

Target Corporate. 2020. Inside Our Stores | Target Corporation. Available at: https://corporate.target.com/about/locations/inside-our-stores. Accessed April 14, 2020

Tecklin J. Pediatric Physical Therapy. 4th ed. Philadelphia: Lippincott Williams & Wilkins; 2008:192–194, 211–214

Thissen D, Liu Y, Magnus B, et al. Estimating minimally important difference (MID) in PROMIS pediatric measures using the scale-judgment method. Qual Life Res. 2016; 25(1):13–23

Vlachou M, Dimitriadis D. Split tendon transfers for the correction of spastic varus foot deformity: a case series study. J Foot Ankle Res. 2010; 3:1–11

Wright M, Palisano RJ. Cerebral palsy. In: Palisano RJ, Orlin MN, Schreiber J. eds. Campbell's Physical Therapy for Children. St. Louis, Missouri: 2017:447–487

Xu N, Matsumoto H, Roye D, Hyman J. Post-operative pain assessment in management of cerebral palsy (CP): a two-pronged comparative study on the experience of surgical patients. J Pediatr Nurs. 2019; 46:e10–e14

Zhou L, Camp M, Gahukamble A, et al. Proximal femoral osteotomy in children with cerebral palsy: the perspective of the trainee. J Child Orthop. 2017; 11(1):6–14

5 Cerebrovascular Accident

General Information	
Case no.	5.A Cerebrovascular Accident
Authors	Ethan Hood, PT, DPT, MBA, Board Certified Clinical Specialist in Geriatrics Physical Therapy, Board Certified Clinical Specialist in Neurologic Physical Therapy Jessica Schwartz, MSPAS, PA-C
Diagnosis	Acute left middle cerebral artery (MCA), cerebrovascular accident (CVA)
Setting	Emergency Department, with transfer to Neurology Ward
Learner expectations	☑ Initial evaluation ☐ Re-evaluation ☐ Treatment session
Learner objectives	1. Recognize the symptoms of stroke and determine most likely location based on presenting symptoms and physical exam. 2. Develop an appropriate rehabilitation plan of care, including the roles of the team members involved. 3. Determine a safe and appropriate discharge plan for a patient who has been diagnosed with a CVA, including any durable medical equipment that may eventually be required. 4. Identify how to work collaboratively with other medical teams when caring for a patient with a CVA (e.g., medicine, neurology, physical therapy, occupational therapy (OT), speech therapy (ST), case management, and nursing).

Medical	
Chief complaint	"Right side weakness and unable to speak properly" for 2 hours
History of present illness	The patient is a 67-year-old right-handed male who presented to the emergency department due to severe right side weakness and speech deficits. He was last seen in his normal state of health the night prior when going to bed. The symptoms started in the morning around 06:00 when the patient woke up. The patient's wife noted weakness on the patient's right side, specifically that he was not using his right upper extremity. She also noted that the patient's right-side face looked "funny." He was having difficulty with his speech, which the wife described as "trouble finding words, can't seem to get the words out." The patient confirmed with shaking his head "no" that he cannot feel his right arm. He denied headache or vision changes. The patient's wife noted that although he had walked this morning, he was still required some assistance. He is typically independent with all mobility. His symptoms have been persistent without change since he woke up 1 hour ago this morning. He has not had any fevers or chills, recent illness, recent travel, or heart palpitations. He has never had symptoms like this in the past.
Past medical history	Hypertension, coronary artery disease, myocardial infarction with drug-eluding stent placement 10 years ago, hypercholesterolemia, diabetes mellitus type 2, smoked for 25 years (1 pack/day)—quit 10 years ago, and obesity—body mass index = 30.1
Past surgical history	Drug-eluding stent placed 10 years ago
Allergies	No known drug allergies
Medications	Lisinopril, Metoprolol tartrate, Aspirin, Atorvastatin, Metformin
Precautions/Orders	Stroke team consult: NPO until cleared by ST Bedrest for 24 hours then activity as tolerated Physical therapy and OT

Social history	
Home setup	• Resides in a split-level house with his wife. • Three steps are there to enter the home with a left railing. • Eight steps to the second floor are with a right railing ascending. • Bedroom and bathroom are on the second floor. • Woodworking shop and den are on the lower level, with eight steps and right rail to descend.
Occupation	• Retired 2 years ago from teaching high school English for 35 years.
Prior level of function	• Independent with functional mobility, activities of daily living (ADLs), and instrumental ADLs. • Walks 1 mile/day with his wife and dog • (+) Drives
Recreational activities	• Fly fish and hunting (bow and arrow) • Woodworking and makes his own furniture • Visits two sons who live locally

Vital signs	Hospital day 0: emergency department
Blood pressure (mmHg)	168/90
Heart rate (beats/minute)	88
Respiratory rate (breaths/minute)	18
Pulse oximetry on room air (SpO$_2$)	97%
Temperature (°F)	96.9

Imaging/Diagnostic test	Hospital day 0: emergency department
Electrocardiogram (ECG)	1. Atrial Fibrillation, no acute ST-T wave changes
Chest X-ray	1. No acute Cardiovascular and pulmonary pathology noted
Computed tomography (CT)—head without contrast	1. No acute masses, hemorrhages, or infarcts noted
Magnetic resonance imaging (MRI)—brain Magnetic resonance angiography (MRA)—head and neck with and without contrast	1. Acute infarction in the left frontal and parietal lobes in the MCA territory (► Fig. 5.1) 2. No hemorrhage or mass noted 3. Moderate occlusion noted at middle one-third of left M1 segment of the left MCA with some collateral flow
Transthoracic two-dimensional echocardiography	1. Left ventricle ejection fraction 65% 2. No wall motion abnormalities 3. Left and right ventricles without any hypertrophy or increased wall thickness 4. Left and right atrial sizes normal, no dilation. No evidence of any valvular stenosis or regurgitation 5. No evidence of clots or vegetation noted based on the limitations of transthoracic approach

Medical management	Hospital day 0: emergency department
Medications	1. Continue aspirin 2. Metformin 3. Hold lisinopril and metoprolol tartrate for first 2–3 days to allow permissive hypertension
Diet	1. Nothing by mouth (NPO) until seen by speech therapy 2. Diet safety to be determined with swallow evaluation
Vitals	1. Every 4 hours with neuro checks 2. Monitor telemetry for arrhythmias

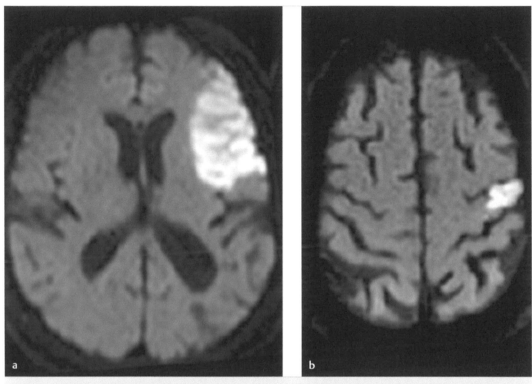

Fig. 5.1 (a,b) Acute infarction in the left frontal and parietal lobes in the MCA territory. (Source: Arterial Ischemia. In: Valdueza Barrios J, Schreiber S, Röhl J, et al, ed. Neurosonology and Neuroimaging of Stroke: A Comprehensive Reference. 2nd ed. Thieme; 2017.)

	Lab	Reference range	Hospital day 0: emergency department
Complete blood cell count	White blood cells	5.0–10.0 × 10⁹/L	7.6
	Hemoglobin	14–17.4 g/dL	14.1
	Hematocrit	42–52%	44
	Platelets	140–400 k/µL	190
Basic metabolic profile	Glucose	60–100 mg/dL	200
	Blood urea nitrogen (BUN)	6–25 mg/dL	21
	Creatinine	0.7–1.3 mg/dL	1.07
	Sodium	135–145 mEq/L	139
	Potassium	3.5–5.0 mEq/L	4.0
	Chloride	98–106 mEq/L	105
	Bicarbonate	21–28 mEq/L	25
	Calcium	8.6–10.3 mg/dL	8.8
Other	Fingerstick glucose	60–100 mg/dL	210
	International normalized ratio (INR)	1.0	0.8–1.2
	Troponin	<0.02 ng/mL	<0.02
	Hemoglobin A1C	4.0–5.6%	8.5%
	Cholesterol	<200 mg/dL	240
	Low-density lipoprotein	65–180 mg/dL	170

(Continued)

(Continued)

Lab	Reference range	Hospital day 0: emergency department
High-density lipoprotein	> 35 mg/dL	55
Triglycerides	< 150 mg/dL	105

Pause points

Based on the above information:
- Is there any significance with the diagnostic tests and measures?
- Who are the members of the stroke team and what are their roles?
- Based on the above findings, describe what should be prioritized for the physical therapy examination.

Hospital Day 1: Physical Therapy Examination
Subjective
"I have difficulty finding the right word." "My right side is weak."
Objective

Vital signs	Pre-treatment			Post-treatment
	Supine	Sitting	Standing	
Blood pressure (mmHg)	136/78	140/80	142/84	144/86
Heart rate (beats/min)	77	76	84	88
Respiratory rate (breaths/min)	12	12	16	16
Pulse oximetry on room air (SpO$_2$)	97%	96%	97%	96%
Modified rate of perceived exertion (RPE) scale (0–10)	1/10	2/10	3/10	4/10
Pain	0/10	0/10	1/10 at right shoulder	1/10 at right shoulder
General	• A 67-year-old male, well developed and well nourished • Supine in bed, awake, and in no acute distress • Lines notable for peripheral Intravenous line, urinary catheter, and telemetry			
Cardiovascular and pulmonary	• Auscultation: Clear lung sounds, irregularly irregular cardiac rhythm • Pulses: 3 + bilateral dorsalis pedis and posterior tibialis			
Gastrointestinal	• Slight abdominal distension, no tenderness to palpation			
Genitourinary	• (+) urinary catheter			
Cognition	• Awake and alert • Oriented once—able to state his name but not his birthdate, location, time, or situation • Speech appears very slow and labored; has difficulty finding correct words to answer questions • Follows one-step commands 100% of the time			
Musculoskeletal	Range of motion	• Passive range of motion of right upper extremity (RUE) and right lower extremity (RLE): within functional limit (WFL). • Active range of motion of left upper extremity (LUE) and left lower extremity (LLE): WFL.		
	Strength	• L shoulder flexion: 5/5 • R shoulder flexion: 1/5 • L elbow flexion: 5/5 • R elbow flexion: 1/5		

(Continued)

(Continued)

		Hospital Day 1: Physical Therapy Examination
		• L wrist extension: 5/5 • R wrist extension: 0/5 • L hip flexion: 5/5 • R hip flexion: 3+/5 • L knee extension: 5/5 • R knee extension: 3+/5 • L ankle dorsiflexion: 5/5 • R ankle dorsiflexion: 3+/5
	Aerobic	• Not tested
Neurological	Balance	• Static unsupported sitting: fair+, requires tactile cues for midline posture. • Static unsupported standing: poor+, requires minimal assist with tactile cues for midline posture. • Berg Balance Scale = 30/56
	Coordination	• L cerebellar function intact with no dysdiadochokinesia • LUE finger to nose intact. Unable to be performed on RUE • Pronator drift unable to be performed due to weakness in RUE • LLE heel to shin intact. RLE ataxic with heel to shin
	Cranial nerves	• II–XII grossly intact except for noted right side facial droop, sparing the forehead • Vision intact, fully tracking with eyes, with no visual field deficits. Denies diplopia.
	Reflexes	• Brachioradialis: 1+L, 2+R • Biceps brachii: 1+L, 2+R • Triceps brachii: 1+L, 2+R • Patellar: 1+L, 2+R
	Sensation	• RUE: loss of sensation to crude touch and pinprick • LUE, RLE, LLE: intact to crude touch and pinprick
	Tone	• RUE flaccid, RLE hypotonic
		Functional status
Bed mobility		• Rolling to left: supervision with bedrails • Supine to sit: minimal assistance once with head of bed elevated ~30 degrees
Transfers		• Sit to/from stand: minimal assistance once with wide base quad cane
Ambulation		• Ambulated 15 feet with minimal assistance and wide base quad cane • Gait deviations notable for right hemiparetic gait, lack of right arm swing and movement requiring physical therapist to support, and poor right weight shift requiring physical therapy verbal and tactile cues to facilitate. • Gait speed 0.20 m/second • ▶ Fig. 5.2
Stairs		• N/A
Other		• Barthel Index: 30/100 • Functional independence measure: 51 total score (35 motor, 16 cognitive)

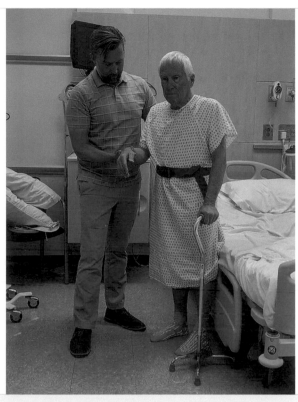

Fig. 5.2 An example of a physical therapist guarding the patient during an ambulation trial.

Assessment	
☑ Physical therapist's	*Assessment left blank for learner to develop.*
Goals	
Patient's	"To walk normal again"
Short term	1.
	Goals left blank for learner to develop.
	2.
Long term	1.
	Goals left blank for learner to develop.
	2.

Plan	
☑ Physical therapist's	Patient is to be seen twice a day for 4–5 days for therapeutic exercise, gait training, transfer training, endurance training, neuromuscular reeducation, patient and family education, positioning to minimize shoulder pathology and pain, and to facilitate discharge to appropriate care level.

Bloom's Taxonomy Level	Case 5.A Questions
Create	1. Synthesizing the medical data and physical examination findings, develop an appropriate physical therapy assessment of the patient.
	2. Develop two short-term physical therapy goals, including an appropriate timeframe.
	3. Develop two long-term physical therapy goals, including an appropriate timeframe.

(Continued)

(Continued)

Bloom's Taxonomy Level	Case 5.A Questions
Evaluate	4. Based on the patient's presentation, what would be the best discharge environment? Why? 5. Based on this patient's current presentation and history, what would be appropriate physical therapy prognosis? 6. How should the physical therapist rate the patient's right hemibody tone?
Analyze	7. What is the significance of the patient's Berg Balance Scale? 8. In terms of function, what is the importance of the patient's gait speed? 9. What outcome measures may assist with functional prognosis? 10. What is the most likely etiology of this patient's infraction based on his clinical presentation and workup thus far?
Apply	11. What cranial nerves are involved with eye function?
Understand	12. Why did medical management withhold blood pressure medications despite the patient's current readings? What is the rationale? 13. What would be the most therapeutic position for this patient while he is in bed? Why?
Remember	14. What is the typical presentation of an MCA infarction? 15. What are some differences in presentation between a right MCA and a left MCA infarct? 16. What affected area of the brain causes expressive aphasia?

Bloom's Taxonomy Level	Case 5.A Answers
Create	1. Patient presents with right hemibody weakness with reduced tone, impaired transfers, gait, and high fall risk on standardized balance testing due to the effects of L MCA distribution stroke impairing ADLs and function. Recommend skilled physical therapist to address the following goals. Recommend assisting once with all mobility while in hospital. Anticipate patient being a good acute inpatient rehabilitation candidate. 2. Short-term goals: • Patient will demonstrate sit to/from stand transfer with contact guard assistance within 3 days to facilitate improved transfer ability. • Patient will ambulate 30 feet on level surfaces with minimal assistance and wide base quad cane, demonstrating step to pattern, within 3 days to improve gait and endurance. 3. Long-term goals: • Patient will ambulate 50 feet on level surfaces with contact guard assistance with wide base quad cane within 7 days to facilitate improve function in home. • Patient will ascend/descend three steps with minimal assistance and left handrail when ascending within 7 days to facilitate getting into and out of his home.
Evaluate	4. Based on the patient's age, prior level of function, past medical history, level of cognition, current functional status, and tolerance to activity, a discharge location of acute inpatient rehab would be most appropriate. 5. Based on the patient's presentation, past medical history, and prior level of function, it is anticipated that the patient will be able to return to independence with functional mobility and community ambulation. He may, however, need adaptive equipment to assist with ADLs depending on his right upper extremity's return. 6. The patient's hemibody tone would be rated as follows: RUE, 0/4; RLE, 1/4.
Analyze	7. The Berg Balance Scale indicated that the patient is a high fall risk. 8. The patient's current speed of 0.20 m/second is extremely slow and not conducive to the patient being a safe community ambulatory at this time. 9. The outcome measures that may assist with functional prognosis are the Functional Independence Measure and the Stroke Rehabilitation Assessment of Movement. 10. This patient most likely has a cardioembolic stroke due to atrial fibrillation. His electrocardiogram suggests evidence of atrial fibrillation, and his cardiac exam reveals an irregularly irregular rhythm. This is an example of a cerebrovascular accident as the initial presentation of new onset atrial fibrillation.
Apply	11. Cranial nerves II, III, IV, VI, and VIII are involved with eye function.

(Continued)

(Continued)

Bloom's Taxonomy Level	Case 5.A Answers
Understand	12. Medical management withheld for antihypertensives to allow the patient to have permissive hypertension in the first 24 hours after his acute ischemic stroke. This allows for adequate perfusion to areas of salvageable brain tissue (penumbra).
	13. The most therapeutic position for this patient while he is in bed is right side lying. This is to maintain glenohumeral joint integrity (▶ Fig. 5.3).
Remember	14. The typical presentation of an MCA infarction is upper extremity, followed by face and lower extremity, respectively.
	15. While the following is not inclusive, a right MCA would have findings on the left side of the body with behavioral changes of impulsivity and minimal insight into deficits. An infarct of the left MCA would have deficits on the right side of the body, with insight into their deficits and tendencies to be extremely cautious.
	16. Broca area (located in the dominant frontal lobe) causes expressive aphasia.

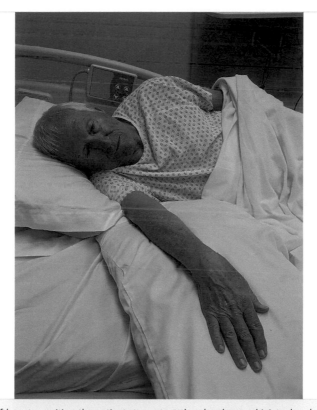

Fig. 5.3 An example of how to position the patient to protect the glenohumeral joint when he is in bed.

Key points

1. MCA distribution stroke typically involves the upper extremity greater than the lower extremity. Based on the side of lesion, very specific characteristics may arise.

2. Based on this patient's presentation, he will need intensive acute inpatient rehabilitation, which is to include physical therapy, OT, and ST, to maximize overall function and quality of life. Durable medical equipment needs will be addressed in acute inpatient rehabilitation, as prescription will be dependent on the patient's level of function at discharge.

(Continued)

(Continued)

Key points
3. To properly care for a patient who has had a stroke, a team approach is required. The team can include physiatry, nursing, rehabilitation therapy, and case management, all of who will ensure the patient's needs are met, education is holistic, and risk factors to reduce a second stroke are discussed. Key risk factors for stroke include hypertension, hyperlipidemia, diabetes, obesity, and smoking history. These risk factors must be addressed by the medical team to help prevent future ischemic events.

General Information	
Case no.	5.B
Authors	Ethan Hood, PT, DPT, MBA, Board Certified Clinical Specialist in Geriatrics Physical Therapy, Board Certified Clinical Specialist in Neurologic Physical Therapy Jessica Schwartz, MSPAS, PA-C
Diagnosis	Acute left middle cerebral artery (MCA), cerebrovascular accident (CVA)
Setting	Acute inpatient rehabilitation
Learner expectations	☑ Initial evaluation ☐ Re-evaluation ☐ Treatment session
Learner objectives	1. Identify how to work collaboratively with other medical teams when caring for a patient with a CVA (e.g., medicine, neurology, physical therapy, occupational therapy (OT), speech therapy, case management, and nursing). 2. Comprehend the integration of setting specific goals of care into a proper physical therapy plan of care. 3. Integrate latest evidence-based treatment ideas into proper physical therapy interventions. 4. Appreciate how changes in medical status can influence patient function and physical therapy care.

Medical	
Chief complaint	"Right side weakness and unable to speak properly"
History of present illness	The patient is a 67-year-old right-handed male admitted to the hospital 5 days ago due to severe one-sided weakness and speech deficits. Imaging confirmed a left MCA infarct with resultant Broca aphasia. Electrocardiogram revealed new onset atrial fibrillation, and this was confirmed on telemetry throughout the patient's hospital stay. He was started on apixaban 5mg PO twice daily to prevent further cardioembolic events. He was also started on sitagliptin 100mg PO daily to help better control his blood glucose levels. His atorvastatin was increased to 80mg PO nightly, given his elevated cholesterol levels and diagnosis of CVA. Consultations in the hospital included speech language pathology, which showed moderate expressive aphasia and dysphagia. A video fluoroscopic swallowing study was performed, and the patient was placed on a level 1 dysphagia puree diet with nectar-thick liquids. He was progressed to a level 2 dysphagia mechanically altered diet with nectar-thick liquids by speech therapy prior to hospital discharge. Other consults include physical therapy and OT. The patient was able to perform transfers and ambulation of 60 feet with minimal assistance and a wide base quad cane. He was seen by physiatry with recommendations for acute inpatient rehabilitation. The patient was admitted to acute inpatient rehabilitation last night.
Past medical history	Hypertension, coronary artery disease, myocardial infarction with drug-eluding stent placement 10 years ago, hypercholesterolemia, diabetes mellitus type 2, and obesity
Past surgical history	Drug-eluding stent placed 10 years ago
Allergies	No known drug allergies (NKDA)
Precautions/Orders	Vitals every 8 hours Activity as tolerated Head of bed (HOB) elevated 30 degrees at all times Dysphagia and thickened liquids diet Assist with all out of bed (OOB) mobility

Social history	
Home setup	• Resides in a split-level house with his wife. • Three steps are there to enter the home with a left railing. • Eight steps are there to the second floor with a right railing ascending. • Bedroom and bathroom are on the second floor. • Woodworking shop and den are on the lower level, with eight steps and right rail to descend.
Occupation	• Retired 2 years ago from teaching high school English for 35 years.
Prior level of function	• Independent with functional mobility, activities of daily living (ADLs), and instrumental ADLs • Walks 1 mile/day with his wife and dog. • (+) Drives
Recreational activities	• Fly fish and hunting (bow and arrow) • Woodworking and makes his own furniture • Visits two sons who live locally

Vital signs	Day 1: acute inpatient rehabilitation
Blood pressure (mmHg)	152/88
Heart rate (beats/minute)	68
Respiratory rate (breaths/minute)	14
Pulse oximetry on room air (SpO$_2$)	99%
Temperature (°F)	98.5

Imaging/Diagnostic test	Day 1: acute inpatient rehabilitation
Patient Health Questionnaire (PHQ-9)	14/27 = moderate depression

Medical management	Day 1: acute inpatient rehabilitation
Medications	1. Lisinopril, Metoprolol tartrate, Aspirin, Clopidogrel, Atorvastatin, Metformin, Sitagliptin 2. Lisinopril to be increased due to elevated blood pressures 3. Start on citalopram for depression
Diet	1. Mechanical soft/nectar thickened liquids
Vitals	1. Every 8 hours with neuro checks

Lab		Reference range	Day 1: acute inpatient rehabilitation
Complete blood cell count	Hemoglobin	14–17.4 g/dL	13.4
	Hematocrit	42–52%	41.5
	White blood cell (WBC)	5.0–10.0 × 10^9/L	9.1
	Platelets	140–400 k/μL	140
Basic metabolic profile	Glucose	60–100 mg/dL	168
	Blood urea nitrogen	7–20 mg/dL	20
	Creatinine	0.4–1.10 mg/dL	0.98
	Sodium	135–145 mEq/L	135
	Potassium	3.5–5.0 mEq/L	3.6
	Chloride	98–106 mEq/L	103
	Bicarbonate	21–28 mEq/L	22
	Calcium	8.6–10.3 mg/dL	8.4
Other	Fingerstick glucose	60–100 mg/dL	182

Pause points
Based on the above information,   • Why were the patient's medications changed/adjusted?   • How should the physical therapy examination be structured? What objective tests and measures seem most appropriate?   • Explain the role of physical therapy, OT, and ST in the rehabilitation of this patient. Explain what specific areas a physical therapist may collaborate.

Day 1, Acute Inpatient Rehabilitation: Physical Therapy Examination				
Subjective				
"I want to get back to a normal life."				
Objective				
Vital signs	Pre-treatment		Post-treatment	
	Supine	Sitting	Standing	Sitting
Blood pressure (mmHg)	150/88	152/86	148/86	150/86
Heart rate (beats/min)	66	66	68	80
Respiratory rate (breaths/min)	13	14	14	18
Pulse oximetry on room air (SpO$_2$)	98%	99%	99%	97%
Modified rate of perceived exertion (RPE) scale (0–10)	0/10	1/10	5/10	6/10
Pain	5/10 at right shoulder	5/10 at right shoulder	6/10 at right shoulder	7/10 at right shoulder
Cognition	• Awake and alert • Oriented three time—able to tell his name, birthdate, location, and current date • Speech appears very slow and labored; had difficulty finding words to answer questions • Follows one-step commands 100% of time			
Musculoskeletal	Range of motion	• Left upper extremity (LUE), active range of motion (AROM): within functional limit (WFL) • Right upper extremity (RUE), passive range of motion (PROM): Shoulder flexion: 0–80 degrees Shoulder abduction: 0–60 degrees Shoulder external rotation: 0–45 degrees Elbow extension: 0–45 degrees Hand: able to extend digits with significant pain *ROM appears to be limited due to increased tone and pain.* • Left lower extremity (LLE), AROM: WFL • Right lower extremity (RLE), PROM: WFL		
	Strength	• L shoulder flexion: 5/5 • R shoulder flexion: 1/5 • L elbow flexion: 5/5 • R elbow flexion: 1/5 • L wrist extension: 5/5 • R wrist extension: 0/5 • L hip flexion: 5/5 • R hip flexion: 3 + /5 • L knee extension: 5/5 • R knee extension: 3 + /5 • L ankle dorsiflexion: 5/5 • R ankle dorsiflexion: 3 + /5		

(Continued)

(Continued)

		Day 1, Acute Inpatient Rehabilitation: Physical Therapy Examination
		Unable to formally assess strength in RUE with Manual Muscle Testing (MMT) due to increased spasticity. The above strength grades are based on functional movements.
	Aerobic	• NuStep for 5 minutes, level 2 • RPE = 15/20. Heart rate: 84 beat/minute post
Neurological	Balance	• Static unsupported sitting: fair +, requires tactile cues for midline posture • Static unsupported standing: poor +, requires minimal assist with tactile cues for midline posture • (+) Romberg Test • Berg Balance Scale = 36/56
	Coordination	• Rapid alternating movements: LUE intact, unable to assess in RUE • Heel to shin—LLE intact, RLE ataxic
	Cranial nerves	• II–XII grossly intact except for noted right-side facial droop, sparing the forehead • Vision intact, fully tracking with eyes, with no visual field deficits • Denies diplopia
	Reflexes	• Brachioradialis: 2 + L, 3 + R • Biceps brachii: 2 + L, 3 + R • Triceps brachii: 2 + L, 3 + R • Patellar: 2 + L, 3 + R
	Sensation	• RUE: loss of sensation to crude touch and pinprick • LUE, RLE, LLE: intact to crude touch and pinprick
	Tone	• RUE: 2 + /4 spasticity on modified Ashworth Scale • RUE: 2 finger sulcus sign on right shoulder • RUE flexor synergy • RLE: hypotonic
	Other	• Stroke Rehabilitation Assessment of Movement (STREAM): 32/70 (6/20 upper extremity; 13/20 lower extremity; 13/30 basic mobility) • Functional Independence Measure: 77 total (52 motor, 25 cognitive) • ▶ Fig. 5.4
		Functional status
Bed mobility		• Rolling to left: supervision with bed rails • Supine to sit: contact guard assist once with HOB elevated ~ 30 degrees and use of bedrails
Transfers		• Sit to/from stand: minimal assistance once with wide base quad cane
Ambulation		• Ambulated 60 feet with minimal assistance and wide base quad cane • Gait deviations notable for right hemiparetic gait with slight right knee hyperextension (genu recurvatum) during midstance and RUE in flexor synergy • Gait speed = 0.25 m/second
Stairs		• Ascend/descend four steps with moderate assistance and left railing ascending. Tactile and verbal cues provided for midline posture • Demonstrated step-to pattern

FIM® Instrument

	7	Complete Independence (timely, safely)		**NO HELPER**
	6	Modified Independence (device)		
L				
E		**Modified Dependence**		
V	5	Supervision (subject = 100%)		
E	4	Minimal Assistance (subject = 75%+)		
L	3	Moderate Assistance (subject = 50%+)		**HELPER**
S		**Complete Dependence**		
	2	Maximal Assistance (subject = 25%+)		
	1	Total Assistance (subject = less than 25%)		

	ADMISSION	DISCHARGE	FOLLOW-UP
Self-Care			
A. Eating			
B. Grooming			
C. Bathing			
D. Dressing: Upper Body			
E. Dressing: Lower Body			
F. Toileting			
Sphincter Control			
G. Bladder Management			
H. Bowel Management			
Transfers			
I. Bed, Chair, Wheelchair			
J. Toilet			
K. Tub, Shower			
Locomotion	W Walk / C Wheelchair / B Both	W Walk / C Wheelchair / B Both	W Walk / C Wheelchair / B Both
L. Walk, Wheelchair			
M. Stairs			
Motor Subtotal Rating			
Communication	A Auditory / V Visual / B Both	A Auditory / V Visual / B Both	A Auditory / V Visual / B Both
N. Comprehension			
O. Expression	V Vocal / N Nonvocal / B Both	V Vocal / N Nonvocal / B Both	V Vocal / N Nonvocal / B Both
Social Cognition			
P. Social Interaction			
Q. Problem Solving			
R. Memory			
Cognitive Subtotal Rating			
TOTAL FIM® RATING			

NOTE: Leave no blanks. Enter 1 if patient is not testable due to risk.

Fig. 5.4 Functional Independence Measure. Copyright @1997 Uniform Data System for Medical Rehabilitation, a division of UB Foundation Activities, Inc. Reprinted with permission.

Assessment	
☑ Physical therapist's	*Assessment left blank for learner to develop.*
Goals	
Patient's	"To be able to walk and talk normal again"
Short term	1.
	Goals left blank for learner to develop.
	2.
Long term	1.
	Goals left blank for learner to develop.
	2.

Plan	
☑ Physical therapist's	Patient to be seen 1–2 hours/day for 5–6 day/week. Treatment to include bed mobility, transfer training, gait training, stair training, therapeutic exercise, endurance activities, neuromuscular reeducation, and patient and family education.

Bloom's Taxonomy Level	Case 5.B Questions
Create	1. Synthesizing the medical data and physical examination findings, develop an appropriate physical therapy assessment of the patient. 2. Develop two short-term physical therapy goals, including an appropriate timeframe. 3. Develop two long-term physical therapy goals, including an appropriate timeframe. 4. Create an appropriate intervention program for this patient in acute inpatient rehab, including dosing.
Evaluate	5. What is the philosophical difference in blood pressure management in the acute phase vs. subacute phase for a patient after stroke?
Analyze	6. Is there anything his physician could prescribe to reduce his spasticity? 7. What is the significance of his PHQ-9 score? 8. Why are different functional measures (i.e. Fugl-Meyer, Functional Independence Measure [FIM], and STREAM) performed? 9. Are there any relationships between the aforementioned functional measures? 10. Can these measures be prognostic? Please explain.
Apply	11. What are the main goals for this patient in the acute inpatient rehab setting? 12. What treatments can be performed to reduce his RUE spasticity?
Understand	13. Given the initial exam findings, are there any concerns for arm positioning or long-term effects of his arm?
Remember	14. Why would the patient present with a flaccid RUE in the hospital and then a spastic RUE in the acute inpatient rehab?

Bloom's Taxonomy Level	Case 5.B Answers
Create	1. Patient presents with right hemibody weakness and abnormal tone, impaired transfers, balance, and gait due to the effects of left MCA infarct impairing ADLs and function. Recommend skilled physical therapist to address goals below. Anticipate successful discharge to home after meeting rehab goals. 2. Short-term goals: • Patient will perform sit to/from stand transfers with supervision within 7 days to facilitate return to independent function. • Patient will ambulate 100 feet with contact guard and wide base quad cane within 7 days to facilitate ability to ambulate around his home. 3. Long-term goals: • Patient will ambulate 300 feet with modified independence and wide base quad cane to facilitate ability to ambulate around his community. • Patient will ascend/descend eight steps with modified independence and one rail to get to second floor of his home where his bedroom and bathroom are located. 4. An appropriate intervention program for this patient in acute inpatient rehab, including dosing, is as follows: • Aerobic: 3–5 days per week; 40–70% VO_2 reserve or heart rate reserve; 20–60 minutes (or 3–10-minute sessions) • Strengthening: 2–3 days per week; 50–80% 1 repetition maximum (RM) (resistance gradually increased over time as tolerated); 1–3 sets of 10–15 repetitions of 8–10 exercises involving the major muscle groups • Balance: dynamic exercises focusing on improving weight shift and coordination of right hemibody
Evaluate	5. In the acute phase of treatment for stroke, the goal is to allow permissive hypertension and keep blood pressure less than 220/120 mmHg. After about 24 hours, permissive hypertension is no longer necessary and goal blood pressure is less than 130/80 mmHg.
Analyze	6. Baclofen can be prescribed by the physician to reduce the patient's spasticity. 7. The patient's PHQ-9 score suggests that the patient is suffering from depression, which is very common after a stroke. 8. Each functional outcome measure looks at different aspects of performance and function. The Fugl-Meyer is a stroke-specific outcome measure that looks at motor function, balance, sensation, movement quality, synergies, and tone. The Functional

(Continued)

(Continued)

Bloom's Taxonomy Level	Case 5.B Answers
	Independence Measure (FIM) is not stroke specific; however, it is used to measure the level of a patient's disability and indicates how much assistance is required for the patient to successfully complete activities. The FIM is popular with many insurance companies to assess level of assistance needed. The Stroke Rehabilitation Assessment of Movement (STREAM) is a stroke-specific outcome measure and designed for physical therapists to assess motor function, as well as functional activities such as transfers and gait.
	9. There is a correlation between the Fugl-Meyer and FIM. A change on the upper or lower extremity, Fugl-Meyer correlates with change in FIM scores. The STREAM also correlates with the Fugl-Meyer and FIM, in addition to numerous functional measures.
	10. Initial scores on standardized measures can be basic prognostic indicators of functional outcomes. The patient's change in FIM from a total of 51 to 77 (26 points) exceeds the MCID of 22 points for a patient who is status post stroke.
Apply	11. The main goal for this patient in the acute inpatient rehab setting is to become as independent as possible with all functional mobility and ADLs to facilitate a safe transition to home.
	12. A treatment that can be performed to reduce the patient's RUE spasticity is positioning the patient on his right side with his right arm extended and shoulder at 90 degrees or positioning on left side with his right arm extended shoulder at 90 degrees, and arm resting on pillow so that his right shoulder is not in horizontal adduction. This positioning schedule should be in collaboration with nursing and occupational therapy. Other treatments include PROM, moist heat, and potential medications, although this would require a discussion with the physician.
Understand	13. Because the patient is experiencing pain and has capsular laxity (as demonstrated by the positive sulcus sign), there are concerns to maintain proper positioning of the glenohumeral joint to prevent long-term negative effects. It is imperative that the right upper extremity is supported at all times to minimize further capsular laxity and assist in the reduction of pain.
Remember	14. Due to cerebral shock, his extremity was flaccid during the acute phase. During recovery, increased spasticity will be realized.

Key points
1. Collaboration among all medical disciplines is imperative to properly care for patients after stroke.
2. The goal of inpatient rehab is to maximize functional independence to facilitate the patient returning home. Afterward, he will receive additional rehabilitation services via home care and/or outpatient settings. The goals of therapy should be designed to reflect the patient's anticipated functional status and needs for returning home.
3. Evidence-based practice is imperative to facilitate maximum improvement with physical therapy.
4. Medical management to control risk factors must continue throughout acute inpatient rehabilitation to prevent secondary sequelae, including a second stroke. Patient and family education regarding upper extremity positioning can assist in reducing pain and improving overall outcomes.

General Information	
Case no.	5.C
Authors	Ethan Hood, PT, DPT, MBA, Board Certified Clinical Specialist in Geriatrics Physical Therapy, Board Certified Clinical Specialist in Neurologic Physical Therapy Jessica Schwartz, MSPAS, PA-C
Diagnosis	Acute left middle cerebral artery (MCA), cerebrovascular accident (CVA)
Setting	Outpatient clinic
Learner expectations	☑ Initial evaluation ☐ Re-evaluation ☐ Treatment session

(Continued)

(Continued)

General Information	
Learner objectives	1. Appreciate the need to monitor vitals and patient performance to identify additional medical sequelae.
	2. Identify appropriate tests and measures that provide information regarding patient function.
	3. Design an appropriate plan of care and interventions based on the patient's needs.

Follow-up visit with primary care provider	
Chief complaint	"Pain, R shoulder"
History of present illness	A 67-year-old right-handed male presents to his primary care provider's office after a 5-day hospitalization and 2-week acute inpatient rehab stay (total 21 days poststroke). He presents with expressive aphasia but is able to make his needs known and answer multistep questions if given time for processing. His wife admits that he does not enjoy drinking thickened liquids and his oral intake is decreased. He still seems somewhat "sad" per the wife, but there is some improvement in his mood and energy levels after starting citalopram at rehab. He has also been continuing to complain of discomfort in his right shoulder that has not improved with usage of baclofen. He describes the pain as sharp, shooting pains that are worse with activity. He would like to discuss this further with physical therapy before any medication adjustments.
Past medical history	Recent right MCA, recent new onset atrial fibrillation. CVA, hypertension, coronary artery disease, myocardial infarction with drug-eluding stent placement 10 years ago, hypercholesterolemia, diabetes mellitus type 2, obesity.
Past surgical history	Drug-eluding stent placed 10 years ago
Allergies	No known drug allergies (NKDA)
Medications	Lisinopril, Metoprolol tartrate, Aspirin, Apixaban, Atorvastatin, Metformin, Sitagliptin, Baclofen, Citalopram

Social history	
Home setup	• Resides in a split-level house with his wife
	• Three steps to enter the home with a left railing
	• Eight steps to the second floor with a right railing ascending
	• Bedroom and bathroom are on the second floor
	• Woodworking shop and den are on lower level, with eight steps and right rail to descend
Occupation	• Retired 2 years ago from teaching high school English x 35 years
Prior level of function	• Independent with functional mobility, activities of daily living (ADLs), and instrumental ADLs
	• Walks 1 mile/day with his wife and dog
	• (+) Drives
Recreational activities	• Fly fish and hunting (bow and arrow)
	• Woodworking and makes his own furniture
	• Visits two sons who live locally

Medical examination by primary care provider	
Vitals	• Blood pressure: 148/88 mmHg
	• Heart rate: 72 beat/min
	• Respiratory rate: 14 breath/min
	• Pulse oximetry: 96% on room air
	• Temperature: 97.2 °F
General	• 67-year-old male, well developed and well nourished
	• Awake and in no acute distress

(Continued)

(Continued)

Medical examination by primary care provider	
Head, ears, eyes, nose, and throat (HEENT)	• Head nontraumatic • Pupils equal, round, reactive to light, accommodation • Extra ocular movement intact • No ptosis or lid lag • Visual fields intact • Mucus membranes appear dry • Neck supple, trachea midline • Thyroid not enlarged • No carotid bruits
Cardiovascular and pulmonary	• Irregularly irregular rhythm, no murmurs/rubs/gallops • Peripheral pulses 2+ with no lower extremity edema • Lungs clear to auscultation bilaterally without wheezes/rhonchi/rales • No accessory muscle use
Abdomen	• Protuberant abdomen • Positive bowel sounds four times • Nontender to palpation with no rigidity, rebound, or guarding
Musculoskeletal	• No noted deformities • Active range of motion of right upper extremity limited secondary to weakness and pain. All other active range of motion intact. • Passive range of motion with significant resistance to movement in right upper extremity. All other passive range of motion intact.
Neurological	• Alert and oriented × 34 • Follows commands without difficulty • Expressive aphasia noted • Cranial nerves II–XII grossly intact except some mild right side facial droop, sparing the forehead • Spasticity in right upper extremity • Left upper extremity (LUE) and left lower extremity (LLE): 5/5 strength. Left hemibody weakness
Other tests	• PHQ 9 = 8 (mild depression)

Medical management	
Medications	• Continue metoprolol tartrate, Aspirin, Apixaban, Atorvastatin, Metformin, Sitagliptin, Baclofen, Citalopram 20 mg PO daily • Increase Lisinopril
Diet	Level 2 mechanical soft diet with nectar-thick liquids
Vitals	As needed with rehab
Lab work	Order complete blood cell count (CBC) and basic metabolic panel (BMP)
Precautions/Orders	• Activity ad libitum • Fall risk • Outpatient physical therapy, occupational therapy (OT), speech-language pathology—evaluate and treat

Pause points

Based on the above information,
• What may be the *best* objective tests to quantify function and fall risk?
• How should the physical therapist best structure the outpatient physical therapy examination?
• How should the physical therapist make the goals of therapy meaningful to the patient?
• What will be the role of family education in making sure teachings are also utilized at home and in the community? How should the physical therapist structure patient and family education?

Physical Therapy Examination				
Subjective				
"I want to get stronger to walk my dogs."				
Objective				
Vital signs	**Pre-treatment**		**Post-treatment**	
	Supine	Sitting	Standing	Sitting
Blood pressure (mmHg)	140/90	138/88	110/60	130/80
Heart rate (beats/min)	72	70	100	84
Respiratory rate (breaths/min)	12	12	18	14
Pulse oximetry on room air (SpO$_2$)	99%	99%	95%	97%
Modified rate of perceived exertion (RPE) scale (0–10)	0/10	0/10	6/10	6/10
Pain	7/10 at right shoulder	7/10 at right shoulder	7/10 at right shoulder	6/10 at right shoulder
Musculoskeletal	Range of motion	• LUE, active range of motion (AROM): within functional limit (WFL) • Right upper extremity (RUE), passive range of motion (PROM): WFL • LLE, AROM: WFL • Right lower extremity (RLE), AROM: within functional limits (WFL)		
	Strength	• L shoulder flexion: 5/5 • R shoulder flexion: 2/5 • L elbow flexion: 5/5 • R elbow flexion: 2/5 • L wrist extension: 5/5 • R wrist extension: 1/5 • L hip flexion: 5/5 • R hip flexion: 4–/5 • L knee extension: 5/5 • R knee extension: 4–/5 • L ankle dorsiflexion: 5/5 • R ankle dorsiflexion: 4–/5		
	Aerobic	• NuStep for 15 minutes, level 3. (RUE secured to handle, with it increased to minimize R shoulder flexion) • RPE =14/20. Post vitals: blood pressure: 132/80 mmHg, heart rate: 86 beat/minute		
Neurological	Balance	• Static sitting unsupported: good • Dynamic standing: good • (–) Romberg eyes closed • Berg Balance Scale = 44/56 • Functional gait assessment = 6/30		
	Cognition	• Alert and oriented x 4 • Follows multistep commands 100% • Limited conversation due to expressive aphasia		
	Coordination	• Finger to nose: LUE intact, unable to perform with RUE due to spasticity and weakness • Heel to shin: LLE intact, RLE ataxic		
	Cranial nerves	• II–XII grossly intact except for noted right side facial droop, sparing the forehead • Vision intact, fully tracking with eyes, with no visual field deficits		

(Continued)

(Continued)

Physical Therapy Examination		
	Reflexes	• Brachioradialis: 2 + L, 3 + R • Biceps brachii: 2 + L, 3 + R • Triceps brachii: 2 + L, 3 + R • Patellar: 2 + L, 3 + R • Achilles: 2 + L, 3 + R
	Sensation	• RUE: loss of sensation to crude touch and pinprick • LUE, RLE, LLE: intact to crude touch and pinprick
	Tone	• RUE increased tone, 2 + /4 MAS • RUE flexor synergy and loss of fractionated movement • RLE hypotonic, 1 + /4 MAS
	Other	• STREAM: 44/70 (6/20 upper extremity, 18/20 lower extremity, 20/30 basic mobility) • Five Times Sit-to-Stand (5xSTS) Test = 35 seconds • Timed Up and Go (TUG) test = 40 seconds • 6-Minute Walk Test—deferred due to symptoms of lightheadedness with prolonged standing
Functional status		
Bed mobility		• Rolling to left: independent on mat table • Supine to/from sit: independent on mat table
Transfers		• Sit to/from stand: modified independent with bilateral upper extremities (BUE) support via armrests. Deficits notable for excessive weight shift to left with sit to stand and touching right knee to chair. When asked to perform sit to stand without knee touching chair, patient requires multiple attempts but able to perform with arm rests. He reports feeling "lightheaded" with standing
Ambulation		• Ambulates 100 feet with modified independence and wide base quad cane • Gait deviations notable for right hemiparetic gait with right upper extremity in flexor synergy, right hip circumduction in swing, right foot flat at initial contact, right knee hyperextension (genu recurvatum) in midstance, and unequal stride length. Ambulation trial stopped due to patient reporting of progressive worsening lightheaded sensation with gait • Gait speed = 0.45 m/second • ▶ Fig. 5.5
Stairs		• Ascend/descend four steps with modified independence, using one rail and wide base quad cane

Assessment	
☑ Physical therapist's	*Assessment left blank for learner to develop*
Goals	
Patient's	"To be able to walk without a cane around town"
Short term	1. *Goals left blank for learner to develop.* 2.
Long term	1. *Goals left blank for learner to develop.* 2.

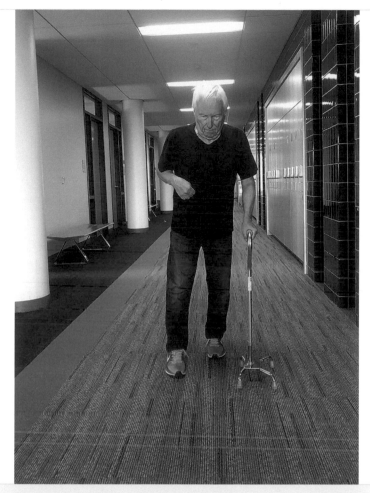

Fig. 5.5 An example of the patient's current gait posture and pattern.

Plan	
☑ Physical therapist's	*Plan left blank for learner to develop.*

Bloom's Taxonomy Level	Case 5.C Questions
Create	1. Synthesizing the medical data and physical examination findings, develop an appropriate physical therapy assessment of the patient.
	2. Develop two short-term physical therapy goals, including an appropriate timeframe for home care.
	3. Develop two long-term physical therapy goals, including an appropriate timeframe for home care.
	4. Create a physical therapy plan of care and specific treatment interventions, including frequency, dosing, and rationale for each intervention.
Evaluate	5. Is there anything abnormal with the patient's vitals and response to activity during the examination? If so, explain.
	6. If so, what should the physical therapist do?
	7. The patient is now almost 30 days' post stroke. Given the current status of their upper extremity function, based on the research, what is the best prognosis for the return of upper extremity function?

(Continued)

(Continued)

Bloom's Taxonomy Level	Case 5.C Questions
Analyze	8. What type of positioning/splinting recommendations should be given to the patient?
	9. What norms on the various tests performed (5xSTS, TUG, functional gait assessment [FGA], Berg Balance Scale) would indicate the patient is at low fall risk?
	10. In this outpatient setting, what will be the frequency of treatment and why?
Apply	11. What gait speed does the patient need to be able to ambulate to cross most streets?
	12. Is it anticipated that this patient will continue to require an assistive device? If so, based on the information, which one and why?
Understand	13. What can be done for the patient's arm pain? What may be the cause(s)?
	14. Describe the concept of fractionated movement.
Remember	15. What criteria does the patient need to meet to be considered an unlimited community walker?

Bloom's Taxonomy Level	Case 5.C Answers
Create	1. The patient presents status post left CVA with right hemiparesis. Physical therapy exam notable for RUE increased spasticity with inability to fractionate movement, RLE weakness resulting in gait deviations, impaired balance with high fall risk as noted across numerous measures (FGA, Berg Balance Scale, TUG, 5xSTS), and reduced endurance due to effects of stroke and prolonged hospitalization. All of the aforementioned impaired the patient's return to independence with ADLs and function. Additionally, during the examination, hypotension with positional changes was noted. The physician was notified, and patient is pending follow-up with PCP—will await physician recommendations before initiating formal exercise regimen. The patient was also complaining of significant shoulder pain. Physical therapist will discuss findings with occupational therapist to optimize positioning to minimize shoulder discomfort. Skilled physical therapist is recommended to address the aforementioned deficits. It is anticipated that the patient should be able to perform all ADLs and ambulate without device.
	2. Short-term goals:
	• Patient will demonstrate independence with home exercise program to improve bilateral lower extremity (BLE) muscle strength and endurance.
	• Patient will ambulate for 5 minutes, five times a day around home to improve endurance.
	• Patient will improve gait speed ≥ 0.60 m/second with least restrictive assistive device to improve safety with community ambulation.
	3. Long-term goals:
	• Patient will score > 51/56 Berg Balance Scale to reduce fall risk with ADLs and functional mobility.
	• Patient will ambulate > 600 meters with least restrictive assistive device to improve safely navigate community distances.
	• Patient will improve gait speed > 0.8 m/second with least restrictive assistive device to improve safety with community ambulation.
	4. The recommended dosing according to the American Stroke Association are as follows:
	• Aerobic: 3–5 days per week; 40–70% VO_2 reserve or heart rate reserve; 20–60 minutes (or 3–10-minute sessions).
	• Strengthening: 2–3 days per week; 50–80% 1 repetition maximum (RM) (resistance gradually increased over time as tolerated); 1–3 sets of 10–15 repetitions of 8–10 exercises involving the major muscle groups.
	• Balance: dynamic exercises focusing on improving weight shift and coordination of right hemibody.
	Focus of the exercise prescription should assist patient to return to independence with all aspects of function. Exercise construction should be centered around tasks that are meaningful to the patient.
Evaluate	5. Patient demonstrated orthostatic hypotension. Lack of fluid intake increase in blood pressure medications, and addition of antidepressant can cause hypotension.
	6. If a patient demonstrates orthostatic hypotension, one or many of the following

(Continued)

Bloom's Taxonomy Level	Case 5.C Answers
	interventions can be implemented: counsel the patient on fluid intake, utilize thrombo-embolus deterrant (TED) stockings, perform therapeutic exercise prior to positional changes, and perform positional changes gradually. Vitals should be monitored throughout treatment. Lastly, the physical therapist should alert any other discipline who may be treating the patient—such as OT and/or ST—of the findings, and depending on the severity contact the physician's office. 7. At 20–30 days after stroke, indicators of poor prognosis include: • No/minimal grip strength → no/minimal hand function later • No/minimal shoulder flexion → no/minimal hand function later
Analyze	8. The patient should lie on his affected side with his right arm at 90 degrees shoulder flexion and elbow extended. The use of a GivMohr Sling, as compared to a traditional sling, would assist with shoulder positioning, reducing pain, and maintaining function of the upper extremity. 9. The norms of the fall risk measures are as follows: • 5xSTS = < 12 seconds • TUG = community dwelling older adults < 13.5 seconds; older patients post stroke < 14 seconds • FGA = > 22/30 (older adults) • Berg Balance Scale = > 45 (out of 56 points) 10. While recent evidence on neuro recovery suggests providing a high dosage of interventions to facilitate neuroplasticity, traditional OP/physical therapy frequency is three times per week, primarily due to insurance coverage. The patient may benefit from an extensive Home exercise program (HEP) and family education/training to supplement his OP/physical therapy.
Apply	11. City planners may use 1.2 m/second as the reference speed to be able to cross the street. However, the speed required to cross at lights may be dependent on local ordinance. 12. It is anticipated that the patient will require SPC use.
Understand	13. A discussion with the patient's PCP regarding the patient's RUE pain is warranted. Potential conservative interventions that physical therapists can provide include positioning, splinting, patient and family education, modalities (including transcutaneous electrical nerve stimulation [TENS]) as needed, and collaboration with our OT colleagues. Pain may be caused by spasticity and/or subluxation of the glenohumeral joint. With that said, the PCP may choose medical management, which could include gabapentin for pain and/or baclofen/Botox injections for spasticity. 14. Fractionated movement is the ability to finely control and coordinate movement across a single joint.
Remember	15. To be an unlimited community ambulator, the patient must be able to independently navigate all home and community activities, including crowds and uneven terrain, and demonstrate complete independence in shopping centers.

Key points
1. Need to monitor vitals with patients after stroke—ischemic strokes are generally caused by cardiovascular pathology. Hypertension and hypercholesterolemia are risk factors for stroke. Medication management may be changing in the outpatient setting and proper monitoring of vitals can assist the health care team with medication dosing. Atrial fibrillation is also a risk factor for stroke, especially if a patient is not already taking an anticoagulant medication.
2. Gait speed is one of the best ways to determine overall functional capability. Gait speed is the "sixth vital sign."
3. When designing physical therapy interventions (especially in the outpatient setting), use the patient's hobbies and interests to develop specific interventions. This will improve their interest in physical therapy and motivation, and potentially lead to improved compliance.

Suggested Readings

6-minute walk test. Available at: https://www.sralab.org/rehabilitation-measures/6-minute-walk-test. Accessed May 1, 2020

Anderson LW, Krathwohl DR. A Taxonomy for Learning, Teaching, and Assessing, Abridged Edition. Boston, MA: Allyn and Bacon; 2001

Armstrong P. Bloom's Taxonomy. Available at: https://cft.vanderbilt.edu/guides-sub-pages/blooms-taxonomy/. Accessed on April 1, 2020

Beebe JA, Lang CE. Active range of motion predicts upper extremity function 3 months after stroke. Stroke. 2009; 40(5):1772–1779

Benjamin EJ, Blaha MJ, Chiuve SE, et al. American Heart Association Statistics Committee and Stroke Statistics Subcommittee. Heart disease and stroke statistics—2017 update: a report from the American Heart Association. Circulation. 2017; 135(10):e146–e603

Billinger SA, Arena R, Bernhardt J, et al. American Heart Association Stroke Council, Council on Cardiovascular and Stroke Nursing, Council on Lifestyle and Cardiometabolic Health, Council on Epidemiology and Prevention, Council on Clinical Cardiology. Physical activity and exercise recommendations for stroke survivors: a statement for healthcare professionals from the American Heart Association/American Stroke Association. Stroke. 2014; 45(8):2532–2553

Chimowitz MI, Lynn MJ, Derdeyn CP, et al. SAMMPRIS Trial Investigators. Stenting versus aggressive medical therapy for intracranial arterial stenosis. N Engl J Med. 2011; 365(11):993–1003

Duim, E., Lebrão, M. L., & Antunes, J. L. F. Walking speed of older people and pedestrian crossing time. Journal of Transport & Health. 2017;5:70–76

Five Times Sit to Stand. Available at: https://www.sralab.org/rehabilitation-measures/five-times-sit-stand-test. Accessed May 1, 2020

Flint AC, Kamel H, Navi BB, et al. Statin use during ischemic stroke hospitalization is strongly associated with improved poststroke survival. Stroke. 2012; 43(1):147–154

Fritz S, Lusardi M. White Paper: "Walking Speed: the Sixth Vital Sign", Journal of Geriatric Physical Therapy. 2009; 32(2):2–5

Holleran CL, Rodriguez KS, Echauz A, Leech KA, Hornby TG. Potential contributions of training intensity on locomotor performance in individuals with chronic stroke. J Neurol Phys Ther. 2015; 39(2):95–102

Hornby TG, Reisman DS, Ward IG, et al. Clinical practice guideline to improve locomotor function following chronic stroke, incomplete spinal cord injury, and brain injury. Journal of Neurologic Physical Therapy. 2020;44(1): 49–100

Lohse KR, Lang CE, Boyd LA. Is more better? Using metadata to explore dose-response relationships in stroke rehabilitation. Stroke. 2014; 45(7):2053–2058

Ottenbacher KJ, Hsu Y, Granger CV, Fiedler RC. The reliability of the functional independence measure: a quantitative review. Arch Phys Med Rehabil. 1996; 77(12):1226–1232

Patient Health Questionnaire (PHQ-9). Available at: https://www.sralab.org/rehabilitation-measures/patient-health-questionnaire-phq-9. Accessed May 1, 2020

Powers WJ, Rabinstein AA, Ackerson T, et al. Guidelines for the early management of patients with acute ischemic stroke: 2019 update to the 2018 Guidelines for the Early Management of Acute Ischemic Stroke: a guideline for healthcare professionals from the American Heart Association/American Stroke Association. Stroke. 2019; 50(12):e344–e418

Rimmer JH, Henley KY. Building the crossroad between inpatient/outpatient rehabilitation and lifelong community-based fitness for people with neurologic disability. J Neurol Phys Ther. 2013; 37(2):72–77

Stroke Rehabilitation Assessment of Movement. Available at: https://www.sralab.org/rehabilitation-measures/stroke-rehabilitation-assessment-movement-measure. Accessed May 1, 2020

Amarenco P, Bogousslavsky J, Callahan A, III, et al. Stroke Prevention by Aggressive Reduction in Cholesterol Levels (SPARCL) Investigators. High-dose atorvastatin after stroke or transient ischemic attack. N Engl J Med. 2006; 355(6):549–559

Timed Up and Go. Available at: https://www.sralab.org/rehabilitation-measures/timed-and-go. Accessed May 1, 2020

van der Kooi E, Schiemanck SK, Nollet F, Kwakkel G, Meijer JW, van de Port I. Falls are associated with lower self-reported functional status in patients after stroke. Arch Phys Med Rehabil. 2017; 98(12):2393–2398

Veerbeek JM, Van Wegen EE, Harmeling-Van der Wel BC, Kwakkel G, EPOS Investigators. Is accurate prediction of gait in nonambulatory stroke patients possible within 72 hours poststroke? The EPOS study. Neurorehabil Neural Repair. 2011; 25(3): 268–274

Veerbeek JM, van Wegen E, van Peppen R, et al. What is the evidence for physical therapy poststroke? A systematic review and meta-analysis. PLoS One. 2014; 9(2):e87987

Whelton PK, Carey RM, Aronow WS, et al. 2017 ACC/AHA/AAPA/ABC/ACPM/AGS/APhA/ASH/ASPC/NMA/PCNA Guideline for the Prevention, Detection, Evaluation, and Management of High Blood Pressure in Adults: a report of the American College of Cardiology/American Heart Association Task Force on Clinical Practice Guidelines. Hypertension. 2018; 71(6):e13–e115

Wing K, Lynskey JV, Bosch PR. Whole-body intensive rehabilitation is feasible and effective in chronic stroke survivors: a retrospective data analysis. Top Stroke Rehabil. 2008; 15(3): 247–255

Winovich DT, Longstreth WT, Jr, Arnold AM, et al. Factors associated with ischemic stroke survival and recovery in older adults. Stroke. 2017; 48(7):1818–1826

Winstein CJ, Stein J, Arena R, et al. American Heart Association Stroke Council, Council on Cardiovascular and Stroke Nursing, Council on Clinical Cardiology, and Council on Quality of Care and Outcomes Research. Guidelines for adult stroke rehabilitation and recovery: a guideline for healthcare professionals from the American Heart Association / American Stroke Association. Stroke. 2016; 47(6):e98–e169

Xu T, Clemson L, O'Loughlin K, Lannin NA, Dean C, Koh G. Risk factors for falls in community stroke survivors: a systematic review and meta-analysis. Arch Phys Med Rehabil. 2018; 99(3):563–573.e5

6 Congestive Heart Failure

General Information	
Case no.	6.A Congestive Heart Failure
Authors	Kelly M. Lindenberg, PT, MSPT, PhD, CSCS Melissa L. Bednarek, PT, DPT, PhD, Board Certified Clinical Specialist in Cardiovascular & Pulmonary Physical Therapy Kala M. Markel, PT, DPT
Diagnosis	Heart failure with atrial fibrillation
Setting	Emergency Department with transfer to Telemetry Unit
Learner expectations	☑ Initial evaluation ☐ Re-evaluation ☐ Treatment session
Learner objectives	1. Explain the pathophysiology of the patient's diagnosis. 2. Relate the pathophysiology of cardiovascular disorders to the clinical manifestations and activity/participation limitations seen in physical therapy practice. 3. Select, implement, and interpret physical therapy interventions based on the medical examination findings. 4. Develop an understanding of medical management and how it influences physical therapy plan of care.

Medical	
Chief complaint	Shortness of breath, fatigue
History of present illness	Patient is a 73-year-old male who presents to the emergency department with increasing severity of shortness of breath over the past 2 days. He reports a decreased tolerance for activity, requiring frequent rest breaks. Patient denies chest pain, nausea, or vomiting. He reports currently having an upper respiratory infection, self-treating with Sudafed. Patient is to be admitted for medical workup and management.
Past medical history	Remote history of ST elevation myocardial infarction (STEMI) with stent placement 5 years ago, atrial fibrillation, hypertension, hyperlipidemia, osteoarthritis, cholecystectomy, anxiety/depression.
Past surgical history	Right total knee arthroplasty
Allergies	Penicillin
Medications	Coumadin, Prinivil, Lopressor, Lipitor, Tylenol
Precautions/Orders	Bed rest

Social history	
Home setup	• Lives in a two-story home with wife. • Flight of steps with unilateral rail to enter home. • Flight of steps with bilateral rails to the second floor. • Has two adult children, one lives nearby; has two grandchildren.
Occupation	• Retired computer analyst.
Prior level of function	• Independent with functional mobility and activities of daily living. • Independent for stairs; however, required increased time. • Spouse manages cooking/cleaning. • Poor tolerance for yard maintenance, hired help. • (+) Driver
Recreational activities	• Vacation planned over summer to celebrate 50th wedding anniversary. • Enjoys reading, watching travel television shows, and fishing.

Vital signs	Hospital day 0: emergency department	Hospital day 1: telemetry unit
Blood pressure (mmHg)	108/58, MAP = 75	134/78, MAP = 97
Heart rate (beat/min)	153, irregular rhythm	102, irregular rhythm
Respiratory rate (breath/min)	26	18
Pulse oximetry (SpO$_2$)	91% on room air	96% on 2 L O$_2$ via nasal cannula
Temperature (°F)	99.1	99.2
Body mass index	31.5	_____

Imaging/Diagnostic test	Hospital day 0: emergency department	Hospital day 1: telemetry unit
EKG	1. Atrial fibrillation with rapid ventricular rate	1. Atrial fibrillation with rapid ventricular rate
Chest X-ray	1. Cardiomegaly, bilateral interstitial and alveolar infiltrates involving predominantly the mid- and lower lung fields ▶ Fig. 6.1	_____
Transesophageal echocardiogram (TEE)	1. Ejection fraction, 40%; no signs of thrombus	1. Ejection fraction, 45%; no signs of thrombus

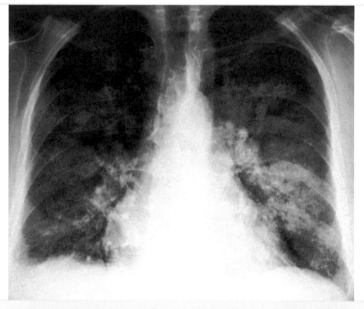

Fig. 6.1 Cardiogenic pulmonary edema. Cardiomegaly, bilateral interstitial, and alveolar infiltrates involving predominantly the mid- and lower lung fields. (*Source*: Burgener F. Disease. In: Burgener F, Kormano M, Pudas T, ed. Differential Diagnosis in Conventional Radiology. 3rd ed. Stuttgart: Thieme; 2007.)

Medical management	Hospital day 0: emergency department	Hospital day 1: telemetry unit
Medications	1. IV Cardizem 2. Coumadin 3. Prinivil 4. Lopressor 5. Lipitor	1. PO Cardizem 2. Coumadin 3. Prinivil 4. Lopressor 5. Lipitor 6. Lasix
Respiratory	1. Supplemental oxygen: 2 L via nasal cannula	1. Supplemental oxygen: 2 L via nasal cannula 2. Incentive spirometer, 10 times/hour
Consults	1. Cardiology	1. Physical therapy 2. Occupational therapy
Precautions	1. Telemetry 2. Fall risk 3. Bed rest	1. Telemetry 2. Fall risk 3. Activity as tolerated

Lab		Reference range	Hospital day 0: emergency department	Hospital day 1: telemetry unit
Complete blood count	WBC	$5.0–10.0 \times 10^9/L$	11.5	11.7
	RBC	4.5–5.5	4.5	4.3
	Hemoglobin	14.0–17.4 d/dL	17	15
	Hematocrit	42–52%	40	39
	Platelet	150–400 k/µL	240	230
Electrolyte panel	Na	134–142 mEq/L	133	130
	K	3.7–5.1 mEq/L	3.7	3.8
	Ca	8.6–10.3 mg/dL	9.0	8.6
	Cl	98–108 mEq/L	107	108
	PO_4	2.3–4.1 mg/dL	2.9	3.2
	Mg	1.2–1.9 mEq/L	1.3	1.5
Lipid panel	HDL	>40 mg/dL	38	————
	LDL	<100 mg/dL	110	————
	Triglyceride	<150 mg/dL	155	————
	Cholesterol	<200 mg/dL	180	————
Bleeding ratio/viscosity	INR	0.8–1.2	2.5	2.3
	Physical therapy	11–13 seconds	11	12
Cardiovascular-specific labs	Troponin—1	<0.03 ng/mL	0.02	————
	BNP	<100 pg/mL	280	650
	CK	30–170 U/L	80	————
Other	Glucose	70–100 mg/dL	120	118
	BUN	6–25 mg/dL	22	26
	Creatinine	0.7–1.3 mg/dL	1.6	1.9

Pause points

Based on the above information, what are the priority
- Examination tests and measures?
- Outcome measures?
- Treatment interventions?

Hospital Day 2, Telemetry Unit: Physical Therapy Examination				
Subjective				
"I am just so tired and have no energy to get up."				
Objective				
Vital signs	Pre-treatment			Post-treatment
	Supine	Sitting	Standing	Sitting
Blood pressure (BP; mmHg)	124/78	118/74	128/76	See post-mobility vital signs below
Heart rate (HR; beat/min)	88	96	104	
Respiratory rate (RR; breath/min)	18	22	24	
Pulse oximetry on 2 L/O$_2$ via nasal cannula (SpO$_2$)	96%	94%	93%	
Modified BORG scale—dyspnea	2/10	2/10	3/10	2/10
Pain	0/10	0/10	0/10	0/10
General	• Patient supine in bed, head of bed elevated at 30 degrees • Lines/tubes/drains notable for telemetry, 2 L/O$_2$ via nasal cannula, IV access via left antecubital, urinary catheter			
Head, ears, eyes, nose, and throat (HEENT)	• Unremarkable			
Cardiovascular and pulmonary	• Normal sinus rhythm • 2 L/min O$_2$ via nasal cannula • Auscultation: mildly diminished breath sounds and fine crackles in bilateral posterior lower lobes, S3 heart sound • Pulse: 1 + bilateral dorsalis pedis • Edema: 2 + foot to 1 inch above lateral malleolus • (+) JVD at 5 cm above sternal angle			
Gastrointestinal	• Reports constipation			
Genitourinary	• Urinary catheter in place • Input and Output (I&O) incongruence per EMR (I>O), now stabilizing			
Musculoskeletal	Range of motion	• Bilateral upper extremity (BUE): within functional limit (WFL) • Bilateral lower extremity (BLE): WFL with the exception of bilateral knees—right knee flexion at 100 degrees, left knee extension limited at 10 degrees		
	Strength	• B shoulder flexion: 4/5 • B elbow flexion: 5/5 • B elbow extension: 5/5 • B wrist extension: 5/5 • B wrist flexion: 5/5 • B hip flexion: 4/5 • B hip abduction: 4/5 • B knee flexion: 4/5 • B knee extension: 4/5 • B ankle dorsiflexion: 5/5 • B ankle plantarflexion: 5/5		
	Aerobic	• Not formally assessed • Reported 3/10 on RPE Scale during transfers		

(Continued)

(Continued)

Hospital Day 2, Telemetry Unit: Physical Therapy Examination		
	Flexibility	• Not formally assessed • On observation, bilateral pectoralis major/minor and bilateral hamstring tightness, rounded shoulder posture.
	Posture	• Sitting: forward head, rounded thoracic spine • Standing: forward head, rounded thoracic spine, flattened lumbar spine
Neurological	Balance	• Static sitting, unsupported: independent • Dynamic sitting, unsupported: supervision • Static standing, unsupported: close supervision • Dynamic standing, unsupported: close supervision
	Cognition	• Alert and oriented x 4
	Coordination	• Finger-to-nose: intact bilaterally • Heel-to-shin: intact bilaterally
	Cranial nerves	• II–XII: intact
	Reflexes	• Biceps: 2 + bilaterally • Patellar: 2 + bilaterally
	Sensation	• BLE dermatomes: intact to light touch
	Tone	• BUE and BLE: normal throughout
Functional status		
Bed mobility		• Supine to left side lying: supervision with head of bed elevated 30 degrees and use of bedrails • Left side lying to sitting: supervision with head of bed elevated 30 degrees and use of bedrails
Transfers		• Sit to/from stand: supervision
Ambulation		• Ambulated 75 feet with close supervision and no assistive device • Gait deviations notable for decreased cadence, decreased heel strike at initial contact bilaterally, and flexed posture • Gait speed: 0.6 m/s Vital signs post ambulation: • BP: 140/78, HR: 116, RR: 28, SpO_2: 91% on 2 L NC • 1-minute recovery: BP: 142/76, HR: 103, RR: 22, SpO_2: 94% on 2 L NC • 3-minute recovery: BP: 132/74, HR: 98, RR: 18, SpO_2: 95% on 2 L NC
Stairs		• Ascend/descend four 6-inch steps with bilateral handrails with contact guard assistance Vital signs post–stair negotiation: • BP: 144/76, HR: 124, RR: 30, SpO_2: 90% on 2 L NC • 1-minute recovery: BP = 130/76, HR: 112, RR: 25, SpO_2: 92% on 2 L NC • Worsening crackles with lung auscultation, (+) mild accessory muscle breathing

Assessment	
☑ Physical therapist's	*Assessment left blank for learner to develop.*
Goals	
Patient's	"I just want to get out of this hospital."
Short term	1. *Goals left blank for learner to develop.* 2.
Long term	1. *Goals left blank for learner to develop.* 2.

	Plan
☑ Physical therapist's	Will treat patient once daily, five days per week at bedside for functional mobility and endurance building activities. Treatment may include lower body ergometer; diaphragmatic breathing training; functional mobility training such as transfers, ambulation, and stair training; and patient education on energy conservation and symptom awareness.

Bloom's Taxonomy Level	Case 6.A Questions
Create	1. Synthesizing the medical data and physical examination findings, develop an appropriate physical therapy assessment of the patient.
	2. Develop two short-term physical therapy goals, including an appropriate timeframe.
	3. Develop two long-term physical therapy goals, including an appropriate timeframe.
Evaluate	4. Interpret the patient's vital sign response to ambulation.
Analyze	5. What does the TEE result on hospital day 0 suggest about the patient's cardiac function?
	6. What does the presence of crackles during auscultation suggest about the patient's condition?
Apply	7. Design two physical therapy interventions that address the patient's goals
Understand	8. What does the jugular venous distention test assess for? What do the results indicate?
	9. What is the relationship between atrial fibrillation and heart failure?
Remember	10. Why does the patient's chest X-ray reveal cardiomegaly?
	11. How is pitting edema quantified?

Bloom's Taxonomy Level	Case 6.A Answers
Create	1. The patient is a 73-year-old male who presented to the hospital with severe shortness of breath. He was diagnosed with atrial fibrillation with rapid ventricular rate. His course was complicated by the new diagnosis of heart failure with reduced ejection fraction (HFrEF) at 40%. Physical therapy evaluation revealed adventitious breath sounds suggesting pulmonary edema along with a positive jugular venous distention test, which further supported the continued presence of heart failure. Mobility assessment revealed that the patient was safe with mobility and transfers at a supervision level but required increased assistance while negotiating stairs with railings. His vital sign response to ambulation and stairs was elevated above expected ranges, suggesting deconditioning. His 1-minute recovery showed appropriate recovery for heart rate; however, his blood pressure recovery ratio at 3 minutes was inadequate at 0.93, suggesting continued complications in cardiovascular function. Self-selected gait speed was less than 1.0 m/s, suggesting an increased risk for falls and diminished community ambulation capacity. The patient would benefit from physical therapy to improve aerobic capacity, safety during stair ambulation, and maximizing functional mobility and safety. The physical therapist will plan to see the patient daily while he is in the acute care hospital. Recommend discharge home with spouse and home health physical therapist when medically stable.
	2. Short-term goals:
	• Patient will ascend/descend 12 steps with single handrail with supervision, demonstrating step to pattern, within 3 days to gain access to his house.
	• Patient will independently demonstrate self-monitoring of heart rate and implementation of RPE Scale to measure intensity in functional mobility within 3 days for safety.
	3. Long-term goals:
	• Patient will recall two methods of self-monitoring for worsening of heart failure symptoms and then to contact physician within 1 week.
	• Patient will independently ambulate for 15 minutes at 1.2 m/s, maintain a heart rate at < 110 beats/min, within 4 weeks to facilitate safe community ambulation.
Evaluate	4. Ambulation on a flat surface at 0.6 m/s (or 1.34 mph) is approximately 2 METS, and sitting at rest is approximately 1 MET. Thus, it is expected that the heart rate should increase to only 10 beat/min and systolic blood pressure should increase to 10 mmHg from the resting state to walking at 0.6 m/s. This patient's heart rate increased to 15 beat/min and systolic blood pressure increased to 18 mmHg. While the heart rate and blood pressure responses were only slightly higher than expected, these results underscore the fluid management issues that exist during heart failure.

(Continued)

(Continued)

Bloom's Taxonomy Level	Case 6.A Answers
	Respiratory rate also increased higher than expected for a low-intensity task, suggesting that the pulmonary system is attempting to bring more oxygen into the body in response to the poor perfusion management. Additionally, the pulmonary edema that is present will decrease alveolar compliance, which will necessitate an increase in respiratory rate to meet the body's oxygen demands. However, there is evidence that oxygenation is still impaired, as this patient's oxygen saturation drops with mobility while on 2 L of supplemental oxygen via nasal cannula.
Analyze	5. The transesophageal echocardiogram shows that the patient's ejection fraction is 40%. Ejection fraction is the percentage of blood that is pumped out of the heart with each ventricular contraction. It is the ratio of the stroke volume to the end-diastolic volume. Normal ejection fraction ranges from 55 to 70%. Therefore, this patient's ejection fraction, currently 40%, is low. This suggests that the heart is not pumping sufficient volumes of blood out of the ventricle during systole. In this case, the resulting diagnosis would be classified as heart failure with reduced ejection fraction (HFrEF). 6. Crackles are often heard over airways that have fluid accumulation. In this patient's case, the presence of crackles may suggest the presence of pulmonary edema. During heart failure, the lack of cardiac output promotes a backlog of fluid into the pulmonary vascular system. As the hydrostatic pressure increases in the capillaries, fluid will filter out of the vessels and into the interstitial space between the capillaries and alveoli. The fluid can further leak into the alveoli. When fluid-filled airways "pop" open toward the end of inspiration, crackles can be heard through a stethoscope.
Apply	7. Two potential physical therapy interventions that address the patient's goals include: a. Ambulation. This activity is functional and can assist with the patient's endurance. Using Frequency, Intensity, Time, and Type (FITT) exercise prescription method, the patient should ambulate: in F: 2–3 times per day I: RPE of 11–12 (maintain HR less than 120 beats/min) T: 5-minute bouts T: ambulation in hallway b. Education on self-monitoring heart rate using the radial pulse. Education should be based on the patient's learning style but should include time to demonstrate and practice with cues as needed. The patient should perform this task daily with the physical therapist checking for accuracy and providing feedback. The heart rate, RPE, and bout time align with recommended guidelines for phase 1 cardiac rehabilitation from the American College of Sports Medicine.
Understand	8. Jugular venous distention (JVD) occurs due to increased pressure in the superior vena cava causing blood to bulge into the jugular vein. A visible pulse is often identifiable. This is indicative of right-side heart failure if the venous distention's highest point is greater than 4 cm above a horizontal line drawn from the sternal angle when the patient is recumbent at a 45-degree angle (▶ Fig. 6.2). 9. The prevalence of atrial fibrillation in patients with heart failure ranges from 6 to 35%. Atrial fibrillation and heart failure share common risk factors including hypertension, diabetes mellitus, ischemic heart disease, and valvular heart disease. Genetic influences, fibrosis of the heart, increased pulmonary vascular pressure, and neuroendocrine activation have all been identified as etiologies linked to both atrial fibrillation and heart failure.
Remember	10. Cardiomegaly, or enlargement of the heart, is associated with hypertrophic changes to the myocardium. This is a common finding in patients diagnosed with heart failure. Underlying cardiac conditions (such as value disease, hypertension, and coronary artery disease) elicit remodeling of the heart that leads to dilated hypertrophy, fibrosis, and contractile malfunction. Over time, these changes result in diminished cardiac output. 11. Pitting edema is quantified by pushing into the patient's skin, holding pressure for 2–3 seconds, then releasing pressure, and measuring the time it takes for depressed skin to return to original appearance. It is graded as follows: 1+: barely perceptible depression 2+: easily identifiable depression with rebound in < 15 seconds 3+: rebound in 15–30 seconds 4+: rebound in > 30 seconds

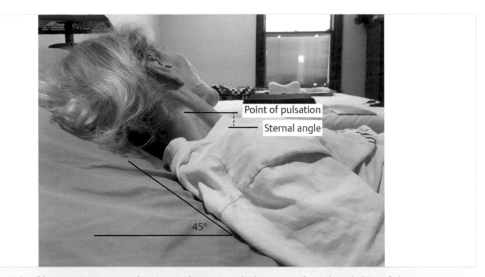

Fig. 6.2 Example of how to measure jugular venous distention, which assesses for right side heart failure.

Key points
1. Synthesizing available medical information (i.e., imaging, lab values, etc.) allows the physical therapist to better understand how pathophysiology influences functional status.
2. Physical therapists must consider how both acute and chronic comorbidities will impact a patient's functional status.
3. Appreciate the insight a physical therapist can gain into the patient's condition when accurate vital sign monitoring is done before, during, and after functional activities.
4. Thorough assessment of available medical data and physical therapy outcome measures will promote the efficiency and effectiveness of a plan of care.

General Information	
Case no.	6.B
Authors	Melissa L. Bednarek, PT, DPT, PhD, Board Certified Clinical Specialist in Cardiovascular & Pulmonary Physical Therapy Kala M. Markel, PT, DPT Kelly M. Lindenberg, PT, MSPT, PhD, CSCS
Diagnosis	Generalized deconditioning
Setting	Home
Learner expectations	☑ Initial evaluation ☐ Re-evaluation ☐ Treatment session
Learner objectives	1. List potential environmental factors that may provide difficulty to the patient.

(Continued)

(Continued)

General Information
2. Identify appropriate outcome measures based on the objective data provided for use in the home environment.
3. Describe psychosocial implications of the patient's condition and implementation strategies for improving his quality of life.
4. Develop a home exercise program based on the patient's body structure and impairments to optimize his participation and quality of life.

Medical	
Chief complaint	Generalized deconditioning and fatigue.
History of present illness	Patient is a 73-year-old male who was recently hospitalized for 5 days with shortness of breath due to atrial fibrillation. His hospital course is notable for conversion to regular rhythm with Cardizem and new development of heart failure. Prior to discharge, the patient was stabilized on current pharmacological management. Patient was discharged to home 1 day ago.
Past medical history	Heart failure with ejection fraction of 40%, remote history of STEMI with stent placement 5 years ago, atrial fibrillation, hypertension, hyperlipidemia, osteoarthritis, cholecystectomy, anxiety/depression.
Past surgical history	Right total knee replacement
Allergies	Penicillin
Medications	Coumadin, Prinivil, Lopressor, Lipitor, Tylenol, Lasix
Precautions/Orders	Activity as tolerated

Social history	
Home setup	• Lives in a two-story home with wife. • Flight of steps with bilateral rails to the second floor • Flight of steps with unilateral rail to enter home • Has two adult children, one lives nearby; has two grandchildren.
Occupation	• Retired computer analyst
Prior level of function	• Independent with functional mobility and activities of daily living • Modified independent for stairs; however, required increased time • Spouse manages cooking/cleaning. • Poor tolerance for yard maintenance, hired help. • (+) Driver
Recreational activities	• Vacation planned over summer to celebrate 50th wedding anniversary. • Enjoys reading, watching travel television shows, and fishing.

Pause points
Based on the above information, what are the priority • Examination tests and measures? • Outcome measures? • Treatment interventions?

Physical Therapy Examination		
Subjective		
"I went into the hospital because I couldn't breathe. Now they tell me my heart isn't doing well."		
Objective		
Vital signs	**Pre-treatment**	**Post-treatment**
Blood pressure (mmHg)	116/70	124/68
Heart rate (beat/min)	85, regular rhythm	92, regular rhythm
Respiratory rate (breath/min)	16	17
Pulse oximetry on room air	96%	96%
Modified BORG scale—dyspnea	2/10	5/10
Pain	0/10	4/10, left knee
General	• Patient sitting in recliner in living room of home • Patient's wife present for session	
Cardiovascular and pulmonary	• Normal sinus rate • Auscultation: fine crackles in posterior lower lobes bilaterally, S3 heart sound • Pulse: 1 + bilateral dorsalis pedis • Edema: 1 + bilateral feet	
Gastrointestinal	• Denies constipation and fecal incontinence	
Genitourinary	• Denies urinary incontinence despite increased frequency	
Musculoskeletal	Range of motion	• BUE: WFL • BLE: WFL with the exception of bilateral knees—right knee flexion at 100 degrees, left knee extension limited at 10 degrees
	Strength	• B shoulder flexion: 4/5 • B elbow flexion: 5/5 • B elbow extension: 5/5 • B wrist extension: 5/5 • B wrist flexion: 5/5 • B hip flexion: 4/5 • B hip abduction: 4/5 • B knee flexion: 4/5 • B knee extension: 4/5 • B ankle dorsiflexion: 5/5 • B ankle plantarflexion: 5/5 • Five Times Sit-to-Stand Test: 16 seconds
	Aerobic	• Seated Step Test. Stage 1 (6-inch step height): BP: 120/72, HR: 95 Modified BORG Scale—dyspnea: 4/10 Stage 2 (12-inch step height): BP: 128/70, HR: 105 Modified BORG Scale—dyspnea: 6/10 Unable to maintain cadence with increasing fatigue; test terminated ▶ Fig. 6.3a–d
	Flexibility	• On observation, bilateral pectoralis major/minor and bilateral hamstring tightness bilaterally, rounded shoulder posture

(Continued)

(Continued)

Physical Therapy Examination		
Neurological	Balance	• Static sitting, unsupported: independent • Dynamic sitting, unsupported: independent • Static standing, unsupported: independent • Dynamic standing, unsupported: supervision • Timed Up and Go: 21 seconds without an assistive device
	Cognition	• Alert and oriented x 4
	Coordination	• Finger-to-nose: intact bilaterally • Heel-to-shin: intact bilaterally
	Cranial nerves	• II–XII: intact
	Reflexes	• Biceps: 2 + bilaterally • Patellar: 2 + bilaterally
	Sensation	• BLE dermatomes: intact to light touch
	Tone	• BUE and BLE: normal throughout
Functional status		
Bed mobility		• Supine to/from sit: independent
Transfers		• Sit to/from stand: modified independent with use of arm rests, required increased time
Ambulation		• Ambulated 100 feet with supervision and no assistive device • Gait deviations notable for decreased cadence, antalgic gait, and flexed posture • Gait speed: 0.8 m/s
Stairs		• Ascend/descend flight of stairs with bilateral rails with supervision • Stair deviations notable for step-to pattern with increased reliance on BUEs, requires increased time Vital signs post stair negotiation: • BP: 120/72, HR: 101, modified BORG Scale—dyspnea: 6/10

Assessment	
☑ Physical therapist's	*Assessment left blank for learner to develop*
Goals	
Patient's	"I want to get stronger."
Short term	1. *Goals left blank for learner to develop.* 2.
Long term	1. *Goals left blank for learner to develop.* 2.

Plan	
☑ Physical therapist's	Plan to see patient twice a week for 6 weeks. Goal of treatment is to ensure medical stability and increase functional independence. Treatment will include therapeutic exercise (i.e., lower extremity strengthening, aerobic conditioning), gait training on even and uneven surfaces, and patient education on signs/symptoms of heart failure.

Bloom's Taxonomy Level	Case 6.B Questions
Create	1. Synthesizing the medical data and physical examination findings, develop an appropriate assessment of the patient. 2. Develop two short-term physical therapy goals, including an appropriate timeframe. 3. Develop two long-term physical therapy goals, including an appropriate timeframe. 4. Develop a home exercise program, including interventions and exercise prescription, and identify how to hold the patient accountable.
Evaluate	5. How does the patient compare to age and sex norms for the Five Times Sit-to-Stand?

(Continued)

(Continued)

Bloom's Taxonomy Level	Case 6.B Questions
	6. How does the patient compare to age and sex norms for the timed up and go?
	7. What are clinical signs and symptoms to monitor for worsening heart failure?
Analyze	8. What are possible reasons for the patient's increased left knee post-treatment?
Apply	9. How might a patient monitor and manage signs and symptoms of worsening heart failure in the home setting?
Understand	10. What options are available to the physical therapist should this patient continue to complain of left knee pain during subsequent treatment sessions?
	11. What are possible side effects of Lasix and how can they be monitored for in the home health setting?
Remember	12. Why is continued use of Coumadin indicated in this patient?

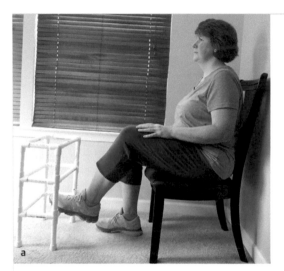
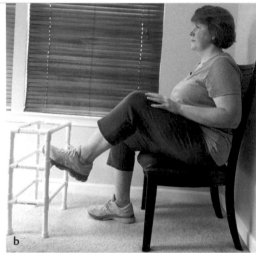
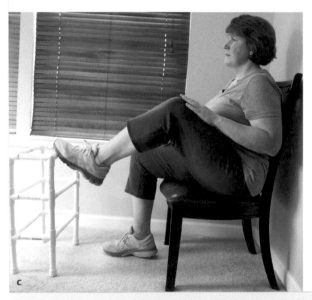
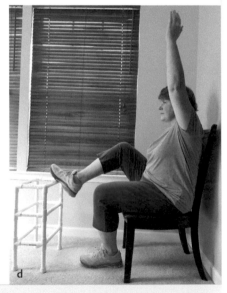

Fig. 6.3 Setup for a patient to perform the Seated Step Test with (**a**) stage 1 at 6-inch step height, (**b**) stage 2 at 12-inch step height, (**c**) stage 3 at 18-inch step height, and (**d**) stage 4 at 18-inch step height with alternating arms. Patient should step at a rate of 60 beats/min.

Bloom's Taxonomy Level	Case 6.B Answers
Create	1. Patient is a 73-year-old male who was recently hospitalized for 5 days with complaints of shortness and breath. He was found to be in rapid atrial fibrillation and subsequently converted to normal sinus rhythm through Cardizem. Hospital course was complicated by development of heart failure which is being managed pharmacologically. Patient was discharged to home yesterday and was seen this date for initial physical therapy evaluation. Patient demonstrated generalized decreased strength and endurance, requiring increased time for completion of ambulation and stair negotiation. Outcome measures for lower extremity strength and balance confirm these impairments as patient's results are below age- and sex-matched norms. Decreased aerobic capacity was evident in his inability to complete all four stages of the Seated Step Test. Patient would benefit from continued physical therapy to improve strength, balance, endurance, and functional mobility, as well as patient education for signs and symptoms of heart failure. Will continue to follow.
	2. Short-term goals:
	• The patient will ascend/descend flight of steps with bilateral handrails and supervision with a modified BORG Scale dyspnea < 3/10 within 1 week to be able to get to/from his second floor bedroom and bathroom safely.
	• The patient will independently recall four signs/symptoms of worsening heart failure (related to breathing, weight gain, lower extremity swelling, and fatigue) within 1 week for independent chronic disease management.
	3. Long-term goals:
	• The patient will perform Five Times Sit-to-Stand in < 13 seconds within 6 weeks for improved BLE strength.
	• The patient will perform timed up and go in < 10 seconds within 6 weeks to decrease risk of falls.
	4. The following are examples of a potential home exercise program. Only three to five exercises should be selected to ensure compliance.
	Strengthening:
	F: 3 × /week;
	I: body weight;
	T: fatigue;
	T: sit to stand from 18-inch chair height
	Aerobic training:
	F: 3 × /day
	I: RPE of 3–4/10 on modified Borg;
	T: 10-minute bouts
	T: Walking program in home
	Breathing training:
	F: 2 × /day;
	I: body weight;
	T: 5 minutes;
	T: diaphragmatic breathing in upright positions
Evaluate	5. The patient performed the Five Times Sit-to-Stand in 16 seconds, which is below age and sex norms. His current score is indicative of lower extremity weakness. For an average or better performance, individuals between ages 70 and 79 should have a time of 12.6 seconds or less.
	6. The patient performed the Timed Up and Go (TUG) in 21 seconds, which is below age and sex norms. His current score is indicative of him being a fall risk. For an average of better performance, community dwelling adults should have a time of 13.5 seconds or less.
	7. Clinical signs and symptoms of worsening left-side heart failure include increased difficulty with breathing, cough, and increased fatigue. Clinical signs and symptoms of worsening right-side heart failure include weight gain, lower extremity swelling, and increased fatigue.
Analyze	8. Differential diagnoses for left knee pain following weight-bearing activity include osteoarthritis, meniscal injury, ligament injury, or trauma. Further special tests could help determine a definitive musculoskeletal diagnosis.

(Continued)

(Continued)

Bloom's Taxonomy Level	Case 6.B Answers
Apply	9. In addition to self-monitoring pulse and adhering to medications as learned in the acute care setting, oftentimes home health care offers the opportunity to provide education on the earlier-listed heart failure symptoms through a green/yellow/red light monitoring system. Green light indicates normal breathing, no significant weight gain, no increase in swelling, and no increase in fatigue. Yellow light indicates some parameters may be worsening and a call and possible visit to the physician is warranted. Red light indicates emergency care is indicated.
Understand	10. With continued complaints of left knee pain, a trial of an assistive device such as a single point cane is warranted. When used in the right hand, this will decrease weight-bearing through the left lower extremity. Referral for continued range of motion/strengthening in the outpatient setting may also be indicated.
	11. With the therapeutic goal of Lasix to reduce fluid volume, there is a risk of fluid depletion and thus dehydration and orthostatic hypotension. Furthermore, as Lasix is a loop diuretic, there is risk of loss of potassium which can result in muscle weakness, muscle cramping, and an arrhythmia with irregular pulse. The patient should be educated on such signs and symptoms so that he can monitor presence, frequency, and intensity.
Remember	12. With a past medical history of a myocardial infarction and recent onset of atrial fibrillation, there is increased risk for blood clots. Coumadin will thus act as an anticoagulant.

Key points
1. Patient education on strategies to manage environmental barriers such as stair negotiation is important.
2. Periodic reassessment of outcome measures during an extended plan of care in home health is important to identify improvement and adjust goals accordingly.
3. Focus on independence with self-management strategies for chronic disease management, including adverse pharmacological side effects.
4. Develop a home exercise program that is feasible and safe within the home environment

General Information	
Case no.	6.C
Authors	Kala M. Markel, PT, DPT Kelly M. Lindenberg, PT, MSPT, PhD, CSCS Melissa L. Bednarek, PT, DPT, PhD, Board Certified Clinical Specialist in Cardiovascular & Pulmonary Physical Therapy
Diagnosis	Left knee pain, generalized deconditioning
Setting	Outpatient clinic
Learner expectations	☑ Initial evaluation ☐ Re-evaluation ☐ Treatment session
Learner objectives	1. Identify appropriate measures based on the subjective data provided for use in the outpatient clinic 2. Correlate the impact of cardiovascular and pulmonary disorders on treatment of an orthopaedic impairment. 3. Develop a treatment program based on the patient's body structure and impairments to optimize his participation and quality of life.

Medical	
Chief complaint	Increased left knee pain for 6 weeks, fatigue.
History of present illness	Patient is a 73-year-old male who presents to an outpatient clinic with left knee pain and fatigue. Of note, the patient was recently hospitalized for New York Heart Association (NYHA) Class II heart failure (ejection fraction = 45%) and an episode of atrial fibrillation. Hospital course notable for a 5-day stay, with follow-up in home health for 6 weeks.
Past medical history	Heart failure with ejection fraction of 40%, remote history of STEMI with stent placement > 5 years, atrial fibrillation, hypertension, hyperlipidemia, osteoarthritis, cholecystectomy, anxiety/depression.
Past surgical history	Right total knee replacement
Allergies	Penicillin
Medications	Coumadin, Prinivil, Lopressor, Lipitor, Tylenol, Lasix
Precautions/Orders	Activity as tolerated

Social history	
Home setup	• Lives in a two-story home with wife. • Flight of steps with unilateral rail to enter home • Flight of steps with bilateral rails to second floor • Has two adult children, one lives nearby; has two grandchildren.
Occupation	• Retired computer analyst
Prior level of function	Prior to hospitalization: • Independent with functional mobility and activities of daily living (ADLs) • Independent for stairs; however, required increased time • Spouse manages cooking/cleaning. • Poor tolerance for yard maintenance, hired help. • (+) Driver Currently: • Independent with bed mobility, transfers (including car), ambulation, and ADLs; however, reports difficulty due to increased left knee pain and thus intermittently using a single point cane. • "Absolutely not" attempting any home or yard maintenance due to fatigue.
Recreational activities	• Vacation planned over summer to celebrate 50th wedding anniversary. • Enjoys reading, watching travel television shows, and fishing.

Pause points
Based on the above information, what are the priority • Examination tests and measures? • Outcome measures? • Treatment interventions?

Physical Therapy Examination
Subjective
"That hospitalization really wrecked my life. I can't do anything I used to be able to do. The home physical therapist helped me a lot, but now my knee is a big problem and I have to use this stupid cane. I'm so frustrated with everything."

Objective			
Vital signs	Pre-6MWT	Post-6MWT—immediately	Post-6MWT—3 minutes
Blood pressure (mmHg)	124/82	124/82	122/80
Heart rate (beat/min)	84	91	86

(Continued)

(Continued)

Physical Therapy Examination			
Respiratory rate (breath/min)	15	19	13
Pulse oximetry on room air (SpO$_2$)	97%	91%	96%
Modified BORG scale—dyspnea	0/10	3/10	1/10
Pain (left knee)	3/10	7/10	7/10
General	• Patient seated in waiting room, single point cane present. • Observed slow transition from sit to stand.		
Cardiovascular and pulmonary	• Auscultation: S1, S2, no S3; no adventitious breath sounds • Pulse: 2 + bilateral dorsalis pedis • Edema: none present in BLEs • Breathing pattern: upper chest breather, shallow breaths		
Gastrointestinal	• Denies constipation and fecal incontinence		
Genitourinary	• Denies urinary incontinence despite increased frequency		
Musculoskeletal	Range of motion	• BUE: WFL • BLE: WFL with the exception of bilateral knees—right: 0–100 degrees, left: 10–114 degrees with pain at end range	
	Strength	• B shoulder flexion: 4/5 • B elbow flexion: 5/5 • B elbow extension: 5/5 • B wrist extension: 5/5 • B wrist flexion: 5/5 • B hip flexion: 4 + /5 • L hip abduction: 4–/5 • R hip abduction: 4/5 • L knee flexion: 4/5* • R knee flexion: 4 + /5 • L knee extension: 4/5* • R knee extension: 5/5 • B ankle dorsiflexion: 5/5 • B ankle plantarflexion: 5/5 *Pain with testing	
	Aerobic	• 6-Minute Walk Test results: Distance = 324 m MET level = 1.46	
	Flexibility	• BLE: moderate restriction in hamstrings and quadriceps, mild restriction in gastrocnemius	
	Other	• Left patellar glides hypomobile superior/inferior, tibial extension hypomobile • 30-Second Chair Rise Test: 10 repetitions with use of upper extremities, HR = 95, SpO$_2$ = 94% on room air, RPE = 3/10 for shortness of breath, 5/10 knee pain.	
Neurological	Balance	• Timed Up and Go = 15 seconds with single point cane	
	Cognition	• Alert and oriented x 4	
	Coordination	• Finger-to-nose: intact bilaterally • Heel-to-shin: intact bilaterally	
	Cranial nerves	• II–XII: intact	
	Reflexes	• Biceps: 2 + bilaterally • Patellar: 2 + bilaterally • Achilles: 2 + bilaterally	

(Continued)

(Continued)

Physical Therapy Examination		
	Sensation	• BLE dermatomes: intact to light touch
	Tone	• BUE and BLE: normal throughout
	Other	• Center for Epidemiologic Studies Depression Scale (CES-D) Questionnaire = 18
Functional status		
Bed mobility	• Supine to/from sit: independent	
Transfers	• Sit to/from stand: modified independent with use of arm rests, required increased time.	
Ambulation	• Ambulated 150 feet with single point cane and supervision. • Gait deviations notable for limited stance time on left lower extremity, lack of heel strike/toe off on left lower extremity, moderate antalgic gait • Gait speed: 0.90 m/s	
Stairs	• Ascend/descend flight of steps bilateral handrails with supervision. • Stair deviations notable for step-to pattern, requires increased time. Vital signs post–stair negotiation: BP: 124/81, HR: 92, SpO_2: 93%, modified BORG Scale—dyspnea: 4/10, pain: 7/10 left knee	

Assessment	
☑ Physical therapist's	*Assessment left blank for learner to develop.*
Goals	
Patient's	"I want to get my life back. I want to travel and fish. I don't want to have to walk with this cane forever."
Short term	1. *Goals left blank for learner to develop.* 2.
Long term	1. *Goals left blank for learner to develop.* 2.

Plan	
☑ Physical therapist's	Plan to see patient 3 × /week for 4 weeks. Treatment will include therapeutic exercise (i.e., generalized upper extremity strengthening, hip/lower extremity strengthening, aerobic conditioning), gait training on even and uneven surfaces, manual therapy techniques to improve knee range of motion and joint mobility, and patient education on signs/symptoms of heart failure.

Bloom's Taxonomy Level	Case 6.C Questions
Create	1. Synthesizing the medical data and physical examination findings, develop an appropriate assessment of the patient. 2. Develop two short-term physical therapy goals, including an appropriate timeframe. 3. Develop two long-term physical therapy goals, including an appropriate timeframe.
Evaluate	4. The patient was given a CES-D questionnaire to complete. What does this questionnaire screen for? What are the normal values associated with it? Why do you think this questionnaire was chosen? 5. Based on the 6-Minute Walk Test (6MWT), is this patient above, at, or below the mean for individuals with heart failure? What is the minimally detectable change that needs to be achieved to show improvement in endurance?
Analyze	6. Analyze the relationship between the patient's pre- and post-6MWT blood pressure results and relate to the current medication regimen.

(Continued)

(Continued)

Bloom's Taxonomy Level	Case 6.C Questions
	7. Analyze the patient's reported dyspnea response to exercise. What interventions can be implemented to decrease dyspnea on exertion?
Apply	8. Design and implement an appropriate aerobic exercise prescription utilizing the FITT components, being mindful of orthopaedic limitations.
	9. Construct a patient education discussion on the importance of pacing and energy conservation.
	10. Plan and implement two strategies to assist in managing this patient's depression symptoms.
Understand	11. Describe the interrelationship between building aerobic capacity and orthopaedic limitations.
Remember	12. What are some common signs of exercise intolerance in heart failure?
	13. What are the NYHA Heart Failure Classes and how do they relate to patient function?

Bloom's Taxonomy Level	Case 6.C Answers
Create	1. Patient is a 73-year-old male with a 6-week occurrence of left knee pain following recent hospitalization, which ultimately resulted in a new diagnosis of NYHA Class II Heart Failure. He was hospitalized for 5 days followed by a course of home health services, including physical therapy for 6 weeks. He now presents to outpatient physical therapy for assessment of his left knee pain and generalized deconditioning. Patient's medical complexity is moderate, given his recent hospitalization and comorbidities. He has left greater than right lower extremity weaknesses, hypomobility of the left knee, and decreased range of motion of the left knee. The patient also has decreased endurance, balance, and gait speed as indicated by outcome measures. He reports a lack of ability to perform prior activities and is concerned about being able to travel for his upcoming wedding anniversary. He has a good support system at home. The patient's condition is stable, with the chance to evolve given his recent diagnosis of heart failure, history of depression, and increased CES-D score. Patient would benefit from continued physical therapy to improve the aforementioned deficits to maximize functional mobility and safety. Will continue to follow.
	2. Short-term goals:
	• The patient will improve left knee MMT by at least ½ grade within 2 weeks to allow for improved ability to ascend/descend stairs.
	• The patient will improve gait speed on level surface to at least 1.2 m/s within 2 weeks to improve independence with community ambulation.
	3. Long-term goals:
	• The patient will improve 30-Second Chair Rise Test repetitions by 5 within 4 weeks, indicating improved lower extremity strength and endurance.
	• The patient will tolerate at least 5.0 METS of activity for 30 minutes with an RPE of 3–5/10 within 4 weeks, showing increased cardiovascular endurance.
Evaluate	4. The CES-D is an instrument that is commonly used to screen for depressive symptoms. It consists of 20 questions, in which the patient rates how often over the past week they experienced symptoms associated with depression. Response options range from 0 to 3 for each item (0 = rarely or none of the time, 1 = some or little of the time, 2 = moderately or much of the time, 3 = most or almost all the time). The total scores range from 0 to 60, with a score ≥ 16 being considered significant for depressive symptoms. The CES-D is an easy-to-administer questionnaire that has been validated for the general public as well as several chronic diseases, including those with cardiac conditions. It is possible that the physical therapist chose this screening due to the patient's history of anxiety and depression, marked with his subjective report on how his current health status is impacting his quality of life.
	5. The 6MWT has been shown to provide reliable information for those with heart failure. A total distance of ≤ 300 m is considered a prognostic marker of mortality in patients with heart failure. This patient's total distance of 324 m places him above the prognostic marker of mortality.
	Research shows that the MCID for this patient population is an improvement of approximately 32 m. Additionally, there is some research on improvement during the 6MWT distance being inversely related to NYHA Heart Failure Class.

(Continued)

(Continued)

Bloom's Taxonomy Level	Case 6.C Answers
Analyze	6. The patient's current medication regimen includes an anticoagulant (Coumadin), ace inhibitor (Prinivil), beta-blocker (Lopressor), lipid-lowering agent (Lipitor), an over-the-counter pain reliever (Tylenol), and diuretic (Lasix). The medications that are likely to have a direct relationship to his blood pressure are the beta-blocker, ace-inhibitor, and diuretic. In this patient, his blood pressure was relatively unchanged throughout mobility. His resting blood pressure was 124/82 mmHg. The patient maintains this level immediately post-test, with a blood pressure of 124/82 mmHg, and slight change to 122/80 mmHg after 3 minutes of rest. Antihypertensive drugs can have the effect of maintaining low blood pressure both at rest and with exercise; so, it is possible to observe a lack of increase during exercise in this patient. It is important to utilize additional measures (i.e., rate of perceived exertion) to capture patient response to exercise in this case. 7. The patient is primarily using secondary inspiratory muscles for breathing. Visually, this presents as an increase in upper chest motion and little motion in the abdominal area. This may be due to known changes of diaphragm positioning in patients with heart failure, which impairs inspiratory muscle strength, and leads to an increase in dyspnea. Instruction in diaphragmatic breathing and implementation of tactile cues would be beneficial for this patient to increase inspiratory muscle strength and endurance, leading to improved ventilation and enhanced exercise tolerance (▶ Fig. 6.4a, b). In conjunction, the patient should be taught pursed-lip breathing. Pursed-lip breathing helps relieve dyspnea by slowing down the breathing rate, keeping the airways open longer, and improving ventilation.
Apply	8. An example of an aerobic exercise for this patient may include the following: Frequency–3–5 day/week. Intensity—moderate (RPE of 2–4 on the 10-point scale). Time—30 minutes (break up into smaller exercise bouts if needed, progressing to 1 bout of 30 minutes). Type—Nu-Step (aerobic machine). 9. For patients with heart failure, fatigue is a common symptom. Therefore, learning appropriate pacing and energy conservation techniques may be beneficial to manage this symptom. First, pacing may help keep fatigue levels lower and position the body in safe ways to minimize injury. Second, energy conservation helps maintain a balance between times of activity and rest, therefore improving overall energy levels. It may be helpful for this patient to prioritize the activities that must get done in a day when energy levels are high. 10. Physical therapists should make referrals for mental health when appropriate. However, physical therapists can implement strategies to assist patients with their overall well-being. Such strategies may include breathing techniques, such as diaphragmatic breathing and pursed-lip breathing, as an effective nonpharmacological treatment for stress, anxiety, and depression. Teaching the patient diaphragmatic breathing not only assists with his abnormal chest movements as discussed earlier but also help calm his thoughts and provide a sense of relaxation. Additionally, positive effects of physical activity and reduction of depression have been shown. Men completing 150 minutes per week of moderate-to-vigorous activity showed lower prevalence of depression. Education on the importance of physical activity and its effect on depression/anxiety is paramount with this patient. By encouraging adherence to the prescribed exercise program, the physical therapist can help the patient benefit both physically and emotionally.
Understand	11. The need to build aerobic capacity and orthopaedic limitations are connected. Orthopaedic limitations have been noted to be a barrier to physical activity, and this barrier is compounded with a past medical history of cardiovascular disease(s). Time and type of aerobic exercise may need to be modified for a patient with an orthopaedic limitation and past medical history of a cardiovascular disease(s). An example of a modification may be performing aerobic training on a Nu-Step machine, instead of an upright bicycle, to decrease stress on the knee joint. It is important to note that physical activity is a means to prevent further decline of many chronic diseases, including osteoarthritis and cardiovascular diseases. When designing intervention strategies, know that comorbid arthritis or joint pain is not necessarily a contraindication.

(Continued)

(Continued)

Bloom's Taxonomy Level	Case 6.C Answers
Remember	12. There are both immediate and delayed signs that may indicate exercise intolerance in patients with heart failure. Immediate signs of exercise intolerance may include a > 10 mmHg drop in systolic blood pressure, presence of S3 heart sound, and/or increased lung sounds (most commonly crackles). Other symptoms, which may occur immediately or several hours postexercise, include peripheral edema, presence of jugular vein distention, or weight gain (2 pounds in 24 hours or 5 pounds in 7 days).
	13. The NYHA Heart Failure Classification system was developed in 1994 as a means to classify patients based on their limitations during physical activity. There are four classifications, with each describing more significant symptoms and restrictions.
	• Class I states that the patient has no limitation of physical activity with ordinary physical activity—not causing undue fatigue, palpitation, or dyspnea.
	• Class II states slight limitations of physical activity, meaning the patient is comfortable at rest and ordinary physical activity results in fatigue, palpitation, or dyspnea.
	• Class III states a marked limitation of physical activity, whereas the patient states still comfortable at rest, but less than ordinary physical activity causes fatigue, palpitation, or dyspnea.
	• Class IV states the patient is unable to carry on any physical activity without discomfort. The patient will have symptoms of heart failure at rest, and any physical activity that occurs will increase their symptoms.

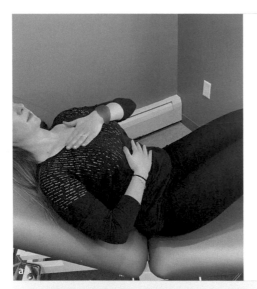 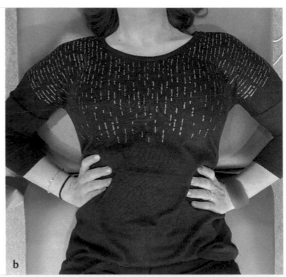

Fig. 6.4 (a) Example of hand placement for diaphragmatic breathing. (b) Hand placement along the lateral rib cage allows for lower lobe lung expansion.

Key points
1. Be conscious of the patient's overall situation, including psychosocial factors, and understand the physical therapist's role in the health care system in identifying needs outside the scope of practice.
2. Recognize the importance of addressing signs and symptoms beyond the primary diagnosis and the interrelationships between body systems as well as their overall impact on rehab performance.
3. Develop appropriate treatment plans that are individualized to each patient's needs and goals.

Suggested Readings

6-Minute Walk Test. Available at: https://www.sralab.org/rehabilitation-measures/6-minute-walk-test. Accessed April 1, 2020

APTA Task Force on Lab Values, 2017. Laboratory Values Interpretation Resource. Academy of Acute Care Physical Therapy

Ainsworth BE, Haskell WL, Herrmann SD, et al. 2011 Compendium of Physical Activities: a second update of codes and MET values. Med Sci Sports Exerc. 2011; 43(8):1575–1581

American Association of Cardiovascular and Pulmonary Rehabilitation. The continuum of care: from inpatient and outpatient cardiac rehabilitation to long-term secondary prevention. In: Guidelines for Cardiac Rehabilitation and Secondary Prevention Programs. 5th ed. Champaign, IL: Human Kinetics; 2013:5–18

American College of Sports Medicine. ACSM's Guidelines for Exercise Testing and Prescription. 10th ed. Baltimore, MD: Lippincott, Williams and Wilkins; 2017

American Heart Association and American Stroke Association. Available at: https://www.heart.org/-/media/files/health-topics/heart-failure/self-check-plan-for-hf-management-477328.pdf?la=en. Accessed September 19, 2020

Arslan S, Erol MK, Gundogdu F, et al. Prognostic value of 6 minute walk test in stable outpatients with heart failure. Tex Heart Inst J. 2007; 34(2):166–169

Bennell K, Hinman R. Exercise as a treatment for osteoarthritis. Curr Opin Rheumatol. 2005; 17(5):634–640

Bohannon RW. Reference values for the five-repetition sit-to-stand test: a descriptive meta-analysis of data from elders. Percept Mot Skills. 2006; 103(1):215–222

Buatois S, Perret, -Guillaume C, Gueguen R, et al. A simple clinical scale to stratify risk of recurrent falls in community-dwelling adults aged 65 years and older. Phys Ther. 2010; 90(4):550–560

Bui AL, Horwich TB, Fonarow GC. Epidemiology and risk profile of heart failure. Nat Rev Cardiol. 2011; 8(1):30–41

Cahalin LP, Arena R, Guazzi M, et al. Inspiratory muscle training in heart disease and heart failure: a review of the literature with a focus on method of training and outcomes. Expert Rev Cardiovasc Ther. 2013; 11(2):161–177

Caruana L, Petrie MC, McMurray JJ, MacFarlane NG. Altered diaphragm position and function in patients with chronic heart failure. Eur J Heart Fail. 2001; 3(2):183–187

Currier D, Lindner R, Spittal MJ, Cvetkovski S, Pirkis J, English DR. Physical activity and depression in men: Increased activity duration and intensity associated with lower likelihood of current depression. J Affect Disord. 2020; 260:426–431

Chua, Chiaco JM, Parikh NI, Fergusson DJ. The jugular venous pressure revisited. Cleve Clin J Med. 2013; 80(10):638–644

Chui K, Hood E, Klima D. Meaningful change in walking speed. Top Geriatr Rehabil. 2012; 28(2):97–103

Dolgin M, Association NYH, Fox AC, Gorlin R, Levin RI, New York Heart Association. Criteria Committee. Nomenclature and Criteria for Diagnosis of Diseases of the Heart and Great Vessels. 9th ed. Boston, MA: Lippincott Williams and Wilkins; March 1, 1994

Five times Sit to Stand. Available at: https://www.sralab.org/rehabilitation-measures/five-times-sit-stand-test. Accessed April 1, 2020

Fletcher GF, Ades PA, Kligfield P, et al. American Heart Association Exercise, Cardiac Rehabilitation, and Prevention Committee of the Council on Clinical Cardiology, Council on Nutrition, Physical Activity and Metabolism, Council on Cardiovascular and Stroke Nursing, and Council on Epidemiology and Prevention. Exercise standards for testing and training: a scientific statement from the American Heart Association. Circulation. 2013; 128(8):873–934

Freedland KE, Carney RM, Rich MW. Effect of depression on prognosis in heart failure. Heart Fail Clin. 2011; 7(1):11–21

Frownfelter D, Dean E. Cardiovascular and Pulmonary Physical Therapy, Evidence to Practice. St. Louis, MO: Saunders Elsevier; 2012

Garfinkel AC, Seidman JG, Seidman CE. Genetic pathogenesis of hypertrophic and dilated cardiomyopathy. Heart Fail Clin. 2018; 14(2):139–146

Giannitsi S, Bougiakli M, Bechlioulis A, Kotsia A, Michalis LK, Naka KK. 6-minute walking test: a useful tool in the management of heart failure patients. Ther Adv Cardiovasc Dis. 2019; 13: 1753944719870084

Goodman CC, Fuller KS. Pathology: Implications for the Physical Therapist. 4th ed. St. Louis, MO: Saunders Elsevier; 2015

Hopper SI, Murray SL, Ferrara LR, Singleton JK. Effectiveness of diaphragmatic breathing for reducing physiological and psychological stress in adults: a quantitative systematic review. JBI Database Syst Rev Implement Reports. 2019; 17(9): 1855–1876

Kandola A, Ashdown-Franks G, Hendrikse J, Sabiston CM, Stubbs B. Physical activity and depression: towards understanding the antidepressant mechanisms of physical activity. Neurosci Biobehav Rev. 2019; 107:525–539

Kato N, Kinugawa K, Shiga T, et al. Depressive symptoms are common and associated with adverse clinical outcomes in heart failure with reduced and preserved ejection fraction. J Cardiol. 2012; 60(1):23–30

Ma X, Yue ZQ, Gong ZQ, et al. The effect of diaphragmatic breathing on attention, negative affect and stress in healthy adults. Front Psychol. 2017; 8:874

Mammen G, Faulkner G. Physical activity and the prevention of depression: a systematic review of prospective studies. Am J Prev Med. 2013; 45(5):649–657

Marzolini S, Candelaria H, Oh P. Prevalence and impact of musculoskeletal comorbidities in cardiac rehabilitation. J Cardiopulm Rehabil Prev. 2010; 30(6):391–400

Noonan V, Dean E. Submaximal exercise testing: clinical application and interpretation. Phys Ther. 2000; 80(8):782–807

Paterson I, Mielniczuk LM, O'Meara E, So A, White JA. Imaging heart failure: current and future applications. Can J Cardiol. 2013; 29 (3):317–328

Ponikowski P, Voors AA, Anker SD, et al. Authors/Task Force Members, Document Reviewers. 2016 ESC Guidelines for the diagnosis and treatment of acute and chronic heart failure: The Task Force for the diagnosis and treatment of acute and chronic heart failure of the European Society of Cardiology (ESC). Developed with the special contribution of the Heart Failure Association (HFA) of the ESC. Eur J Heart Fail. 2016; 18(8):891–975

Rocha JA, Allison TG, Santoalha JM, Araújo V, Pereira FP, Maciel MJ. Musculoskeletal complaints in cardiac rehabilitation: Prevalence and impact on cardiovascular risk factor profile and functional and psychosocial status. Rev Port Cardiol. 2015; 34(2): 117–123

Rocklin DM. The role of the clinical examination in patients with heart failure: E-Z CVP. JACC Heart Fail. 2018; 6(11):972–973

Sharkey NA, Williams NI, Guerin JB. The role of exercise in the prevention and treatment of osteoporosis and osteoarthritis. Nurs Clin North Am. 2000; 35(1):209–221

Shoemaker MJ, Curtis AB, Vangsnes E, Dickinson MG. Clinically meaningful change estimates for the six-minute walk test and daily activity in individuals with chronic heart failure. Cardiopulm Phys Ther J. 2013; 24(3):21–29

Shumway-Cook A, Brauer S, Woollacott M. Predicting the probability for falls in community-dwelling older adults using the timed up & go test. Phys Ther. 2000; 80(9):896–903

Steffen TM, Hacker TA, Mollinger L. Age- and gender-related test performance in community-dwelling elderly people: six-minute walk test, berg balance scale, timed up & go test, and gait speeds. Phys Ther. 2002; 82(2):128–137

Stiell IG, Macle L, CCS Atrial Fibrillation Guidelines Committee. Canadian Cardiovascular Society atrial fibrillation guidelines 2010:

management of recent-onset atrial fibrillation and flutter in the emergency department. Can J Cardiol. 2011; 27(1):38–46

Tanai E, Frantz S. Pathophysiology of heart failure. Compr Physiol. 2015; 6(1):187–214

Timed Up and Go. Available at: https://www.sralab.org/rehabilitation-measures/timed-and-go. Accessed April 1, 2020

Yap J, Lim FY, Gao F, Teo LL, Lam CSP, Yeo KK. Correlation of the New York Heart Association Classification and the 6-minute walk distance: a systematic review. Clin Cardiol. 2015; 38(10):621–628

7 Cystic Fibrosis

General Information	
Case no.	7.A Cystic Fibrosis
Authors	Laura Friedman, PT, DPT, Board Certified Clinical Specialist in Cardiovascular & Pulmonary Physical Therapy Margot Miller, PT, DPT
Diagnosis	Cystic fibrosis (CF)
Setting	Outpatient pulmonary rehab
Learner expectations	☑ Initial evaluation ☐ Re-evaluation ☐ Treatment session
Learner objectives	1. Explain the pathophysiology of the patient's diagnosis. 2. Relate the pathophysiology and progression of pathology from a chronic pulmonary disorder to the clinical manifestations and activity/participation limitations seen in physical therapy practice. 3. Select, implement, and interpret physical therapy interventions based on the medical examination findings. 4. Develop an understanding of medical management and how it influences physical therapy plan of care.

Medical	
Chief complaint	Shortness of breath, decreased activity tolerance, and lower extremity weakness
History of present illness	The patient is a 32-year-old man with CF diagnosed at birth referred to pulmonary rehabilitation (PR) to optimize conditioning as recently listed for lung transplant. He reports performing airway clearance with vest two times a day and utilizing positive expiratory pressure device. He was last hospitalized 2 weeks ago for 5 days due to infection and remains on intravenous (IV) antibiotics with peripherally inserted central catheter (PICC) line in place. He is also status post (s/p) gastric tube placement 6 months ago due to malnutrition.
Past medical history	CF, pancreatic insufficiency, osteoporosis, type II diabetes mellitus (DM), and malnutrition
Past surgical history	Gastric tube (6 months ago)
Allergies	None
Medications	Albuterol metered-dose inhaler (MDI), Hypertonic saline 7% (nebulized), Pulmozyme, Azithromycin, Tobramycin (nebulized), Symdeko, Advair, IV cefepime and Tobramycin since recent hospital discharge
Precautions/orders	Contact precautions Titrate oxygen to maintain ≥ 90% Activity as tolerated

Social history	
Home setup	• Lives in a two-story home with his wife. • Three steps + one handrail to enter. • One flight of steps + one handrail to the second floor, where bedroom and full bathroom are located. • Half bath is on the first floor.
Occupation	• Works as accountant, primarily sedentary.
Prior level of function	• Independent with all mobility, activities of daily living (ADLs), instrumental ADLs (IADLs), and driving.
Recreational activities	• Played soccer until about 3 years ago, but reports it became too hard on his breathing. • Has a treadmill at home but hasn't used it in over a month. • Enjoys hiking with his wife.

Imaging/diagnostic test	Results
Pulmonary function tests (test performed at pulmonary clinic visit 1 week ago)	Forced vital capacity (FVC): 1.73 Forced expiratory volume in 1 second (FEV1): 0.55 FEV1/FVC: 32 Findings/impression: FVC and FEV1 severely reduced (<35%); FEV1/FVC is reduced; flow volume curve demonstrates both an obstructive and a restrictive pattern; very severe obstructive defect is present.
Chest computed tomography (CT; imaging performed at pulmonary clinic visit 1 week ago; ▶ Fig. 7.1; ▶ Fig. 7.2)	Impression: 1. Bronchial wall thickening, cylindrical and early varicose bronchiectasis, lung hyper-inflation, and multifocal areas of segmental and subsegmental atelectasis. Findings represent changes secondary to known CF. 2. Multiple clustered nodules and focal nodular airspace opacities particularly in the right lower lobe could be secondary to airway obstruction or related to infection. No large consolidation seen. 3. Severe atrophy of the pancreas (not unusual with CF)
Chest X-ray (imaging performed at pulmonary clinic visit 1 week ago; ▶ Fig. 7.3)	Findings: Cardiomediastinal silhouette: stable size and contour Lungs: hyperinflated with underlying emphysema and biapical pleural–parenchymal scarring. Coarse somewhat linear opacities in both mid lungs also likely underlying scarring from emphysema. No lobar consolidation, large pleural effusion, or pneumothorax.

Pause points

Based on the above information, what are the priorities?
- Diagnostic tests and measures?
- Outcome measures?
- Treatment interventions?

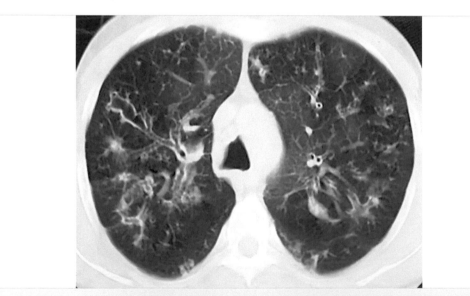

Fig. 7.1 A 32-year-old man with wheezing, dyspnea, and productive cough. Unenhanced chest CT (lung window). Demonstrates extensive bronchiectasis in the right upper lobe. (Parker M, Rosado-de-Christenson M, Abbott G. Radiologic Findings. In: Abbott G, Parker M, Rosado-de-Christenson M, ed. Teaching Atlas of Chest Imaging. 1st Edition. New York: Thieme; 2005).

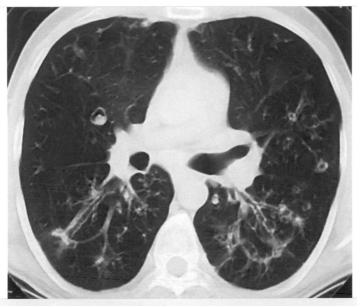

Fig. 7.2 A 32-year-old man with wheezing, dyspnea, and productive cough. Unenhanced chest CT (lung window) Note cystic bronchiectasis with internal mucous plug in right upper lobe. (Parker M, Rosado-de-Christenson M, Abbott G. Radiologic Findings. In: Abbott G, Parker M, Rosado-de-Christenson M, ed. Teaching Atlas of Chest Imaging. 1st Edition. New York: Thieme; 2005).

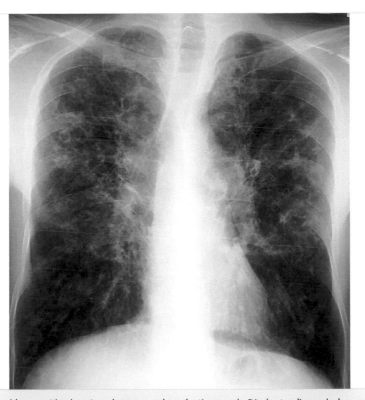

Fig. 7.3 A 32-year-old man with wheezing, dyspnea, and productive cough. PA chest radiograph demonstrates increased lung volumes and extensive bilateral bronchiectasis manifesting as ring, tram track, nodular, and reticular opacities most severe in the upper lungs. (Parker M, Rosado-de-Christenson M, Abbott G. Radiologic Findings. In: Abbott G, Parker M, Rosado-de-Christenson M, ed. Teaching Atlas of Chest Imaging. 1st Edition. New York: Thieme; 2005).

Physical Therapy Examination			
Subjective			
"I want to be able to run around again without shortness of breath."			
Objective			
Vital signs	Resting	Maximum with exercise	Postexercise
Blood pressure (mmHg)	122/64	140/66	124/64
Heart rate (beats/min)	102	136	112
Respiratory rate (breaths/min)	28	44	28
Oxygen saturation (SpO$_2$) on 4L/min O$_2$ via nasal cannula (NC)	97%	91%	96%
Modified Borg Dyspnea Scale	2/10	6/10	2/10
Pain	0/10	0/10	0/10
General	• Walked into the clinic independently. • Lines notable for NC, right upper extremity (RUE) PICC line, gastric tube. • Observations: thin male, rounded shoulders, mild thoracic kyphosis, barrel chest, moderate clubbing noted to fingers (▶ Fig. 7.4) and toes, no cyanosis.		
Head, ears, eyes, nose, and throat (HEENT)	• Patient wears contacts/glasses. Otherwise intact.		
Cardiovascular and pulmonary	• Auscultation: mild to coarse crackles throughout, no adventitious heart sounds. • No edema noted in upper or lower extremities. • Cough: strong, currently nonproductive. Patient reports performed airway clearance prior to arrival. • Breathing pattern: symmetrical, minimal accessory muscle use noted at rest and increased with activity.		
Gastrointestinal	• Gastric tube intact, no signs of infection. • Patient reports nightly feeding through tube.		
Genitourinary	• Patient reports no current issues.		
Musculoskeletal	Range of motion	• Bilateral upper extremity (BUE): within functional limit (WFL) • Bilateral lower extremity (BLE): WFL	
	Strength	• Bilateral upper extremities (BUE): 5/5 • Bilateral hip flexion: 4/5 • Bilateral hip abduction: 3 + /5 • Bilateral knee flexion: 5/5 • Bilateral knee extension: 5/5 • Bilateral Ankle Dorsiflexion: 5/5 • Five Times Sit-to-Stand: 13.2 seconds	
	Aerobic	• 6-Minute Walk Test: 1,140 feet (347 m) on 6 L/min via NC	
	Flexibility	• Mild hamstring tightness bilaterally	
Neurological	Balance	• Static sitting, unsupported: independent • Dynamic sitting, unsupported: independent • Static standing: independent • Dynamic standing: independent	
	Cognition	• Alert and oriented (A&O) × 4	
	Coordination	• Finger to nose: intact bilaterally • Heel to shin: intact bilaterally	
	Cranial nerves	• II– XII: intact	
	Reflexes	• Patellar: 2 + bilaterally • Achilles: 2 + bilaterally	
	Sensation	• BUE/BLE: intact to light touch and proprioception	
	Tone	• BUE and BLE: normal tone throughout	

(Continued)

(Continued)

Physical Therapy Examination	
Functional status	
Bed mobility	• Supine to/from sit: independent
Transfers	• Sit to/from stand: independent
Ambulation	• Ambulated × 1,140 feet independently • Gait deviations: unremarkable
Stairs	• Ascend/descend 12 steps + 1 rail independently, demonstrated reciprocal stepping pattern

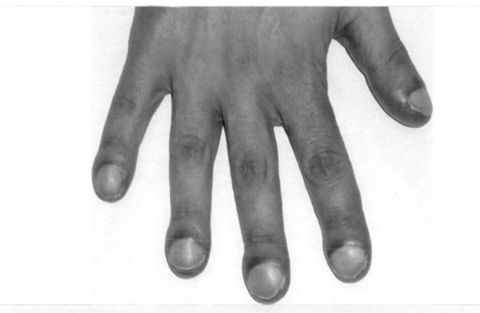

Fig. 7.4 Digital clubbing.

Assessment	
☑ Physical therapist's	*Assessment left blank for learner to develop*
Goals	
Patient's	"I want to get stronger, get a lung transplant, and return to normal."
Short term	1. *Goals left blank for learner to develop.* 2.
Long term	1. *Goals left blank for learner to develop.* 2.

	Plan
☐ Physician's ☑ Physical therapist's ☐ Other's	Will continue to see patient 3 times per week for 6 weeks. Treatment will include therapeutic exercises (proximal lower extremity and upper extremity strengthening, stretching, postural exercises, aerobic conditioning, breathing exercises), airway clearance as indicated, and energy conservation strategies.

Bloom's Taxonomy Level	Case 7.A Questions
Create	1. Synthesizing the medical data and physical examination findings, develop an appropriate physical therapy assessment of the patient. 2. Develop two short-term physical therapy goals, including an appropriate timeframe. 3. Develop two long-term physical therapy goals, including an appropriate timeframe.
Evaluate	4. Determine potential referral sources to other health care providers. 5. Explain why malnutrition is seen commonly in patients with CF. 6. Explain why an airway clearance routine is critical for patients with CF.
Analyze	7. Based on the 6-Minute Walk Test, is the patient above, at, or below the mean for individuals with CF? Is the patient above or below age-matched individuals? What is the minimally detectable change that needs to be achieved to show improvement in endurance? 8. Analyze the relationship between the primary diagnosis of CF and postural dysfunction. 9. Analyze the patient's posture during sitting and gait.
Apply	10. Design and implement two interventions to improve the patient's aerobic capacity. 11. Design and implement two interventions—one stretching and one strengthening—to improve cervical and shoulder posture. 12. Design and implement two interventions to improve endurance/activity tolerance. 13. Describe the purpose of the patient's Aerobika. Describe two other interventions that could be utilized to improve airway clearance during pulmonary rehab.
Understand	14. Describe the purpose of the medications this patient is currently taking. Will these medications have any physical therapy implications?
Remember	15. Based on the patient's medical diagnosis of type II DM, is it important to measure the patient's blood glucose before, during, or after pulmonary rehab sessions? What would be signs the blood glucose level may be too low or too high? 16. Why are contact precautions in place for CF patients across all settings? What personal protective equipment (PPE) should be donned by the clinicians treating this population?

Bloom's Taxonomy Level	Case 7.A Answers

Create	1. The patient is a 32-year-old man with CF recently listed for bilateral lung transplant s/p recent hospitalization for infection and now presents for outpatient pulmonary rehab evaluation. Upon initial evaluation, the patient presents with impaired aerobic capacity, bilateral proximal lower extremity muscular weakness, postural dysfunction, and impaired endurance, which contribute to inability to walk long distances or for long durations and to engage in usual exercise and sport activities. The patient is at risk for increased hospital readmissions and further deconditioning without physical therapy interventions. The patient is a good candidate for skilled physical therapy services as motivated to optimize strength and conditioning in preparation for future lung transplant.
	2. Short-term goals:
	  • Patient will increase hip flexor strength to >/=4+/5 manual muscle testing (MMT) grade within 3 weeks to allow for independent reciprocal stair negotiation without rail for 12 steps.
	  • Patient will increase 6-Minute Walk Test by 150 feet within 3 weeks to demonstrate improved endurance.
	3. Long-term goals:
	  • Patient will decrease Five Times Sit-to-Stand time to < 10 seconds within 6 weeks to show improved BLE strength.
	  • Patient will increase 6-Minute Walk Test by 300 feet within 6 weeks to demonstrate improved endurance and ability to return to leisure/sports activities.

Evaluate	4. Fortunately, since this patient is now active on the lung transplant list, he has routine visits with a lung transplant dietician to ensure he is gaining weight appropriately. The

(Continued)

(Continued)

Bloom's Taxonomy Level	Case 7.A Answers
	patient also has routine visits with a pulmonologist and endocrinologist to manage CF and diabetes, respectively. Any patient with CF would benefit from referral to a dietician as weight loss is very common, as well as to ensure on right regimen of vitamins due to associated pancreatic insufficiency with CF. Also, a referral to a psychiatrist or psychologist may be beneficial to help the individual cope with chronic illness, possible anxiety, depression, and potential life-changing events, such as lung transplantation.
	5. The main reason malnutrition is common in patients with CF is a buildup of mucus in the digestive tract making it difficult to digest and absorb nutrients, malabsorption due to pancreatic insufficiency, and increased resting energy expenditure. Other attributing factors include CF-related diabetes, decreased appetite, and behavioral feeding problems.
	6. An airway clearance routine is critical for patients with CF as it is a genetic disease that primarily affects the lungs and characterized by dehydration of airway surface liquid and impaired mucociliary clearance. Airway clearance is necessary to clear pathogens from the lungs to limit pulmonary infections and inflammation.
Analyze	7. This patient appears to be below the mean for patients with CF as the largest study looking at CF patients had a mean of 1,725 feet (526 m). There is an additional study with CF patients with moderate airflow limitation that had a mean of 2,053 feet (626 m), but this study only had a sample size of 25 patients. One additional study in 2004 had 109 subjects but of varying airway restrictions and the mean distance was 1,049 feet (320 m). There is limited research looking at the 6-Minute Walk Test in the CF population. The patient is well below age-matched individuals as the predicted value for males of his height and weight is 2,468 feet (752.2 m). The minimally detectable change to show improved endurance that is most closely related to CF is that for chronic obstructive pulmonary disease (COPD), which is 177 feet (54 m).
	8. The risk factors that can lead to postural dysfunction in individuals with CF include reduced FEV1, low lean body mass, CF-related diabetes, corticosteroid treatments, pancreatic insufficiency, physical inactivity, low vitamin D, chronic pulmonary conditions, delayed puberty, and Delta F508 genotype. There is ongoing research as to whether the CF transmembrane conductance regulator (CFTR) defect, which causes CF and which has been identified in bone and muscle cells, is a primary cause of bone complications, especially low bone mineral density, or whether postural problems are a secondary complication of the CF disease process. It may be the altered cough and breathing patterns plus inflammatory processes, as well as decreased activity levels with pulmonary infections, as the main cause of postural dysfunction. Also, the muscles of the trunk work to facilitate breathing while also supporting posture, and therefore the more demand placed on them for breathing, the less ability they have to support your posture.
	9. The patient's posture includes rounded shoulders, mild thoracic kyphosis, and a barrel chest. The kyphosis is more prominent during ambulation. In sitting, a slumped posture is noted. Unfortunately, the chest wall muscles have likely shortened due to the chronic manifestations of CF.
Apply	10. To improve the patient's aerobic capacity, the patient could coordinate deep breathing with upper extremity D2 proprioceptive neuromuscular facilitation (PNF) pattern. The patient will inhale through his nose while raising arms and exhale through pursed lips as they lower the arms. This will aid in chest expansion and will be a great exercise to carry over to the post lung transplant phase. A second intervention would be to utilize an inspiratory muscle trainer.
	11. To improve cervical and shoulder posture, address shortened anterior muscles, such as pectoralis minor, via stretches, as well as strengthen the scapular retractors (middle trapezius, rhomboids). The pectoralis minors can be gently self-stretched in supine, aided by gravity. The patient flexes shoulders and elbows to 90 degrees ("goal post" position) and then slides arms toward the head of the bed until a gentle stretch is felt. The patient can hold this stretch for 10 to 20 seconds at a time, increasing duration to tolerance, up to 10 minutes total per day. Shoulder retraction exercises can be initiated in supine, with attention given to proper form; progress the exercises by performing in upright, as well as introducing a resistance band for increased resistance and strengthening. As the shoulder retractors

(Continued)

(Continued)

Bloom's Taxonomy Level	Case 7.A Answers
	are postural stabilizers, emphasize strength training for endurance, that is, lower load, higher repetitions.
	Overall flexibility exercises can also improve posture, and strength and yoga and Tai Chi can have a positive impact on posture, strength, and flexibility.
	12. To improve endurance, the patient could utilize the treadmill to increase duration and intensity of walking. For example, the patient could start with 10 to 15 minutes for three trials at a light to moderate intensity (30 to < 60% of peak work rates). The goal would be to first increase duration to get to 30 to 45 minutes of continuous activity. Once this is achieved, intensity can be increased to vigorous (60–80% of peak work rates). This could be initiated in pulmonary rehab and then continued as part of home program. The upper body ergometer or NuStep machine could be utilized in addition to the treadmill to incorporate upper extremity work. Again, duration would be increased first, followed by intensity.
	13. The Aerobika is an oscillatory positive expiratory pressure (OPEP) device that is utilized to improve mucus clearance by providing resistance as exhale into the device. The acapella is another commonly used OPEP device. Both of these devices have the ability to be combined with a nebulizer treatment, with the medication being administered prior to use of the device.
	Two other interventions that could be performed are percussion and postural drainage and active cycle of breathing therapy (ACBT). The percussion and postural drainage would especially be indicated if specific area(s) of lungs sound more congested during auscultation. The ACBT is an ideal intervention as it can be done independently by the patient and requires no equipment. ACBT includes three phases: breathing control, chest expansion exercises, and forced expiratory technique or huff coughing. The patient starts by taking slow, relaxed breaths ideally through pursed lip breathing technique and once breath control is achieved, the patient moves to taking deep breaths in which the patient tries to hold inhalation for 2 to 3 seconds for three to five deep breaths. The final phase is to take two to three huff coughs to try and remove secretions as the huff cough is more effective than regular coughing in removing mucus from the smaller airways to the larger airways. The cycle can be repeated as many times as necessary to clear secretions (▶ Fig. 7.5a,b).
Understand	14. The purpose of the medications are as follows:
	• Albuterol: a bronchodilator and utilized to relax muscles in the airways and increase airflow to the lungs. Tachycardia is a potential side effect that could impact physical therapy.
	• Hypertonic saline: helps lung function and decreases risk for infection by thinning mucus in the airways.
	• Pulmozyme: a synthetic protein that breaks down excess deoxyribonucleic acid (DNA) in the mucus and therefore improves lung function and reduces risk of infection.
	• Azithromycin, tobramycin, and cefepime: antibiotics used to fight infection. Patients with CF can be on oral and/or IV antibiotics based on severity and strain of infection. Common side effects that could impact physical therapy are diarrhea and nausea.
	• Symdeko: a CFTR modulator that is taken to correct the malfunctioning protein made by the CFTR gene. Side effects that could impact physical therapy include dizziness, nausea, headaches, and liver problems.
	• Advair: a combination medicine that has a steroid and a bronchodilator and therefore prevents inflammation as well as relaxes the muscles in the airways to improve breathing. The side effect that would most likely impact physical therapy is tachycardia, which occurs in 1 to 10% of patients taking Advair.
Remember	15. It is important to measure an individual with diabetes blood glucose before, during, and after exercise to ensure safe tolerance of exercise/activity. It is important to note how the patient's body responds to exercise in terms of potential fluctuations in blood glucose. Exercise can cause the patient's blood glucose to decrease and therefore it is ideal for the blood glucose to be higher than 100 mg/dL prior to starting exercise. It is also dangerous if blood glucose is elevated above 250 mg/dL as it puts the patient at risk for ketoacidosis. It is recommended to check the patient's blood sugar every 30 minutes during exercise, especially if starting a new exercise

(Continued)

(Continued)

Bloom's Taxonomy Level	Case 7.A Answers
	program. Symptoms of hyperglycemia include increased thirst, dry mouth, increased urination, blurry vision, fatigue, difficulty concentrating, and headaches. Symptoms of hypoglycemia include feeling shaky/weakness, sweating, chills, irritability, confusion, anxiety, dizziness, tachycardia, and fatigue.
	16. Individuals with CF have decreased ability to clear bacteria/pathogens from their lungs and many of these pathogens are drug resistant and some strains may always be present. Contact precautions are in place to prevent the spread of infection. It is important to keep CF patients separated from one another in all clinical settings and individuals with CF should always be wearing face masks to cover their mouth and nose when in health care settings. Clinicians treating individuals with CF should wear the following PPE at all times: gown and gloves. They should also practice good hand hygiene regardless of respiratory tract culture results of their patient.

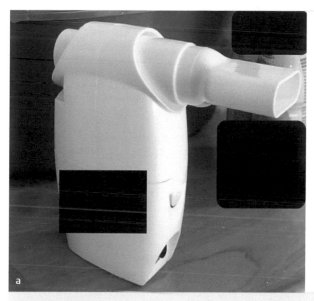 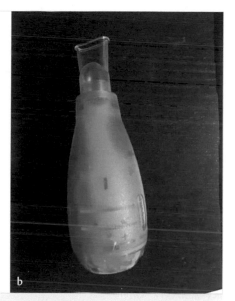

Fig. 7.5 (a) Aerobika. (b) Acapella.

Key points
1. It is important for the physical therapist to understand what interventions will best prepare the patient for lung transplant surgery.
2. It is important to understand all the systems, especially the pulmonary, gastrointestinal, and musculoskeletal systems, can be impacted by CF.
3. Ensure, that early on, a physical therapist provides a home exercise program that highlights primary impairments, such as quad strength and endurance in this case, and educate on appropriate use of home treadmill for endurance training that compliments versus hinders pulmonary rehab.

General Information	
Case no.	7.B
Authors	Margot Miller, PT, DPT Laura Friedman, PT, DPT, Board Certified Clinical Specialist in Cardiovascular & Pulmonary Physical Therapy
Diagnosis	Cystic fibrosis (CF)

(Continued)

(Continued)

General Information	
Setting	Acute care hospital—cardiothoracic intensive care unit (CICU)
Learner expectations	☑ Initial evaluation ☐ Re-evaluation ☐ Treatment session
Learner objectives	1. Identify the benefits of early mobilization in the ICU setting following lung transplant. 2. Understand common side effects of immunosuppressive/posttransplant drugs. 3. Select and implement physical therapy interventions based on the physical therapy examination findings in the context of the acute care setting and patient goals. 4. Develop an understanding of medical management and how it influences physical therapy plan of care.

Medical	
Chief complaint	Postoperative day (POD) 1 bilateral lung transplant (clamshell incision; ▸ Fig. 7.6).
History of present illness	The patient is a 32-year-old man with CF diagnosed at birth. He completed a comprehensive workup for lung transplant listing about 10 months ago. Shortly thereafter, his listing was made temporarily inactive, as he was determined to be "too well" for active listing. His listing was reactivated 8 weeks ago due to worsening health status documented during a routine pulmonary clinic visit. He had been participating in outpatient pulmonary rehab 3 times a week up until approximately 6 weeks ago when his supplemental oxygen demands increased, and it became too cumbersome to transport additional tanks to rehab. Additionally, he endorses decreased tolerance for activity. He was admitted to the hospital yesterday for possible lung transplant.
Past medical history	CF, pancreatic insufficiency, osteoporosis, type II diabetes mellitus, malnutrition status post (s/p) gastric tube placement, multiple respiratory infections—most recently 3 months ago, necessitating hospitalization, peripherally inserted central catheter (PICC) line placement, and intravenous (IV) antibiotics.
Past surgical history	Gastric tube (placed 9 months ago)
Allergies	None
Medications	Albuterol metered-dose inhaler (MDI), Hypertonic saline 7% (nebulized), Pulmozyme, Azithromycin, Tobramycin (nebulized), Symdeko, and Advair
Precautions/Orders	Activity as tolerated Weight bearing as tolerated (WBAT) bilateral lower extremities (BLE) Contact precautions—immunocompromised Fall precautions

Social history	
Home setup	• Lives in a two-story home with his wife. • Three steps + one handrail to enter. • One flight of steps + one handrail to the second floor, where bedroom and full bathroom are located. • Half bath is on the first floor. • Most recently, the patient has been sleeping on the ground floor living room to avoid stair climbing due to increased shortness of breath.
Occupation	• Works as an accountant, primarily sedentary.
Prior level of function	• Previously, independent with all mobility, activities of daily living (ADLs), instrumental ADLs (IADLs), driving. • More recently, he is ambulating household distances and independent/modified independent with basic ADLs (BADLs), utilizing a shower chair and increased time due to shortness of breath He has an active license but has not been driving for the last 6 weeks.
Recreational activities	• Played soccer until about 3 years ago, but reports it became too hard on his breathing. • Has a treadmill at home, which he tried to begin using after discontinuing participation in pulmonary rehab. He reports tolerating 3 to 4 minutes of continuous walking before needing a seated rest break to catch his breath.

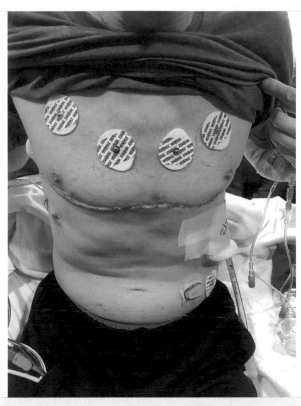

Fig. 7.6 Example of a patient with a clamshell incision, commonly utilized in bilateral lung transplant surgeries. Additionally, note the chest tube at the patient's left lateral rib cage which is connected to a water seal chest drain (out of frame).

Vital signs	Hospital day 1, POD 0: CICU	Hospital day 2, POD 1: CICU
Blood pressure (mmHg)	92/55	110/58
Heart rate (beats/min)	106	95
Respiratory rate (breaths/min)	22	18
Oxygen saturatio (SpO_2)	93% on 4 L/min O_2 via nasal cannula (NC)	94% on 2 L/min O_2 via NC

Imaging/diagnostic test	Hospital day 1, POD 0: CICU	Hospital day 2, POD 1: CICU
Electrocardiogram (ECG)	1. Sinus tachycardia	1. Normal sinus rhythm and rate\
Chest X-ray	1. Stable bilateral chest tubes 2. Stable cardiomediastinal silhouette 3. Lungs: bibasilar interstitial opacities, atelectasis, grossly stable. No evidence of focal consolidation. No pleural effusions. Trace left apical pneumothorax.	- Unchanged
Tansesophageal echocardiogram (TEE)	1. Ejection fraction 45% (unchanged from pre-surgical baseline), dilated right ventricle with mildly decreased systolic function.	- Unchanged

Medical management	Hospital day 1, POD 0: CICU	Hospital day 2, POD 1: CICU
Medications	Wean pressors (norepinephrine) as tolerated while maintaining mean arterial pressure (MAP) > 60. Albuterol, Acetaminophen, Furosemide, Heparin, Insulin, Lidocaine patch, Lorazepam, Metoprolol, Oxycodone, Miralax, Sertraline, Prednisone, Bactrim, Tacrolimus (Prograf), Tramadol, Voriconazole (Vfend).	Continued per medical plan of care
Respiratory	1. Extubated this morning, currently on 4 L via NC. 2. Chest tubes × 2; left chest tube maintained to low suction (▶ Fig. 7.7).	1. Incentive spirometer, 10 times per hour. 2. Wean supplemental oxygen as tolerated while maintaining SpO_2 > 92%. 3. Monitor chest tube output.
Consults	1. Infectious disease 2. Pharmacology	1. Physical therapy 2. Occupational therapy 3. Speech-language pathology

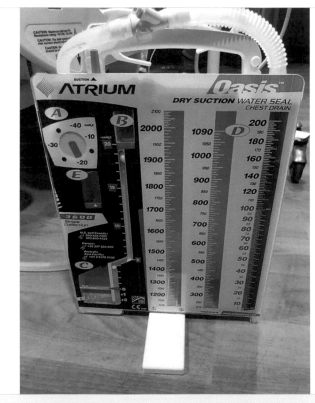

Fig. 7.7 Water seal chest drain. This drain may be connected to wall or portable suction device.

Lab		Reference range	Hospital day 1, POD 0: CICU	Hospital day 2, POD 1: CICU
Arterial blood gas	pH	7.36–7.46	7.31	7.45
	PaCO$_2$	32–46	50	38
	PaO$_2$	83–108	136	142
	HCO$_3^-$	21–29	24	25
Complete blood count	White blood cell (WBC)	$5.0–10.0 \times 10^9$/L	14.0	21.0
	Red blood cell (RBC)	4.5–5.5	2.57	3.21
	Hemoglobin	14.0–17.4 d/dL	8.5	9.9
	Hematocrit	42–52%	29.6	28.7
	Platelet	150–400 k/µL	164	160
Electrolytes	Sodium	134–142 mEq/L	136	134
	Potassium	3.7–5.1 mEq/L	4.5	4.6
	Chlorine	98–108 mEq/L	100	103
	Calcium	8.6–10.3 mg/dL	8.6	8.2
Other	Tacrolimus	8–12 ng/mL	< 1.0	1.8
	Glucose	70–100 mg/dL	205, 220, 168	188, 170
	Blood urea nitrogen (BUN)	6–25 mg/dL	18	16
	Creatinine	0.7–1.3 mg/dL	1.3	1.1

Pause points

Based on the above information, what are the priorities?
• Diagnostic tests and measures?
• Outcome measures?
• Treatment interventions?

Hospital Day 2, POD 1: Physical Therapy Examination

Subjective

"How am I supposed to move with all of these tubes?"

Objective

Vital signs	Pre-treatment			Post-treatment
	Supine	Sitting	Standing	Sitting (bedside chair)
Blood pressure (mmHg)	119/59	118/72	108/70	124/65
Heart rate (beats/min)	88	105	131	112
Respiratory rate (breaths/min)	18	22	32	20
Oxygen saturation (SpO$_2$) on 2L/min O$_2$ via NC	92%	96%	98%	98%
Modified Borg Dyspnea Scale	0/10	1/10	4/10	2/10
Pain	3/10 (incisional site, chest tube sites)	5/10 (immediately following transfer, improved with rest)	3/10	3/10

(Continued)

(Continued)

Hospital Day 2, POD 1: Physical Therapy Examination		
General		• Patient seated at the edge of the bed. • Posture notable for rounded shoulders, mild thoracic kyphosis, barrel chest. • Lines/tubes/drains notable for telemetry, central venous pressure (CVP) monitor, arterial line, blood pressure cuff, bilateral chest tubes with left (L) chest tube to low suction, NC, pulse oximeter, central line, peripheral IV, PICC line, gastric tube, wound manager, service dressings, urinary catheter, sequential compression devices. • No evident distress, though noted to move gingerly.
Head, ears, eyes, nose, and throat (HEENT)		• Patient wears glasses. Otherwise, unremarkable.
Cardiovascular and pulmonary		• Normal sinus rhythm. Normal S1, S2 • 2 L/min O_2 via NC • Clear and equal breath sounds; no wheezing, rales, or rhonchi • Shallow breathing pattern, increased use of accessory muscles • Tachycardia and tachypnea with transfers and standing edge of bed, though improved with verbal cueing.
Gastrointestinal		• Gastric tube • No abdominal discomfort or bloating reported • Denies bowel movement since surgery • NPO until swallow evaluation with speech-language pathologist.
Genitourinary		• Urinary catheter is in place.
Musculoskeletal	Range of motion (ROM)	• Cervical: within functional limit (WFL) • Bilateral upper extremity (BUE): WFL with the exception of bilateral shoulder flexion, which is limited by pain at surgical site. • Thoracic/lumbar: WFL, mildly limited by pain at surgical site. • Bilateral lower extremity (BLE): WFL
	Strength	• Bilateral shoulder flexion: 3 + /5 • Bilateral elbow flexion: 3 + /5 • Bilateral elbow extension: 3 + /5 *Proximal BUE strength primarily limited by pain* • Left wrist extension: 5/5 • Right wrist extension: not performed due to arterial line • Bilateral hip flexion MMT: 3+/5 • Bilateral hip abduction: 3 + /5 • Bilateral knee flexion: 4/5 • Bilateral knee extension: 4/5 • Bilateral ankle dorsiflexion: 5/5 • Bilateral ankle plantar flexion: 5/5
	Aerobic	• Reported 4/10 on Rate of Perceived Exertion (RPE) Scale during transfers • Plan for 6-Minute Walk Test as soon as able.
	Flexibility	• Not formally assessed • On observation, minimally limited cervical rotation and lateral flexion bilaterally, suspect secondary to shortened scalenes, and sternocleidomastoids. • Trunk ROM limited by pain at surgical and chest tube sites
Neurological	Balance	• Static sitting, unsupported: supervision • Dynamic sitting, unsupported: stand by assistance for weight shifting within base of support (BOS); contact guard assistance for weight shifting excursions outside BOS. Patient's tolerance for weight shifting outside BOS limited by incisional pain.

(Continued)

(Continued)

		Hospital Day 2, POD 1: **Physical Therapy Examination**
		• Static standing: contact guard assistance with rolling walker. • Dynamic standing: contact guard assistance with rolling walker, patient demonstrates difficulty reaching across midline without upper extremity support.
	Cognition	• Alert and oriented (A&O) × 4 • Richmond Agitation–Sedation Scale (RASS): 0 • Confusion assessment method for the ICU (CAM-ICU): negative
	Coordination	• Finger to nose: intact bilaterally • Heel to shin: intact bilaterally
	Cranial Nerves	• II–XII: intact
	Reflexes	• Patellar: 2 + bilaterally • Achilles: 2 + bilaterally
	Sensation	• Light touch intact in all four extremities. • Patient does endorse intermittent numbness and tingling in bilateral feet; however, this was reported pre-op as well.
	Tone	• Normal tone throughout BUE, BLE
	Other	• N/A
		Functional status
Bed mobility		• Rolling either direction: moderate assistance using log roll technique • Supine to/from sit: moderate assistance *For all mobility, head of bed elevated ~30 degrees and use of bed rails. Pain and lines/tubes/drains were primary reasons for assistance.*
Transfers		• Sit to/from stand: minimal assist, use of upper extremity support on bedrail/chair armrests • Stand pivot transfer: minimal assistance with rolling walker
Ambulation		• Ambulated 20 feet × 2 with contact guard assistance and rolling walker; took seated rest break between trials. • Gait deviations notable for decreased cadence, irregular step placement, shortened step length, positive Trendelenburg bilaterally.
Stairs		• Deferred due to patient reporting fatigue with ambulation.
Other		• Functional Status Score for the ICU (FSS-ICU): 16

Assessment	
☑ Physical therapist's	*Assessment left blank for learner to develop*
Goals	
Patient's	"I want to get back home and sleep in my upstairs bedroom again."
Short term	1 *Goals left blank for learner to develop.* 2.
Long term	1. *Goals left blank for learner to develop.* 2.

Plan	
☐ Physician's ☑ Physical therapist's ☐ Other's	Plan to see patient five to six times per week to progress functional mobility and ambulation, address present (and limit additional) proximal upper extremity/lower extremity weakness, improve gait stability, and improve activity tolerance and endurance. Additionally, address breathing mechanics for improved efficiency.

Bloom's Taxonomy Level	Case 7.B Questions
Create	1. Synthesizing the medical data and physical examination findings, develop an appropriate physical therapy assessment of the patient. 2. Develop two short-term physical therapy goals, including an appropriate timeframe. 3. Develop two long-term physical therapy goals, including an appropriate timeframe.
Evaluate	4. Explain the physical therapy findings and expected discharge disposition to the lung transplant team.
Analyze	5. Explain the importance of encouraging upright activity and positional changes following surgery and while remaining hospitalized. 6. Explain the impact chest tubes may have on a patient's breathing pattern. 7. Explain why the patient's blood glucose is elevated, despite previously well-controlled diabetes.
Apply	8. Design and implement two interventions to improve energy conservation. 9. Design and implement two interventions to address the patient's gait instability.
Understand	10. What are the physical therapy implications for the patient's immunosuppressive medication regimen? 11. Interpret the chest X-ray findings and relate them to the medical management, as well as the chosen physical therapy interventions.
Remember	12. When mobilizing and actively monitoring blood pressure via an arterial line, what should be kept in mind? 13. What precautions should be considered due to the patient's immunocompromised status?

Bloom's Taxonomy Level	Case 7.B Answers

Create	1. The patient is a 32-year-old man POD 1 s/p bilateral lung transplant. Significant past medical history (PMH) includes cystic fibrosis, pancreatic insufficiency, type II diabetes mellitus, osteoporosis, and malnutrition s/p gastric tube placement. Patient demonstrates impaired BLE/BUE strength (proximal > distal), pain with mobility due to surgical incision and chest tube placement, decreased endurance (seated rest break required following ~20 feet of ambulation at rolling walker), mild gait instability suspect due to decreased hip girdle strength, and impaired posture due to prolonged use of accessory muscles for respiration prior to transplant, all of which are contributing to decreased functional mobility. The patient will benefit from continued skilled physical therapy to address the aforementioned impairments, which currently limit the patient's independence with mobility tasks, as well as to counteract negative effects of the patient's prolonged use of corticosteroids and new immunosuppressive drug regimen on strength and bone health. Will continue to follow.
	2. Short-term goals:
	  • Patient will independently perform supine to/from sit via logroll technique within 5 days to get in/out of bed upon discharge (d/c) to home.
	  • Patient will demonstrate improved breathing mechanics with no more than three verbal cues (decreased use of accessory muscles, decreased respiratory rate, etc.) in a therapy session within 5 days for improved energy conservation with daily activities.
	3. Long-term goals:
	  • Patient will ascend/descend 12 steps, utilizing one handrail, with supervision within 10 days to facilitate safe negotiation of stairs at home and use of patient's bedroom on the second floor.

(Continued)

(Continued)

Bloom's Taxonomy Level	Case 7.B Answers
	• Patient will ambulate > 500 feet with supervision and least restrictive assistive device (vs. none) with ≤ 2 standing rest breaks within 10 days for improved activity endurance upon d/c to home.
Evaluate	4. At initial evaluation (POD 1), the patient requires physical assistance with all mobility; however, the physical therapist suspects that pain and lines/tubes/drains are primary limiting factors. It is anticipated that with improved pain management and removal of chest tubes patient will require decreased physical assist for mobility. The physical therapist anticipates seeing the patient five to six times a week, with emphasis on functional mobility training, BUE/BLE strengthening, and endurance training. Assuming no major medical complications and improved oral/nutritional intake, the patient will be able to discharge to home with family support and home physical therapy to continue progressing strength, balance, and endurance training, as well as intermittent assistance with IADLs/BADLs.
Analyze	5. Body positioning can have profound effects on physiologic function. Changes in positioning and mobility are preferable to remaining in any one position, which can have negative effects on the cardiovascular and pulmonary systems, as well as the integumentary and musculoskeletal systems. Upright positioning promotes greater gravitational stress, challenging the body's fluid/blood volume regulation. It also offers a more advantageous position to the lungs, unimpeded by the weight of one's chest/abdomen in supine; additionally, when upright, the downward movement of the diaphragm is gravity assisted, allowing for deeper inhalation and optimized lung volumes. Mobility further perturbs the body's various regulatory systems. These perturbations promote increased oxygen transport in response to increased energy demands, regulate circulation and cardiac output, aid in airway clearance and cough production, improve arousal, and can encourage return of normal bowel and bladder function, among other benefits.
	6. Commonly, following cardiothoracic surgeries, chest tubes are inserted into the pleural or mediastinal spaces to drain excess fluid or blood. They are inserted between the ribs, requiring incisions to the internal and external intercostal muscles. The external intercostals are principal muscles of inspiration. Therefore, a person who has a chest tube may experience discomfort with inhalation/chest expansion, resulting in more shallow breathing patterns to limit pain. The use of a pillow held snuggly against the chest ("splinting") may alleviate some pain experienced with coughing, laughing, etc. Most patients will find considerable pain relief with the removal of chest tubes.
	7. Following transplant, it is necessary for the patient to take antirejection drugs to protect the patient's transplanted organ. A side effect of immunosuppressive medications, such as tacrolimus or prednisone, is increased blood sugar. Medical management will involve adjusting the patient's medications to provide sufficient protection against rejection while minimizing side effects. The patient's drug regimen to address elevated blood sugars may similarly need to be adjusted.
Apply	8. Two interventions to address energy conservation include pursed lip breathing and utilization of the Modified Borg Dyspnea Scale to assist with activity pacing Pursed lip breathing entails inhalation through the nose, followed by exhalation through the mouth. Emphasize a 1:2 ratio of inhalation to exhalation duration (for example, 2 second inhale, 4 second exhale). Progress the intervention by pairing exhalation with exertional effort, that is, breathing out as one performs a sit to stand transfer. The Modified Borg Dyspnea Scale asks the patient to identify his perceived degree of breathlessness (using a numerical scale) during any given activity. The clinician can instruct the patient to perform activities within a specified range, cueing for rest breaks if the patient's degree of breathlessness begins to exceed the prescribed range. Through activity pacing, the patient can limit excess fatigue and the need for extended recovery times, as well as enable himself to perform an activity for an increased duration. Commonly, in the acute care setting, 3/10 or "moderate" degree of breathlessness is a good target for activity intensity.

(Continued)

(Continued)

Bloom's Taxonomy Level	Case 7.B Answers
	9. In the acute care setting, hallway ambulation is vital in improving overall gait stability. The physical therapist should emphasize normalizing gait pattern (step length, step clearance, cadence, base of support [BOS] width, etc.), as well as the progression of duration and contiguous distance. Initial utilization of assistive devices, such as a rolling walker, may be beneficial. The use of an assistive device, can provide increased stability and activity confidence, allowing the patient to devote greater attention to optimizing gait mechanics. As the patient's gait mechanics improve, the device can be weaned. Side stepping, backward stepping, and diagonal stepping are other interventions that can promote improved gait stability. Side and diagonal stepping, in particular, encourage movement outside of the sagittal plane, recruiting hip girdle muscles that aid in upright stabilization. The use of a resistance band at the ankles or just about the knees can progress this intervention for increased challenge.
Understand	10. Pretransplant drug regimens of patients with CF commonly include corticosteroids. Prolonged use of corticosteroids, in conjunction with impaired nutrition (specifically decreased protein intake), contributes to decreased bone and muscle mass. As a result, these patients are at increased risk of compression fractures. They will benefit from education and instruction in body mechanics, posture, and safe lifting techniques, as well as careful introduction of resistance training. Tacrolimus and other posttransplant antirejection drugs are similarly found to impair skeletal muscle function, contributing to posttransplant sarcopenia. Additionally, many immuno-suppressive medications can cause kidney damage.
	11. The chest X-ray indicates atelectasis, as well as a trace left apical pneumothorax. Atelectasis—the collapse and/or fluid infiltration of alveoli—is a common complication following surgeries. It is mitigated by using an incentive spirometer, which promotes reinflation of the alveoli. Additionally, upright positioning and mobility will encourage improved secretion clearance and deep breathing, reducing atelectasis. The trace pneumothorax is the result of air leaking into the pleural space, which, in serious situations, can result in the lung collapsing. Here, a chest tube has been inserted to address the air leak; the connection to suction aids in encouraging air flow out of the pleural space in order to restore normal pleural pressures. Again, ambulation and out-of-bed activity can additionally promote lung re-expansion.
Remember	12. The patient's blood pressure readings are via an (intra)arterial line, which is connected to a transducer. The transducer's output, that is, measure of blood pressure, is position dependent. The transducer should be located at the level of the right atrium to ensure accurate readings. The transducer's level will have an inverse effect on the blood pressure reading. If the transducer is too high, the blood pressure will read low. If the transducer is too low, the blood pressure will read high. Additionally, the physical therapist will want to ensure a good waveform when accurately assessing blood pressure. The waveform can be impacted by positioning of the limb. For example, the arterial line is commonly placed in the radial artery; wrist flexion can disrupt blood flow (vessel patency), impacting the waveform and pressure reading; ▶ Fig. 7.8).
	13. Following transplant, special precautions should be taken to limit risk of infection, given the patient's immunocompromised status. The patient should don a surgical mask when ambulating outside of his hospital room; subsequently, he will need to wear masks in public places following his discharge from the hospital. He should avoid sick contacts and pay close attention to hand hygiene. Additionally, following transplant, the patient should practice safe food handling and make smart food choices to limit the risk of food-borne infections.

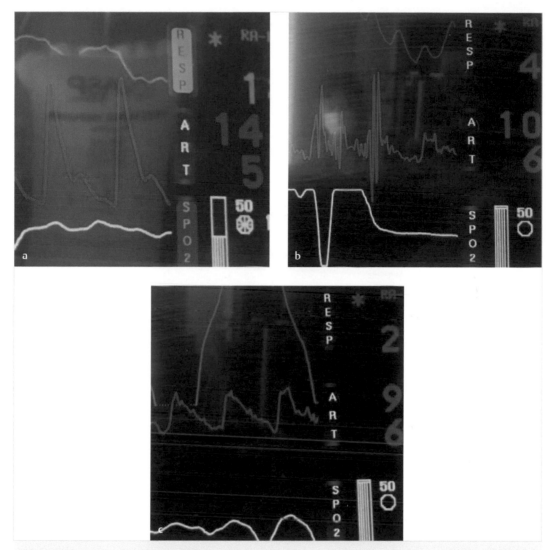

Fig. 7.8 Examples of arterial line waveforms (*red lines*) on a central monitor. **(a)** Good waveform. **(b)** Poor waveform (*artifact*). **(c)** Poor waveform (*overdamped, artifact*).

Key points
1. Following lung transplant, upright positioning and early mobility are essential for promoting gravitational and energetic stressors to the body (which encourage normal physiologic function of the body's systems), as well as limiting deleterious effects of immobility.
2. Inpatient physical therapy interventions should acknowledge and address the negative side effects of immunosuppressive drug regimens (commonplace in patients following transplants) on large proximal muscles groups in the upper and lower extremities.
3. Breathing mechanics should be addressed early and often, following transplant, to promote improved efficiency and decreased work of breathing.

General Information	
Case no.	7.C
Authors	Laura Friedman, PT, DPT, Board Certified Clinical Specialist in Cardiovascular & Pulmonary Physical Therapy Margot Miller, PT, DPT
Diagnosis	Cystic fibrosis (CF) status post (s/p) bilateral lung transplant
Setting	Home
Learner expectations	☑ Initial evaluation ☐ Re-evaluation ☐ Treatment session
Learner objectives	1. List the patient's body structure and impairments. 2. Identify appropriate physical therapy interventions to be performed in the home care setting based on the examination. 3. Understand the overall impact of lung transplant and diagnosis of CF on all body systems.

Medical	
Chief complaint	Generalized deconditioning, dyspnea on exertion
History of present illness	The patient is a 32-year-old man with CF diagnosed at birth. He is s/p bilateral sequential lung transplant via clamshell incision 18 days ago. He was in surgical intensive care unit (ICU) for 6 days and spent the remainder of hospital course on step-down/telemetry unit. He was discharged home from the hospital 2 days ago. Hospitalization surrounding lung transplant was relatively uncomplicated except for difficulty with blood glucose control.
Past medical history	CF, pancreatic insufficiency, osteoporosis, type II diabetes mellitus (DM), malnutrition
Past surgical history	Bilateral sequential lung transplant 18 days ago, gastric tube placement ~10 months ago
Allergies	None
Medications	Acetaminophen, Oxycodone, Prednisone, Bactrim, Tacrolimus (Prograf), Cellcept, Voriconazole (VFend), Valcyte, Folic acid, Vitamin D, Multivitamin, Pancreatic enzymes, Melatonin, Magnesium oxide, Protonix, Senokot, Miralax, Bactrim, Noxafil, Insulin (Lantus), Atrovent
Precautions/orders	Contact precautions; immunocompromised precautions; physical therapy to evaluate and treat; titrate oxygen to maintain $SpO_2 \geq 92\%$

Social history	
Home setup	• Lives in a two-story home with his wife. • Three steps + one handrail to enter. • One flight of steps + one handrail to the second floor, where bedroom and full bathroom are located. • Half bath is on the first floor.
Occupation	• Works as an accountant, primarily sedentary.
Prior level of function	Pretransplant: • Independent with all mobility but primarily limited to household distances. • Independent/modified independent with basic activities of daily living (BADLs), utilizes a shower chair, and reports increased time to complete tasks like dressing and grooming due to shortness of breath with activity. • Wife has largely been handling household chores. • Has active driver's license, but hasn't driven in ~2 months. Posttransplant: • Modified independent for BADLs and functional mobility. • Has been sleeping on the first floor, has not negotiated flight of steps to master bedroom since returning home. • On room air at rest, 1 to 2 L/min for activity.
Recreational activities	• Played soccer until about 3 years ago, but reports it became too hard on his breathing. • Has a treadmill at home, but only able to walk for 2- to 3-minute bouts prior to transplant. • Enjoys hiking with his wife.

Imaging/diagnostic test	Results (from day of hospital discharge)
Pulmonary function tests	Forced vital capacity (FVC): 3.78 Forced expiratory volume in 1 second (FEV1): 2.54 FEV1/FVC: 67 Findings/impression: FVC is moderately reduced (60–69%); FEV1 is moderate to severely reduced (50–59%); FEV1/FVC is normal; a mild obstructive defect is present.

Pause points
Based on the above information, what are the priorities? • Diagnostic tests and measures? • Outcome measures? • Treatment interventions?

Physical Therapy Examination
Subjective
"I want to be able to easily climb stairs so able to sleep upstairs with my wife again."

Objective			
Vitals	**Resting**	**Maximum with exercise**	**Postexercise**
Blood pressure (mmHg)	124/66	140/66	128/66
Heart rate (beats/min)	110	134	114
Respiratory rate (breaths/min)	18	36	20
Pulse oximetry (SpO$_2$)	96% on room air	99% on 2 L/min via nasal cannula	95% on room air
Modified Borg Dyspnea Scale	0/10	5/10	1/10
Pain	2/10 (chest incisional pain)	3/10 (chest incisional pain)	2/10 (chest incisional pain)
General	• Patient on room air sitting in a chair at the kitchen table. • Patient has no ancillary equipment; however, a portable oxygen tank is noted to be in the room, with an oxygen concentrator in the master bedroom. • Observations: thin male, rounded shoulders, mild thoracic kyphosis, barrel chest, moderate clubbing noted to fingers and toes, and no cyanosis. Clamshell incision and previous chest tube sites intact, healing well and open to air, and patient reports no drainage.		
Head, ears, eyes, nose, and throat (HEENT)	• Patient wears contacts/glasses (otherwise intact) and reports no vision changes since transplant.		
Cardiovascular and pulmonary	• Normal rate and rhythm. Normal S1, S2 • Lung auscultation: clear throughout • No edema noted in upper or lower extremities • Cough: strong, currently nonproductive. Patients reports minimal clear secretions throughout the day • Breathing pattern: symmetrical, no accessory muscle use noted at rest		
Gastrointestinal	• Gastric tube intact. Patient reports that he hasn't used it in over a week and hopeful will be removed in a couple months). • Patient reports occasional nausea, which attributes to meds.		
Musculoskeletal	Range of motion	• Bilateral shoulder flexion: 0 to ~100 degrees • Bilateral shoulder abduction: 0 to ~100 degrees • Bilateral elbow flexion/extension: within functional limit (WFL) • Bilateral wrist flexion/extension: WFL • Bilateral lower extremity (BLE): WFL	

(Continued)

(Continued)

Physical Therapy Examination		
	Strength	• Bilateral shoulder flexion: 3 + /5 • Bilateral shoulder abduction: 3 + /5 • Bilateral elbow flexion: 4 + /5 • Bilateral elbow extension: 4 + /5 • Bilateral wrist flexion: 4 + /5 • Bilateral wrist extension: 4 + /5 • Bilateral grip strength: 4 + /5 • Bilateral hip flexion: 3 + /5 • Bilateral hip abduction: 3 + /5 • Bilateral hip extension: 3 + /5 • Bilateral knee flexion: 4/5 • Bilateral knee extension: 4/5 • Bilateral ankle dorsiflexion: 5/5 • Bilateral knee plantar flexion: 5/5 • Five Times Sit-to-Stand: 14.5 seconds
	Aerobic	• 6-Minute Walk Test: 865 feet (264 m) (completed day of discharge from hospital)
	Flexibility	• Decreased flexibility throughout trunk noted • Bilateral hamstring tightness noted
Neurological	Balance	• Sitting, static, and dynamic: independent • Standing, static: independent • Standing, dynamic: supervision • Single leg stance: < 5 seconds bilaterally
	Cognition	• Alert and oriented (A&O) × 4 • Follows 100% of one-step commands
	Coordination	• Finger to nose: intact bilaterally • Heel to shin: intact bilaterally
	Cranial Nerves	• II–XII: intact
	Reflexes	• Patellar: 2 + bilaterally • Achilles: 2 + bilaterally
	Sensation	• Bilateral upper extremity (BUE) and BLE: intact to light touch intact—reported numbness to areas of anterior chest since transplant surgery.
	Tone	• Normal throughout BUEs and BLEs
Functional status		
Bed mobility		• Rolling either direction: independent • Supine to/from sit: independent
Transfers		• Sit to/from stand: modified independent, utilizes upper extremities from low surfaces • Stand pivot transfer: supervision
Ambulation		• Ambulated 175 feet with supervision, able to push portable oxygen tank independently. • Gait deviations notable for decreased cadence, decreased step length, decreased heel strike; minimal kyphosis also noted.
Stairs		• Ascend/descend 12 steps + 1 handrail with supervision, demonstrating step-to pattern.

Assessment	
☑ Physical therapist's	*Assessment left blank for learner to develop*
Goals	
Patient's	"To be able to go hiking this summer with wife"
Short term	1.
	Goals left blank for learner to develop.
	2.
Long term	1.
	Goals left blank for learner to develop.
	2.

Plan	
☐ Physician's ☑ Physical therapist's ☐ Other's	Will continue to see the patient two to three times a week × 4 weeks. Treatment will include gait and stair training, therapeutic exercises (proximal lower extremity and upper extremity strengthening, stretching, postural exercises), dynamic standing balance exercises, endurance training, breathing exercises, and energy conservation strategies.

Bloom's Taxonomy Level	Case 7.C Questions
Create	1. Synthesizing the medical data and physical examination findings, develop an appropriate physical therapy assessment of the patient. 2. Develop two short-term physical therapy goals, including an appropriate timeframe. 3. Develop two long-term physical therapy goals, including an appropriate timeframe.
Evaluate	4. What clinical signs and symptoms should the physical therapist monitor for that could be indicative of organ rejection? 5. How should the physical therapist evaluate the patient's need for continued oxygen? How should the physical therapist educate the patient to monitor need for oxygen use throughout the day?
Analyze	6. When comparing the Pulmonary Function Test from pretransplant, has it improved? Why is the patient's Pulmonary Function Test still abnormal? Will it ever be normal again?
Apply	7. Design and implement two interventions to improve dynamic standing balance. 8. Design and implement five therapeutic exercises to improve the patient's quadriceps strength. 9. Once the surgical incision is well healed, what are scar management strategies that the patient can perform?
Understand	10. How should the physical therapist educate the patient on the difference between hypoxia and decreased endurance/activity tolerance to aid in weaning oxygen use? 11. Will there be pulmonary manifestations of CF post lung transplant? Will the patient still need to use his Aerobika and vest for airway clearance?
Remember	12. Does a lung transplant cure CF? 13. Is it important for patients post lung transplant to live a healthy lifestyle and participate in an exercise routine for their life's duration? What is the survival rate for patients with CF post lung transplant?

Bloom's Taxonomy Level	Case 7.C Answers
Create	1. The patient is a 32-year-old man with CF s/p bilateral sequential lung transplant discharged from hospital 2 days ago. Upon initial evaluation, the patient presents with bilateral proximal lower extremity muscular weakness, postural dysfunction, impaired dynamic standing balance, and impaired endurance as demonstrated by the 6-Minute Walk Test, which was performed on the day of hospital discharge. All of these impairments contribute to the patient's inability to walk for long distances or duration, increased difficulty with stair negotiation, and inability to engage in usual

(Continued)

Bloom's Taxonomy Level	Case 7.C Answers
	exercise and sport activities. The patient would benefit from continued physical therapy to optimize strength, balance, and endurance to maximize return to functional independence and eventual return to work and sports. The patient is an excellent candidate for skilled physical therapy services as motivated to optimize strength and conditioning to "return to normal." 2. Short-term goals: • The patient will increase hip flexor strength to >/=4/5 manual muscle testing (MMT) grade within 2 weeks to allow for modified independent reciprocal stair negotiation of 12 steps. • The patient will decrease Five Times Sit-to-Stand time to < 11 seconds within 2 weeks to show improved strength. 3. Long-term goals: • Patient will be able to tandem walk for 20 feet within 4 weeks to demonstrate improved dynamic standing balance. • Patient will increase 6-Minute Walk Test by 200 feet within 4 weeks to demonstrate improved endurance and ability to return to leisure/sports activities.
Evaluate	4. Signs and symptoms of organ rejection include fever, feeling of general malaise/lethargy, new onset of dyspnea on exertion or shortness of breath, decline in functional activity tolerance, increasing oxygen requirements, decrease in Pulmonary Function Test values, change in sputum, incisional redness or new onset of drainage from incision, nausea, vomiting, or diarrhea. If these signs or symptoms occur, the physical therapist should call the patient's physician or lung transplant coordinator immediately. 5. The best way to monitor the patient's oxygen saturation in the home care setting is through the use of a finger pulse oximeter. The continuous supplemental oxygen should be increased or decreased to maintain the oxygen saturation ≥ 92% per the physician order. The patient should have his own pulse oximeter to evaluate his oxygen throughout the day to ensure receiving appropriate amounts. The pulse oximeter should have a heart rate on it as well and this heart rate should correlate with the patient's actual pulse (i.e., radial pulse) to ensure accuracy of the pulse oximeter readings. The pulse oximeters are not always accurate if there is decreased blood flow to fingers for any reason or during exercise.
Analyze	6. The pulmonary function tests did improve from the pretransplant pulmonary function tests but are still abnormal. The tests are still abnormal because this individual's respiratory status is still recovering from the recent lung transplant surgery. The Pulmonary Function Test values of this patient can return to a normal value; however, it may take up to a year post lung transplant. Pulmonary function tests and home spirometry are important tests to not only show improved lung function in the first year but also to show possible rejection or infection. A decrease in FVC > 11% and a decrease in FEV1 > 12% are considered significant indicators of rejection or infection in bilateral lung transplant recipients.
Apply	7. Two interventions to improve dynamic standing balance are single leg stance and tandem stance progressing to tandem walking. For single leg stance, the patient should stand in front of the counter or stable surface to allow for upper extremity support initially and progress to no upper extremity support and increased time on each lower extremity. The goal is for 30 seconds on each lower extremity without upper extremity support. For tandem stance, have the heel of one foot in front of the toes of the other foot (feet touching) and maintain this position for up to 30 seconds. Repeat with the opposite foot in front. Once successful in maintaining static tandem stances, progress to walking with the heel of one foot touching the toes of the other foot with each step. 8. To improve quad strengthening, five potential exercises the patient could perform are wall slides, mini squats, straight leg raises, step-ups, and lunges. Exercises could be progressed with external weights, number of repetitions (for endurance), and/or step height for step-ups. 9. Scar management is important once the incision itself is well healed to prevent abnormal scar formation and improve skin elasticity Typically, it takes 4 to 6 weeks of healing prior to initiation of scar massage. Scar massage is meant to loosen any deeper adhesions and decrease sensitivity. With scar massage, you can use the index

(Continued)

Bloom's Taxonomy Level	Case 7.C Answers
	and middle finger to perform circular, up-and-down, and side-to-side motions directly on the incision. Cocoa butter, lotion, or petroleum jelly can be used in conjunction with the massage. Silicone gel in sheets or liquid is also commonly used to help with optimal scar healing. Finally, stretching exercises can be utilized to enhance elasticity of the entire thoracic cavity.
Understand	10. It is very common for individuals post lung transplant to have difficulty weaning from supplemental oxygen. Hypoxia occurs when the body does not receive adequate oxygen supply at the tissue level and is seen in patients with chronic lung disease. The best way to measure hypoxia is through arterial blood gases and the use of finger pulse oximeters. Individuals after lung transplant will feel short of breath due to deconditioning associated with the surgery and chronic illness, but this does not necessarily mean the individual is hypoxic. It is important to explain the difference to these individuals and teach them to continue to utilize their pulse oximeters so that they are able to determine when there is a true need for oxygen. Shortness of breath and dyspnea on exertion are common for anybody starting a new exercise program (i.e., training for a marathon) or recovering from a major surgery, but it does not necessarily correlate with hypoxia and a need for supplemental oxygen. 11. After this patient received a lung transplant, he no longer has CF in his lungs. Therefore, the routine airway clearance that was indicated prior to transplant is no longer indicated. However, immediately postoperatively, and anytime there is a pulmonary infection, airway clearance will likely be indicated. Airway clearance devices, such as the Aerobika, acapella, and/or vest, may be utilized in the immediate postoperative period or during infections, but no longer mandated multiple times a day when an infection is not present.
Remember	12. CF is a disease that affects the lungs, digestive system, sweat glands, and the reproductive tract. Patients with CF have abnormal transport of chloride and sodium across secretory epithelia, resulting in thickened, viscous secretions in the bronchi, biliary tract, pancreas, intestines, and reproductive system. A lung transplant does not cure the individual of CF, but the individual should be cured of the pulmonary manifestation associated with CF. However, the individual can still have pulmonary manifestations in the setting of infection or rejection. Treatment will need to continue posttransplant to manage the CF in the other organs. Liver failure is also common in individuals with CF and some individuals require liver transplants. There all also health risks associated with transplant such as malignancy and renal failure due to immunosuppressive medications. 13. It is extremely important that individuals, post lung transplant, maintain a healthy and active lifestyle to optimize survival and stave off the side effects associated with all the transplant meds. It has been shown that despite normal lung function in many post lungs transplants, exercise capacity never returns to normal due to peripheral muscle dysfunction. It is important to ensure aerobic and strengthening exercises are part of daily routine to maximize function and overall health. Individuals with CF have improved survival rate compared to lung transplants for other diseases as measured by median survival (8.3 years for CF; 5.7 years for all transplants) or median survival conditional on survival to 1 year (10.5 years for CF; 7.9 years for all transplants). The International Society for Heart and Lung Transplantation (ISHLT) 2019 data reports indicate the survival rate for adults s/p lung transplant as follows: 1-year survival is ~87%; 5-year survival is ~65%; and 10-year survival is ~50% (▶ Fig. 7.9).

Key points

1. Consider what impairments are related to CF and can be improved upon, as well as impact on lung transplant surgery on these impairments, especially posture and proximal strength.

2. When able and appropriate, utilize the same outcome measures across settings to track progression versus regression and can often utilize electronic medical records to review outcome measures (i.e., 6-Minute Walking Test) previously performed.

3. Consider physical therapy interventions that can be implemented within the home that the patient enjoys and provide appropriate progressions to allow for independent continuation throughout their life span.

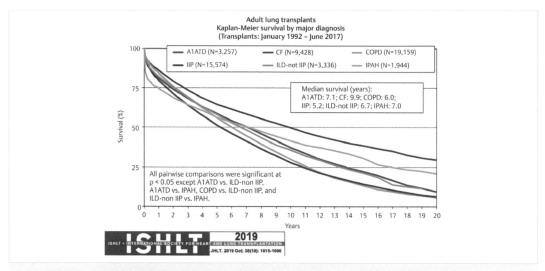

Fig. 7.9 Adult lung transplants Kaplan-Meier survival by major diagnosis. Adapted from ISHLT, 2019 https://ishltregistries.org/registries/slides.asp.

Suggested Readings

6-minute walk test. Available at: https://www.sralab.org/rehabilitation-measures/6-minute-walk-test. Accessed June 1, 2020

Bartels MN, Armstrong HF, Gerardo RE, et al. Evaluation of pulmonary function and exercise performance by cardiopulmonary exercise testing before and after lung transplantation. Chest. 2011; 140(6):1604–1611

Belle-van Meerkerk G, van de Graaf EA, Kwakkel-van Erp JM, et al. Diabetes before and after lung transplantation in patients with cystic fibrosis and other lung diseases. Diabet Med. 2012; 29(8):e159–e162

Button BM, Wilson C, Dentice R, et al. Physiotherapy for cystic fibrosis in Australia and New Zealand: a clinical practice guideline. Respirology. 2016; 21(4):656–667

Chowdhury TA. Post-transplant diabetes mellitus. Clin Med (Lond). 2019; 19(5):392–395

Currie S, Greenwood K, Weber L, et al. Physical activity levels in individuals with cystic fibrosis-related diabetes. Physiother Can. 2017; 69(2):171–177

Five Times Sit to Stand. Available at: https://www.sralab.org/rehabilitation-measures/five-times-sit-stand-test. Accessed June 1, 2020

Flume PA, Robinson KA, O'Sullivan BP, et al. Clinical Practice Guidelines for Pulmonary Therapies Committee. Cystic fibrosis pulmonary guidelines: airway clearance therapies. Respir Care. 2009; 54(4):522–537

Frownfelter DL, Dean E, eds. Cardiovascular and Pulmonary Physical Therapy: Evidence to Practice. 5th ed. St Louis, MO: Elsevier/Mosby; 2012

Fuller LM, Button B, Tarrant B, et al. Longer versus shorter duration of supervised rehabilitation after lung transplantation: a randomized trial. Arch Phys Med Rehabil. 2017; 98(2):220–226.e3

Gloeckl R, Halle M, Kenn K. Interval versus continuous training in lung transplant candidates: a randomized trial. J Heart Lung Transplant. 2012; 31(9):934–941

Goodman CC, Fuller KS. Pathology: Implications for the Physical Therapist. Philadelphia, PA: WB Saunders; 2015

Gulve EA. Exercise and glycemic control in diabetes: benefits, challenges, and adjustments to pharmacotherapy. Phys Ther. 2008; 88(11):1297–1321

Gupta A, Gupta Y. Glucocorticoid-induced myopathy: pathophysiology, diagnosis, and treatment. Indian J Endocrinol Metab. 2013; 17(5):913–916

Hackman KL, Bailey MJ, Snell GI, Bach LA. Diabetes is a major risk factor for mortality after lung transplantation. Am J Transplant. 2014; 14(2):438–445

Hatt K, Kinback NC, Shah A, Cruz E, Altschuler EL. A review of lung transplantation and its implications for the acute inpatient rehabilitation team. PM R. 2017; 9(3):294–305

Hirche TO, Knoop C, Hebestreit H, et al. ECORN-CF Study Group. Practical guidelines: lung transplantation in patients with cystic fibrosis. Pulm Med. 2014; 2014:621342

Knols RH, Fischer N, Kohlbrenner D, Manettas A, de Bruin ED. Replicability of physical exercise interventions in lung transplant recipients; a systematic review. Front Physiol. 2018; 9:946

Li M, Mathur S, Chowdhury NA, Helm D, Singer LG. Pulmonary rehabilitation in lung transplant candidates. J Heart Lung Transplant. 2013; 32(6):626–632

Lynch JP, III, Sayah DM, Belperio JA, Weigt SS. Lung transplantation for cystic fibrosis: results, indications, complications, and controversies. Semin Respir Crit Care Med. 2015; 36(2):299–320

Mailhot G, Dion N, Farlay D, et al. Impaired rib bone mass and quality in end-stage cystic fibrosis patients. Bone. 2017; 98:9–17

Martin C, Chapron J, Hubert D, et al. Prognostic value of six minute walk test in cystic fibrosis adults. Respir Med. 2013; 107(12):1881–1887

Mitchell MJ, Baz MA, Fulton MN, Lisor CF, Braith RW. Resistance training prevents vertebral osteoporosis in lung transplant recipients. Transplantation. 2003; 76(3):557–562

Orava C, Fitzgerald J, Figliomeni S, et al. Relationship between physical activity and fatigue in adults with cystic fibrosis. Physiother Can. 2018; 70(1):42–48

Pêgo-Fernandes PM, Abrão FC, Fernandes FLA, Caramori ML, Samano MN, Jatene FB. Spirometric assessment of lung transplant patients: one year follow-up. Clinics (São Paulo). 2009; 64(6):519–525

Radtke T, Nevitt SJ, Hebestreit H, Kriemler S. Physical exercise training for cystic fibrosis. Cochrane Database Syst Rev. 2017; 11 (11):CD002768

Rovedder PME, Borba GC, Anderle M, et al. Peripheral muscle strength is associated with lung function and functional capacity in patients with cystic fibrosis. Physiother Res Int. 2019; 24(3):e1771

Saiman L, Siegel JD, LiPuma JJ, et al. Cystic Fibrous Foundation, Society for Healthcare Epidemiology of America. Infection prevention and control guideline for cystic fibrosis: 2013 update. Infect Control Hosp Epidemiol. 2014; 35 Suppl 1:S1–S67

Sheppard E, Chang K, Cotton J, et al. Functional tests of leg muscle strength and power in adults with cystic fibrosis. Respir Care. 2019; 64(1):40–47

Shoemaker MJ, Hurt H, Arndt L. The evidence regarding exercise training in the management of cystic fibrosis: a systematic review. Cardiopulm Phys Ther J. 2008; 19(3):75–83

Six-minute walk test. Available at: https://www.sralab.org/rehabilitation-measures/6-minute-walk-test#pulmonary-diseases. Accessed May 28, 2020

Stephenson AL, Sykes J, Berthiaume Y, et al. Clinical and demographic factors associated with post-lung transplantation survival in individuals with cystic fibrosis. J Heart Lung Transplant. 2015; 34(9):1139–1145

Tarrant BJ, Holland A, Le Maitre C, et al. The timing and extent of acute physiotherapy involvement following lung transplantation: an observational study. Physiother Res Int. 2018; 23(3): e1710

Walsh JR, Chambers DC, Davis RJ, et al. Impaired exercise capacity after lung transplantation is related to delayed recovery of muscle strength. Clin Transplant. 2013; 27(4):E504–E511

Ward N, Stiller K, Holland AE, Australian Cystic Fibrosis Exercise Survey group. Exercise is commonly used as a substitute for traditional airway clearance techniques by adults with cystic fibrosis in Australia: a survey. J Physiother. 2019; 65(1):43–50

Wickerson L, Mathur S, Brooks D. Exercise training after lung transplantation: a systematic review. J Heart Lung Transplant. 2010; 29(5):497–503

Wickerson L, Mathur S, Singer LG, Brooks D. Physical activity levels early after lung transplantation. Phys Ther. 2015; 95(4):517–525

8 Diabetes Mellitus

General Information	
Case no.	8.A Diabetes Mellitus
Authors	Sheena MacFarlane, PT, DPT, Board Certified Clinical Specialist in Cardiovascular & Pulmonary Physical Therapy Melissa Brown MSPAS, PA-C
Diagnosis	Type 2 diabetes mellitus (DM) with peripheral neuropathy
Setting	Outpatient clinic
Learner expectations	☑ Initial evaluation ☐ Re-evaluation ☐ Treatment session
Learner objectives	1. Explain the pathophysiology of the patient's diagnosis. 2. Relate the pathophysiology and progression of pathology to clinical manifestations and activity/participation limitations seen in physical therapy practice. 3. Select, implement, and interpret physical therapy interventions based on the medical examination findings.

Medical	
Chief complaint	Loss of balance and bilateral foot pain
History of present illness	The patient is a 68-year-old woman with a long-standing history of uncontrolled type 2 diabetes. She was referred to outpatient physical therapy for evaluation and treatment of balance deficits and bilateral foot pain. She has been experiencing bilateral foot pain for the past 5 years. She describes the pain as an intermittent burning sensation of both feet, which she rates as a 6/10. She also notes worsening left ankle pain over the past month. She describes the ankle pain as a "nagging" 4/10 pain. She has been feeling unsteady on her feet and fallen three times in the past 3 months. She fell once in the shower, outside on uneven surfaces, and when ascending stairs to enter the home. She is intermittently compliant with medications and does not follow a diabetic diet.
Past medical history	Type 2 DM—uncontrolled with peripheral neuropathy, nephropathy, and retinopathy; hypertension (HTN), hyperlipidemia, coronary artery disease (CAD) with a myocardial infarction (MI) 6 years ago.
Past surgical history	Coronary artery bypass grafting (CABG) × 4 vessels 6 years ago
Allergies	Penicillin: rash
Medications	Metformin, Sitagliptin, Glipizide, Dapagliflozin, Lisinopril, Amlodipine, Metoprolol, Simvastatin, Aspirin
Precautions/orders	Activity as tolerated

Social history	
Home setup	• Resides in a single-level home alone. • Two steps without handrail to enter. • Flight of stairs + one handrail to basement where laundry is located. • No grab bars in the bathroom.
Occupation	• Part-time librarian, reduced hours from full time 6 years ago.
Prior level of function	• Independent with functional mobility and activities of daily living (ADLs); however, he admits to being a "furniture walker." • Modified independence for stairs, required increased time. • Leans on a shopping cart when grocery shopping. • (+) driver
Recreational activities	• Primarily reading and knitting • Previously enjoyed shopping but fatigues quickly.

Lab		Reference range	Results (from outpatient visits 2 weeks ago)
Complete blood count	Hemoglobin	14.0–17.4 d/dL	13.2 g/dL
	Hematocrit	42–52%	41.8%
	White blood cell	5.0–10.0 × 10⁹/L	9,200/µL
	Platelets	140,000–400,000/µL	284,000/µL
Electrolytes	Calcium	8.6–10.3 mg/dL	10.1
	Chloride	98–108 mEq/L	104
	Magnesium	1.2–1.9 mEq/L	1.4
	Phosphate	2.3–4.1 mg/dL	3.8
	Potassium	3.7–5.1 mEq/L	4.8
	Sodium	134–142 mEq/L	141
	Blood urea nitrogen	7–20 mg/d	20
	Creatinine	0.5–1.4	1.8
Other	Glucose	60–110 mg/dL	268
	Hemoglobin A1C	<5.7%	8.9%
	Total cholesterol	<200 mg/dL	180
	High-density lipoprotein (HDL)	>35 mg/dL	32
	Low-density lipoprotein (LDL)	<130 mg/dL	128
	Triglycerides	<150 mg/dL	254

Pause points
Based on the above information, what are the priorities? • Lab values? • Outcome measures? • Treatment interventions?

Physical Therapy Examination
Subjective
"Can you help me with my feet? I don't want to fall again."
Objective

Vital signs	Pre-treatment			Post-treatment
	Supine	Sitting	Standing	Sitting
Blood pressure (mmHg)	140/86	142/84	138/86	138/82
Heart rate (beats/min)	62	64	60	68
Respiratory rate (breaths/min)	16	18	16	18
Pulse oximetry on room air (SpO₂)	100	97	98	99
Borg Scale	1/10	2/10	3/10	2/10
Pain	3/10 bilateral feet			4/10 bilateral feet
General	• The patient is sitting comfortably in the waiting room. • The patient does not appear to be in distress. • Observations notable for obese body habitus.			

(Continued)

(Continued)

Physical Therapy Examination		
Head, ears, eyes, nose, and throat (HEENT)	• Normocephalic, atraumatic • Pupils equal, round, responsive to light • Mucous membranes are moist	
Cardiovascular and pulmonary	• Auscultation: normal heart rate. No murmurs, rubs, or gallops • Lungs clear to auscultation • Pulses: dorsalis pedis and posterior tibial: left: 1+, right: 2+ Femoral: bilateral: 2+ • Left foot and ankle appear pale, cool to touch	
Gastrointestinal	• Rounded, no hepatosplenomegaly	
Musculoskeletal	Range of motion (ROM)	• Bilateral upper extremity (BUE): within functional range • Bilateral lower extremity (BLE): within functional range except bilateral dorsiflexion: 5 degrees
	Strength	• Bilateral shoulder flexion: 4+/5 • Bilateral elbow flexion: 5/5 • Bilateral wrist extension: 4/5 • Bilateral hip flexion: 4+/5 • Bilateral knee extension: 5/5 • Right ankle dorsiflexion: 4/5 • Left ankle dorsiflexion: 3+/5
	Aerobic	• 6-Minute Walk Test: 90 feet (27 m) in 2 minutes and 12 seconds. • Patient experienced two losses of balance with second loss of balance requiring a chair.
	Flexibility	• Not assessed
	Other	• Left forefoot collapse • 2-cm callus metatarsal head of left foot
Neurological	Balance	• Timed Up and Go (TUG): 22.4 seconds • Five Times Sit-to-Stand Test: 12.2 seconds
	Cognition	• Alert and oriented × 4
	Coordination	• Finger to nose: intact bilaterally • Heel to shin: intact bilaterally
	Cranial nerves	• II–XII: intact
	Reflexes	• Patellar: 2+ bilaterally • Achilles: 1+ bilaterally

	Sensation	• Proximal L4: intact to vibratory sensation bilaterally (17 seconds)
		• Distal L4 and L5: decreased bilateral vibratory sensation at great toe (5 seconds) and medial malleolus (7 seconds) bilaterally
		• Distal L4/L5/S1: absent to crude touch bilaterally
		• Monofilament testing (▶ Fig. 8.1a):
		  ○ Intact at proximal L4 bilaterally; tested at patella
		  ○ Absent at L4/L5/S1 bilaterally; tested at distal phalanges (1–5; ▶ Fig. 8.1b), hallux, navicular, and plantar aspect calcaneus

	Tone	• BUE and BLE: normal

(Continued)

(Continued)

Physical Therapy Examination	
Functional status	
Bed mobility	• Supine to/from sit: independent
Transfers	• Sit to/from stand: modified independent with use of hands
Ambulation	• Ambulates 50 feet with supervision with no assistive device. • Gait deviations notable for decreased cadence, decreased bilateral step length, (+) loss of balance using a stepping strategy to correct.
Stairs	• Ascend/descend four steps with modified independence using one handrail. • Step-to pattern noted

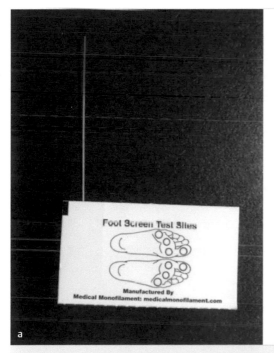 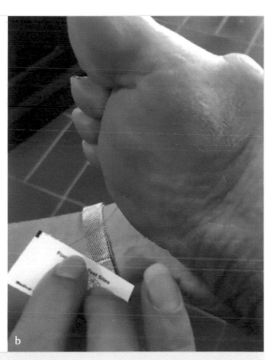

Fig. 8.1 (a,b) ADA diabetic foot screening test with 10 g monofilament.

Assessment	
☑ Physical therapist's	*Assessment left blank for learner to develop.*
Goals	
Patient's	"I would like to never fall again."
Short term	1. *Goals left blank for learner to develop.* 2.
Long term	1. *Goals left blank for learner to develop.* 2.

Plan	
☐ Physician's ☑ Physical therapist's ☐ Other's	Will treat patient thrice a week with balance and endurance interventions to progress functional mobility and safety.

Bloom's Taxonomy Level	Case 8.A Questions
Create	1. Synthesizing the medical data and physical examination findings, develop an appropriate physical therapy assessment of the patient. 2. Develop two short-term physical therapy goals, including an appropriate timeframe. 3. Develop two long-term physical therapy goals, including an appropriate timeframe.
Evaluate	4. For a patient with DM, what pathology contributes to gait dysfunction? Give specific gait deviations. 5. List at least three other health care providers that the patient should be referred to optimize management and the rationale.
Analyze	6. Explain the pathophysiology and clinical manifestations of decreased palpable dorsalis pedis and posterior tibial pulses. 7. Interpret the results of TUG, Five Times Sit-to-Stand Test, and 6-Minute Walk Test.
Apply	8. Design and implement two interventions to improve this patient's balance and decrease her fall risk. 9. Design and implement an intervention to address this patient's endurance deficits. 10. Based on lab values, pertinent past medical history, and physical therapy findings, what educational interventions should be provided to this patient?
Understand	11. What are the physical therapy implications of the above medications?
Remember	12. Which of the patient's medication causes a low heart rate? 13. What is the difference between type 1 DM and type 2 DM? 14. What balance strategies are there (aside from the stepping strategy)?

Bloom's Taxonomy Level	Case 8.A Answers

Create	1. The patient is a 68-year-old woman with a past medical history of type 2 DM complicated by peripheral neuropathy, HTN, CAD with resultant MI, and CABG, presenting to the clinic today with bilateral foot pain described as "burning" and three falls in the past 3 months. She ambulates without an assistive device but reports using furniture/shopping carts to stabilize herself as needed. The patient presents with ankle weakness, limited ankle dorsiflexion ROM, decreased sensation in BLE, and impaired balance. All of these contribute to impaired functional mobility and decreased safety. The patient would benefit from physical therapy to address her ROM, strength, endurance, balance, function, and safety. Will continue to follow.
	2. Short-term goals:
	  • Patient will improve her dynamic standing balance as evident by a score of 15 seconds on the TUG within 8 sessions to improve safety.
	  • Patient will ambulate 250 feet with a least restrictive assistive device independently without loss of balance within 8 sessions to improve functional mobility and safety.
	3. Long-term goals:
	  • Patient will ambulate 540 meters with least restrictive assistive device on the 6MWT without loss of balance within 16 sessions to demonstrate improved endurance.
	  • Patient will independently ascend/descend 13 steps with a single handrail, demonstrating reciprocal step pattern, within 16 sessions to improve safety at home.

Evaluate	4. DM presents with various polyneuropathies, including autonomic nervous system neuropathies (vestibular and visual), diabetic peripheral neuropathy, affecting sensory and muscle strength. Diabetic peripheral neuropathy is the progressive loss of peripheral sensation in BUEs and BLEs, with a stocking glove presentation as the distal component most impaired. Individually or collectively, loss of peripheral sensation, limb proprioception, and/or vestibular and visual input can lead to gait deviations. Such gait deviations may include decreased speed, impaired swing phase with shorter step length, impaired terminal stance phase with decreased force production, and/or wide base of support.

(Continued)

(Continued)

Bloom's Taxonomy Level	Case 8.A Answers
	5. Other health care providers that the patient should be referred to include, but not limited to, podiatrist, primary care physician, nutritionist, ophthalmologist, and/or diabetic educator. A podiatrist could address her pain and peripheral neuropathy via custom shoes and education, as well as provide proper nail care. Her primary care physician could address her uncontrolled HTN, her uncontrolled type 2 DM, and her undiagnosed decreased pulses, pain, and pale lower extremities. A nutritionist could address dietary intake for weight loss and improving her lab values (specifically fasting glucose, hemoglobin A1C, cholesterol, and triglycerides). An ophthalmologist screens annually for diabetic retinopathy. Diabetic educators are a great resource for overall education about the disease and appropriate self-care.
Analyze	6. The patient has bilateral + 1 dorsalis pedis and posterior tibial pulses. + 1 is defined as a "thready" pulse or easily obliterated with slight pressure. Individuals with DM tend to have earlier onset atherosclerotic changes effecting peripheral arteries. Atherosclerosis leads to peripheral arterial disease (PAD), which presents with decreased distal pulses, lower extremity pain that worsens with lower extremity elevation, and pale skin of the affected distal extremities. Lower extremity hair loss, claudication, and arterial ulcerations can also be seen with PAD. 7. • The patient's TUG score of 22.4 seconds is slower than the age-based norm of 15 seconds for community-dwelling adults with comorbidities, indicating impaired balance, positive fall risk, and impaired walking ability. • The patient's Five Times Sit-to-Stand Test score of 12.2 seconds is slower than the age-based norm of 11.4 seconds for community-dwelling geriatric adults, indicating impaired strength, transfer function, and increased fall risk. • The patient's 6MWT of 27 meters prior to loss of balance and termination of the test is well below age-based normative data for geriatric women, 538 feet.
Apply	8. Since the patient is currently falling one time per month for the last 3 months, has balance deficits as identified on the TUG score and Five Times Sit-to-Stand Test, and ankle weakness, addressing lower extremity strength and balance should be prioritized. Two potential interventions are: • Standing heel raises while holding a stable object: This weight-bearing activity would focus on ankle strength and dynamic balance. • Single leg stance static balance: This would emphasize ankle muscle strengthening in weight-bearing position and assist in activation of ankle strategy for balance. 9. Since the patient is currently only ambulating household distances and endurance deficits as identified on the 6MWT, endurance interventions are indicated. Two potential interventions are: • Seated (recumbent or upright) bicycle 30 to 50% of peak work rates for 10 minutes with rest breaks as needed. • Upper body ergometer (UBE) 30 to 50% of peak work rates for 5 to 10 minutes with rest breaks as needed. Both of these interventions have her in a seated position and therefore optimize safety until standing balance is improved. 10. • Due to physical therapy findings of fall risk TUG score and Five Times Sit-to-Stand Test score, physical therapy should educate on methods to decrease her risk of falls while she improves her balance via ongoing physical therapy: environmental modifications at home, benefits of a rollator for household ambulation to allow for seated rest breaks as needed, benefits of a commode to utilize at night next to the bed, and requesting family assistance with community-based ADL. • Due to past medical history of type 2 DM with hemoglobin A1C of 8.9%, the physical therapist should educate on methods to prevent skin breakdown on her feet: daily diabetic skin checks, diabetics socks, and appropriately fitted shoes. • Due to past medical history of CAD and MI with lab values of triglycerides 254 and LDL 128, and type 2 DM with correlating lab values, the physical therapist should educate on benefits of exercise to decrease cardiac risk factors (triglycerides, HDL, LDL, cholesterol, inactivity) and optimize her glucose metabolism, as well as timing exercise around meals and DM medication.

(Continued)

(Continued)

Bloom's Taxonomy Level	Case 8.A Answers
Understand	11.
	• Metformin, sitagliptin, glipizide, dapagliflozin are all medications for control of glucose in the bloodstream. Glipizide promotes glucose-independent insulin release, which places the patient at high risk of developing hypoglycemia. The physical therapy implications are timing meals, medication administration, and exercise to prevent hypoglycemia.
	• Lisinopril and amlodipine can cause orthostatic hypotension.
	• Metoprolol causes a blunted heart rate response to exercise or any activation of the sympathetic nervous system. The physical therapist should utilize rate of perceived exertion (Borg rating of perceived exertion) for exercise intensity assessment, instead of heart rate.
	• Simvastatin is to decrease LDL level in the bloodstream, which causes statin-induced myopathy (muscle weakness, muscle pain, and muscle inflammation) in 5 to 10% of patients taking statins. Screening for statin-induced myopathy is an important part of physical therapy evaluation and physical therapy treatment sessions. Progression of statin-induced myopathy to rhabdomyolysis is another adverse effect of statins.
	• Aspirin inhibits platelet aggregation and is utilized post-MI to maintain coronary artery perfusion but can cause hemorrhaging.
Remember	12. Metoprolol is a selective beta-blocker, and therefore can lower heart rate.
	13. Type 1 DM is categorized by little to no endogenous insulin production requiring exogenous insulin to treat; onset is usually abrupt prior to 20 years of age and is most often associated with autoimmune destruction of pancreatic beta cells. Type 2 DM is categorized by varying insulin production linked to obesity-associated insulin resistance with a gradual onset. Incidence of type 2 DM increases with age. Type 2 DM can be treated with weight loss, lifestyle modifications, oral medications, and exogenous insulin. Type 2 DM is much more prevalent compared to type 1 DM.
	14. The balance strategies utilized by the body to maintain the center of mass over the base of support are ankle, hip, and stepping strategies. Ankle strategy is movement occurring at the ankle joint with the gastrocnemius soleus and anterior tibialis muscles initially activated. The hip strategy is the movement occurring at the hip joint with abdominals, paraspinals, and hip musculature initially activated. Ankle strategy is typically utilized for low disturbances, then hip strategy is utilized for larger disturbances, and stepping strategy is utilized for fast and large disturbances.

Key points
1. It is important for the physical therapist to synthesize all components of a physical therapy examination and physical therapy evaluation to determine how the primary diagnosis is affecting the patient's overall function.
2. Consider the pathophysiology and progression of chronic disease (CAD and type 2 DM) to analyze the patient's findings.
3. When prescribing the frequency, intensity, and duration of exercise, prioritize the patient's overall safety but do not "under-dose" the exercise prescription.
4. Always remember as a physical therapist, you are an integral part of a patient's interdisciplinary team, even if you are working alone in an outpatient physical therapy clinic.

General Information	
Case no.	8.B
Authors	Sheena MacFarlane, PT, DPT, Board Certified Clinical Specialist in Cardiovascular & Pulmonary physical therapy Melissa Brown MSPAS, PA-C
Diagnosis	Type 2 diabetes mellitus (DM) with peripheral neuropathy, Charcot foot, and diabetic wound
Setting	Acute care hospital

(Continued)

(Continued)

General Information	
Learner expectations	☑ Initial evaluation ☐ Re-evaluation ☐ Treatment session
Learner objectives	1. Identify signs, symptoms, and complications of diabetic neuropathy. 2. Develop an understanding of medical management of wounds and how it influences physical therapy plan of care. 3. Relate progression of diabetes to clinical manifestations and activity limitations seen in physical therapy practice.

Medical	
Chief complaint	Wound healing and difficulty ambulating.
History of present illness	The patient is a 68-year-old woman with a long-standing history of uncontrolled type 2 DM who was admitted 2 days ago with osteomyelitis of the left foot. She had participated in physical therapy as an outpatient for signs and symptoms related to diabetic neuropathy, including balance training. She has fallen once in the past 2 months. At that time, she was also diagnosed with a Charcot foot (neuropathic arthropathy). Despite conservative management, the patient developed an ulceration of the left foot 1 month ago that has progressively worsened. She has completed two courses of oral antibiotics as well as received a heel off-loading shoe. She currently notes intermittent "burning" pain in bilateral feet, which she rates at a 4/10. In the emergency department, intravenous (IV) antibiotics, IV insulin, and IV fluids were started. Oral diabetic medications were discontinued.
Past medical history	Uncontrolled type 2 diabetes with peripheral neuropathy, nephropathy, and retinopathy, hypertension (HTN), hyperlipidemia, coronary artery disease (CAD) with a myocardial infarction 6 years ago.
Past surgical history	Coronary artery bypass grafting (CABG) × 4 vessels 6 years ago
Allergies	Penicillin: rash
Medications (home)	Metformin, Sitagliptin, Glipizide, Dapagliflozin, Lisinopril, Amlodipine, Metoprolol, Simvastatin, Aspirin, Vancomycin, Ceftriaxone
Precautions/orders	Non–weight bearing (NWB) on left lower extremity (LLE) Activity as tolerated

Social history	
Home setup	• Resides in a single-level home alone. • Two steps without handrail to enter. • Flight of stairs + one handrail to basement where laundry is located. • No grab bars in the bathroom.
Occupation	• Part-time librarian, reduced hours from full time 6 years ago.
Prior level of function	• Independent with functional mobility and activities of daily living (ADLs), however, admits to being a "furniture walker." • Modified independence for stairs, required increased time. • Leans on a shopping cart when grocery shopping. • (+) driver
Recreational activities	• Primarily reading and knitting • Previously enjoyed shopping but fatigues quickly.

Vital signs	Hospital day 0: emergency department	Hospital day 1: medical/surgical ward
Blood pressure (mmHg)	150/92	136/84
Heart rate (beats/min)	66	64
Respiratory rate (breaths/min)	16	14
Pulse oximetry on room air (SpO$_2$)	98%	99%
Temperature (°F)	101.8 (oral)	100.8 (oral)

Imaging/Diagnostic tests	Hospital day 0: emergency department
Left foot X-ray	▶ Fig. 8.2 a. Weight-bearing radiograph b. Oblique radiograph c. Lateral radiograph
Wound culture left foot	• Positive for *Staphylococcus aureus (S. aureus)*
Blood cultures	• Negative

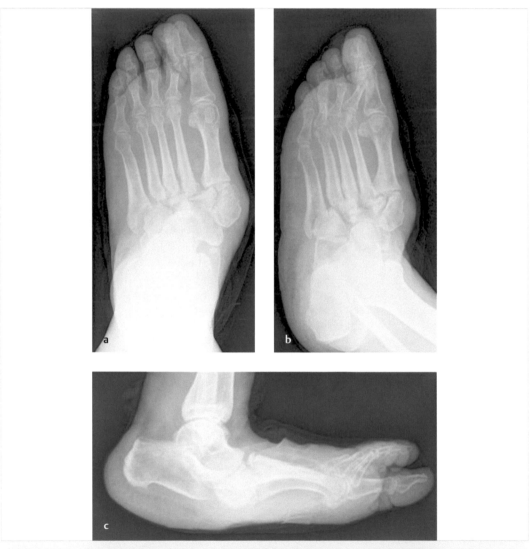

Fig. 8.2 (a-c) An example of Charcot arthropathy. (Adapted from Kessler S, Staebler A. Diabetic osteoarthropathy, Charcot arthropathy. In: Szeimies U, Stäbler A, Walther M, ed. Diagnostic Imaging of the Foot and Ankle. 1st ed. New York, NY: Thieme; 2014.)

Medical management	Hospital day 0: emergency department	Hospital day 1: medical/surgical ward
Medications	1. Vancomycin IV 2. Ceftriaxone IV 3. Insulin glargine 4. Insulin lispro 5. Amlodipine 6. Metoprolol 7. Simvastatin 8. Gabapentin 9. Enoxaparin 10. Acetaminophen: pro re nata (PRN) pain/fever 11. Tramadol: PRN for pain	1. Continued per medical plan of care
Procedures	N/A	1. Left foot wound irrigation and debridement by hospital podiatrist.

Lab		Reference range	Hospital day 0: emergency department	Hospital day 1: medical/surgical ward
Complete blood count	White blood cell	$5.0–10.0 \times 10^9$/L	14.8	16.2
	Hemoglobin	14.0–17.4 d/dL	14.6	14.1
	Hematocrit	42–52%	43.1	42.6
	Red blood cell	4.5–5.5	4.7	4.6
	Platelet	140,000–400,000/µL	388	392
Metabolic panel	Calcium	8.6–10.3 mg/dL	10.1	10.2
	Chloride	98–108 mEq/L	101	103
	Magnesium	1.2–1.9 mEq/L	1.3	1.4
	Phosphate	2.3–4.1 mg/dL	3.9	3.8
	Potassium	3.7–5.1 mEq/L	5.1	4.9
	Sodium	134–142 mEq/L	135	138
	Blood urea nitrogen	7–20 mg/dL	22	16
	Creatinine	0.7–1.3 mg/dL	2.02	1.96
Other	Glucose	60–110 mg/dL	302	186
	Hemoglobin A1C	<5.7%	9.2	Not reordered
	C-reactive protein	<3.0	24	
	International normalization rate	0.8–1.2	0.8	
	Lactate	<2 mmol	1.4	

Pause points
Based on the above information, what are the priorities? • Diagnostic tests and measures? • Wound presentations? • Treatment interventions?

Hospital day 2, Medical surgical ward: Physical Therapy Examination				
Subjective				
"Thank you for coming to see me today. I am looking forward to working with you."				
Objective				
Vital signs	**Pre-treatment**			**Post-treatment**
	Supine	**Sitting**	**Standing**	**Sitting**
Blood pressure (mmHg)	128/78	130/80	126/74	132/80
Heart rate (beats/min)	58	62	60	60
Respiratory rate (breaths/min)	14	16	26	14
Pulse oximetry on room air (SpO$_2$)	99%	97%	98%	99%
Borg Scale	1/10	3/10	7/10	3/10
Pain	0/10			0/10
General	• Patient is lying comfortably in bed, in no acute distress. • Observations are notable for obese body habitus. • Lines are notable for IV in left hand. • Left foot: gauze roll as secondary dressing around foot and ankle ▶ Fig. 8.3a, b			
Cardiovascular and pulmonary	• Auscultation: normal rate. No murmurs, rubs, or gallops • Lungs clear to auscultation • Pulses: dorsalis pedis and posterior tibial: left: 1 +, right: 2 + Femoral: bilateral: 2 + • Left foot and ankle appear pale, cool to touch • Ankle brachial index (ABI) results: Right: 125/132 = 0.95 Left 93/132 = 0.70			
Gastrointestinal	• Rounded, no hepatosplenomegaly			
Musculoskeletal	Range of motion	• Bilateral upper extremity (BUE): within functional range • Bilateral lower extremity (BLE): within functional range except ankle dorsiflexion; left: 0 degrees, right: 5 degrees		
	Strength	• Bilateral shoulder flexion: 4/5 • Bilateral elbow flexion: 4 + /5 • Bilateral wrist extension: 4/5 • Bilateral hip flexion: 3 + /5 • Bilateral knee extension: 4 + /5 • Right ankle dorsiflexion: 3/5 • Left ankle dorsiflexion: not tested due to recent debridement/ bandages • Five Times Sit-to-Stand Test: patient attempted; however, she was unable to perform secondary to assistance needed on sit to stand transfer.		
	Aerobic	• Dyspnea on exertion: 7/10 on Borg rate of perceived exertion with respiratory rate 25 breaths per minute when completing stand pivot transfer.		
	Flexibility	• Not assessed		
	Other	• Left forefoot collapse		
Neurological	Balance	• Unsupported sitting, static: good, independent × 1 minute • Unsupported sitting, dynamic: good, independent × 1 minute • Supported standing: fair, minimal assistance with rolling walker (RW) × 30 seconds; able to maintain left lower extremity (LLE) NWB		

(Continued)

(Continued)

Hospital day 2, Medical surgical ward: Physical Therapy Examination		
	Cognition	• Alert and oriented × 4
	Coordination	• Finger to nose: intact bilaterally • Heel to shin: intact bilaterally
	Cranial nerves	• II–XII: intact
	Reflexes	• Patellar: 2 + bilaterally • Achilles: 1 + bilaterally

	Sensation	• Proximal L4: intact to vibratory sensation bilaterally (17 seconds)
		• Distal L4 and L5: decreased bilateral vibratory sensation at great toe (5 seconds) and medial malleolus (7 seconds)
		• Distal L4/L5/S1: absent bilateral crude touch
		• Monofilament testing:
		  ○ Intact at proximal L4 bilaterally; tested at patella
		  ○ Absent at L4/L5/S1 bilaterally; tested at distal phalanges (1–5), hallux, navicular, and plantar aspect calcaneus

	Tone	• BUE and BLE: normal
Integumentary	Skin	• Location: plantar aspect of the navicular bone • Minimal surrounding periwound erythema • Minimal serous drainage • 4 cm × 4 cm stage 4 ulceration • 2-cm tunneling noted at the 2 o'clock position • Dry purulent material covering wound base
	Dressing change	• Applied: antibacterial topical • Applied: hydrogel as primary dressing • Applied gauze roll as secondary dressing
Functional status		
Bed mobility	• Supine to sit: moderate assistance for LLE • Sit to supine: moderate assistance for LLE • Scooting up in bed: moderate assistance × 1 with bed in Trendelenburg position and mattress setting on "maximum inflation."	
Transfers	• Sit to stand: minimal assistance with an RW • Stand pivot transfer: moderate assistance with an RW • Stand to sit: minimal assistance with an RW Verbal cues provided throughout all transfers for proper hand placement.	
Ambulation	• Hopped ~3 steps from bed to chair using moderate assistance and RW • Able to maintain NWB status throughout	

Assessment	
☑ Physical therapist's	*Assessment left blank for learner to develop*
Goals	
Patient's	"I really want to get walking again."
Short term	1. <p align="center">*Goals left blank for learner to develop.*</p>2.
Long term	1. <p align="center">*Goals left blank for learner to develop.*</p>2.

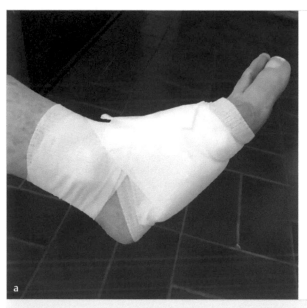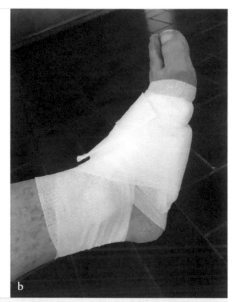

Fig. 8.3 (a,b) Gauze roll on left foot.

Plan	
☐ Physician's ☑ Physical therapist's ☐ Other's	Will treat the patient three to five times a week to improve functional mobility as tolerated through strength, balance, and endurance interventions. For wound healing, will continue with wound care dressing changes in conjunction with nursing (removal of dressing, cleaning wound, applying antibacterial topical, hydrogel, and gauze roll) to assure daily dressing changes.

Bloom's Taxonomy Level	Case 8.B Questions
Create	1. Synthesizing the medical data and physical examination findings, develop an appropriate physical therapy assessment of the patient. 2. Develop two short-term physical therapy goals, including an appropriate timeframe. 3. Develop two long-term physical therapy goals, including an appropriate timeframe.
Evaluate	4. Based on the patient's past medical history, prior level of function, and current impairments, what next level of care is recommended for the patient upon hospital discharge?
Analyze	5. Name two factors that contribute to developing hyperglycemia and hypoglycemia. Identify four signs and/or symptoms of each. 6. What is the interpretation of the ABI? 7. Interpret the description of the wound above. What presentation would indicate wound healing?
Apply	8. Design and implement two interventions to improve the patent's aerobic capacity while maintaining NWB status. 9. Design and implement two interventions to improve the patient's proximal muscle strength to optimize functional independence while maintaining NWB status.
Understand	10. Why might you observe a blunted heart rate and systolic blood pressure (SBP) response to therapeutic interventions?
Remember	11. What is Charcot foot (neuropathic arthropathy)? Consider what radiographic evidence supports this diagnosis. 12. List the characteristics of an arterial wound, venous wound, and diabetic wound. 13. What is osteomyelitis? 14. What is the difference between the following lab values: hemoglobin 1AC and blood glucose?

Bloom's Taxonomy Level	Case 8.B Answers
Create	1. The patient is a 68-year-old woman with past medical history of HTN, CAD with resultant MI and CABG, and type 2 DM (hemoglobin 1AC of 9.2) complicated by peripheral diabetic neuropathy and left Charcot foot, who presents to the hospital with nonhealing/infected diabetic wound on the plantar aspect of the left midfoot. Yesterday, she underwent a left foot wound irrigation and debridement. As a result, she is NWB on LLE. Physical examination reveals general weakness, absent sensation bilateral toes, dressing on left ankle/foot, decreased balance, and decreased endurance. All of these, combined with NWB LLE, lead to impaired functional mobility requiring minimal to moderate assistance. Patient would benefit from physical therapy to address her above to maximize functional mobility and safety. Will continue to follow. Recommend nursing complete daily (or twice a day) dressing changes: removal of dressing, cleaning wound, applying antibacterial topical, hydrogel, and gauze roll. 2. Short-term goals: • Patient will increase her lower extremity strength by half grade to perform a sit to stand transfer with contact guard within five sessions to improve functional mobility. • Patient will ambulate 25 feet with RW and minimal assistance, with a Borg score of 3/10 to demonstrate increased endurance within five sessions. 3. Long-term goals: • Patient will ambulate (maintaining NWB status) 50 feet with an RW and supervision within 10 sessions to demonstrate progressive independence. • Patient's wound will display signs of healing with >50% granulated tissue and <1 cm tunneling within 10 sessions.
Evaluate	4. Patient has significant past medical history with systemic pathology, deconditioned prior level of function (which includes a fall history and warranted use of an assistive device), and her current level of function is minimal to moderate assistance required for transfers and ambulation of 3 feet. Based on this information, it not expected for her to be able to achieve safe, independent mobility and household ambulation by hospital discharge. Therefore, another level of rehabilitation—likely acute inpatient rehabilitation—would be recommended.
Analyze	5. • Hyperglycemia in individuals with type 2 DM occurs secondary to excessive carbohydrate/food intake, inadequate insulin response, increased stress response, or high-intensity exercise. Increased stress response can be the result of illness or physical/emotional stress that causes elevation of cortisol and other counter-regulatory hormones. Signs of marked hyperglycemia include severe dehydration and increased serum osmolality, fatigue, changes in vision, polyuria, polydipsia, polyphagia, and weakness. Individuals with type 1 DM are more likely to also have ketonuria and metabolic acidosis with extreme hyperglycemia. • Hypoglycemia in individuals with type 2 DM occurs secondary to inadequate nutritional intake with endogenous insulin administration or certain oral medications as well as long-duration moderate-intensity exercise. Signs of hypoglycemia include rapid onset of nervousness, diaphoresis, tachycardia, palpitations, nausea, feeling shaky, and headache. As hypoglycemia becomes more severe, symptoms include irritability, confusion, loss of consciousness, and possibly seizures. • It is important to control glucose and minimize both hyper- and hypoglycemia. 6. Normal ABI result is around 1.0. The patient's ABI results are 0.95 for the right LE (RLE) and 0.70 for the LLE. The patient's left ABI results indicate inadequate perfusion to the LLE. Physical examination findings that support poor perfusion include decreased distal LLE pulses, pale presentation and cool to touch in left ankle and foot, and presence of wound and impaired wound healing. 7. Physical therapists' examination/evaluation of wounds should include location, size, tissue type, exudate, and periwound. The patient's wound assessment includes all five components: • Location = midfoot: plantar aspect of the navicular bone of the left foot • Size = 4 cm × 4 cm with tunneling • Tissue type = dry, purulent material • Exudate = minimal serous drainage • Periwound = (+) erythema The presentation of this wound is typical for an individual with peripheral arterial disease and diabetes. Diabetic and arterial ulcers tend to be over bony prominences, size

(Continued)

(Continued)

Bloom's Taxonomy Level	Case 8.B Answers
	depends on extent of injury, but presentation tends to be round, and exudate tends to be minimal with a dry wound bed. In addition, diabetic ulcers tend to be in areas of impaired sensation (peripheral neuropathy) and have a high infection rate. Granulated tissues, lack of infection, decreasing size of wound and of tunneling, and moist wound bed would all indicate wound healing.
Apply	8. Since the patient has a rate of perceived exertion of 7/10 (Modified Borg Scale) with stand pivot transfers and is only able to ambulate 3 feet with an RW, endurance deficits have been identified and interventions are indicated. Two potential interventions are: • Upper body ergometer (UBE) 30 to 40% of peak work rates for 5 to 10 minutes with rest breaks as needed. • Wheelchair propulsion on even surface at controlled, consistent rate, with the goal of a continuous 5 to 10 minutes. 9. Patient has 3 + /5 hip strength and requires minimal assistance with RW to complete sit to stand transfers. Therefore, proximal muscle strengthening is indicated to optimize function. Two potential interventions are: • Side-lying hip abduction "clam shells": lay on left side with both hips and knees flexed. Keeping heels together, lift right knee up toward the ceiling. Coordinate with ankle dorsiflexion and plantar flexion. Perform on both sides. Add theraband resistance once able to perform three to four sets of 15 to 20 reps. • Mini-squats with elevated hospital bed (or elevated chair height): stand in front of elevated bed or chair standing on RLE holding onto RW, perform a mini-squat resting on elevated bed or chair as needed. Height should be high enough that the patient can perform exercise with contact guard/supervision (not minimal assistance). If able, simultaneously perform ankle pumps with left ankle.
Understand	10. Patient is on metoprolol, which is in the class of medication called beta blockers. The medication is used to treat numerous conditions including HTN, stable angina, tachycardia, and/or chronic heart failure. Side effects of the medication include a lower resting heart rate and blunted heart rate response during exercise. With therapeutic interventions, a blunted heart rate and SBP response would be a stable heart rate and SBP response despite increases in exercise intensity, tachypnea, and Borg rate of perceived exertion during exercise.
Remember	11. Charcot foot (neuropathic arthropathy) is a result of repeated microtrauma on a foot without sensation and with impaired arterial blood flow (both symptoms of diabetes) that leads to bone and joint destruction. The radiograph above correlates with Charcot foot: midfoot collapse, flattening of the calcaneus, navicular drop, and downward displacement of the tarsometatarsal joint. The rigid rocker-bottom deformity is evident. 12. • Arterial wounds tend to be located in distal lower extremity and foot, be painful, have minimal exudate, regular round shape to the wound, and blanched or pale color periwound. • Venous wounds tend to be located on the medial aspect of the distal leg and foot, be painful, have large amount of exudate with wet wound beds, have irregular edges of the wound, with edematous periwound and distal extremity. • Diabetic wounds tend to be located in areas of peripheral neuropathy and pressure points (plantar aspect of the foot, toes, heel and plantar aspect of the talus and navicular bones for a Charcot foot), not be painful, minimal exudate, regular round shape to the wound, and have a high infection rate. 13. Osteomyelitis is an infection of the bone. 14. • Blood glucose testing represents the amount of glucose in the bloodstream when the sample was obtained. It indicates normal (70–100 mg/dL), hypoglycemia (<70 mg/dL), and hyperglycemia (>200 mg/dL) at the time the sample was obtained. • Hemoglobin 1AC represents the amount of glucose in the bloodstream over ~100 to 120 days prior to when the sample was obtained. It assists with diagnosis of DM: normal (<5.7%), pre-DM (5.7–6.4%), and DM (>6.5%) and assists in lifestyle recommendation and pharmaceutical management.

Key points	
1. Not only is it essential for the physical therapist to complete chart reviews to obtain necessary information, such as weight-bearing status, but it is also important to review medical data (imaging, lab values, presence of an infection, medication, medical interventions, or surgeries).	
2. The skin is the largest organ in the body and the integumentary system may be directly (providing wound care) or indirectly (providing education or scar tissue management) involved in our physical therapist's assessment and plan of care.	
3. Be creative with exercise prescription, even if a patient has precautions (weight-bearing precautions) and is in the inpatient setting.	

General Information	
Case no.	8.C
Authors	Sheena MacFarlane, PT, DPT, Board Certified Clinical Specialist in Cardiovascular & Pulmonary Physical Therapy Melissa Brown MSPAS, PA-C
Diagnosis	Type 2 diabetes mellitus (DM) status post left transtibial amputation (TTA)
Setting	Acute inpatient rehabilitation
Learner expectations	☑ Initial evaluation ☐ Re-evaluation ☐ Treatment session
Learner objectives	1. Discuss preventative measures that should be implemented in a patient with a recent TTA to decrease complications and functional limitations. 2. Develop a physical therapy plan to prepare a patient for prosthetic fitting and training as well as transition a patient with a TTA from an acute rehab to a home setting. 3. Understand the equipment required in a patient with a TTA in acute rehab and home settings.

Medical	
Chief complaint	Gait training and functional mobilization
History of present illness	The patient is a 68-year-old woman with a long-standing history of uncontrolled type 2 diabetes. The patient had a left Charcot foot, with chronic nonhealing wound and osteomyelitis. The wound progressed over the last 6 months. Conservative management with physical therapy, heel off-loading shoe, and local dressing changes by home nursing was unsuccessful. The patient did receive intravenous (IV) antibiotics for treatment of *Staphylococcus aureus*. Surgical debridement three times over two separate hospitalizations were unsuccessful as the wound continued to worsen in size with no signs of granulation. As a result, the decision was made to undergo a left TTA, which was performed 5 days ago. After medical stabilization, the patient was transferred to acute inpatient rehabilitation. Her most recent hospitalization was 25 days. She has been on morphine and gabapentin for pain control. She is currently experiencing 8/10 pain at the left residual limb.
Past medical history	Uncontrolled type 2 diabetes with peripheral neuropathy, nephropathy, and retinopathy, hypertension (HTN), hyperlipidemia, coronary artery disease with a myocardial infarction 6 years ago.
Past surgical history	Left TTA 5 days ago Coronary artery bypass grafting × 4 vessels 6 years ago
Allergies	Penicillin: rash
Precautions/orders	Non–weight bearing (NWB) left lower extremity (LLE) Activity as tolerated Rigid dressing to LLE when out of bed

Social history	
Home setup	• Resides in a single-level home alone. • Temporarily living with her adult son with a first floor setup and one step to enter with bilateral railings.
Occupation	• Retired librarian
Prior level of function	• Independent with functional mobility and activities of daily living (ADLs) until 6 months ago. • Past 6 months, she has had repeat hospitalizations and discharges to skilled nursing facilities. She has been ambulating 50 to 100 feet with a rolling walker (RW) at contact guard level of assistance, unable to ascend/descend stairs, and remains sedentary the majority of the day.
Recreational activities	• Primarily reading and knitting • Previously enjoyed shopping but fatigues quickly.

Vital signs	Day 1: acute inpatient rehabilitation
Blood pressure (mmHg)	132/80
Heart rate (beats/min)	64
Respiratory rate (breaths/min)	14
Pulse oximetry on room air (SpO$_2$)	99%
Temperature (°F)	97.4 (oral)

Medical management	Day 1: acute inpatient rehabilitation
Medications	1. Insulin glargine 2. Insulin lispro 3. Gabapentin 4. Lisinopril 5. Amlodipine 6. Metoprolol 7. Simvastatin 8. Enoxaparin 9. Morphine: pro re nata (PRN) for pain 10. Acetaminophen: PRN pain/fever

Lab		Reference range	Day 1: acute inpatient rehabilitation
Complete blood count	White blood cell (WBC)	5.0–10.0 × 10^9/L	14.6
	Hemoglobin	14.0–17.4 d/dL	12.0
	Hematocrit	42–52%	40.1
	Red blood cell	4.5–5.5	4.3
	Platelet	140,000–400,000/µL	398
Metabolic panel	Calcium	8.6–10.3 mg/dL	10.0
	Chloride	98–108 mEq/L	102
	Potassium	3.7–5.1 mEq/L	4.6
	Sodium	134–142 mEq/L	139

(Continued)

(Continued)

Lab		Reference range	Day 1: acute inpatient rehabilitation
Other	Blood urea nitrogen	7–20 mg/d	14
	Creatinine	0.7–1.3 mg/dL	1.62
	Glucose	60–110 mg/dL	164
	Hemoglobin A1C	<5.7%	
	C-reactive protein	<3.0	
	International normalization rate	0.8–1.2	Not reordered
	Lactate	<2 mmol	

Pause points

Based on the above information, what are the priorities?
• Diagnostic tests and measures?
• Common postoperative TTA impairments?
• Treatment interventions?

Day 1, Acute inpatient rehabilitation: Physical Therapy Examination

Subjective

"How can I go home like this?"

Objective

Vital signs	Pre-treatment		Post-treatment	
	Supine	Sitting	Ambulating	Sitting
Blood pressure (mmHg)	122/76	126/74	128/78	130/82
Heart rate (beats/min)	60	62	62	60
Respiratory rate (breaths/min)	16	18	24	20
Pulse oximetry on room air (SpO$_2$)	100%	100%	98%	98%
Borg Scale	2/10	3/10	6/10	4/10
Pain	8/10 left residual limb			9/10 left residual limb
General	• Patient is sitting in wheelchair in no acute distress. • Observations notable for obese body habitus. • Lines notable for peripherally inserted central catheter (PICC) access. • Removable rigid dressings over left residual limb. ▶ Fig. 8.4			
Cardiovascular and pulmonary	• Auscultation: normal rate. No murmurs, rubs, or gallops • Lungs clear to auscultation • Pulses: dorsalis pedis and posterior tibial: right: 2 + Femoral: bilateral: 2 + • Edema: + 1 left residual limb			
Musculoskeletal	Range of motion (ROM)	• Bilateral upper extremity (BUE): within functional range • Bilateral lower extremity (BLE):		

(Continued)

(Continued)

		Day 1, Acute inpatient rehabilitation: Physical Therapy Examination
		Hips: bilateral hip flexion contractures present, able to achieve approximately neutral hip extension with passive range of motion (PROM), hip abduction limited to 10 degrees with PROM Knees: within functional range. Right ankle: within functional range except dorsiflexion, 5 degrees.
	Strength	• Bilateral shoulder flexion: 4/5 • Bilateral elbow flexion: 4/5 • Bilateral wrist extension: 4/5 • Bilateral hip flexion: 2 + /5 • Bilateral knee extension: 2 + /5 • Bilateral knee flexion: 2 + /5 • Right ankle dorsiflexion: 2 + /5
	Aerobic	• Dyspnea on exertion: 6/10 on Borg rate of perceived exertion with respiratory rate of 24 breaths per minute when completing ambulation
	Flexibility	• BUE musculature within normal limit • BLE: decreased muscle flexibility in iliopsoas, hip adductors, and right gastrocnemius soleus muscles
Neurological	Balance	• Unsupported sitting, static: close supervision with BUE support × 5 minutes • Unsupported sitting, dynamic: moderate assistance with BUE support • Supported standing, static: not assessed
	Cognition	• Alert and oriented × 4
	Coordination	• Finger to nose: intact bilaterally
	Cranial Nerves	• II–XII: intact
	Reflexes	• Patellar: 2 + right lower extremity (RLE) • Achilles: 1 + RLE

	Sensation	• Proximal L4: intact to vibratory sensation bilaterally (17 seconds)
		• Right distal L4/L5/S1: absent to crude touch
		• Monofilament testing:
		  ○ Intact at proximal L4 bilaterally; tested at patella
		  ○ Right distal L4/L5/S1: absent at distal phalanges (1–5), plantar aspect of calcaneus, medial and lateral tibia, and medial and lateral gastrocnemius soleus complex

	Tone	• BUE and BLE: normal
Integumentary	Skin	• Observations: removable rigid dressing, figure 8 bandage, and nonadhesive sterile gauze primary dressing all removed from left residual limb to assess skin • Skin intact, incision dry, sutures in place
	Dressing change	• Applied: nonadhesive sterile gauze as primary dressing • Reapplied elastic bandage figure-of-eight pattern and removable rigid dressing
		Functional status
Bed mobility		• Supine to sit: maximal assistance • Sit to supine: moderate assistance • Scooting up in bed: moderate assistance × 2 with bed in Trendelenburg position and mattress setting on "maximum inflation."

(Continued)

(Continued)

Day 1, Acute inpatient rehabilitation: Physical Therapy Examination	
Transfers	• Sit to/from stand: unsuccessful attempt from wheelchair with assist × 2 • Sit to/from stand: utilized assistive technology with knee block, forearm prop, and foot plate; two persons present to operate lift and provide contact guard
Ambulation	• Patient ambulated 10 feet with partial body weight support system with sling and forearm prop with hand grips; two persons present to operate assistive technology and provide contact guard.
Wheelchair mobility	• 100-feet wheelchair propulsion on level surfaces with BUE utilization with minimal assistance to negotiate around obstacles. • RLE on-foot plate. Left residual limb on wheelchair residual limb support.

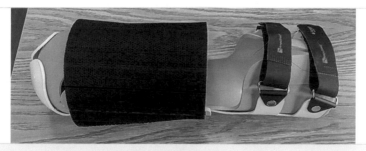

Fig. 8.4 An example of a removable rigid dressing for a residual limb.

Assessment	
☑ Physical therapist's	*Assessment left blank for learner to develop.*
Goals	
Patient's	"Do you really think I will be able to walk with a prosthetic? I really want to go back to work part-time."
Short term	1. *Goals left blank for learner to develop.* 2.
Long term	1. *Goals left blank for learner to develop.* 2.

	Plan
☐ Physician's ☑ Physical therapist's ☐ Other's	Will treat patient 1 to 2 hours a day six to seven times a week to progress functional mobility as tolerated through ROM, stretching, strengthening, balance, endurance, and wound care interventions.

Bloom's Taxonomy Level	Case 8.C Questions
Create	1. Synthesizing the medical data and physical examination findings, develop an appropriate physical therapy assessment of the patient. 2. Develop two short-term physical therapy goals, including an appropriate timeframe. 3. Develop two long-term physical therapy goals, including an appropriate timeframe.
Evaluate	4. Anticipating the patient will remain in acute inpatient rehab for 3 to 4 weeks, and considering the patient's home setup, determine equipment and services that the patient will require for safe discharge home.
Analyze	5. Interpret the laboratory findings from day 1: acute inpatient rehabilitation. Do any lab values require holding physical therapy evaluation or modifying the session?
Apply	6. Design and implement two interventions to address this patient's bilateral LE ROM deficits. 7. Design and implement two interventions to address this patient's gait deviation and ambulation deficits. 8. Based on knowledge of the integumentary system and endocrine system, what education should be provided to the patient to limit her chances of RLE amputation?
Understand	9. What are the physical therapy implications of morphine and gabapentin? 10. What is the purpose of the removable rigid dressing (▶ Fig. 8.4) status post TTA? 11. What benefits for the physical therapist (or health care worker) are there to utilizing assistive technology for transfers and ambulation?
Remember	12. What are K-levels for prosthetics? What does each mean?

Bloom's Taxonomy Level	Case 8.C Answers
Create	1. The patient is a 68-year-old woman admitted to acute rehab facility yesterday after a complicated hospital course for *S. aureus*, diabetic/arterial nonhealing wound with osteomyelitis, and subsequent left TTA (postoperative day 6). She presents with global weakness, decreased ROM of BLE, decreased sensation of RLE, decreased endurance, decreased balance, and dressing and removable rigid dressings over left residual limb. All of these contribute to impaired mobility, for which she requires moderate-dependent assist. She would benefit from physical therapy to address her above deficits, prevention of negative sequela, and maximize functional mobility and safety. Will continue to follow. 2. Short-term goals: • Patient will perform moderate assistance transfers within 12 sessions to improve functional mobility. • Patient will increase her hip ROM by 10 degrees and maintain her knee ROM to optimize future success with prosthetic limb within 12 sessions. • Patient will independently propel wheelchair × 150 feet on level surface, avoiding 100% of obstacles, within 12 sessions to become more independent. 3. Long-term goals: • Patient will demonstrate improved endurance by performing bike ergo-meter × 15 minutes with normal vital sign response within 24 sessions. • Patient will ambulate 40 feet with an RW with contact guard assist within 24 sessions to improve mobility around home. • Patient will ascend/descend one step with bilateral railings with contact guard assist within 24 sessions to be able to enter/exit her son's house.
Evaluate	4. Patient lives with her son with a first-floor setup and one step to enter. Patient is expected to achieve contact guard functional mobility prior to discharge home within 3 to 4 weeks. For safe discharge home, it is anticipated that the patient will need home physical therapy to address continued deficits, RW for safe ambulation, bedside commode, shower chair, and manual wheelchair for community distances.

(Continued)

(Continued)

Bloom's Taxonomy Level	Case 8.C Answers
Analyze	5. In regard to lab values on day 1: acute inpatient rehabilitation, the following are notable: • WBC: 14.6. This is above normal (> 10.0) indicating leukocytosis. It is most likely elevated due to wound infection and osteomyelitis. It is trending down from 15.4 toward normal range. • Glucose: 164. This is above normal (110 mg/dL) nonfasting glucose level indicating hyperglycemia. It is trending down as compared to prior lab draws. Neither lab value requires physical therapy session modification.
Apply	6. Since the patient presents with limited hip extension and hip abduction ROM with (+) hip flexion contracture, stretching exercises are indicated. Due to the technique for surgical securement of muscle and postoperative immobility (typically in seated or elevated head of bed supine), hip flexion, hip abduction, and knee flexion contractures are common. The presence of contractures delays fitting of a prosthetic and alters rehabilitation potential. Two potential interventions are: • Prone positioning with neutral hip extension, neutral knee extension, and mild hip abduction. This stretch should be held for 30 minutes, twice a day for static prolonged stretch of hip flexors, hip adductors, and knee flexors. • Supine hip abduction (windshield wipers) on mat with towels under heel to decrease friction, 4 sets of 5 repetition with focus on full ROM. 7. This patient utilized partial body weight support system with sling and forearm prop with hand grips to ambulate × 10 feet. During this, she demonstrated a hop-to pattern with subsequent WB into BUE forearm prop and sling to compensate for trunk and proximal hip gluteus maximus weakness. This indicates the need for training to improve her gait. Two potential interventions are: • Glut squeezes, 4 sets of 5 repetition. • Prone hip extensions, 4 sets of 5 repetition. As the patient is able to tolerate more endurance and standing, exercises could progress to ambulation training with assistive technology and person(s) assist with focus on decreasing body support, minimizing gait deviations, and increasing distance. 8. People with DM are at a higher risk of amputation due to impaired vascularization and sensation. Patients who have had an amputation are at a high risk of requiring further amputations. Physical therapists are frequently very involved in prevention of subsequent ipsilateral amputations and prevention of uninvolved LE amputations. The patient should be educated on the following techniques: • daily diabetic foot care (keep clean and dry, use moisturizer to prevent cracking). • regular adherence to medical appointments and pharmaceutical management. • frequent foot skin checks with a mirror to inspect all surfaces. • wearing appropriate shoes to distribute pressure points. • minimizing skin trauma. • early identification of skin breakdowns and wounds. • early identification of infection (warmth, redness, edema).
Understand	9. Both gabapentin and morphine have side effects of decreased arousal, sedation, drowsiness, and fatigue. Decreased respiratory drive is a serious adverse effect of the medications being taken together. Physical therapists should routinely take vitals, check artery bypass grafting (if available), and assess level of arousal throughout the physical therapy session. 10. A removable rigid dressing is applied to the postoperative residual limb to protect the residual limb from trauma, decrease postoperative edema, prevent contractures, and allow for ease of skin assessment/incision assessment. 11. The majority of physical therapists will experience workplace injuries during their career. The incidence of workplace injuries among physical therapists is 16.9% per year of full-time employment with the highest reported work-related musculoskeletal disorder being low back pain. Additionally, many physical therapists have changed jobs previously and/or are considering changing positions due to workplace injury. It is important on an individual level to prioritize one's health as a physical therapist as well as support a culture of safe patient handling. Assistive technologies (sit to stand devices to assist with transfers and partial body weight support systems) are useful in mitigating workplace injuries.

(Continued)

(Continued)

Bloom's Taxonomy Level	Case 8.C Answers
Remember	12. According to O'Sullivan et al, the K-levels are as follows: • Functional level 0/K-level 0: with (or without) a prosthetic, patient does not have the potential to transfer or ambulate. Patients tend to be wheelchair bound. • Functional level 1/K-level 1: with a prosthetic, patient has the potential to transfer or ambulate on level surfaces. Patients tend to be household ambulators. • Functional level 2/K-level 2: with a prosthetic, patient has the potential to ambulate and transverse low-level environmental barriers (ramps, curbs, uneven ground, etc.). Patients tend to be limited community ambulators. • Functional level 3/K-level 3: with prosthetic, patient has potential to ambulate with variable cadence and transverse high-level environmental barriers (stairs, lifting, etc.). Patients tend to be able to resume vocation, recreation, and exercise. • Functional level 4/K-level 4: with prosthetic, patient has the potential to exceed basic ambulation and complete high-impact activities. Patients tend to be children or athletes and return to full activity participation.

Key points
1. Be aware of pathophysiology as well as postoperative risks of surgical procedures to ensure frequent evidence-based physical therapy assessment (ROM, incision healing).
2. With short length of stays in hospitals and rehabilitation facilities, it is important to start addressing discharge needs and plans during the first physical therapy session.
3. Physical therapy exercise prescription in patient status post LE amputation should address the combination of preventative, specific impairments (endurance, ROM, strength, function), as well as preprosthetic training.

Suggested Readings

Adeletti K, Bryan C, Brown-Crowell M, et al. Laboratory Values Interpretation Resource. Pittsburgh, PA: Academy of Acute Care Physical Therapy – APTA Task Force of Lab Values; 2017:1–42

Alam U, Riley DR, Jugdey RS, et al. Diabetic neuropathy and gait: a review. Diabetes Ther. 2017; 8(6):1253–1264

American College of Sports Medicine. ACSM's Guidelines for Exercise Testing and Prescription. 10th ed. Baltimore, MD: Lippincott, Williams and Wilkins; 2017

Anderson LW, Krathwohl DR. A Taxonomy for Learning, Teaching, and Assessing, Abridged Edition. Boston, MA: Allyn and Bacon; 2001

Armstrong P. Bloom's Taxonomy. Available at: https://cft.vanderbilt.edu/guides-sub-pages/blooms-taxonomy/. Accessed on April 1, 2018

Bohannon RW. Reference values for the five-repetition sit-to-stand test: a descriptive meta-analysis of data from elders. Percept Mot Skills. 2006; 103(1):215–222

Church TS, Blair SN, Cocreham S, et al. Effects of aerobic and resistance training on hemoglobin A1c levels in patients with type 2 diabetes: a randomized controlled trial. JAMA. 2010; 304(20):2253–2262

Ciccone CD. Pharmacology in Rehabilitation. 5th ed. Philadelphia, PA: FA Davis; 2015

Communications E. Diagnostic imaging of the foot and ankle. Medone-radiology.thieme.com. Available at: https://medone-radiology.thieme.com/ebooks/1563267?fromSearch=true#/ebook_1563267_SL64712420. Accessed March 11, 2020

da Cruz Anjos DM, de Souza Moreira B, Pereira DS, et al. Impact of type-2 diabetes time since diagnosis on elderly women gait and functional status. Physiother Res Int. 2017; 22(2):e1651

Darragh AR, Huddleston W, King P. Work-related musculoskeletal injuries and disorders among occupational and physical therapists. Am J Occup Ther. 2009; 63(3):351–362

Deschamps K, Matricali GA, Roosen P, et al. Comparison of foot segmental mobility and coupling during gait between patients with diabetes mellitus with and without neuropathy and adults without diabetes. Clin Biomech (Bristol, Avon). 2013; 28(7):813–819

Eraydin Ş, Avşar G. The effect of foot exercises on wound healing in type 2 diabetic patients with a foot ulcer: a randomized control study. J Wound Ostomy Continence Nurs. 2018; 45(2):123–130

Ghazali MF, Abd Razak NA, Abu Osman NA, Gholizadeh H. Awareness, potential factors, and post-amputation care of stump flexion contractures among transtibial amputees. Turk J Phys Med Rehabil. 2018; 64(3):268–276

Goodman CC, Fuller KS. Pathology-E-Book: Implications for the Physical Therapist. 4th ed. St. Louis, MO: Saunders Elsevier Health Sciences; 2015

Griffin KJ, Rashid TS, Bailey MA, Bird SA, Bridge K, Scott JD. Toe amputation: a predictor of future limb loss? J Diabetes Complications. 2012; 26(3):251–254

Highsmith MJ, Kahle JT, Miro RM, et al. Prosthetic interventions for people with transtibial amputation: systematic review and meta-analysis of high-quality prospective literature and systematic reviews. J Rehabil Res Dev. 2016; 53(2):157–184

Hillegass E. Essentials of Cardiopulmonary Physical Therapy. 4th ed. St. Louis, MO: Elsevier Health Sciences; 2017

Ites KI, Anderson EJ, Cahill ML, Kearney JA, Post EC, Gilchrist LS. Balance interventions for diabetic peripheral neuropathy: a systematic review. J Geriatr Phys Ther. 2011; 34(3):109–116

Izumi Y, Satterfield K, Lee S, Harkless LB. Risk of reamputation in diabetic patients stratified by limb and level of amputation: a 10-year observation. Diabetes Care. 2006; 29(3):566–570

Jette DU, Grover L, Keck CP. A qualitative study of clinical decision making in recommending discharge placement from the acute care setting. Phys Ther. 2003; 83(3):224–236

Keylock KT, Young H. Delayed wound healing: can exercise accelerate it? Int J Exerc Sci. 2010; 3(3):2

Keylock T, Meserve L, Wolfe A. Low-intensity exercise accelerates wound healing in diabetic mice. Wounds. 2018; 30(3): 68–71

Kluding PM, Bareiss SK, Hastings M, Marcus RL, Sinacore DR, Mueller MJ. Physical training and activity in people with diabetic peripheral neuropathy: paradigm shift. Phys Ther. 2017; 97(1): 31–43

McCulloch JM, Kloth LC. Wound Healing: Evidence-Based Management. 4th ed. Philadelphia, PA: FA Davis; 2010

Nawijn SE, van der Linde H, Emmelot CH, Hofstad CJ. Stump management after trans-tibial amputation: a systematic review. Prosthet Orthot Int. 2005; 29(1):13–26

O'Sullivan SB, Schmitz TJ, Fulk G. Physical Rehabilitation. 7th ed. Philadelphia, PA: FA Davis; 2019

Schafer ZA, Perry JL, Vanicek N. A personalised exercise programme for individuals with lower limb amputation reduces falls and improves gait biomechanics: a block randomised controlled trial. Gait Posture. 2018; 63:282–289

Shirley Ryan AbilityLab. 2020. Five Times Sit-to-Stand test. Available at: https://www.sralab.org/rehabilitation-measures/five-times-sit-stand-test#older-adults-and-geriatric-care. Accessed May 21, 2020

Shirley Ryan AbilityLab. 2020. Timed Up and Go. Available at: https://www.sralab.org/rehabilitation-measures/timed-and-go#older-adults-and-geriatric-care. Accessed May 21, 2020

Skoutas D, Papanas N, Georgiadis GS, et al. Risk factors for ipsilateral reamputation in patients with diabetic foot lesions. Int J Low Extrem Wounds. 2009; 8(2):69–74

Smith BA, Fields CJ, Fernandez N. Physical therapists make accurate and appropriate discharge recommendations for patients who are acutely ill. Phys Ther. 2010; 90(5):693–703

Steffen TM, Hacker TA, Mollinger L. Age- and gender-related test performance in community-dwelling elderly people: six-minute walk test, Berg balance scale, timed up & go test, and gait speeds. Phys Ther. 2002; 82(2):128–137

Waters TR, Rockefeller K. Safe patient handling for rehabilitation professionals. Rehabil Nurs. 2010; 35(5):216–222

Wong CK, Ehrlich JE, Ersing JC, Maroldi NJ, Stevenson CE, Varca MJ. Exercise programs to improve gait performance in people with lower limb amputation: a systematic review. Prosthet Orthot Int. 2016; 40(1):8–17

9 Intertrochanteric Fracture

General Information	
Case no.	9.A Intertrochanteric Fracture
Authors	Julie M. Skrzat, PT, DPT, PhD, Board Certified Clinical Specialist in Cardiovascular & Pulmonary Physical Therapy Sean Griech, PT, DPT, PhD, COMT, Board Certified Clinical Specialist in Orthopaedic Physical Therapy
Diagnosis	Intertrochanteric fracture
Setting	Acute care setting, postoperative floor
Learner expectations	☑ Initial evaluation ☐ Re-evaluation ☐ Treatment session
Learner objectives	1. To appreciate the importance of taking vital signs with positional changes in a patient who is postoperative. 2. To understand the underlying mechanism of injury, especially as it pertains to falls, to prevent further adverse events. 3. To articulate efficient and effective communication between health care providers to optimize the patient's plan of care. 4. Relate the pathophysiology and progression of pathology of an orthopaedic injury to the clinical manifestations and activity/participation limitations seen in physical therapy practice. 5. Select, implement, and interpret physical therapy interventions based on the medical examination findings and plan of care. 6. Develop an understanding of the medical management of a patient with an orthopaedic injury.

Medical	
Chief complaint	Status post (s/p) fall
History of present illness	The patient is a 60-year-old woman who presents to the emergency department s/p fall. She reports tripping over cat while walking to the bathroom. She was able to crawl to the phone to dial 911, but was unable to stand and bear weight on the right lower extremity (RLE). She denies striking her head or loss of consciousness.
Past medical history	Hypertension, coronary artery disease, type 2 diabetes mellitus, obesity (body mass index [BMI] = 31.05), diabetic neuropathy
Past surgical history	Hysterectomy
Allergies	No known drug allergies
Medications	Lisinopril, Atorvastatin, Pregabalin, Metformin

Social history	
Home setup	• Resides in a multilevel home with her husband. • Three steps with no rail to enter. • Half bath is on the first floor. • Bedroom and bathroom are located on the second floor. • Flight of stairs + one handrail to the second floor.
Occupation	• Employed as a fifth-grade elementary school teacher.
Prior level of function	• Independent with functional mobility and activities of daily living (ADLs). • Denies any functional limitations. • (+) driver
Recreational activities	• Enjoys playing with her grandchildren (2 and 3 years old) and reading for leisure.

Vital signs	Hospital day 0: emergency department	Hospital day 1: postoperative, on the ward
Blood pressure (mmHg)	149/82	128/72
Heart rate (beats/min)	116	78
Respiratory rate (beats/min)	18	16
Pulse oximetry on room air (SpO$_2$)	97%	98%
Temperature (°F)	98.6	98.8

Hospital day 0: emergency department	
General	Well-nourished woman, appears to have discomfort in right hip, cognitively intact, answering questions appropriately.
Constitutional	(-) fever, chills, or weight loss
Head, ears, eyes, nose, and throat (HEENT)	(-) congestion, sore throat or otalgia, denies head injury in fall
Cardiovascular and pulmonary	(-) chest pain, palpitations, dyspnea on exertion, edema, syncope, aspiration, shortness of breath, orthopnea (-) cough, congestion, wheezing or sputum production
Gastrointestinal	(-) abdominal pain, hematemesis, melena, nausea, vomiting, diarrhea
Genitourinary	(-) dysuria, frequency, urgency, blood in urine
Musculoskeletal	(+) right thigh and hip pain secondary to fall (-) involvement of any other joint via swelling or warmth
Integumentary	(-) rash, open sores, cuts, bruises
Neurological	(-) headache, dizziness, weakness, numbness in extremities (+) generalized tingling in both feel, which at times, becomes painful
Hematology/lymph	(-) abnormal bleeding or bruising; bumps or lumps

Imaging /diagnostic test	Hospital day 0: emergency department	Hospital day 1: postoperative, ward
X-ray (right hip and pelvis)	1. Displaced intertrochanteric fracture of right femur 2. Marked osteoarthritic changes in the pelvis, acetabulum, and right hip joint	
Electrocardiogram (ECG)	1. ▶ Fig. 9.1	1. Normal sinus rate and rhythm

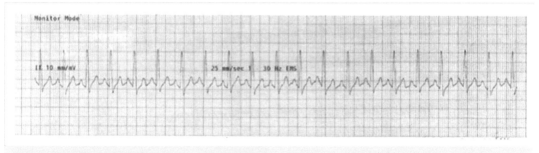

Fig. 9.1 The patient's electrocardiogram on hospital day 0.

Medical management	Hospital day 0: emergency department	Hospital day 1: postoperative, ward
Medications	1. Morphine sulfate 2 prn pain 2. Acetaminophen prn pain 3. Ondansetron prn nausea, vomiting 4. 0.9% sodium chloride 500 mL intra-venous (IV) bolus	1. Acetaminophen prn pain 2. Ibuprofen prn pain 3. Oxycodone prn pain
Orthopaedic team	1. Recommend open reduction internal fixation to repair intertrochanteric fracture	1. Post-op hemoglobin has dropped from 11.6 to 9.2 g/dL. Start ferrous sulfate, ascorbic acid; monitor hemoglobin and hematocrit with complete blood count (CBC) tomorrow morning. 2. Pain well controlled, continue current regimen 3. Incision clear/dry/intact
Precautions	• Bed rest • Fall risk • Non–weight bearing (NWB) RLE • Telemetry	• Activity as tolerated • Fall risk • Weight bearing as tolerated (WBAT) RLE • Telemetry

Pause points
Based on the above information, what are the priorities? • Diagnostic tests and measures? • Outcome measures? • Treatment interventions?

Hospital Day 2, Post-Op Day 1, Ward: Physical Therapy Examination
Subjective
"Am I allowed to get out of bed?"
Objective

Vital signs	Pre-treatment			Post-treatment
	Supine	Sitting	Standing	
Blood pressure (mmHg)	110/78	90/50		108/80
Heart rate (beats/min)	84	86		89
Respiratory rate (breaths/min)	16	17		18
Pulse oximetry (SpO$_2$)	94% on room air	94% on room air	Not attempted due to safety concerns	93% on 2 L/min O$_2$ via nasal cannula (NC)
Borg Scale	0/10	3/10		0/10
Pain	1/10, incision site	5/10, incision site		3/10, incision site
General	• Well-nourished woman • Appears to have discomfort in right hip			
Cardiovascular and pulmonary	• Denies chest pain • Normal S1, S2 • Normal rate and rhythm • Bilateral lung bases with decreased breath sounds • Strong, nonproductive cough			
Gastrointestinal	(+) reports constipation			
Genitourinary	(+) urinary catheter ▶ Fig. 9.2			
Integumentary	▶ Fig. 9.3			

(Continued)

(Continued)

Hospital Day 2, Post-Op Day 1, Ward: Physical Therapy Examination		
Musculoskeletal	Range of motion (ROM)	• Bilateral upper extremity (BUE): within functional limit (WFL) • Left lower extremity (LLE): WFL • RLE: hip with empty end feels in all directions due to pain, knee WFL, ankle WFL
	Strength	• BUE: grossly 5/5 • LLE: grossly 5/5 • Right hip: not formally test tested • Right knee flexion/extension: 4/5 • Right anterior tibialis and evertors: 1/5
	Aerobic	• Unable to test
	Flexibility	• Good appropriate hamstring length as shown by long sit to get out of bed
	Other	• N/A
Neurological	Balance	• Unsupported sitting edge of bed: maximal assistance
	Cognition	• Alert and oriented × 4, somewhat drowsy
	Coordination	• Finger to nose: intact BUE
	Cranial nerves	• II–XII: intact
	Reflexes	• Left patellar: 2+ • Right patellar: not tested
	Sensation	• Impaired sensation to light touch and vibration stocking distribution • Decreased tactile sense in peroneal distribution right leg and foot
	Tone	• Normal throughout BUEs and BLEs
	Other	• N/A
Functional status		
Bed mobility		• Rolling to left: supervision with moderate assistance to support RLE • Rolling to right: attempted, but was unable to complete due to increased pain in the right hip • Scooting up in bed: maximal assistance × 2 • Supine to/from sit via long sit: moderate assistance • When sitting edge of bed, patient reported mild dizziness and lightheadedness Interventions were provided, with no resolutions of symptoms.
Transfers		• N/A
Ambulation		• N/A
Stairs		• N/A

Assessment	
☑ Physical therapist's	*Assessment left blank for learner to develop.*
Goals	
Patient's	"I want to get back to work."
Short-term	1. *Goals left blank for learner to develop.* 2.
Long-term	1. *Goals left blank for learner to develop.* 2.

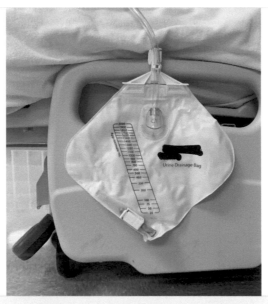

Fig. 9.2 An example of a urinary catheter.

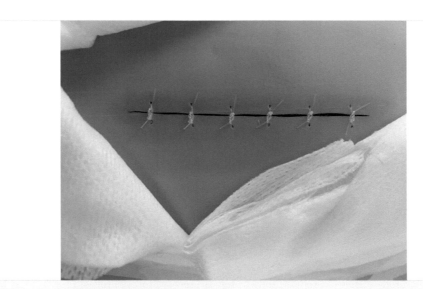

Fig. 9.3 An example of the patient's incision.

Plan
☑ Physical therapist's   Will continue to see patient twice a day × 2 to 3 days. Will progress functional mobility within confines of weight-bearing status in preparation for discharge.

Bloom's Taxonomy Level	Case 9.A Questions
Create	1. Synthesizing the medical data and physical examination findings, develop an appropriate physical therapy assessment of the patient. 2. Develop two short-term physical therapy goals, including an appropriate timeframe. 3. Develop two long-term physical therapy goals, including an appropriate timeframe. 4. Develop a home exercise program for this patient. It should consistent of four exercises.
Evaluate	5. What member of the health care team would the physical therapist immediately communicate with about the patient's hemodynamic response to sitting on the edge of the bed? Why is this important? 6. Should the physical therapist consult an orthotist to fabricate a molded ankle–foot orthosis (MAFO) if by post-op day 5 she still had foot drop?
Analyze	7. What is the rate and rhythm of the ECG strip on the day of presentation? 8. What is the interpretation of the patient's incision?
Apply	9. If the patient did not eat her breakfast but did take the prescribed Metformin, would the physical therapist expect her blood sugar to be higher, lower, or the same as her normal, and how would this change the physical therapist's plan of care? 10. Why does the patient have decreased breath sounds in bilateral lung fields? Is there anything physical therapists can do to remedy this? 11. Provide two therapeutic treatment recommendations for orthostatic hypotension.
Understand	12. Are there any precautions for mobility related to the urinary catheter? If so, what are they? 13. Describe the Wells Criteria for deep vein thrombosis (DVT). What is its indication and why might this be indicated with this patient?
Remember	14. State the purpose for the patient's home medications: Atorvastatin, Pregabalin, Metformin, Lisinopril. 15. Define orthostatic hypotension. Identify common signs and symptoms.

Bloom's Taxonomy Level	Case 9.A Answers
Create	1. The patient is a 60-year-old woman s/p mechanical fall, resulting in displaced intertrochanteric fracture of the right femur. She is s/p right open reduction internal fixation. Medical precautions include RLE WBAT, activity as tolerated, fall risk, and telemetry. From a mobility perspective, she demonstrates increased pain and signs and symptoms associated with orthostatic hypotension (systolic blood pressure dropped 20 mmHg when sitting on the edge of the bed). Diaphragmatic breathing and lower extremity therapeutic exercise did not resolve symptoms; therefore, patient was returned to supine with resolution of symptoms and return of stable vitals. Resident nurse (RN) informed. She would benefit from continued physical therapy to improve endurance, strength, and ROM to maximize functional mobility and safety. Will continue to follow and progress as tolerated. 2. Short-term goals: • Patient will perform supine to/from sit with head of bed flat and supervision to get in and out of bed at home within 4 days. • Patient will perform sit to/from stand transfers with RW and supervision to get on/off toilet within 4 days. 3. Long-term goals: • Patient will ascend/descend three steps with minimal assistance from family member to enter and exit home within 7 days. • Patient will ambulate 50 feet with RW and supervision within 4 days to navigate within home. 4. Four exercises the patient can perform at home are: • ankle pumps • long arc quads • mini-squats with external support (i.e., countertop) • standing hip flexion/extension/abduction/adduction with external support

(Continued)

(Continued)

Bloom's Taxonomy Level	Case 9.A Answers
Evaluate	5. Upon noticing that the patient develops signs and symptoms of orthostatic hypotension, the first step should be ensuring the patient's safety. If necessary, she should be returned to supine with interventions to relieve signs and symptoms. Additionally, vitals should be monitored. After, the nurse should be notified of the patient's vitals (including heart rate), signs and symptoms, and event that precipitated signs and symptoms. The physical therapist or nurse should also notify the physician.
	6. If the patient still had foot drop 5 days postsurgery, the physical therapist should not consult an orthotist to fabricate an MAFO. The issue may be neuropraxic and resolve itself shortly. If necessary, an inexpensive ACE wrap or toe lift can be used.
Analyze	7. The patient's heart rate is 110 beats/min and the heart rhythm is sinus tachycardia.
	8. The patient's wound is clear, dry, and intact.
Apply	9. If the patient did not eat her breakfast but did take the prescribed Metformin, the physical therapist would expect the patient's blood sugar to be lower.
	10. The patient may have decreased breaths sounds in bilateral lung fields due to surgery and taking shallow breaths. To promote inhalation, the physical therapist can educate the patient on the use of an incentive spirometer. The patient should give a return demonstration to ensure proper technique.
	11. Two therapeutic treatment recommendations for orthostatic hypotension include (a) implementation of lower extremity exercises (ankle pumps, long arc quads, etc.) and (b) gradual progression of the head of bed being elevated to promote hemodynamic stability in upright positions.
Understand	12. When mobilizing a patient with a urinary catheter, the catheter bag should remain below the patient's bladder. This helps prevent backflow into the patient.
	13. The Wells Criteria are utilized to stratify the risk or likelihood of lower extremity DVT across patient populations and settings. The Wells Criteria for DVTs include: • active cancer • bedridden recently > 3 days or major surgery within 12 weeks • calf swelling > 3 cm compared to the other leg • collateral superficial veins present • entire leg swollen • localized tenderness along the deep venous system • pitting edema, confined to sympathetic leg • paralysis, paresis, or recent plaster immobilization of the lower extremity • previously documented DVT It is important to implement the Wells Criteria in this patient because of her orthopaedic surgery.
Remember	14. Atorvastatin: treats high cholesterol and triglyceride levels. Pregabalin: treats nerve and muscle pain. Metformin: treats high glucose levels as a result of type 2 diabetes mellitus. Lisinopril: treats hypertension.
	15. Orthostatic hypotension is defined as a decrease in systolic blood pressure of 20 mmHg or a decrease in diastolic blood pressure of 10 mmHg within 3 minutes of standing when compared with blood pressure from sitting or supine position. It could result from venous pooling or a decrease in hemoglobin postsurgery. Common symptoms include dizziness, lightheadedness, blurred vision, weakness, fatigue, nausea, heart palpitations, and headaches.

Key points
1. Especially postoperatively, it is important to monitor vitals throughout all positional changes to assess for adverse reactions.
2. If a patient presents with falls, it is important for the physical therapist to understand the reason for the fall to assist with fall prevention in the future.
3. Efficient and effective communication between team members is imperative to optimize the patient' s plan of care.

General Information

Case no.	9.B
Authors	Julie M Skrzat, PT, DPT, PhD, Board Certified Clinical Specialist in Cardiovascular & Pulmonary Physical Therapy Sean Griech, PT, DPT, PhD, COMT, Board Certified Clinical Specialist in Orthopaedic Physical Therapy
Diagnosis	Intertrochanteric fracture
Setting	Home
Learner expectations	☑ Initial evaluation ☐ Re-evaluation ☐ Treatment session
Learner objectives	1. To emphasize the importance of "yellow flags" and "red flags" regardless of clinical setting. 2. To understand the appropriate course of action when an unexpected finding is present. 3. To take into consideration the role of patient's family member/caregiver when designing a home exercise program.

Medical

Chief complaint	Status post (s/p) fall with open reduction and internal fixation (ORIF).
History of present illness	The patient was recently admitted to the acute care hospital for a mechanical fall. X-ray revealed a right intertrochanteric fracture. Orthopaedic surgery was consulted and an ORIF was performed to repair the intertrochanteric fracture. Postoperatively, the patient had two bouts of orthostatic hypotension—one with the physical therapist and one with the resident nurse—but resolved. The patient was in the hospital for 3 days then discharged to her home. The patient's husband transported the patient home without incident. Home physical therapy is starting on day 2 of being home (5 days after surgery).
Past medical history	Hypertension, coronary artery disease, type 2 diabetes mellitus, obesity (body mass index [BMI] = 31.05), diabetic neuropathy
Past surgical history	Hysterectomy
Allergies	No known drug allergies
Medications	Lisinopril, Atorvastatin, Pregabalin, Metformin, Acetaminophen pro re nata (prn) pain, Ibuprofen prn pain, Oxycodone prn pain
Precautions/orders	Weight bearing as tolerated (WBAT) right lower extremity (RLE)

Social history

Home setup	• Resides in a multilevel home with her husband. • Three steps with no rail to enter. • Half bath is on the first floor. • Bedroom and bathroom are located on the second floor. • Flight of stairs + one handrail to the second floor.
Occupation	• Employed as a fifth-grade elementary school teacher
Prior level of function	Currently: • Modified independent with bed mobility • Supervision for transfers and ambulation with a rolling walker (RW) • Assistance × 1: supervision to ascend/descend steps • Otherwise, primarily been watching TV while sitting in the recliner. Prior to hospitalization: • Independent with functional mobility and activities of daily living (ADLs). • Denies any functional limitations. • (+) driver
Recreational activities	• Enjoys playing with her grandchildren (2 and 3 years old) and reading for leisure.

Pause points

Based on the above information, what are the priorities?
• Diagnostic tests and measures?
• Outcome measures?
• Treatment interventions?

Physical Therapy Examination			
Subjective			
"My leg is more swollen today."			
Objective			

Vital signs	Pre-treatment			Post-treatment
	Supine	Sitting	Standing	
Blood pressure (mmHg)	123/85	125/83	124/88	135/87
Heart rate (beats/min)	88	90	91	101
Respiratory rate (breaths/min)	12	14	13	16
Pulse oximetry on room air (SpO$_2$)	98	97	96	99
Borg Scale	7/20	8/20	9/20	10/20
Pain (throughout right hip/ incision site)	2/10	4/10	6/10	4/10
General	• Patient seated in kitchen chair. She is displaying no signs or symptoms of distress. RW is nearby. Patient's husband in present.			
Cardiovascular and pulmonary	• Denies chest pain • Normal S1, S2 • Normal rate and rhythm • Bilateral lung bases with mild decrease in breath sounds • Peripheral pulses: Left lower extremity (LLE): 2 + dorsalis pedis (DP) RLE: 1 + DP • Wells Criteria: ▶ Fig. 9.4			
Gastrointestinal	• Unremarkable			
Genitourinary	• Unremarkable			
Musculoskeletal	Range of motion	• Bilateral upper extremity (BUE): within functional limit (WFL) • LLE: WFL • RLE: functional range of motion, knee WFL, ankle WFL		
	Strength	• BUE: 5/5 • LLE: 5/5 • Right hip flexion: 3 + /5 • Right hip abduction 3/5 • Right knee flexion / extension: 4/5 • Right anterior tibialis and evertors: 1/5		
	Aerobic	• 14/20 on the Rate of Perceived Exertion (RPE) Scale when ascending the stairs		
	Flexibility	• Tight right hip flexors and right hamstrings noted		
	Edema	• Calf circumferential measurements: 3.75-cm difference between left and right calves, with right being larger • Pitting edema in RLE: 3 +		
Neurological	Balance	• Sitting, static, and dynamic: independent • Standing, static: modified independent with RW • Standing, dynamic: modified independent—supervision; requires assistance if not external support		
	Cognition	• Alert and oriented × 4		
	Coordination	• LLE: intact heel to shin • RLE: difficult to perform due to pain		
	Cranial Nerves	• II–XII: intact		
	Reflexes	• Patellar: 2 + bilaterally		

(Continued)

(Continued)

Physical Therapy Examination		
	Sensation	• LLE: intact • RLE: decreased to light touch in L3, L4, L5 dermatome distribution
	Tone	• Unremarkable
	Other	• N/A
Functional status		
Bed mobility		• Supine to sit: independent using long-sit technique • Sit to supine: modified independent with use of long-handled leg lifter and long-sit technique
Transfers		• Sit to/from stand: supervision with RW
Ambulation		• Ambulates × 75 feet with RW supervision • Gait deviations notable for decreased cadence, steppage gait ▸ Fig. 9.5
Stairs		• Outside: ascend/descend three stairs with assistance × one due to lack of railings • Inside: ascend/descend 12 steps with supervision single heart rate and both upper extremities, using step-to method, increased WB through BUE

Clinical characteristic	Score
Active cancer (patient either receiving treatment for cancer within the previous 6 months or currently receiving palliative treatment)	1
Paralysis, paresis, or recent cast immobilization of the lower extremities	1
Recently bedridden for $\geq$ 3 days, or major surgery within the previous 12 weeks requiring general or regional anesthesia	1
Localized tenderness along the distribution of the deep venous system	1
Entire leg swelling	1
Calf swelling at least 3 cm larger than that on the asymptomatic side (measured 10 cm below tibial tuberosity)	1
Pitting edema confined to the symptomatic leg	1
Collateral superficial veins (non-varicose)	1
Previously documented deep vein thrombosis	1
Alternative diagnosis at least as likely as deep vein thrombosis	−2

[a] Wells scoring system for DVT: −2 to 0: low probability, 1 to 2 points: moderate probability, 3 to 8 points: high probability

Fig. 9.4 Wells Criteria for the prediction of deep vein thrombosis (DVT) (Adapted from Modi S, Deisler R, Gozel K, et al. Wells Criteria for DVT is a reliable clinical tool to assess the risk of deep venous thrombosis in trauma patients. World J Emerg Surg 2016;11:24.)

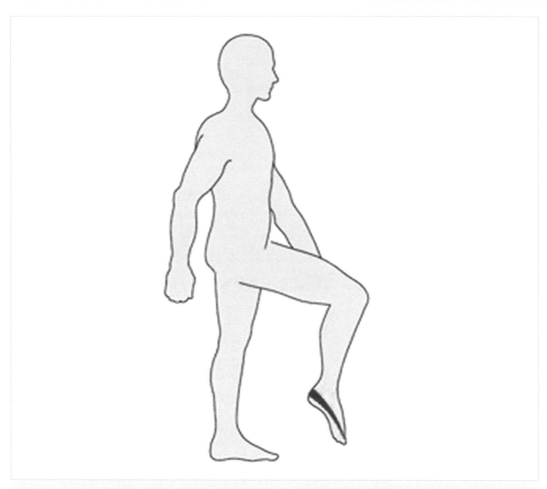

Fig. 9.5 Steppage gait with foot drop (Adapted from Stance and Gait. In: Mattle H, Mumenthaler M, Taub E, ed. Fundamentals of Neurology: An Illustrated Guide. 2nd ed. New York, NY: Thieme; 2017.)

Assessment	
☑ Physical therapist's	*Assessment left blank for learner to develop.*
Goals	
Patient's	"To decrease the swelling; be able to walk without the RW."
Short term	1.
	Goals left blank for learner to develop.
	2.
Long term	1.
	Goals left blank for learner to develop.
	2.

Plan	
☐ Physician's ☑ Physical therapist's ☐ Other's	Upon medical clearance, will continue to follow two to three times a week to progress strength, balance, and endurance to maximize functional mobility and safety.

Bloom's Taxonomy Level	Case 9.B Questions
Create	1. Synthesizing the medical data and physical examination findings, develop an appropriate physical therapy assessment of the patient. 2. Develop two short-term physical therapy goals, including an appropriate timeframe. 3. Develop two long-term physical therapy goals, including an appropriate timeframe.
Evaluate	4. Name two different diagnoses for the etiology of the lower motor neuron foot drop.
Analyze	5. Identify which criteria, if any, the patient meets for the Wells Criteria for DVT. Interpret. 6. If a DVT is suspected, what is the physical therapist's most immediate course of action?
Apply	7. How would the physical therapist educate the patient's husband to assist the patient with functional mobility to optimize his body mechanics?
Understand	8. What objective findings contribute to the suspicion of a DVT? 9. This patient has a steppage gait. Interpret what it means and explain why the patient may have this gait deviation.
Remember	10. State the purpose for the patient's home medications: Atorvastatin, Pregabalin, Metformin, Lisinopril, Acetaminophen, Ibuprofen, Oxycodone.

Bloom's Taxonomy Level	Case 9.B Answers

Create	1. The patient is a 60-year-old woman s/p mechanical fall, resulting in displaced intertrochanteric fracture of the right femur. She is now 5 days post right ORIF. Hospitalization was complicated by orthostatic hypotension. She has since been discharged home with home physical therapy. Upon initial evaluation, she demonstrates decreased strength in RLE, most notable in anterior tibialis and evertors, mildly decreased RLE dorsalis pedis pulse, increased right calf circumferential measures, right pitting edema, and decreased RLE sensation. The above objective findings are concerning for a DVT. Wells Criteria score was 3, indicating a high probability of a DVT. Suggest the patient follow up with primary care provider. Will continue physical therapy once medically cleared.
	2. Short-term goals:
	    • The patient will be independent with bilateral lower extremity home exercise program for strength and endurance within 4 days to aid in functional mobility improvement.
	    • The patient will ascend/descend three steps with single point cane and supervision within 4 days to enter/exit home.
	3. Long-term goals:
	    • The patient will ambulate 985 feet with an RW independently to ambulate within the community within 10 days.
	    • The patient will ascend/descend 12 steps with a single handrail independently within 10 days to get to/from the second floor.

Evaluate	4. Two different diagnoses for the etiology of the lower motor neuron foot drop are (a) pressure neuropathy to the common peroneal nerve at the level of the fibular head and (b) diabetic mononeuropathy.
Analyze	5. When looking at the Wells Criteria, the patient is positive for having major surgery within the past 12 weeks, calf swelling > 3 cm compared to the other leg, and pitting edema, which is greater in the symptomatic leg. The patient does not have an alternative diagnosis that could lead to these signs and symptoms. Therefore, the patient scored a 3, indicating a high probability of having a DVT. 6. If a DVT is suspected, the physical therapist's most immediate course of action will be to call the primary care physician. The physical therapist should be prepared to report the objective findings and results and interpretation from the Wells Criteria.

(Continued)

(Continued)

Bloom's Taxonomy Level	Case 9.B Answers
Apply	7. To educate the patient's husband on how to physically assist the patient, the physical therapist should demonstrate proper body mechanics. Additionally, the patient's husband should be taught to bend with his legs and not his back.
Understand	8. The objective findings that contribute to the suspicion of a DVT are recent surgery, swelling > 3 cm, and pitting edema in surgical extremity. 9. This patient has weakness of the tibialis anterior muscle as determined by a manual muscle testing (MMT) grade of 1/5 for ankle dorsiflexion. During the swing phase of gait, the patient's dorsiflexors (including tibialis anterior) are needed for foot and toe clearance. To compensate for this weakness, the patient overactives his right hip flexors, which allows clearance during the swing phase. The patient also likely demonstrates right foot flat or foot flap at initial contact due to their inability to initiate heel strike.
Remember	10. Atorvastatin: treats high cholesterol and triglyceride levels. Pregabalin: treats nerve and muscle pain. Metformin: treats high glucose levels as a result of type 2 diabetes mellitus. Lisinopril: treats hypertension. Acetaminophen: treats minor aches and pain, reduces fever. Ibuprofen: nonsteroidal anti-inflammatory drug [NSAID], treats minor aches and pains. Oxycodone: narcotic, treats moderate to severe pain.

Key points
1. Do not underestimate the patient's medical acuity. Just because the patient is not in the hospital does not mean ignorance of "red flags."
2. Be mindful of the effects of an orthopaedic injury on body systems outside of the musculoskeletal system.
3. When designing a home exercise program, consider not only the patient's needs, but also those of the family members and/or caregivers.

General Information	
Case no.	9.C
Authors	Julie M. Skrzat, PT, DPT, PhD, Board Certified Clinical Specialist in Cardiovascular & Pulmonary Physical Therapy Sean F. Griech, PT, DPT, PhD, COMT, Board Certified Clinical Specialist in Orthopaedic Physical Therapy
Diagnosis	Generalized deconditioning
Setting	Outpatient clinic
Learner expectations	☑ Initial evaluation ☐ Re-evaluation ☐ Treatment session
Learner objectives	1. List the patient's body structure and impairments. 2. Identify appropriate outcome measures based on the objective data provided for use in the outpatient clinic. 3. Correlate the impact of a deep vein thrombosis (DVT). 4. Develop a home exercise program based on the patient's body structure and impairments to optimize his or her participation and quality of life.

Medical	
Chief complaint	Right hip pain and gait dysfunction status post (s/p) open reduction and internal fixation (ORIF).
History of present illness	The patient is a 60-year-old woman who presents to an outpatient clinic with right hip pain and gait dysfunction following an ORIF of her right hip. She had a normal hospital course and was discharged home healthy. Home physical therapy was initiated; however, during the initial evaluation, a DVT was suspected. She was referred to the emergency

(Continued)

(Continued)

Medical	
	department where a DVT was diagnosed using a duplex ultrasound. She was discharged home the same day on apixaban. She received an additional four home physical therapy visits. She is now presenting to an outpatient clinic for further strength and conditioning (6 weeks postoperatively).
Past medical history	Hypertension, coronary artery disease, type 2 diabetes mellitus, obesity (body mass index [BMI] = 31.05), diabetic neuropathy
Past surgical history	Hysterectomy
Allergies	No known drug allergies
Medications	Lisinopril, Atorvastatin, Pregabalin, Metformin, Apixaban, Acetaminophen pro re nata (prn) pain, Ibuprofen prn pain, Oxycodone prn pain
Precautions/orders	• Weight bearing as tolerated (WBAT) right lower extremity (RLE) • Activity as tolerated

Social history	
Home setup	• Resides in a multilevel home with her husband • Three steps with no rail to enter. • Half bath i on the first floor. • Bedroom and bathroom are located on the second floor. • Flight of stairs + one handrail to the second floor.
Occupation	• Employed as a fifth-grade elementary school teacher.
Level of function	Currently: • Independent with bed mobility, transfers, self-care activities of daily living (ADLs). • Modified independent for ambulation with use of single point cane (SPC) on level surfaces, requires supervision from husband for stairs. She is using a rolling walker for community distances. • (-) driver Prior to hospitalization: • Independent with functional mobility and ADLs • Denies any functional limitations • (+) driver
Recreational activities	• Enjoys playing with her grandchildren (2 and 3 years old) and reading for leisure.

Pause points
Based on the above information, what are the priorities? • Diagnostic tests and measures? • Outcome measures? • Treatment interventions?

Physical Therapy Examination
Subjective
"I feel like I was really making progress with the home physical therapy, but the clot really seemed to set me back. I really want to get stronger so I can get upstairs by myself and play with my grandkids."

Objective		
Vital signs	Pre-treatment	Post-treatment
Blood pressure (mmHg)	128/81	133/83
Heart rate (beats/min)	76	86
Respiratory rate (breaths/min)	12	14
Pulse oximetry on room air (SpO$_2$)	98%	97%
Pain (right hip)	5/10	6/10

(Continued)

(Continued)

Physical Therapy Examination		
General	• Patient sitting in waiting room with rolling walker. Patient's husband accompanied her to visit.	
Cardiovascular and pulmonary	• Blood pressure, heart rate, and SaO_2 all were within normal limits (WNLs) at the time of examination. • No apparent distress was noted at rest. • Normal increased heart rate with activity is noted.	
Gastrointestinal	• Opioid-related constipation	
Genitourinary	• Unremarkable	
Musculoskeletal	Range of motion (ROM)	• Bilateral upper extremity (BUE): WNL • Left lower extremity (LLE): WNL • RLE: ↓ hip flexion (95 degrees), hip abduction (30 degrees), hip external rotation (ER; 35 degrees), internal rotation (IR; 20 degrees), and knee flexion (125 degrees)
	Strength	• BUE: 5/5 throughout • LLE: 5/5 throughout • RLE: hip flexion: 4/5 Hip extension (gluteus maximus): 3/5 Hip abduction: 3/5 Hip adduction: 5/5 Hip ER and IR: 4/5 Knee flexion (HS): 5/5 Knee extension: 4/5
	Aerobic	• 2-Minute Walk Test: 150 m • 30-Second Sit to Stand Test: 10
	Flexibility	• Tight hamstrings B/L (popliteal angle > 20 degrees) • Thomas Test + for tight hip flexors on right
	Other	• Residual swelling/edema of right calf from DVT • Surgical incision: no sign of infection or inflammation
Neurological	Balance	• Timed Up and Go (TUG) Test: 12 seconds
	Cognition	• Alert and oriented × 4
	Coordination	• Intact finger to nose bilaterally
	Cranial Nerves	• II–XII: intact
	Reflexes	• Patellar: 2 + bilaterally
	Sensation	• Intact to light touch throughout bilateral lower extremity (BLE)
	Tone	• Normal throughout BUE and BLE
	Other	• N/A
Functional status		
Bed mobility	• Supine to sit: independent	
Transfers	• Sit to/from stand: independent, frequently uses arms for assistance	
Ambulation	• Ambulates ~500 feet with modified independence and SPC. **Video 9.1.**	
Stairs	• Outside: ascend/descend three stairs with minimal assistance × 1 due to lack of railings. • Inside: ascend/descend 12 steps with single heart rate using both upper extremities, step-to method with supervision.	

Assessment	
☑ Physical therapist's	*Assessment left blank for learner to develop*

Goals	
Patient's	"I want to be able to go up and down the stairs by myself and sit on the floor (and get back up) to play with my grandkids."
Short term	1. *Goals left blank for learner to develop.* 2
Long term	1. *Goals left blank for learner to develop.* 2.

Plan	
□ Physician's ☑ Physical therapist's □ Other's	Will continue to see patient twice a week × 4 weeks. Treatment will include therapeutic exercise (proximal hip and RLE strengthening, aerobic conditioning), gait training on level surfaces and stairs, and functional mobility training.

Bloom's Taxonomy Level	Case 9.C Questions
Create	1. Synthesizing the medical data and physical examination findings, develop an appropriate assessment of the patient. 2. Develop two short-term physical therapy goals, including an appropriate timeframe. 3. Develop two long-term physical therapy goals, including an appropriate timeframe.
Evaluate	4. Explain how the recent hospitalization and DVT may affect this patient's course of care to her and her husband.
Analyze	5. Analyze the patient's gait. 6. Interpret the patient's 2-Minute Walk Test results. What is the minimal detectable change for this patient? 7. What is the appropriate interpretation of the TUG Test for this patient?
Apply	8. Design and implement two interventions to improve the patient's ability to walk community distance with an SPC. 9. Design and implement two interventions to improve the patient's ability to negotiate stairs independently. 10. Design and implement two interventions to improve lower extremity mobility and ROM. 11. Explain appropriate patient education topics for enhancing the patient's functional status.
Understand	12. Explain in patient-friendly terms any specific signs and symptoms the patient should be cautious of due to her history of DVT.
Remember	13. Based on the patient's diagnosis, what precautions (if any) should be observed?

Bloom's Taxonomy Level	Case 9.C Answers
Create	1. The patient is a 60-year-old woman s/p ORIF of her right hip. She had a normal hospital course and was discharged to home physical therapy; however, during this time she was diagnosed with a DVT. She was treated with apixaban and received an additional four home physical therapy visits. She currently presents with limited mobility and endurance, hip weakness (especially hip extensors), and postoperative pain. The patient lives in a two-story home and would like to improve her ability to go upstairs. The patient is a good candidate for skilled physical therapy.

(Continued)

(Continued)

Bloom's Taxonomy Level	Case 9.C Answers
	2. Short-term goals: • The patient will improve her 2-Minute Walk Test distance by 12.2 m (40 feet) within 2 weeks to mobilize more efficiently throughout the community. • The patient will ascend/descend 12 steps with a single handrail, using one upper extremity, and step-to method independently within 2 weeks to be able to get to/from the second floor of her home. 3. Long-term goals: • The patient will complete 15 sit to stands in 30 seconds within 4 weeks to demonstrate improved endurance and functional strength. • The patient will improve TUG score to less than 10 seconds with a SPC in 4 weeks to demonstrate improved mobility and decreased fall risk.
Evaluate	4. Due to the patient's recent DVT, she is now prescribed the anticoagulant apixaban. A side effect of this medication is the risk of bleeding. Because of this, her balance should thoroughly be assessed, especially since a fall was the initial cause of her femur fracture. She should be educated on signs and symptoms of bleeding, as well as signs and symptoms of another clot.
Analyze	5. The patient presents with a Trendelenburg gait due to her gluteus medius weakness. 6. The 2-Minute Walk Test is a measure of endurance. The patient's distance during administration of the test is 150 m, which is considered in the normal range for older adults. The minimal detectable change is 12.2 m (40 feet). 7. For community-dwelling adults, the cutoff score for risk of falling is > 13.5 seconds. This patient took 12 seconds to complete the test; therefore, she is not a fall risk.
Apply	8. Two interventions to improve the patient's ability to walk community distance with an SPC include (a) endurance training (i.e., walking on a treadmill with a gradual increase in time) and (b) balance training with a unilateral device (i.e., walking in the parallel bars with a single support). Eventually, the physical therapist should incorporate dual tasks and obstacles to ensure safety in the community. 9. Two interventions to improve the patient's ability to negotiate stairs independently include (a) exercises to improve hip flexion (i.e., tying a theraband at stair height around the parallel bars and having the patient attempt to step over) and (b) exercises to strengthen hip abductors (i.e., single limb stance exercises). 10. Two interventions to improve lower extremity mobility and ROM include (a) standing mini-squats with external support (i.e., countertop) and (b) supine heel slides, which can be active assisted with a sheet if necessary. 11. Because the catalyst for the intertrochanteric fracture was a mechanical fall, education on fall prevention and balance interventions should be primary. This includes review of home setup and fall prevention modifications. Additionally, education should include how to screen for DVT and infection at the surgical site.
Understand	12. "Because of your recent surgery, you are at risk of developing blood clots, also known as DVT, in your leg. Signs and symptoms to monitor for include swelling > 3 cm, pitting edema, or localized tenderness along your leg. Should any of these signs or symptoms arise, you should contact your primary care physician immediately. To prevent the development of a DVT, I encourage you to keep your legs moving. Do ankle pumps and walk around frequently. The muscle activity pumps the blood towards your heart and prevents it from becoming stagnant."
Remember	13. Based on the patient's diagnosis, the patient is WBAT on her right lower extremity.

Suggested Readings

2-minute walk test. Available at: https://www.sralab.org/rehabilitation-measures/2-minute-walk-test. Accessed October 30, 2019

30 second chair stand. Available at: https://www.cdc.gov/steadi/pdf/STEADI-Assessment-30Sec-508.pdf. Accessed October 31, 2019

American College of Sports Medicine. ACSM's Guidelines for Exercise Testing and Prescription. 10th ed. Baltimore, MD: Lippincott, Williams and Wilkins; 2017

Connelly DM, Thomas BK, Cliffe SJ, Perry WM, Smith RE. Clinical utility of the 2-minute walk test for older adults living in long-term care. Physiother Can. 2009; 61(2):78–87

Drugs@FDA: FDA-Approved Drugs. Available at: https://www.accessdata.fda.gov/scripts/cder/daf/index.cfm?event=overview.process&ApplNo=202155. Accessed on April 1, 2020

Drug Approval Package. Eliquis (Apixaban). Available at: https://www.accessdata.fda.gov/drugsatfda_docs/nda/2012/202155Orig1s000TOC.cfm. Accessed April 1, 2020

Goodman CC, Fuller KS. Pathology: Implications for the Physical Therapist. 4th ed. St. Louis, MO: Saunders Elsevier; 2015

Hillegass E. Essentials of Cardiopulmonary Physical Therapy. 4th ed. St. Louis, MO: Elsevier; 2017

Hillegass E, Puthoff M, Frese EM, Thigpen M, Sobush DC, Auten B, Guideline Development Group. Role of physical therapists in the management of individuals at risk for or diagnosed with venous thromboembolism: evidence-based clinical practice guideline. Phys Ther. 2016; 96(2):143–166

Lanier JB, Mote MB, Clay EC. Evaluation and management of orthostatic hypotension. Am Fam Physician. 2011; 84(5):527–536

Modi S, Deisler R, Gozel K, et al. Wells criteria for DVT is a reliable clinical tool to assess the risk of deep venous thrombosis in trauma patients. World J Emerg Surg. 2016; 11:24

Perry J, Burnfield J. Gait Analysis: Normal and Pathological Function. 2nd ed. Thorofare, NJ: Slack Incorporated; 2010

Timed Up and Go. Available at: https://www.sralab.org/rehabilitation-measures/timed-and-go. Accessed October 30, 2019

10 Low Back Pain

General Information	
Case no.	10.A Low Back Pain
Author(s)	David Gillette, PT, DPT, Board Certified Clinical Specialist in Geriatrics Physical Therapy Bhavana Raja, PT, PhD Todd Davenport, PT, DPT, MPH, Board Certified Clinical Specialist in Orthopaedic Physical Therapy
Diagnosis	Low back pain without radiculopathy
Setting	Outpatient clinic
Learner expectations	☑ Initial evaluation ☐ Re-evaluation ☐ Treatment session
Learner objectives	1. Explain the processes of examination and evaluation for referral in an individual with low back pain related to medical pathology. 2. Discuss the general referral pattern for retroperitoneal abdominal structures. 3. Create a physical therapy plan of care for an individual with low back pain secondary to a medical condition across care settings.

Medical	
Chief concern	Pain in lower back and abdomen, nausea
History of present illness	The patient is a 72-year-old man who self-referred to outpatient physical therapy with worsening low back pain. The patient reports first onset of low back pain in his 20s while playing a game of baseball. Since that time, he has had intermittent episodes of pain that have "come and gone" on its own. He has self-managed his symptoms over the years with Tylenol, rest, and use of a heating pad. Episodes usually last 2 weeks. He noted current episode of pain beginning 3 days ago, beginning with an insidious onset. This is not unusual based on his prior pain presentations. Yet, this time, the pain has become very severe in a very short period of time. His symptoms are worsened with standing, walking, sitting, and laying supine. Tylenol, rest, and heating pad have not been helpful to alleviate symptoms.
Past medical history	Hypertension, chronic obstructive pulmonary disease (COPD), diabetes mellitus type 2, right hip osteoarthritis, hypercholesterolemia, obesity Tobacco: 1 pack per day for 40 years, expresses desire to quit Caffeine: 2 cups of coffee per day; recently quit soda Alcohol: occasionally
Past surgical history	Right total knee arthroplasty: 5 years ago; left rotator cuff repair: 2 years ago
Allergies	No known drug allergies.
Medications	Lisinopril, Atorvastatin, Metoprolol, Naproxen, Aspirin, Hyzaar *Patient reports being noncompliant with medications*
Precautions/orders	Activity as tolerated

Social history	
Home setup	• Resides in a multilevel home with wife. • Two steps to enter, rail is on the left. • Half bath + guest room are on the first floor. • Bedroom and bathroom are located on the second floor. • Flight of stair + right handrail to the second floor.
Occupation	• Retired as research scientist 2 years ago; now drives Uber for extra income and volunteers at a local homeless shelter.
Prior level of function	• Independent with functional mobility and activities of daily living (ADLs). • No assistive device prior to recent hospitalization but has rolling walker and single point cane from prior surgery.

(Continued)

(Continued)

Social history	
	• Two noninjurious falls in the last year: one at night going to the bathroom quickly and one when walking on uneven sidewalk during the day. • Spouse works full-time as a partner at a regional law firm; currently on a case that requires them to be gone during the week. • Has estranged son and daughter from first marriage.
Recreational activities	• Primarily watching TV and reading. • Enjoys fishing from a boat, but now is limited due to back ache.

Pause points
Based on the above information, what are the priority: • Diagnostic tests and measures? • Outcome measures? • Treatment interventions?

Physical Therapy Examination
Subjective
"This is the worst back pain I've ever had. Nothing Is helping and it's not going away. In fact, it's getting a lot worse, quickly. I wanted to see you before I go to my doc."

Objective

Vital signs	Pre-treatment	Post-treatment
Blood pressure (mmHg)	131/88	128/84
Heart rate (beats/min)	112	115
Respiratory rate (breaths/min)	26	25
Pulse oximetry on room air (SpO_2)	98%	97%
Pain	"12/10" per patient report	"12/10" per patient report
Temperature (°F)	97.7	–
General	• Presents seated in clinic waiting room, appears slightly pale. • Reports mild nausea.	
Cardiovascular and pulmonary	• Tachycardia • No adventitious cardiac and lung sounds. • Pulsatile mass noted superior to the umbilicus, which is more noticeable. The lateral margins of the mass increase from superior to inferior from 3.5 to 9 cm apart at its widest point just superior to the umbilicus. The pulsatile mass is not painful with palpation. • Auscultation positive for bruits over the abdominal aorta.	
Gastrointestinal	• Mild nausea • Eating a normal diet. • Bowel habit has not changed.	
Musculoskeletal	Range of motion	• Bilateral upper extremity (BUE): not apparently restrictive to functional mobility, though not formally tested. • Bilateral lower extremity (BLE): not apparently restrictive to functional mobility, though not formally tested.
	Strength	• BUE: grossly > 3 + /5 for the major antigravity muscle groups as demonstrated through functional mobility, not formally tested. • BLE: grossly > 3 + /5 for the major antigravity muscle groups as demonstrated through functional mobility, not formally tested.

(Continued)

(Continued)

Physical Therapy Examination		
	Inspection	• Patient stands in trunk and hip flexion. He has discomfort when asked to stand erect. A pulsatile mass is noted superior to the umbilicus.
Neurological	Balance	• Sitting, static: independent • Sitting, dynamic: independent • Standing, static: independent • Standing, dynamic: independent
	Cognition	• Alert and oriented × 4
Functional status		
Bed mobility		• Rolling either direction: independent • Supine to/from sit: independent, increased time to perform
Transfers		• Sit to/from stand: independent
Ambulation		• Ambulates from waiting room to/from treatment room (~150 feet) independently with no assistive device. • Gait deviations notable for decreased cadence and stride length, with persistent trunk flexion throughout the gait cycle and limited hip extension and ankle dorsiflexion in terminal stance.
Stairs		• Not assessed at this time

Pause points
Based on the above information: • What is the best decision regarding the appropriateness of physical therapy (retain, refer, or comanage)? • What are features of the case that are consistent with a decision to refer the emergency department?

Assessment	
☑ Physical therapist's	*Assessment left blank for learner to develop*
Goals	
Patient's	"I want to understand what is happening with me and then go back to being able to fish without pain."
Short term	1. *Goals left blank for learner to develop* 2.
Long term	1. *Goals left blank for learner to develop* 2.

Plan	
☑ Physical therapist's	The plan for this patient is to be referred to the emergency department for additional medical evaluation, including diagnostic imaging to either confirm or disconfirm a suspected abdominal aortic aneurysm (AAA).

Bloom's Taxonomy Level	Case 10.A Questions
Create	1. Synthesizing the medical data and physical examination findings, develop an appropriate physical therapy assessment of the patient. 2. Develop two short-term physical therapy goals, including an appropriate timeframe. 3. Develop two long-term physical therapy goals, including an appropriate timeframe.

(Continued)

(Continued)

Bloom's Taxonomy Level	Case 10.A Questions
Evaluate	4. What is the best synthesis of this patient's findings in order to establish a provisional diagnosis that guides additional patient care and case management?
Analyze	5. What palpation findings would suggest the presence of AAA?
Apply	6. What is the reliability of physical examination findings to determine the potential presence of AAA?
Understand	7. Is it safe to palpate the abdominal aorta in the presence of a possible dissection?
Remember	8. Where is the abdominal aorta located? 9. What is the frequency of AAA in the United States? 10. What is an aneurysm?

Bloom's Taxonomy Level	Case 10.A Answers
Create	1. The patient is a 72-year-old man who presents with low back pain and pulsatile mass, which raises the index of clinical suspicion for AAA. This physical therapy assessment requires referral for additional testing and consultation to confirm, as may be considered medically appropriate. Recommend holding physical therapy at this time pending additional referral and consultation with the emergency department. 2. Short-term goals: • Patient will follow up with emergency department immediately to evaluate for AAA. • Patient will verbally demonstrate understanding of the plan for physical therapy to refer out to the emergency department at this time. 3. Long-term goals: • Patient will follow up with outpatient physical therapist when medically appropriate to complete physical therapy evaluation.
Evaluate	4. According to the literature, the pretest probability of AAA is high in this patient secondary to the presence of two main risk factors. The odds ratios associated with male gender and age 70 years are 5.71 (95% confidence interval [CI]; 95% CI: 5.57–5.81) and 14.46 (95% CI: 13.45–15.55) for AAA. This means that (a) men are over 5 times more likely than women to present with AAA and (b) people aged ≥ 70 years are almost 15 times more likely than people aged 50 years to present with AAA. The patient's previous history of smoking also places him at elevated risk of vascular pathology.
Analyze	5. AAA are defined as 3.0-cm enlargements of the abdominal aorta. The clinician uses their fingertips to assess the lateral margins of the abdominal aortic pulse, and then the distance is measured as an approximation of the diameter of the abdominal aorta. The advantages of using the fingertips instead of thumbs are (a) broader palpation surface for more patient comfort and (b) a decrease in likelihood of mistaking one's own digital pulse for the patient's pulse. Palpation distances may be greater as palpated from the abdomen, because pulsatile waves are transmitted through the abdominal tissues. (▶ Fig. 10.1) Diagnostic ultrasound or computed tomography is required to confirm the diagnosis and characterize the size of an AAA.
Apply	6. Palpation to approximate the width of the abdominal aorta demonstrates moderate diagnostic accuracy overall to determine the presence of an AAA. According to Fink and colleagues, palpation yielded sensitivity of 68% (95% CI: 60–76%), specificity of 75% (95% CI: 68–82%), positive likelihood ratio of 2.7 (95% CI: 2.0–3.6), and negative likelihood ratio of 0.43 (95% CI: 0.33–0.56) with respect to diagnostic ultrasound. Sensitivity was increased for larger AAA (>5.0 cm). In addition to size of the AAA, additional factors that affect diagnostic accuracy of palpation reduce as abdominal girth and abdominal wall stiffness increase.
Understand	7. It is safe to palpate a suspected case of AAA; there are no documented cases of dissection related to palpation.

(Continued)

(Continued)

Bloom's Taxonomy Level	Case 10.A Answers
Remember	8. The abdominal aorta begins at the diaphragm, generally at the T12 level, and is located to the left of the lumbar spine. The abdominal aorta bifurcates into the common iliac arteries at the level of the umbilicus.
	9. AAA affects ~1.1 million older adults in the United States (1.4%). Rupture rates from natural history studies are ~5.3 to 6.3% per year but may be as high as 33%. Rupture rates increase positively with aneurysm size.
	10. An aneurysm is a weakness of the arterial wall. There is no universally accepted mechanism for how aneurysms occur, but there are many well-characterized risk factors.

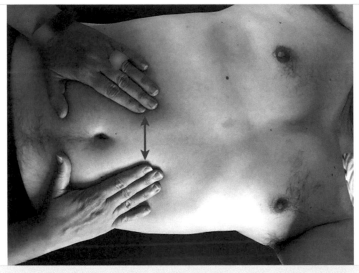

Fig. 10.1 Assessment of abdominal aorta. With the patient lying supine, the clinician stands at the side of the patient. Place fingertips over the epigastrium to determine the presence of a pulse, and with palms down and index fingers on either side of aorta slowly track laterally from the midline. Width of the aorta can be estimated by measurement of the finger distance from one another once the pulse disappears. An abdominal aortic aneurysm (AAA) is defined as 3.0-cm enlargements of the abdominal aorta. (Adapted from Chaikof EL, Dalman RL, Eskandari MK, et al. The Society for Vascular Surgery practice guidelines on the care of patients with an abdominal aortic aneurysm. J Vasc Surg. 2018;67(1):2–77 e72.)

Key points
1. Low back pain may arise from causes that are not amenable to physical therapy interventions.
2. AAA is more common in men than in women and in individuals older than 55 years, with increasing relative incidence over time.
3. Referral decisions should be made in a manner that considers a cautious interpretation of the patient's subjective and objective findings. Thus, in the case of this symptomatic patient, emergent referral is necessary to exclude the possibility of AAA.

General Information	
Case no.	10.B
Author(s)	David Gillette, PT, DPT, Board Certified Clinical Specialist in Geriatrics Physical Therapy Bhavana Raja, PT, PhD Todd Davenport, PT, DPT, MPH, Board Certified Clinical Specialist in Orthopaedic Physical Therapy
Diagnosis	Abdominal aortic aneurysm (AAA)
Setting	Emergency Department, with transfer to the Intensive Care Unit
Learner expectations	☑ Initial evaluation ☐ Re-evaluation ☐ Treatment session
Learner objectives	1. Explain the pathophysiology of the patient's diagnosis. 2. Relate the pathophysiology and progression of pathology from low back pain to the acute condition and its impact on activity/participation limitations seen in physical therapy practice. 3. Select, implement, and interpret physical therapy interventions based on the medical examination findings. 4. Develop an understanding of medical management and how it influences physical therapy plan of care.

Medical	
Chief concern	Pain in lower back and abdomen, nausea.
History of present illness	The patient is a 72-year-old man who was referred to the emergency department today from outpatient physical therapy with a primary complaint of chronic low back pain and secondary complaints of nausea and abdominal pain that have been worsening over last few days. He denies any falls, or trauma. He was seen by his primary care physician 2 weeks ago and was referred to outpatient physical therapy for management of what was thought to be mechanical low back pain. However, during the physical therapy evaluation, the physical therapist noticed a pulsating mass in the patient's abdomen and recommended the patient to go to the emergency department immediately. The patient drove from the physical therapist's clinic to the emergency department of the hospital, where he was subsequently admitted for surgical intervention.
Past medical history	Hypertension, chronic obstructive pulmonary disease (COPD), diabetes mellitus type 2, right hip osteoarthritis, hypercholesterolemia, obesity Tobacco: 1 pack per day for 40 years, expresses desire to quit Caffeine: 2 cups of coffee per day; recently quit soda Alcohol: occasionally
Past surgical history	Right total knee arthroplasty: 5 years ago; left rotator cuff repair: 2 years ago.
Allergies	No known drug allergies.
Medications	Lisinopril, Atorvastatin, Metoprolol, Naproxen, Aspirin, Hyzaar. *Patient reports being noncompliant with medications.*
Precautions/orders	Bedrest

Social history	
Home setup	• Resides in a multilevel home with his wife. • Two steps to enter, rail is on the left. • Half bath + guest room are on the first floor. • Bedroom and bathroom are located on the second floor. • Flight of stairs + right handrail to the second floor. • Spouse works full-time as a partner at a regional law firm; currently on a case that requires them to be gone during the week. • Has estranged son and daughter from first marriage.
Occupation	• Retired as research scientist 2 years ago; now drives Uber for extra income and volunteers at a local homeless shelter.

(Continued)

(Continued)

Social history	
Prior level of function	• Independent with functional mobility and activities of daily living (ADLs). • No assistive device prior to recent hospitalization but has rolling walker and single point cane from prior surgery. • Two noninjurious falls in the last year: one at night going to the bathroom quickly and one when walking on uneven sidewalk during the day.
Recreational activities	• Primarily watching TV and reading. • Fishing from a boat, but now is limited due to back ache.

Vital signs	Hospital day 0: emergency department	Hospital day 1: intensive care unit
Blood pressure (mmHg)	120/78	118/74
Heart rate (beats/min)	125	84
Respiratory rate (breaths/min)	20	16
Pulse oximetry (SpO$_2$)	91% on room air	95% on 4 L nasal cannula (NC)
Temperature (°F)	101.2	–

Imaging/diagnostic test	Hospital day 0: emergency department	Hospital day 1: intensive care unit
Computed tomography (CT) scan with contrast	1. Widened aortic lumen measuring ~5.8 cm. 2. Mural thrombus surrounding the contrast material. 3. No contrast material in peritoneal cavity.	–
Abdominal X-ray	–	1. ▶ Fig. 10.2
Ultrasound	1. A 5.7-cm dilation of distal abdominal aorta.	–

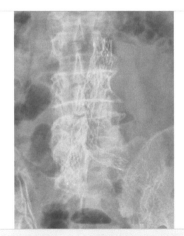

Fig. 10.2 Post-EVAR, a plain abdominal radiograph can help serve as a baseline for future stent graft follow-up. (Adapted from Gover D, ed. Case 50. In: Top 3 Differentials in Vascular and Interventional Radiology: A Case Review. 1st ed. New York, NY: Thieme; 2018.)

Medical management	Hospital day 0: emergency department	Hospital day 1: intensive care unit
Medications	1. Intravenous (IV) fluids 2. Ceftriaxone IV 3. Metoprolol 4. Acetaminophen 1,000 mg 5. Aspirin 6. Morphine 15 mg (PRN)	Continued per medical plan of care
Procedures	1. Endovascular repair of the AAA	–
Lines/tubes/drains	1. Telemetry 2. IV placed on left forearm 3. Central line 4. Urinary catheter	Continued per medical plan of care
Consults	1. Vascular surgery	1. Physical therapy 2. Occupational therapy
Precautions/orders	• Bedrest	• Activity as tolerated • Fall risk

Lab		Reference range	Hospital day 0: emergency department	Hospital day 1: intensive care unit
Arterial blood gas	pH	7.35–7.45	7.32	7.37
	PaCO$_2$	37–43	38	39
	PaO$_2$	80–95	96	96
	HCO$_3^-$	20–30	23	25
Complete blood count	White blood cell	5.0–10.0 × 10^9/L	9.6	8.3
	Hemoglobin	14.0–17.4 g/dL	10.8	8.6
	Hematocrit	42–52%	36.5	32.2
	Red blood cell	4.5–5.5	3.5	3.0
	Platelet	140,000–400,000/μL	240	115
Electrolytes	Calcium	8.6–10.3 mg/dL	8.9	9.1
	Chloride	98–108 mEq/L	98	100
	Magnesium	1.2–1.9 mEq/l	1.8	1.9
	Phosphate	2.3–4.1 mg/dL	2.9	2.8
	Potassium	3.7–5.1 mEq/L	4.2	4.5
	Sodium	134–142 mEq/L	141	140
Other	Cholesterol	<200 mg/dL	260	
	High-density lipoprotein	≥35 mg/dL	67	
	Low-density lipoprotein	65–180 mg/dL	198	Not reordered
	Triglycerides	<150 mg/dL	210	
	Blood urea nitrogen	7–20 mg/d	24	
	Creatinine	0.5–1.4	1.6	1.6
	Glucose	60–110 mg/dL	198	176
	B-type natriuretic peptide	<100 pg/mL	98	Not reordered
	D-dimer	<400 ng/mL	58	
	International normalized ratio	0.8–1.2	2.1	2.0

(Continued)

(Continued)

Lab		Reference range	Hospital day 0: emergency department	Hospital day 1: intensive care unit
	Lactate	<2 mmol	3.0	1.2
	Troponin - 1		0.02	
	Troponin - 2	<0.03 ng/mL	0.01	Not reordered
	Troponin - 3		0.02	

Pause points
Based on the above information, what are the priority: • Diagnostic tests and measures? • Outcome measures? • Treatment interventions?

Hospital Day 2, Post-Op Day 2, Intensive Care Unit: Physical Therapy Examination
Subjective
"My back and abdomen hurt. It's difficult to sit or move around."

Objective				
Vital signs	Pre-treatment			Post-treatment
	Supine	Sitting	Standing	Sitting
Blood pressure (mmHg)	110/73	100/70	99/74	115/79
Heart rate (beats/min)	70	73	84	90
Respiratory rate (breaths/min)	18	18	18	20
Pulse oximetry on 4 L NC (SpO$_2$)	100%	98%	97%	95%
Modified Borg Scale for shortness of breath	4/10		2/10, improved with upright posture and rest	
Pain	5/10, right abdomen/groin		7/10, right abdomen/groin	
	Pain worsens with coughing, sneezing, and taking deep breaths.			
General	• Patient supine in bed, Fowler's position, (+) abdominal guarding with pillow. • Lines notable for telemetry, NC, central line, urinary catheter.			
Cardiovascular and pulmonary	• Normal heart rate and rhythm. • Auscultation: no adventitious heart or lung sounds. • Pulses: 2 + bilateral dorsalis pedis			
Gastrointestinal	• Abdomen slightly distended, surgical incision on lower abdomen/groin, covered with dressing.			
Genitourinary	• (+) urinary catheter			
Musculoskeletal	Range of motion	• Bilateral upper extremity (BUE): within functional range • Bilateral lower extremity (BLE): within functional range with the exception of bilateral hip flexion, which has contracture of ~10 degrees.		
	Strength	• B shoulder motions all: 4 + /5 • B elbow flexion: 4/5 • B elbow extension: 4/5 • B wrist extension: 4/5 • B hip flexion: 3 + /5 • B knee flexion: 4/5 • B knee extension: 4/5 • B ankle dorsiflexion: 4/5		

(Continued)

(Continued)

Hospital Day 2, Post-Op Day 2, Intensive Care Unit: **Physical Therapy Examination**		
		• B ankle plantar flexion: 4/5 • 30-Second Sit to Stand: unable to complete one repetition of sit to stand without assistive device and minimum assistance from physical therapist.
	Aerobic	• Unable to perform standardized test at this time
	Flexibility	• On observation, tight bilateral pectoralis major and minor was demonstrated by rounded shoulder posture. • Additionally, tight hip flexors was demonstrated by increased lumbar lordosis. • Otherwise, formal flexibility tests not performed due to inability to lie flat, side lying, or prone due to surgical incision and pain.
Neurological	Balance	• Static sitting, unsupported: minimal assistance • Dynamic sitting, unsupported: minimal assistance • Static standing, supported: minimal assistance with rolling walker • Dynamic standing, supported: minimal assistance with rolling walker
	Cognition	• Alert and oriented × 4 • Richmond Agitation-Sedation Scale (RASS): 0 • Confusion Assessment Method for the ICU (CAM-ICU): negative
	Coordination	• Finger to nose: intact bilaterally
	Cranial nerves	• II–XII: intact
	Reflexes	• Patellar: 2 + bilaterally
	Sensation	• BLE: intact to light touch
	Tone	• BUE and BLE: normal throughout
Functional status		
Bed mobility	• Supine to sit: moderate assistance with head of bed elevated ~45 degrees	
Transfers	• Sit to/from stand: minimal assistance with rolling walker	
Ambulation	• Ambulated 5 feet from bed to chair with minimal assistance and rolling walker.	
Stairs	• N/A	

Assessment	
☑ Physical therapist's	*Assessment left blank for learner to develop*
Goals	
Patient's	"I want to get back home safely."
Short term	1. *Goals left blank for learner to develop* 2.
Long term	1. *Goals left blank for learner to develop* 2.

Plan	
☑ Physical therapist's	Will continue to see patient, once daily, five times a week. Will continue to progress functional mobility as tolerated through strengthening and endurance interventions. Introduce safe mobility techniques to minimize pain and soreness at the incision site and postural reeducation to minimize low back pain.

Bloom's Taxonomy Level	Case 10.B Questions
Create	1. Synthesizing the medical data and physical examination findings, develop an appropriate physical therapy assessment of the patient.
	2. Develop two short-term physical therapy goals, including an appropriate timeframe.
	3. Develop two long-term physical therapy goals, including an appropriate timeframe.
Evaluate	4. Explain the physical therapy findings and expected discharge disposition to the resident physician.
Analyze	5. Develop a differential diagnosis plan for a patient with low back pain to reach an AAA diagnosis.
Apply	6. What are two potential interventions to maximize functional mobility and reduce pain during physical therapy sessions?
	7. What are two potential interventions—one stretching and one strengthening—to improve posture?
Understand	8. What are the physical therapy implications for the patient's home medications?
Remember	9. For this patient, what are modifiable risk factors for the development of his aneurysm?
	10. What is a potential neurological complication associated with an endovascular repair of an AAA?

Bloom's Taxonomy Level	Case 10.B Answers
Create	1. The patient is a 72-year-old man who presented to the emergency department with low back pain, abdominal pain, and nausea. He was diagnosed with an AAA, requiring urgent surgical intervention. From a mobility perspective, he demonstrated fatigue, weakness, and reduced endurance. This is likely due to decreased activity levels from prolonged lower back pain and abdominal pain, and his occupational history. As a result, he is unable to complete functional mobility independently. He would benefit from continued physical therapy to improve posture and endurance to maximize functional mobility and safety. Will continue to follow.
	2. Short-term goals:
	• Patient will perform supine to/from sit with head of bed flat with supervision within 4 days to get in and out of bed at home.
	• Patient will ambulate × 100 feet with rolling walker and supervision within 4 days to navigate within home.
	3. Long-term goals:
	• Patient will ascend/descend 13 steps with a single handrail and supervision within 7 days to get to the second floor bedroom.
	• Patient will perform Five Times Sit-to-Stand Test in < 12.6 seconds within 7 days to improve BLE strength.
Evaluate	4. During the physical therapy initial evaluation, the patient demonstrated a decrease in systolic blood pressure and mild increase in heart rate. This is thought to be due to a prolonged supine position. The above, in combination with post-op pain, contribute to decreased functional mobility requiring minimal assistance and a rolling walker. With recovery postsurgery and continued inpatient physical therapy, it is anticipated that the patient will return to his baseline functional status (with or without an assistive device) and therefore will likely be able to return home with assistance and home physical therapy. This is, however, dependent on his ability to perform stairs since he has three steps to enter.
Analyze	5. The causes for low back pain can be grouped into three categories: mechanical, nonmechanical, and visceral.
	• Mechanical causes of low back pain: associated with a specific mechanism of injury (e.g., a fall), has specific aggravating and relieving factors.
	• Nonmechanical causes of low back pain (e.g., malignancy or infection): malignant back ache is most likely associated with history of cancer, unexplained weight loss, pain not responding to conservative treatments, age > 50 years; infection is usually accompanied by fever, malaise, and fatigue.

(Continued)

(Continued)

Bloom's Taxonomy Level	Case 10.B Answers
	• Visceral causes of low back pain: heartburn, nausea, indigestion, changes in appetite, difficulty swallowing, constipation, and changes in frequency of bowel movements or changes in urination or changes in urinary frequency. However, complaints of pain worsening with deep breaths and coughing and bending, lifting and twisting movements, and presence of pulsating mass in the abdomen are significant signs of AAA.
Apply	6. Two interventions to improve this patient's functional mobility may be: • Promotion and maintenance of upright posture during upright activities, including ambulation, to promote hemodynamic stability and respirations, and reduce stress on back muscles. • Scheduling therapy sessions/functional mobility around the time of his pain medications to get maximum effort. 7. Therefore, two potential interventions to improve this patient's posture may be: • Stretching: chin tucks, posterior shoulder rolls, pectoral stretches. • Strengthening: standing hip extension, scapular retractions, and posterior pelvic tilts.
Understand	8. Ceftriaxone: cephalosporin antibiotic, works to fight bacteria in the body Acetaminophen: used to treat mild to moderate and pain Morphine: an opiate, relieves moderate to severe pain Aspirin: anticoagulant Metoprolol: beta blocker, lowers blood pressure and heart rate
Remember	9. For this patient, he could modify his diet, exercise, and smoking habits. These changes could contribute to a reduction in hypertension, hypercholesterolemia, and weight. 10. A potential neurological complication associated with an endovascular repair of an AAA is a spinal cord injury. This is thought to be due to spinal cord ischemia.

Key points

1. It is important for the physical therapist to synthesize all medical data (i.e., patient's signs and symptoms, past medical history, vital signs, imaging, lab values, etc.) to understand how the patient's pathophysiology can affect functional status.

2. During activity, including low-level functional mobility, it is important to monitor the patient's pain and Rate of Perceived Exertion (RPE) since the patient might have reduced endurance postsurgery.

3. Early mobilization postsurgery facilitates better functional recovery, reduced length of stay, and higher likelihood of return to prior level of function.

General Information

Case no.	10.C
Authors	David Gillette, PT, DPT, Board Certified Clinical Specialist in Geriatrics Physical Therapy Bhavana Raja, PT, PhD Todd Davenport, PT, DPT, MPH, Board Certified Clinical Specialist in Orthopaedic Physical Therapy
Diagnosis	Status post (s/p) endovascular aneurysm repair (EVAR) for abdominal aortic aneurysm (AAA)
Setting	Home
Learner expectations	☑ Initial evaluation ☐ Re-evaluation ☐ Treatment session
Learner objectives	1. Identify and prioritize relevant impairments and functional limitations for a patient with an AAA repair and related comorbidities. 2. Select appropriate outcome measures for this patient population. 3. Choose and prioritize appropriate interventions for this patient population.

Medical	
Chief concern	Abdominal incision pain, weakness, fatigue, shortness of breath (SOB)
History of present illness	The patient is a 72-year-old man who initially presented to outpatient physical therapy for mechanical low back pain. During the evaluation, the physical therapist noticed a pulsating mass in the patient's abdomen (groin area) and recommended the patient to go to the Emergency Department immediately. The patient was admitted and is now 6 days s/p transabdominal EVAR. Upon hospital discharge, a home physical therapy consult was placed.
Past medical history	Hypertension, chronic obstructive pulmonary disease (COPD), diabetes mellitus type 2 (A1c in hospital was 8%), hypercholesterolemia, obesity, right hip osteoarthritis Tobacco: 1 pack per day for 40 years, expresses desire to quit Caffeine: 2 cups of coffee per day; recently quit soda Alcohol: occasionally
Past surgical history	Right total knee arthroplasty: 5 years ago; left rotator cuff repair: 2 years ago
Allergies	No known drug allergies.
Medications	Atorvastatin, Metoprolol, Acetaminophen, Aspirin, Senna, Tiotropium (Spiriva), Metformin Patient reports improved compliance with medications.
Precautions/orders	Activity as tolerated

Social history	
Home setup	• Resides in a multilevel home with his wife. • Two steps to enter, rail is on the left. • Half bath + guest room are on the first floor. • Bedroom and bathroom are located on the second floor. • Flight of stairs + right handrail to the second floor.
Occupation	• Retired as research scientist 2 years ago; now drives Uber for extra income and volunteers at a local homeless shelter.
Prior level of function	• Independent in all activities of daily living (ADLs) • Intermittently uses an assistive device—either rolling walker or single point cane—but did not use one prior to surgery. • Two noninjurious falls in the last year: one at night going to the bathroom quickly and one when walking on uneven sidewalk during the day. • Spouse works full-time as a partner at a regional law firm; currently on a case that requires them to be gone during the week. • Has estranged son and daughter from first marriage.
Recreational activities	• Fishing from a boat, watching TV

Imaging/diagnostic test	Results (from day of hospital discharge)
Computed tomography (CT) scan	• Repair area shows decrease from 5.8 to 2.7 cm.

Medical management	
Home health registered nurse (RN)	• Medication management/instruction, wound management
Vascular surgeon	• Follow-up for post-op check-up 6 weeks after surgery

Pause points
Based on the above information, what are the priority: • Diagnostic tests and measures? • Outcome measures? • Treatment in terventions?

Physical Therapy Examination
Subjective
"I feel like crap. I get winded and tired just getting around my house, and I don't want to do anything. The pain is okay."
Objective

Vital signs	Pre-treatment			Post-treatment
	Supine	Sitting	Standing	Sitting
Blood pressure (mmHg)	110/82	104/78	100/79	139/84
Heart rate (beats/min)	70	72	75	80
Respiratory rate (breaths/min)	16	16	16	22
Pulse oximetry on room air (SpO_2)	95%	93%	91%	92%
Modified Borg Scale for shortness of breath (0–10)	0/10	1/10	1/10	6/10
Pain	0/10	2/10 R abdomen/groin	4/10 R abdomen/groin	3/10 R abdomen/groin
General	• Well-nourished male in no apparent distress, on room air, lying in guest bed propped up on pillows.			
Cardiovascular and pulmonary	• Normal heart rate and rhythm. • No adventitious breath sounds. • Diaphragmatic breathing with no accessory muscle use.			
Gastrointestinal	• Constipation postsurgery. • Bowel sounds present but reduced in all quadrants. • Groin wound demonstrates no redness or drainage.			
Genitourinary	• Able to void; stress incontinence with coughing since surgery.			
Musculoskeletal	Range of motion	• Bilateral upper extremity (BUE): within functional limit (WFL). • Bilateral lower extremity (BLE). WFL with the exception of bilateral hip flexion contractures at 10 degrees.		
	Strength	• B shoulder flexion: 4/5 • B elbow flexion: 4/5 • B elbow extension: 4/5 • B wrist extension: 4/5 • L hip flexion: 4/5 • R hip flexion: 4/5 • L knee flexion: 4/5 • R knee flexion: 4/5 • L knee extension: 4/5 • R knee extension: 4/5 • B ankle dorsiflexion: 4/5 • B ankle plantar flexion: 4/5 • 30-Second Sit to Stand: unable to perform without use of upper extremities.		
	Aerobic	• 6-Minute Walk Test: 350 feet with 10 standing rest breaks.		

(Continued)

(Continued)

Physical Therapy Examination		
Neurological	Balance	• Timed Up and Go (TUG): 18.9 seconds • Berg Balance Scale: 40/56
	Cognition	• Alert and oriented × 4
	Coordination	• Finger to nose: intact bilaterally
	Cranial nerves	• II–XII: intact
	Reflexes	• Patellar: 1 + bilaterally • Achilles: 1 + bilaterally
	Sensation	• Intact to light touch to BLE; reduced protective sensation to 5.07 Semmes Weinstein monofilament on soles of B feet
	Tone	• BUE and BLE: normal throughout
	Other	• Proprioception and kinesthetic awareness reduced in B great toes and ankles

Functional status	
Bed mobility	• Supine to/from sit: contact guard assistance with increased time and effort
Transfers	• Sit to/from stand: stand by assist with increased time and use of bilateral upper extremities, required multiple attempts to achieve full upright position.
Ambulation	• Ambulate × 50 feet with rolling walker and stand by assist. • Gait deviations notable for reduced step length bilaterally, reduced toe clearance bilaterally while using front wheeled walker (FWW) with forward flexed posture. • Gait speed is 0.4 m/s
Stairs	• Ascend/descend two steps with minimal assistance, demonstrating step-to pattern, required increased time. • Reported dyspnea on exertion

Assessment	
☑ Physical therapist's	*Assessment left blank for learner to develop*

Goals	
Patient's	"I want to return to fishing, and to be more active so I don't have further medical problems."
Short term	1. *Goals left blank for learner to develop* 2.
Long term	1. *Goals left blank for learner to develop* 2.

Plan	
☑ Physical therapist's	Plan of care will include therapeutic exercise, neuromuscular reeducation, endurance training, postural retraining, and functional mobility training for twice a week for 2 weeks, once a week for 2 weeks.

Bloom's Taxonomy Level	Case 10.C Questions
Create	1. Synthesizing the medical data and physical examination findings, develop an appropriate physical therapy assessment of the patient. 2. Develop two short-term physical therapy goals, including an appropriate timeframe.

(Continued)

(Continued)

Bloom's Taxonomy Level	Case 10.C Questions
	3. Develop two long-term physical therapy goals, including an appropriate timeframe.
	4. Create a list of educational interventions for this patient.
Evaluate	5. Based on the case information, which impairment(s) should be the focus of the plan of care?
Analyze	6. What can the physical therapist conclude about the patient based on the gait speed?
	7. If the patient progresses and scores a 47/56 and 11 seconds on the Berg Balance Scale and TUG, respectively, at physical therapy discharge from home, should he continue to use an assistive device? Why or why not?
Apply	8. What impairments might be contributing to his TUG and Berg scores?
Understand	9. Does this patient have orthostatic hypotension? Why or why not?
	10. Is this patient at risk of falls? Provide data to support the decision.
	11. What are the effects of smoking for this patient?
Remember	12. What is the effect of a beta blocker on physical activity?
	13. What does A1c measure?
	14. What is COPD?

Bloom's Taxonomy Level	Case 10.C Answers
Create	1. The patient is a 72-year-old man s/p EVAR, with complex past medical history. He presents with reduced functional strength, reduced endurance, reduced proprioception and kinesthetic awareness BLE, stress incontinence, and reduced balance in static and dynamic standing. These factors are limiting his independent and safety with transfers, gait and stair negotiation, independence in his own home and community, as well as increasing risk of rehospitalization and falls. He would benefit from continued physical therapy to address above impairments to maximize independence and safety, restore to prior level of function, and return him to the community while working toward his personal goals of fishing and of becoming more active to reduce his risk of further medical events. Will continue to follow.
	2. Short-term goals:
	• Patient will be able to perform supine to/from sit independently within 4 days to increase independence within the home and reduce caregiver burden.
	• Patient will demonstrate modified independence with least restrictive assistive device with sit to/from stand within 4 days to increase independence within the home.
	• Patient will demonstrate independence in a home exercise program (HEP), which will focus on BLE strength and endurance, within 4 days to maintain and increase functional gains within the home.
	3. Long-term goals:
	• Patient will improve his 30-Second Sit to Stand Test score to 8 repetitions within 4 weeks to increase independence within the home and return him to accessing the community.
	• Patient will increase his 6MWT distance to 900 feet within 4 weeks to demonstrate an improvement in cardiovascular endurance.
	• Patient will demonstrate modified independence when ascending/descending 12 stairs + R handrail ascending within 4 weeks to allow patient to access and sleep in his own bedroom.
	4. Educational interventions that can be addressed with this patient are related to the following topics:
	• Home exercise program (HEP): instruction on the modified Borg Scale for Rating of Perceived Exertion and for Dyspnea on Exertion, strengthening and stretching, breathing, and pelvic floor training.
	• Functional training: the importance of posture, appropriate use of an assistive device, and techniques to optimize function while minimizing pain.
	• Self-care: the importance of smoking cessation and diabetes management, medication management.

(Continued)

(Continued)

Bloom's Taxonomy Level	Case 10.C Answers
Evaluate	5. Based on the case information, the patient present's impairments include reduced strength, reduced endurance, reduced balance, and reduced sensation. The focus of the plan of care should be on strength and endurance to return him to independence within the home and community. The ultimate goal should be to get the patient in well enough condition that he can attend outpatient physical therapy, where his balance and back pain can be further addressed.
Analyze	6. The patient's gait speed of 0.4 m/s is indicative of being dependent in ADLs, increased risk of hospitalization, increased risk of falls, and limited community ambulatory. 7. Based on the patient's Berg Balance Scale score of 47/56 and TUG score of 11 seconds, the patient should continue to use an assistive device. The use of an assistive device can help reduce his fall risk and conserve energy. He can reduce reliance on it and eliminate the need for it as he progresses through outpatient therapy.
Apply	8. Impairments contributing to his Berg Balance Scale and TUG scores are reduced strength, reduced endurance, reduced proprioception and kinesthetic awareness, reduced sensation, and forward flexed posture.
Understand	9. The patient does not have orthostatic hypotension. Orthostatic hypotension is defined as a drop in systolic blood pressure of a minimum of 20 mmHg or a drop in diastolic blood pressure of a minimum of 10 mmHg within 3 minutes of standing or > 60 degree head-up tilt. This patient had a drop in systolic blood pressure of 10 mmHg and a drop in diastolic blood pressure of 3 mmHg, which does not meet the criteria for orthostatic hypotension. 10. The patient is at risk of falls based on his TUG and Berg Balance Scale scores. Additionally, he has risk factors for falls including use of an assistive device, inability to perform the 30-Second Sit to Stand Test, reduced sensation/proprioception/kinesthetic awareness in his feet, and reduced gait speed. 11. Smoking will reduce his activity tolerance, slow his rate of healing from surgery, increase his blood pressure, increase his symptoms of COPD, and make his diabetes more difficult to control. It also increases his risk of stroke and cancer.
Remember	12. A beta blocker lowers blood pressure and heart rate and reduces strain on the heart. However, it should be noted that during exercise or physical activity, beta blockers blunt the heart rate response. Therefore, heart rate cannot be used as an indicator of exercise intensity. Instead, the Borg Scale for Rating of Perceived Exertion (▶ Fig. 10.3). 13. A1c measures the average blood sugar over the past 90 to 120 days and is an indication of how well diabetes is being managed. His A1c of 8% indicates his diabetes has not been well managed in this period of time; metformin can help manage blood sugars. 14. COPD is a progressive disease of the lungs where the airway and alveoli become less elastic, the airway becomes inflamed and generate more mucus, and the walls of alveoli collapse, all of which make it harder to breathe.

Key points
1. Patients postsurgery may have multiple impairments that need to be addressed by physical therapy treatment and should be prioritized accordingly.
2. Vital signs and RPE should be assessed during all activities and exercises.
3. Manual muscle tests are not indicative of functional strength, and goals should involve functional outcome measures.

How you might describe your exertion	Borg rating of your exertion	Examples (for most adults <65 years old)
None	6	Reading a book, watching television
Very, very light	7 to 8	Tying shoes
Very light	9 to 10	Chores like folding clothes that seem to take little effort
Fairly light	11 to 12	Walking through the grocery store or other activities that require some effort but not enough to speed up your breathing
Somewhat hard	13 to 14	Brisk walking or other activities that require moderate effort and speed your heart rate and breathing but don't make you out of breath
Hard	15 to 16	Bicycling, swimming, or other activities that take vigorous effort and get the heart pounding and make breathing very fast
Very hard	17 to 18	The highest level of activity you can sustain
Very, very hard	19 to 20	A finishing kick in a race or other burst of activity that you can't maintain for long

Fig. 10.3 An example of the Borg Scale for Rating of perceived exertion that can be used with patients receiving beta blockers. (Adapted from https://www.hsph.harvard.edu/nutritionsource/borg-scale/.)

Suggested Readings

6-minute walk test. Available at: https://www.sralab.org/rehabilitation-measures/6-minute-walk-test. Accessed September 1, 2020

30 Second Chair Stand. Available at: https://www.cdc.gov/steadi/pdf/STEADI-Assessment-30Sec-508.pdf. Accessed September 1, 2020

Academy of Acute Care Physical Therapy-APTA Taskforce on Lab Values. Laboratory Values Interpretation Resource. Pittsburgh, PA: APTA; 2017

American Heart Association. What is an aneurysm? Available at: https://www.heart.org/en/health-topics/aortic-aneurysm/what-is-an-aneurysm. Accessed September 29, 2020

Arnold AC, Raj SR. Orthostatic hypotension: a practical approach to investigation and management. Can J Cardiol. 2017; 33(12):1725–1728

Atlas SJ, Deyo RA. Evaluating and managing acute low back pain in the primary care setting. J Gen Intern Med. 2001; 16(2):120–131

Berg Balance Scale. Available at: https://www.sralab.org/rehabilitation-measures/berg-balance-scale. Accessed September 1, 2020

Chaikof EL, Dalman RL, Eskandari MK, et al. The Society for Vascular Surgery practice guidelines on the care of patients with an abdominal aortic aneurysm. J Vasc Surg. 2018; 67(1):2–77.e2

Clancy K, Wong J, Spicher A. Abdominal aortic aneurysm: a case report and literature review. Perm J. 2019; 23:18–218

Daye D, Walker TG. Complications of endovascular aneurysm repair of the thoracic and abdominal aorta: evaluation and management. Cardiovasc Diagn Ther. 2018; 8 Suppl 1:S138–S156

Fink HA, Lederle FA, Roth CS, Bowles CA, Nelson DB, Haas MA. The accuracy of physical examination to detect abdominal aortic aneurysm. Arch Intern Med. 2000; 160(6):833–836

Fritz S, Lusardi M. White paper: "walking speed: the sixth vital sign.". J Geriatr Phys Ther. 2009; 32(2):46–49

Goodman CC, Fuller KS. Pathology: Implications for the Physical Therapist. 4th ed. St. Louis, MO: Saunders Elsevier; 2015

Hillegass E. Essentials of Cardiopulmonary Physical Therapy. 4th ed. St. Louis, MO: Elsevier; 2017

Mechelli F, Preboski Z, Boissonnault WG. Differential diagnosis of a patient referred to physical therapy with low back pain: abdominal aortic aneurysm. J Orthop Sports Phys Ther. 2008; 38(9):551–557

McDaniel JC, Browning KK. Smoking, chronic wound healing, and implications for evidence based practice. J Wound Ostomy Continence Nurs. 2014; 41(5):415–423, quiz E1–E2

Morisaki K, Matsumoto T, Matsubara Y, et al. A rare complication of spinal cord ischemia following endovascular aneurysm repair of an infrarenal abdominal aortic aneurysm with arteriosclerosis obliterans: report of a case. Ann Vasc Dis. 2016; 9(3):255–257

Moulakakis KG, Alexiou VG, Karaolanis G, et al. Spinal cord ischemia following elective endovascular repair of infrarenal aortic aneurysms: a systematic review. Ann Vasc Surg. 2018; 52:280–291

Timed Up and Go. https://www.sralab.org/rehabilitation-measures/timed-and-go. Accessed March 19, 2020

Van Wyngaarden JJ, Ross MD, Hando BR. Abdominal aortic aneurysm in a patient with low back pain. J Orthop Sports Phys Ther. 2014; 44(7):500–507

11 Non-Small Cell Lung Cancer

General Information	
Case no.	11.A Non-Small Cell Lung Cancer
Authors	Rachel Pata, PT, DPT, CHSE, Board Certified Clinical Specialist in Cardiovascular & Pulmonary Physical Therapy Karen Blood, PT, DPT, Board Certified Clinical Specialist in Geriatrics Physical Therapy Sarah Ferrero, PT, DPT, Board Certified Clinical Specialist in Geriatrics Physical Therapy
Diagnosis	Non–small cell lung cancer (NSCLC), status post (s/p) left upper lobectomy
Setting	Medical Intensive Care Unit, transfer to Medical Oncology Floor
Learner expectations	☑ Initial evaluation ☐ Re-evaluation ☐ Treatment session
Learner objectives	1. Describe the patient's history in progress and discuss physical therapy implications of an acute thoracotomy procedure. 2. Prioritize the acute care evaluation of this patient. 3. Discuss patient monitoring and hemodynamic response. 4. Create a patient-centered discharge plan.

Medical	
Chief complaint	Difficulty breathing
History of present illness	The patient is an 82-year-old man with a diagnosis of NSCLC. He initially sought medical attention from his primary care physician 1 month ago secondary to persistent cough and hemoptysis. Chest computed tomography (CT) revealed a mass in the left hilar region. Fiberoptic bronchoscopy was performed and biopsy confirmed non–small cell squamous cell carcinoma. A positron emission tomography (PET) scan revealed no metastatic disease. The patient was referred to an oncologist and the decision was made to proceed with a left upper lobectomy with lymph node dissection via thoracotomy. The cancer was classified as stage IIB (T2b N1 M0).
Past medical history	Osteoarthritis, benign prostatic hypertrophy, diabetes mellitus
Past surgical history	s/p left total hip arthroplasty 6 years ago
Allergies	No known drug allergies
Medications	Flomax, Metformin, Glucosamine sulfate
Precautions/orders	Physical therapy, evaluate and treat Out of bed (OOB) as tolerated Titrate O_2 to maintain saturation > 90% Fall precautions

Social history	
Home setup	• Lives with his wife in assisted living facility (ALF). • One-bedroom apartment is on the second floor. • Elevator access to apartment (~1,000 feet from the apartment to the elevator) • Congregate meals on the first floor, but can also be delivered to apartments or prepared in unit kitchenettes. • Assisted living has transport wheelchairs available.
Occupation	• Retired; owned a dry-cleaning business for 50 years
Prior level of function	• Independent in all functional mobility and activities of daily living (ADLs) without supplemental O_2; used a cane for community ambulation. • Participated in instrumental ADLs (IADLs) with his wife, such as shopping and light meal prep; ate breakfast and dinner in congregate dining room. • + Driving

(Continued)

(Continued)

Social history	
Recreational activities	• Participates in weekly bridge club at ALF. • Goes to daughter's home every Thursday with his wife to babysit two grandkids (ages 5 and 7). • Participates in group exercise classes thrice a week at ALF.

Vital signs	Hospital day 0	
	Preoperative	Postoperative
Blood pressure (mmHg)	118/68	108/62
Heart rate (beats/min)	72	80
Respiratory rate (breaths/min)	15	12
Pulse oximetry (SpO$_2$)	96% on room air	93% Intubated via endotracheal tube, on assist control mode
Temperature (°F)	98.8	98.7

Imaging/diagnostic test	Hospital day 0: surgery/postanesthesia care unit (PACU)	Hospital day 1: intensive care unit (ICU)	Hospital day 2: ICU
Chest CT	▶ Fig. 11.1	1. s/p left upper lobectomy. Chest tube in intrapleural space, small left pleural effusion.	1. s/p left upper lobectomy, pleural effusion improved from previous study.

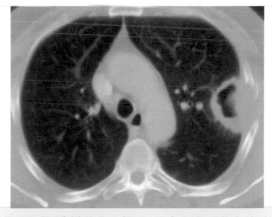

Fig. 11.1 Chest CT showing a mass in the left hilar region. (Source: Parker M, Rosado-de-Christenson M, Abbott G. In: Abbott G, Parker M, Rosado-de-Christenson M, ed. Teaching Atlas of Chest Imaging. 1st Edition. New York: Thieme; 2005.)

Medical management	Hospital day 0: surgery/PACU	Hospital day 1: ICU	Hospital day 2: ICU
Procedure/surgery	1. Patient sedated and intubated via endotracheal tube in preparation for surgery. 2. Internal jugular (IJ) central venous line placed. 3. Foley catheter placed. 4. Left thoracotomy and left upper lobectomy performed. 5. Chest tube placed in left intrapleural space.	1. IJ central venous line remains in place. 2. Foley catheter remains in place. 3. Bandage in place with minimal drainage. 4. Chest tube in place.	1. Patient extubated to 6L O$_2$ by nasal cannula (NC). 2. Central venous line removed. 3. Foley catheter removed. 4. Incision healing well and bandage in place. 5. Chest tube removed.

(Continued)

Medical management	Hospital day 0: surgery/PACU	Hospital day 1: ICU	Hospital day 2: ICU
Additional medication	1. Heparin (subcutaneous) daily 2. Oxycodone 3. Intravenous (IV) fluids	1. Continue per medical orders	
Respiratory	1. Intubated on assist control mode, FiO_2 60%, positive end-expiratory pressure (PEEP) 5 cm H_2O.	1. Weaning from ventilator, on synchronized intermittent mandatory ventilation (SIMV), FiO_2 40%, PEEP 5 cm H_2O 2. DuoNeb q.i.d.	1. 6 L O_2 by NC 2. Continue DuoNeb q.i.d.

Lab		Reference range	Hospital day 0: post-op	Hospital day 1: ICU	Hospital day 2: ICU
Complete blood count (CBC)	White blood cell (WBC)	$5.0–10.0 \times 10^9$/L	6.8	8.2	10.1
	Red blood cell (RBC)	4.1–5.3 million/mm^3	4.0	3.8	3.6
	Hemoglobin	14–17.4 g/dL	14	11	10
	Hematocrit	42–52%	42%	36%	33%
	Platelets	140,000–400,000/μL	260	245	240
ABG	PaO_2	80–95 mmHg	78	75	82
	$PaCO_2$	37–43 mmHg	40	38	38
	PH	7.35–7.45	7.4	7.41	7.41
	HCO_3	20–30 mmol/L	24	25	24
Basic metabolic panel (BMP)	Glucose (fast)	70–100 mg/dL	156	164	152
	Hemoglobin A1C	<5.7%	6.2%	—	—
	Cholesterol	<200 mg/dL	185	—	—
	Low-density lipoprotein (LDL)	<70 mg/dL	120	—	—
	High-density lipoprotein (HDL)	>60 mg/dL	65	—	—
	Blood urea nitrogen (BUN)	6–25 mg/dL	25	26	27
	Creatinine	0.7–1.3 mg/dL	1.2	1.4	1.3
	Potassium	3.7–5.1 mEq/L	4.2	4.0	4.1
	Sodium	134–142 mEq/L	138	140	138
	Chloride	98–108 mEq/L	99	100	102
	Calcium	8.6–10.3 mg/dL	8.7	8.5	8.7
	Magnesium	1.2–1.9 mEq/L	1.4	1.5	1.3

Pause points

Based on the above information, what are:
- Anticipated patient impairments?
- Examination priorities?
- Patient precautions/monitoring strategies?

Who is on the interprofessional team and what are the roles of the team members?

Hospital Day 3, Step-Down Unit: Physical Therapy Examination					
Subjective					
"I just transferred to the Medical Oncology floor this morning. They want to get me up but it is hard to move due to pain 6/10 on my left side."					
Objective					
Vital signs	Pre-treatment			During ambulation	Post-treatment
	Supine	Sitting	Standing		Sitting
Blood pressure (mmHg)	112/76	110/72	118/78	120/80	126/80
Heart rate (beats/min)	87	92	102	117	110
▸ Fig. 11.2 *Electrocardiography during activity*					
Respiratory rate (breath/min)	16	18	22	26	24
Pulse oximetry on 2 L NC (SpO$_2$)	94%	95%	95%	92%	96%
Borg rate of perceived exertion (RPE) scale	10/20	11/20	13/20	14/20	11/20
Pain	6/10 Left side of thorax	6/10 Left side of thorax	7/10 Left side of thorax	8/10 Left side of thorax	6/10 Left side of thorax
General	• Patient found supine in bed with head of bed (HOB) elevated 45 degrees and arms resting on a pillow in her lap. • No apparent distress or difficulty breathing. • Bandage in place over left thorax with minimal serosanguineous drainage from incision. • Lines/equipment notable for telemetry, right upper extremity (RUE) peripheral IV, 4L O$_2$ by NC.				
Cardiovascular and pulmonary	• Inspection: no accessory muscle use, left lateral trunk lean with decreased left thoracic expansion. • Palpation: reduced expansion left upper lobe (L UL). 2+pedal pulses bilateral lower extremity (BLE). • Auscultation: diminished breath sounds L UL, no adventitious sounds.				
Gastrointestinal	• Normal bowel movement this morning				
Genitourinary	• Voiding independently on bed pan, clear, yellow urine				
Musculoskeletal	Range of motion (ROM)	• Left shoulder: flexion and abduction (ABD): 120 degrees • Left elbow, wrist, and hand: within functional limit (WFL) • Right upper extremity (RUE): WFL throughout • BLE: WFL throughout			
	Strength	• Left shoulder flexion and ABD: 3–/5 and limited by pain • Left elbow, wrist, and hand: 3+/5 • RUE: 3+/5 throughout • BLE:>3+/5 throughout as demonstrated through functional mobility			
	Aerobic	• Unable to perform standardized assessment at this time. • Refer to patient vital signs and signs and symptoms.			
	Flexibility	• Not assessed at this time			
	Other	• N/A			
Neurological	Balance	• Static sitting: good • Dynamic sitting: good • Supported static standing: fair • Supported dynamic standing: fair			

(Continued)

(Continued)

Hospital Day 3, Step-Down Unit: Physical Therapy Examination		
	Cognition	• Alert and oriented (A&O) × 4
	Coordination	• Finger to nose: intact BUE • Toe tapping: intact BLE
	Cranial nerves	• II–XII: intact
	Reflexes	• Not tested at this time
	Sensation	• BUE: intact to light touch • BLE: intact to light touch
	Tone	• BUE: within normal limit (WNL) • BLE: WNL
	Other	• N/A
Functional status		
Bed mobility		• Scooting: independent • Bridge: independent • Right rolling: minimal assistance • Supine to/from sit: minimal assistance
Transfers		• Sit to/from stand: minimal assistance with rolling walker (RW) • Bed to/from chair: minimal assistance with RW
Ambulation		• Ambulate × 40 feet with contact guard assistance (CGA) and RW
Stairs		• Unable to assess secondary to pain and fatigue.
Posture		• Maintaining slight left side bend in all positions.
Other		• AM-PAC Basic Mobility Inpatient Short Form: 14/24

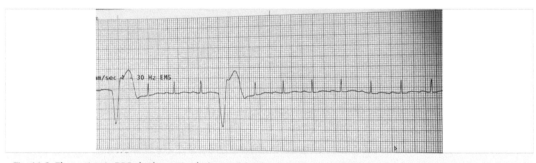

Fig. 11.2 The patient's ECG rhythm strip during activity.

Assessment	
☑ Physical therapist's	*Assessment left blank for learner to develop.*
Goals	
Patient's	"I want to take care of myself at home."
Short term	1. *Goals left blank for learner to develop.* 2.
Long term	1. *Goals left blank for learner to develop.* 2.

	Plan
☐ Physician's ☑ Physical therapist's ☐ Other's	Patient will be seen 3 to 5 days per week for skilled physical therapy including bed mobility, transfer training, gait training, therapeutic exercise, and education on pacing and self-monitoring to improve strength, ROM, functional mobility, and endurance.

Bloom's Taxonomy Level	Case 11.A Questions
Create	1. Synthesizing the medical data and physical examination findings, develop an appropriate physical therapy assessment of the patient. 2. Develop two short-term physical therapy goals, including an appropriate timeframe. 3. Develop two long-term physical therapy goals, including an appropriate timeframe.
Evaluate	4. Describe the physical therapist's discharge recommendation and the factors that contribute to this. 5. Identify information that should be gathered from the patient that is not in his medical record. 6. Discuss this patient's medical prognosis.
Analyze	7. Describe why this patient is posturing in this manner. 8. Discuss this patient's hemodynamic response to mobility.
Apply	9. Discuss how the physical therapist should teach this patient to self-monitor. 10. Implement strategies for pain management.
Understand	11. Interpret this patient's trend in hemoglobin values.
Remember	12. What is a lateral thoracotomy? 13. Is this patient on high- or low-flow oxygen at this time?

Bloom's Taxonomy Level	Case 11.A Answers
Create	1. The patient is an 82-year-old man admitted to the hospital with NSCLC, now s/p thoracotomy and left upper lobectomy. He presents with impaired strength, ROM, functional mobility, posture, and endurance associated with hospitalization due to above procedure, in addition to his past medical history of osteoarthritis and non–insulin-dependent diabetes mellitus (NIDDM). He would benefit from skilled physical therapy services to improve strength, ROM, functional mobility, posture, and endurance. 2. Short-term goals: • Patient will perform sit to/from stand transfers with CGA of 1 with RW within 1 week to safely transfer at home with his wife. • Patient will ambulate 100 feet with RW and CGA of 1, keeping O_2 saturation > 90%, within 1 week to ambulate around his apartment. 3. Long-term goals: • Patient will perform sit to/from stand transfers with modified independence with RW within 2 weeks to safely transfer at home. • Patient will ambulate 200 feet with RW and supervision, keeping O_2 saturation > 90%, within 2 weeks in order to walk into his doctor's office.
Evaluate	4. Discharge to home with home services with assistance of the patient's wife is the optimal discharge plan. For equipment, the patient will need an RW for ambulation, use of a manual wheelchair to get from his parking lot to the apartment, and potentially supplemental oxygen. Currently, the maximum assistance he needs to complete functional mobility is assistance of 1. It is anticipated that his mobility will continue to improve during his hospital stay and this physical assistance may not be needed upon discharge. His wife will need to be trained on safe mobility techniques. A discharge home will also minimize risk of infection in this patient. Additionally, it will allow for this patient to start chemotherapy treatments. 5. The patient's goals for therapy, as well as him and his wife's concerns. Cancer can significantly impact mental health and patient well-being. Depression and anxiety may hinder recovery as well as quality of life. Ensuring a patient-centered plan of care will likely improve participation and progress with therapy. 6. This patient's prognosis is fair. NSCLC has a better prognosis than small cell lung cancer. The 5-year survival rate of stage 2b small cell lung cancer is 31 to 40%.

(Continued)

(Continued)

Bloom's Taxonomy Level	Case 11.A Answers
Analyze	7. The patient is leaning toward the side of the thoracotomy to reduce pain and stretching on the incision. Although this is a more comfortable position for the patient, it can lead to increased adhesion, reduced trunk and LUE ROM, and reduced inspiratory volumes of the remaining left lung. If this is not addressed in the acute phase, the patient is at increased risk of long-term impaired posture, ROM, ventilation, and functional mobility. The patient should be educated in maintaining a normal posture and performing active ROM (AROM) frequently to tolerance.
	8. This patient presents with a normal hemodynamic response to exercise. Systolic blood pressure rises proportionate to activity and diastolic blood pressure does not fluctuate more than 10 mmHg. Heart rate rises from 87 to 117. The 30-beat increase is normal given that this patient is reporting an RPE of 14 (somewhat hard). The patient is having occasional premature ventricular contractions (PVCs) and the therapist should confirm with nursing that this is the patient's baseline. This will not significantly affect cardiac output and hemodynamics. The patient has a mild desaturation in response to activity but remains > 90%.
Apply	9. This patient should self-monitor using signs and symptoms as well as vital signs. Using a 6 to 20 PRE Scale, 14 is at the high end of moderate intensity and a good cutoff point for activity. Using the 1 to 4 subjective rating of dyspnea, 2/4, or moderate, is the recommended cutoff point. The patient should also stop activity with any dizziness, lightheadedness, or other adverse events. Teaching the patient to self-monitor heart rate and oxygen saturation with a home finger monitor can also be helpful. If this is not possible, palpation of pulse can be taught. Oxygen saturation should remain ≥ 90%. Given that the patient was at an RPE of 14 at 117 beats per minute (beats/min; 85% of age-adjusted maximum), this heart rate is a good rest point for this patient.
	10. Pain management strategies may include premedication prior to mobilization, deep breathing and relaxation techniques, and education in a splinted cough or huff technique for airway clearance.
Understand	11. The patient's hemoglobin declined from 14 g/dL preoperatively to 10 g/dL on postoperative day 2. Even though this is outside of the normal reference range, it is an anticipated response after surgery. This patient may be mobilized while monitoring signs and symptoms as well as vital signs.
Remember	12. A lateral thoracotomy involves an incision to the lateral chest, usually at the fourth, fifth, or sixth intercostal space. The incision typically extends from the nipple line to the scapula. The latissimus dorsi muscle is retracted and the serratus anterior and intercostal muscles are incised. The ribs are then retracted to reach the underlying lungs.
	13. This patient is on 4 L of oxygen by NC, which is a low-flow oxygen device. Low-flow oxygen devices deliver oxygen below the patient's inspiratory flow rate, entrain room air, and provide a variable FiO_2. Four liter of oxygen will deliver approximately 40% FiO_2.

Key points
1. Consider the prior level of function, goals of the patient, and benefits of early mobilization when formulating a physical therapy plan of care.
2. Strategies to monitor hemodynamic response and patient pacing will assist in decreasing short of breath and will improve participation in early mobilization.
3. Early patient education on postsurgical mobility, postural correction, and ROM can improve long-term outcomes.

General Information	
Case no.	11.B
Authors	Karen Blood, PT, DPT, Board Certified Clinical Specialist in Geriatrics Physical Therapy
	Rachel Pata, PT, DPT, CHSE, Board Certified Clinical Specialist in Cardiovascular & Pulmonary Physical Therapy
	Sarah Ferrero, PT, DPT, Board Certified Clinical Specialist in Geriatrics Physical Therapy
Diagnosis	Non–small cell lung cancer; stage IIB (T2b N1 M0); status post (s/p) left upper lobectomy

(Continued)

(Continued)

General Information	
Setting	Home
Learner expectations	☑ Initial evaluation ☐ Re-evaluation ☐ Treatment session
Learner objectives	1. Recall features of the patient's pathology including common progression of disease process. 2. Describe positive and negative prognostic factors that may influence the rehabilitation potential of the patient. 3. Interpret the patient's performance on functional outcome measures. 4. Develop a home exercise program based on the patient's body structure and impairments to optimize his participation and quality of life.

Medical	
Chief complaint	"I can't walk to the dining room like I want."
History of present illness	The patient is an 82-year-old man who was recently hospitalized for 6 days following left upper lobectomy for new diagnosis of non–small cell lung cancer. Hospital course notable for a 3-day intensive care unit (ICU) stay. Initial medical management included single chest tube, which was removed on postoperative day 3. The patient was discharged home 2 days ago on 2 L O_2 via nasal cannula. He reports that he will return to the oncologist in 2 weeks for port-a-cath placement for chemotherapy.
Past medical history	Osteoarthritis, benign prostatic hypertrophy, diabetes mellitus
Past surgical history	s/p left total hip arthroplasty 6 years ago
Allergies	No known drug allergies
Medications	Flomax, Albuterol inhaler, Metformin, Glucosamine sulfate
Precautions/orders	Physical therapy, evaluate and treat as indicated Activity as tolerated Oxygen 0 to 2 L via nasal cannula to maintain $SpO_2 > 90\%$

Social history	
Home setup	• Lives with his wife in assisted living facility (ALF). • One-bedroom apartment is on the second floor. • Elevator access to apartment (1,000 feet from the apartment to the elevator). • Congregate meals on the first floor, but can also be delivered to apartments or prepared in unit kitchenettes. • Assisted living has transport wheelchairs available.
Occupation	• Retired; owned a dry-cleaning business for 50 years
Prior level of function	• Independent in all functional mobility and activities of daily living (ADLs) without supplemental O_2; used a cane for community ambulation. • Participated in instrumental ADLs (IADLs) with his wife, such as shopping and light meal prep; ate breakfast and dinner in congregate dining room. • + Driving.
Recreational activities	• Participates in weekly bridge club at ALF. • Goes to daughter's home every Thursday with his wife to babysit two grandkids (ages 5 and 7). • Participates in group exercise classes thrice a week at ALF.

Pause points
Based on the above information, what are the priorities? • Diagnostic tests and measures? • Outcome measures? • Treatment interventions?

Physical Therapy Examination		
Subjective		
"I still feel tired when I try to do anything. I keep tripping on this darn tubing."		
Objective		
Vital signs	**Pre-treatment**	**Post-treatment**
Blood pressure (mmHg)	122/78	128/84
Heart rate (beats/min)	90	115
Respiratory rate (breaths/min)	18	24
Pulse oximetry (SpO$_2$)	94% 2 L O$_2$ via NC	92% 2 L O$_2$ via NC
Borg scale	8/20	12/20
Pain	2/10—incision site	4/10—incision site
General	• Patient found sitting in recliner chair with feet elevated. • Oxygen being delivered by concentrator unit. • Rolling walker (RW) is nearby with urinal hanging from it. • Wife is present for session.	
Cardiovascular and pulmonary	• Inspection (at rest): no accessory muscle use • Palpation: reduced expansion left upper lobe; 2+ pedal pulses bilateral lower extremity (BLE) • Auscultation: absent breath sounds left upper lobe; diminished breath sounds bilateral bases	
Gastrointestinal	• Patient reports that he had a normal bowel movement this morning.	
Genitourinary	• Clear yellow urine in urinal	
Musculoskeletal	Range of motion (ROM)	• Left shoulder: flexion and abduction limited to 120 degrees • Left elbow, wrist, and hand: within functional limit (WFL) • Right upper extremity (RUE): WFL • BLE: decreased terminal knee extension, decreased ankle dorsiflexion
	Strength	• Bilateral hip flexion: >3+/5 as demonstrated through functional mobility • Bilateral knee extension: 4/5 • Bilateral ankle dorsiflexion: 4/5 • Five Times Sit-to-Stand Test: 22.5 seconds
	Aerobic	• 6-Minute Walk Test: 200 m (656 feet) with RW
	Flexibility	• Not assessed at this time.
	Other	• Kyphotic posture, forward heard, rounded shoulders. ▶ Fig. 11.3.
Neurological	Balance	• Timed Up and Go (TUG): 12.5 seconds with RW
	Cognition	• Alert and oriented (A&O) × 4
	Coordination	• Finger to nose: intact bilateral upper extremity (BUE) • Heel to shin: intact BLE
	Cranial nerves	• I–XII: intact
	Reflexes	• Patellar: 2+ bilaterally
	Sensation	• BLE: intact to light touch
	Tone	• BUE: WNL • BLE: WNL
	Other	N/A
Functional status		
Bed mobility	• Patient reports that he has slept in recliner chair since coming home from hospital. • Supine to sit: minimal assistance for trunk management • Sit to supine: minimal assistance for BLE management	
Transfers	• Sit to/from stand: modified independent with BUE use from recliner chair, requires increased time and effort to complete.	
Ambulation	• Ambulated 100 feet with supervision and RW; requires assistance for safe management of oxygen tubing.	
Stairs	• N/A	

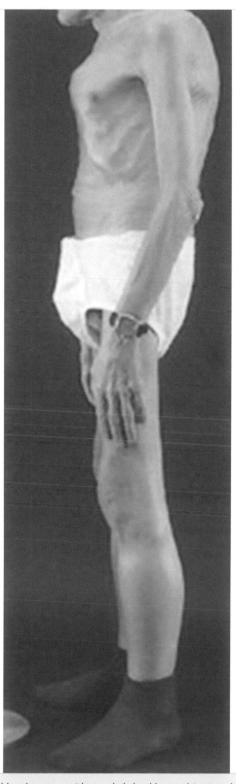

Fig. 11.3 Lateral view of forward head posture with rounded shoulders and increased thoracic kyphosis. (Source: Siegenthaler W. Differential Diagnosis in Internal Medicine: From Symptom to Diagnosis. 1st ed. Thieme; 2007.)

Assessment	
☑ Physical therapist's	*Assessment left blank for learner to develop.*

Goals	
Patient's	"I want to get back to just using my cane."
Short term	1.
	Goals left blank for learner to develop.
	2.
Long term	1.
	Goals left blank for learner to develop.
	2.

Plan	
☐ Physician's ☑ Physical therapist's ☐ Other's	Patient will be seen for twice a week × 4 weeks for physical therapy including therapeutic exercise, bed mobility training, transfer training, gait training, balance training, and instruction in breathing techniques to improve strength, ROM, functional mobility, and endurance.

Bloom's Taxonomy Level	Case 11.B Questions
Create	1. Synthesizing the medical data and physical examination findings, develop an appropriate physical therapy assessment of the patient. 2. Develop two short-term physical therapy goals, including an appropriate timeframe. 3. Develop two long-term physical therapy goals, including an appropriate timeframe.
Evaluate	4. Discuss positive prognostic indicators for this patient. 5. Compare the patient's prognosis with what it would be if he had been diagnosed with small-cell lung cancer.
Analyze	6. Analyze how this patient's surgical procedure may affect his endurance. 7. What are some reasons that the patient is sleeping in the recliner chair instead of the bed? 8. Based on the Five Times Sit-to-Stand Test, is the patient above, at, or below normative values for individuals his age? 9. What is the appropriate interpretation of the patient's 6-Minute Walk Test? Are his results considered normal for a community-dwelling male of his age?
Apply	10. Design a walking program to improve the patient's 6-Minute Walk Test distance. 11. The patient does not have access to a pulse oximeter in the home. Explain how the wife will be able to determine if the patient is experiencing hypoxia.
Understand	12. Based on the results of TUG, would the physical therapist classify the patient at risk of falling?
Remember	13. What does the T2b N1 M0 classification tell the physical therapist about the stage of the patient's cancer? 14. What are the most common sites of metastases for non–small cell lung cancer? 15. Besides smoking, what are the risk factors for development of lung cancer?

Bloom's Taxonomy Level	Case 11.B Answers
Create	1. The patient is an 82-year-old man who was recently hospitalized for 6 days following left upper lobectomy for new diagnosis of non–small cell lung cancer. Hospital course notable for a 3-day ICU stay. He is now being seen by a physical therapist at home. He currently presents with impaired BLE strength, impaired bilateral ankle dorsiflexion ROM, impaired left upper extremity (LUE) ROM, and requires 2 L O_2 via NC at rest and with activity. In addition, results of the 6-Minute Walk Test indicate that he has decreased functional mobility tolerance and results of the Five Times Sit-to-Stand Test indicate decreased functional strength. He presents below his baseline level of functional mobility as indicated by his need for assistance with bed mobility, need for use of assistive device for ambulation, impaired ambulation distance, and need for increased time and effort with transfers. He is at risk of decline in functional mobility and independence, which may lead to decline in quality of life and need for increased caregiver burden. He requires skilled physical therapy twice a week for 4 weeks to address these impairments and functional limitations to maximize functional outcomes and promote return to prior level of function. 2. Short-term goals: • The patient will independently perform sit to/from supine within 1 week to be able to sleep in his bed again. • The patient will independently ambulate 200 feet with RW including safe management of O_2 tubing within 1 week to safely negotiate in his home environment. 3. Long-term goals: • The patient will independently ambulate 1,000 feet with cane without supplemental O_2 and Borg of 8/20 within 4 weeks to reintegrate into community by eating meals in the dining room. • The patient will demonstrate independence with written/pictorial home exercise program (HEP) for BLE strengthening within 4 weeks to maximize functional mobility.
Evaluate	4. Positive prognostic indicators for this patient include presence of social support (wife), uncomplicated hospital course, no evidence of metastatic disease, intact cognition, and activity level prior to hospitalization. 5. Small-cell lung cancer grows much more rapidly than non–small cell lung cancer. Small-cell lung cancer is associated with very early metastases and is often not amenable to surgical resection. If this patient had been diagnosed with small-cell lung cancer, it would be anticipated that he would have a poorer prognosis as well as increased susceptibility to paraneoplastic syndromes. It would be highly likely that the patient would not have opted to undergo a surgical resection given no clear benefits of surgery.
Analyze	6. Surgical resection via lobectomy can decrease a patient's vital capacity by 15%. Vital capacity includes inspiratory reserve volume, tidal volume, and expiratory reserve volume. When this capacity is decreased, the patient may have trouble maximally inspiring and then maximally exhaling, which in turn could affect oxygenation to major muscle groups. 7. Lying flat may impair the patient's ability to ventilate optimally due to a rise of the diaphragm, decreasing space in the thoracic cavity. When this happens, the lungs are not able to expand fully. Additionally, the thoracotomy incision may be painful, and the patient may not feel comfortable lying on his side. 8. The patient's current Five Times Sit-to-Stand score (22.5 seconds) is below the mean for community-dwelling older adults aged 80 to 89 (14.8 seconds). This indicates that the patient has decreased lower extremity functional strength. 9. For community-dwelling males age 80 to 89, the average 6-Minute Walk Test distance is 417 m (1,368 feet). Based on the patient's distance of 200 m (656 feet), he demonstrates significantly decreased distance as compared to age- and gender-matched peers.
Apply	10. Initial speed of the patient's 6-Minute Walk Test can be decreased by 20% initially with the goal of increasing the patient's total walking time to 15 to 20 minutes. One calculation that can be used is the actual 6-Minute Walk Test distance multiplied by 3.33 m and then multiplied by 0.80. This can then be increase in intensity to 0.90 as tolerated. 11. A person with hypoxia may present with impaired judgment, loss of cognitive and motor functions, decreased exercise tolerance, headache, breathlessness, palpitations, chest pain, restlessness, or tremors. The wife should be educated to watch for signs and symptoms of worsening hypoxia as well as what to do in an emergency.

(Continued)

(Continued)

Bloom's Taxonomy Level	Case 11.B Answers
Understand	12. Based on the patient's score of 12.5 seconds for the TUG, the patient would not be classified as at risk for falls.
Remember	13. T2b indicates tumor size greater than 4 cm and ≤ 5 cm; N1 indicates regional lymph node involvement; M0 indicates no distant metastases. The patient would be given a staging of IIB
	14. The most common sites for non–small cell lung cancer to metastasize to include the adrenals, brain, bone, and liver
	15. Risk factors for developing lung cancer include exposure to second-hand smoke, marihuana use, occupational exposure, previous lung disease, decreased intake of fruits and vegetables, consuming a diet high in saturated fat, genetic susceptibility, and low levels of physical activity. Specific occupational risks include exposure to paint thinners, welding equipment, and smoke soot or exhaust.

Key points
1. A knowledge of pathology including prognosis is important for establishing a physical therapy plan of care and reasonable goals.
2. In addition to pathology and age, many factors including prior level of function, social support, and cognition will impact overall prognosis.
3. When reporting on outcome measures, refer to age, gender, and/or condition-specific normative values to produce defensible documentation.
4. An HEP needs to be specific to patient's impairments and activity/participation limitations to maximize adherence.

General Information	
Case no.	11.C
Authors	Sarah Ferrero, PT, DPT, Board Certified Clinical Specialist in Geriatrics Physical Therapy Karen Blood, PT, DPT, Board Certified Clinical Specialist in Geriatrics Physical Therapy Rachel Pata, PT, DPT, CHSE, Board Certified Clinical Specialist in Cardiovascular & Pulmonary Physical Therapy
Diagnosis	Non–small cell lung cancer; stage IIB (T2b N1 M0); status post (s/p) left upper lobectomy
Setting	Outpatient clinic
Learner expectations	☑ Initial evaluation ☐ Re-evaluation ☐ Treatment session
Learner objectives	1. Categorize risk factors for falling. 2. Interpret the patient's performance on functional outcome measures related to fall risk. 3. Synthesize examination data to create a plan of care that addresses the patient's risk for falls.

Medical	
Chief complaint	History of two falls in the last month.
History of present illness	The patient is an 82-year-old man who was referred by MD secondary to complaints of weakness and frequent falls at a recent follow-up appointment. Four months ago, he underwent left upper lobectomy secondary to non–small cell lung cancer; hospital stay was 6 days. He was then discharged home where he had eight home physical therapy visits. Three weeks ago, he completed chemotherapy treatment that consisted of a combination of cisplatin-vinorelbine.
Past medical history	Osteoarthritis (OA), benign prostatic hypertrophy (BPH), diabetes mellitus (DM)
Past surgical history	s/p left total hip arthroplasty 6 years ago, left upper lobectomy 3 months ago
Allergies	No known drug allergies
Medications	Metformin, Flomax, Glucosamine, Iron
Precautions/orders	"Evaluate and treat secondary to weakness and falls."

Social history	
Home setup	• Lives with his wife in assisted living facility (ALF). • One-bedroom apartment is on the second floor. • Elevator access to apartment (1,000 feet from the apartment to the elevator). • Congregate meals on the first floor, but can also be delivered to apartments or prepared in unit kitchenettes. • Assisted living has transport wheelchairs available.
Occupation	• Retired; owned a dry-cleaning business for 50 years
Prior level of function	• Independent in all functional mobility and activities of daily living (ADLs) without supplemental O_2; used a cane for community ambulation. • Participated in instrumental ADLs (IADLs) with his wife, such as shopping and light meal prep; ate breakfast and dinner in congregate dining room. • + Driving
Recreational activities	• Participates in weekly bridge club at ALF. • Goes to daughter's home every Thursday with his wife to babysit two grandkids (ages 5 and 7). • Participates in group exercise classes thrice a week at ALF.

Medical management	
Per wife's report	Workup for infection negative

Pause points
Based on the above information, what are the priorities? • Diagnostic tests and measures? • Outcome measures? • Treatment interventions?

Physical Examination
Subjective
"I keep falling and it's getting annoying." Per wife, patient with two falls in past month. The first time was at night; patient tripped ambulating to the bathroom without his walker; the second time "he was trying to get up from his easy chair."

Objective			
Vital signs	Pre-treatment		Post-treatment
	Sitting	Standing	
Blood pressure (mmHg)	116/76	110/76	118/78
Heart rate (beats/min)	82	86	85
Respiratory rate (breaths/min)	17	20	18
Pulse oximetry on room air (SpO_2)	92	92	93
Borg scale	1	3	2
Pain	2/10, left shoulder, end range of motion (ROM)		
General	• Patient sitting in standard chair with arms in waiting room with rolling walker (RW) in front of him. • Wife present and reports out most background information. • Patient pleasant but defers to wife to answer questions.		

(Continued)

(Continued)

Physical Examination		
Cardiovascular and pulmonary	• Pedal pulses: 2 + bilaterally • No use of accessory muscles at rest • Skin color normal at nail beds	
Gastrointestinal/ Genitourinary	• Wife reports frequent night-time urination	
Integumentary	• Port placed left upper chest wall	
Musculoskeletal	ROM	• Left shoulder flex/abduction: 120-degree active ROM (AROM) • Right upper extremity (RUE): within functional limit (WFL) • Bilateral lower extremity (BLE): hip extension to neutral, decreased terminal knee extension, decreased ankle dorsiflexion.
	Strength	• Right shoulder flex/abduction: 4/5 • Left shoulder flex/abduction: 3–/5 • Bilateral elbow flexion/extension: 4/5 • Grip strength: equal bilaterally • Bilateral hip flexion 4–/5 • Bilateral hip abduction: 4–/5 • Bilateral knee extension: 4/5 • Bilateral dorsiflexion: 3 + /5
	Aerobic	• 6-Minute Walk Test: 755 feet with RW
	Flexibility	• Kyphotic posture • Decreased trunk ROM all planes • Tight hamstrings
	Other	• 30-Second Chair Rise = 0 • Modified 30-Second Chair Rise = 2
Neurological	Balance	• Timed Up and Go (TUG) 12.5 seconds with RW; 16.2 seconds with a straight cane. • Tinetti Test: 18/28 (10/16 balance, 8/12 gait) • Four-stage balance test: 1. feet side by side: 10 seconds 2. Feet staggered: 8 seconds 3. Tandem: 4 seconds 4. Single leg: 1 second
	Cognition	• Alert and oriented (A&O) × 4 • Communicated appropriately
	Coordination	• Heel to shin: decreased accuracy bilaterally
	Cranial nerves	• I–XII: intact
	Reflexes	• Patellar reflex: 2 + bilaterally
	Sensation	• Bilateral toes: diminished light touch, complaints of burning and cramping
	Tone	• BUE: WNL • BLE: WNL
	Other	• Gait speed: 0.8 m/s with RW 0.45 m/s with straight cane
Functional status		
Bed mobility	• Rolling either direction: independent • Supine to/from sit: independent Of note, patient requires increased time to complete all bed mobility.	
Transfers	• Sit to/from stand: independent; uses BUE, required two attempts to complete task with noted decreased forward flexion of the trunk. ▶ Fig. 11.4.	

(Continued)

(Continued)

Physical Examination	
	• Stand pivot transfer: independent, increased time to complete.
Ambulation	• Ambulated 40 feet with straight cane and contact guard assistance (CGA). • Gait deficits notable for slow cadence, short stride length, minimal heel strike on initial contact; two losses of balance during turns requiring minimal assistance for recovery. Of note, patient independently ambulated 50 feet with RW from the car to the clinic.
Stairs	• Ascend/descend four 6-inch steps with bilateral handrails and supervision, requires increased time. Of note, patient reports that he only has stairs at his daughter's home.
Task specific	Reports most difficulty with sit to stand; "Once I'm up, I'm fine."

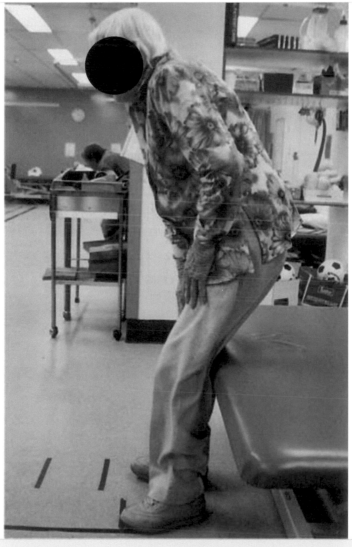

Fig. 11.4 Decreased forward trunk flexion demonstrated with sit to stand movement. (Adapted from Mehrholz J, ed. Maximizing Muscle Endurance and Physical Fitness. In: Physical Therapy for the Stroke Patient: Early Stage Rehabilitation. 1st ed. New York, NY: Thieme; 2012.)

Assessment	
☑ Physical therapist's	*Assessment left blank for learner to develop.*
Goals	
Patient's	"I want to get back to just using my cane."
Short term	1.
	Goals left blank for learner to develop.
	2.
Long term	1.
	Goals left blank for learner to develop.
	2.

Plan	
☐ Physician's ☑ Physical therapist's ☐ Other's	Patient would benefit from skilled physical therapy services twice a week × 4 weeks, with treatment to include therapeutic exercise (proximal hip and core strengthening, aerobic conditioning), standing balance retraining, gait training on level surfaces and stairs, and education on energy conservation strategies and management of fall risk.

Bloom's Taxonomy Level	Case 11.C Questions
Create	1. Synthesizing the medical data and physical examination findings, develop an appropriate physical therapy assessment of the patient. 2. Develop two short-term physical therapy goals, including an appropriate timeframe for outpatient. 3. Develop two long-term physical therapy goals, including an appropriate timeframe for outpatient. 4. Generate a list of follow-up questions needed to ask the patient to further assess fall risk.

Evaluate	5. Discuss lab tests appropriate for this patient:
	  a) What lab tests would the physical therapist expect the patient to have undergone for the wife to report that "workup for infection was negative"?
	  b) What other lab tests would the physical therapist expect the physician to order given his underlying medical condition?
	6. Categorize the patient's risk factors for falling into intrinsic and extrinsic factors:
	  a) Which of these risk factors warrant referral to another member of the interdisciplinary team?

Analyze	7. Analyze the relationship between the history of lung cancer and the chief complaint for this episode of care.
	8. Analyze the patient's movement from sit to stand:
	  a) Which aspect of the task is most difficult?
	  b) What impairments are contributing to the patient's difficulty with this movement?

Apply	9. Design a plan of care to address the patient's impairments that are contributing to his increased risk of falling. 10. What recommendations can be made to modify the task of sit to stand?
Understand	11. How does the patient's gait speed fit into the patient's current functional status? Is he a "community ambulator"?
Remember	12. What are intrinsic risk factors for falling? What are extrinsic risk factors for falling?

Bloom's Taxonomy Level	Case 11.C Answers
Create	1. The patient is an 82-year-old man who presents with impaired lower extremity strength, diminished distal lower extremity sensation, and decreased endurance that all result in impaired standing balance, difficulty with sit to stand transfers, and inefficiency of gait. He is at increased risk of falling as demonstrated by a TUG of 16. 2 seconds with straight cane, and a Tinetti score of 18/28.
	2. Short-term goals:
	• Patient will ambulate with straight cane 75 feet with supervision with no loss of balance with gait speed of 0.6 m/s within 2 weeks.
	• Patient will complete four repetitions during the 30-Second Chair Rise Test to improve lower extremity strength and decrease risk of falls within 2 weeks.
	3. Long-term goals:
	• Patient will ambulate community distances with straight cane at a gait speed of .8 m/s within 4 weeks.
	• Patient will complete TUG in 12 seconds with straight cane in order to decrease risk of falls within 4 weeks.
	• Patient will complete 10 repetitions of 30-Second Chair Rise to decrease risk of falls within 4 weeks.
	4. Follow-up questions include:
	• Describe the circumstances of each fall
	• Do you feel unsteady when walking or standing?
	• Do you worry about falling?
	• Any lightheadedness or dizziness when changing position?
	• Any recent changes in medications?
	• Any recent changes in vision?
	• What do you typically use for footwear?
	• Any throw rugs or other obstacles in the environment?
Evaluate	5. It is expected that the patient would have had a complete blood count (CBC) ordered to evaluate the white blood cell (WBC) count. The CBC would also have given information regarding the red blood cell (RBC) and platelets, both cell types that are impacted by chemotherapy agents. The patient also would have likely had a basic metabolic panel (BMP) done as part of a routine follow-up to assess electrolyte balance as fluid status can fluctuate post chemotherapy. A BMP also would allow for monitoring of blood glucose/A1C given diagnosis of DM.
	6. This patient's intrinsic risk factors include impaired sensation leading to impaired balance as a chief contributor as well as decreased ROM and strength of the trunk and lower extremity; deconditioning postsurgery, fatigue. Extrinsic risk factors include poor lighting at night and obstacles.
	Other members of the interdisciplinary team that could be involved include physician or pharmacist (to review medication list), optometrist (to reassess vision), occupational therapist (to assess ADLs and environmental issues), nurse manager at ALF (to assess for need for add-on services available at the ALF).
Analyze	7. The patient has undergone treatment for lung cancer, including chemotherapy. Side effects of chemotherapy agents can include peripheral neuropathy. Sensory input is a crucial element in the complex task of maintaining balance. Falling is a multifaceted problem, but impaired sensory input and balance can be contributing factors. Chemotherapy also impacts blood cells; chemo can destroy RBC leading to anemia. Symptoms of anemia include fatigue and shortness of breath. This along with other side effects of chemotherapy including nausea and vomiting can contribute to a decreased activity level in general, which can lead to deconditioning.
	8. The patient is having the most difficulty with forward trunk flexion to initiate the sit to stand movement. The patient's limited trunk ROM related to guarding due to pain post-op, which developed into an abnormal movement pattern. The patient may not be able to compensate with the use of upper extremity due to decreased shoulder ROM and strength. Looking down the chain, consideration must be given to the fact that this is a geriatric patient. The patient also has decreased proximal hip strength and decreased ROM at the hips, knees, and ankles, which are contributing to impairments with this task.

(Continued)

(Continued)

Bloom's Taxonomy Level	Case 11.C Answers
Apply	9. Interventions to address the patient's increased risk for falls can be categorized into exercise interventions or environmental adaptations. Specific to this patient, interventions that address his strength impairments and trunk/lower extremity ROM limitations, as well as introduction of exercise programs such as Otago Exercise program or Tai Chi, are appropriate. Environmental adaptations can include ensuring that pathways are uncluttered, pathways are well lit, chairs are sturdy with arm rests, commonly used items are within arm's reach. 10. Recommendations to modify the task could include raising the height of the surface or using a firmer surface. Education on proper setup of the task (scooting to edge of surface, ensuring feet aligned under knees vs. farther out, use of upper extremity) to improve mechanical advantages to complete task.
Understand	11. The patient's gait speed of 0.8 m/s with an RW puts him on the border of limited community ambulator and community ambulator according to Fritz and Lusardi. This matches his presentation in that he can ambulate into the clinic independently with an RW. His gait speed of 0.45 m/s with a straight cane categorizes him as household walker with increased dependence in ADLs. Both gait speeds categorize him as being discharged to home versus skilled nursing facility (SNF), but both speeds require interventions to reduce risk of falls.
Remember	12. Falls are multifactorial. In this patient's case, impaired sensation leading to impaired balance is a chief contributor as well as decreased ROM and strength of the trunk and lower extremity. Standardized testing revealed an increased fall risk due to impaired balance and strength (30-Second Chair Rise Test norm for males 80–84 > 10; four-stage balance test tandem stance time < 10 seconds; TUG > 12 seconds). Other intrinsic potential factors include deconditioning following surgery and chemo treatment related to decreased physical activity compared to his norm presurgery; fatigue related to anemia due to chemo agents destroying RBC; electrolyte imbalances could lead to fluid imbalances, which could result in orthostatic hypotension; frequency of urination. Potential environmental contributors include poor lighting, or possible cluttering of the environment leading to obstacles. Intrinsic risk factors for falling are those factors that are internal to the patient and include advanced age, previous falls, muscle weakness, gait and balance problems, poor vision, postural hypotension, chronic conditions (i.e., arthritis, incontinence, diabetes, etc.), and/or fear of falling Extrinsic risk factors for falling are those factors that are external to the patient and include lack of stair handrails, lack of grab bars in the bathroom, dim lighting or glare, obstacle and/or tripping hazards, slippery or uneven surfaces, psychoactive medications, and/or improper use of assistive device.

Key points
1. Fall risk assessment relies on assessment of multiple factors, including medical factors, social supports, and physical capabilities. 2. A person's past medical history can have a significant impact on current body structure and function impairments, activity limitations, and participation. 3. A thorough analysis of a task is important to prioritize impairments to address in a plan of care.

Suggested Readings

Academy of Acute Care Physical Therapy-APTA Taskforce on Lab Values. Laboratory Values Interpretation Resource. Pittsburgh, PA: APTA; 2017

Ahmad AM. Essentials of physiotherapy after thoracic surgery: what physiotherapists need to know. A narrative review. Korean J Thorac Cardiovasc Surg. 2018; 51(5):293–307

Aksu NT, Erdogan A, Ozgur N. Effects of progressive muscle relaxation training on sleep and quality of life in patients with pulmonary resection. Sleep Breath. 2018; 22(3):695–702

American College of Sports Medicine. ACSM's Guidelines for Exercise Testing and Prescription. 10th ed. Baltimore, MD: Lippincott, Williams and Wilkins; 2017

Anderson LW, Krathwohl DR. A Taxonomy for Learning, Teaching, and Assessing, Abridged Edition. Boston, MA: Allyn and Bacon; 2001

Armstrong P. Bloom's Taxonomy. Available at: https://cft.vanderbilt.edu/guides-sub-pages/blooms-taxonomy/. Accessed on April 1, 2018

Borg GA. Psychophysical bases of perceived exertion. Med Sci Sports Exerc. 1982; 14(5):377–381

Borg Rating of Perceived Exertion. Available at: https://www.sralab.org/rehabilitation-measures/borg-rating-scale-perceived-exertion#older-adults-and-geriatric-care. Accessed March 11, 2020

CDC. Materials for Healthcare Providers | STEADI - Older Adult Fall Prevention | CDC Injury Center. Available at: https://www.cdc.gov/steadi/materials.html. Published September 5, 2019. Accessed March 28, 2020

Chandrasekaran B, Reddy KC. Six-minute walk test as a guide for walking prescription for patients with chronic obstructive pulmonary diseases. I J Respiratory Care. 2018; 7:73–76

Fritz S, Lusardi M. White paper: "walking speed: the sixth vital sign.". J Geriatr Phys Ther. 2009; 32(2):46–49

Fruth SJ. Fundamentals of the Physical Therapy Examination: Patient Interviews and Tests & Measures. Burlington, MA: Jones & Bartlett Learning; 2014

Goodman CC, Fuller KS. Pathology: Implications for the Physical Therapist. 4th ed. St. Louis, MO: Saunders Elsevier; 2015

Hillegass E. Essentials of Cardiopulmonary Physical Therapy. 4th ed. St. Louis, MO: Elsevier; 2017

Hillegass E, Fick A, Pawlik A, et al. Supplemental oxygen utilization during physical therapy interventions. Cardiopulm Phys Ther J. 2014; 25(2):38–49

Jette DU, Stilphen M, Ranganathan VK, Passek SD, Frost FS, Jette AM. AM-PAC. AM-PAC "6-Clicks" functional assessment scores predict acute care hospital discharge destination. Phys Ther. 2014; 94(9):1252–1261

Niedzwiedz CL, Knifton L, Robb KA, Katikireddi SV, Smith DJ. Depression and anxiety among people living with and beyond cancer: a growing clinical and research priority. BMC Cancer. 2019; 19(1):943

Postmus PE, Kerr KM, Oudkerk M, et al. Early and locally advanced (non-metastatic) non-small-cell lung cancer: ESMO Clinical Practice Guidelines for diagnosis, treatment and follow-up. Ann Oncol. 2017; 28(Suppl 4):iv1–iv21

Quinn L, Gordon J. Documentation for Rehabilitation. 3rd ed. Maryland Heights, MO: Elsevier; 2016

Shirley Ryan AbilityLab. Activity Measure for Post Acute Care. Available at: https://www.sralab.org/search?contains=AMPAC. Accessed March 11, 2020

Shirley Ryan AbilityLab. Five Times Sit to Stand Test. Available at: https://www.sralab.org/rehabilitation-measures/five-times-sit-stand-test. Accessed March 9, 2020

Shirley Ryan AbilityLab. Timed Up and Go. Available at: https://www.sralab.org/rehabilitation-measures/timed-and-go. Accessed March 19, 2020

Van Mieghem W, Demedts M. Cardiopulmonary function after lobectomy or pneumonectomy for pulmonary neoplasm. Respir Med. 1989; 83(3):199–206

Watchie J. Cardiovascular and Pulmonary Physical Therapy. 2nd ed. St. Louis, MO: Elsevier; 2010

Weinberger SE, Cockrill BA, Mandel J. Principles of Pulmonary Medicine. Philadelphia, PA: Saunders; 2008

Yano T, Haro A, Shikada Y, Maruyama R, Maehara Y. Non-small cell lung cancer in never smokers as a representative "non-smoking-associated lung cancer": epidemiology and clinical features. Int J Clin Oncol. 2011; 16(4):287–293

12 Multi Trauma

General Information	
Case no.	12.A Multi Trauma
Authors	Rachel Pata, PT, DPT, CHSE, Board Certified Clinical Specialist in Cardiovascular & Pulmonary Physical Therapy Tracy Wall, PT, PhD Erin Lampron, PT, DPT, Board Certified Clinical Specialist in Neurologic Physical Therapy
Diagnosis	Multitrauma status post (s/p) 50-foot fall, multiple right rib fractures, moderate right pneumothorax, open right tibial/fibular fracture with internal fixation.
Setting	Emergency Department to Trauma Intensive Care Unit (ICU).
Learner expectations	☑ Initial evaluation ☐ Re-evaluation ☐ Treatment session
Learner objectives	1. Describe the pathophysiology of the patient's history in progress. 2. Discuss the impact of patient comorbidities on activity tolerance and healing. 3. Interpret examination components for this patient. 4. Formulate a safe and evidence-based plan of care.

Medical	
Chief complaint	Right lower extremity (RLE) pain and difficulty breathing
History of present illness	The patient is a 62-year-old man brought to hospital by ambulance. The patient is s/p a work-related trauma in which he fell 50 feet from a scaffold. He presented to the Emergency Department with acute shortness of breath, hypoxemia, and laceration of the RLE. He was diagnosed with multiple right-sided rib fractures, a moderate right pneumothorax and open right distal tibial/fibular fracture. He was stabilized with right chest tube placement and then underwent open reduction internal fixation (ORIF) of his RLE.
Past medical history	Chronic obstructive pulmonary disease (COPD), obesity, non–insulin-dependent diabetes mellitus, hypertension, anxiety
Past surgical history	s/p appendectomy 30 years ago
Allergies	None
Medications	Ambien, Lisinopril, Xanax, Albuterol, Metformin
Precautions/orders	Activity as tolerated Non–weight bearing (NWB) RLE No range of motion (ROM) of right ankle/Controlled Ankle Motion (CAM) boot at all times ▶ Fig. 12.1

Social history	
Home setup	• Lives alone in a ranch-style home. • Four steps to enter from the front door; two steps to enter from the garage. • Flight of steps to basement, where laundry is located.
Occupation	• Works full time as a commercial painter.
Prior level of function	• Independent in all functional mobility and activities of daily living (ADLs) without supplemental O_2. • Fatigue with prolonged community ambulation. • (+) Driving
Recreational activities	• Primarily sedentary during his time off, watches TV. • Meets up with friends at the bar twice a week. • Walks his dog around the block daily.

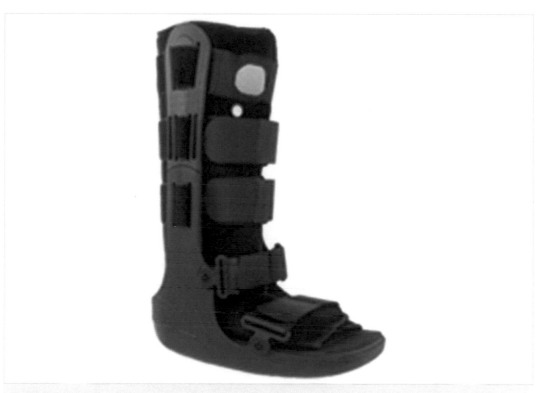

Fig. 12.1 An example of a CAM boot.

Hospital day 0: Emergency Department		
Vital signs	**Presentation**	**Corrected**
Blood pressure (mmHg)	150/92	132/84
Heart rate (beats/min)	110	95
Respiratory rate (breaths/min)	36	23
Pulse oximetry (SpO$_2$)	82% 4 L nasal cannula (NC)	91% 2 L NC
Temperature (°F)	98.7	98.6

Imaging/diagnostic tests	Hospital day 0: Emergency Department	Hospital day 1: ICU
Chest X-ray	1. Impression: fracture to right ribs 3 to 5 at the costal angle, moderate right pneumothorax.	1. Impression: chest tube in place with small right pneumothorax, improved from last study.
RLE X-ray	1. Impression: comminuted open fracture of the distal right tibia and fibula	1. Impression: ORIF in place with good alignment of tibia and fibula ▶ Fig. 12.2

Medical management	Hospital day 0: Emergency Department	Hospital day 1: ICU
Procedure	1. Right chest tube placed	1. Chest tube remains in place
Additional medications	1. Percocet 5 mg/325 mg every 12 hours 2. Lovenox 40 mg subcutaneous daily 3. Intravenous (IV) fluids	1. Continue per medical orders

(Continued)

(Continued)

Medical management	Hospital day 0: Emergency Department	Hospital day 1: ICU
Respiratory	1. Oxygen: 4 L O_2 by NC in ambulance, reduced to 2 L after chest tube placement and stabilization of hypoxic respiratory failure.	1. Continue 2 L O_2 by NC to keep O_2 saturation ≥ 90% 2. Duonebs q.i.d.
Surgery	_____	1. s/p ORIF right distal tibial/fibular fracture in the operating room

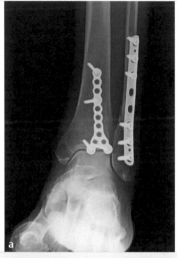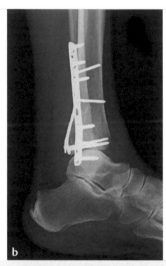

Fig. 12.2 (a,b) Radiologic evaluation of lower leg, ankle, and foot fracture fixation hardware. (Adapted from Mar W, Schilling J, Lomasney L et al. Radiologic evaluation of lower leg, ankle, and foot fracture fixation hardware. Semin Musculoskelet Radiol 2019;23(02):36–55.)

	Lab	Reference range	Hospital day 0: Emergency Department	Hospital day 1: ICU	Hospital day 2: ICU
Complete blood count	White blood cell (WBC)	5.0–10.0 × 10^9/L	6.4	8.7	12.2
	Red blood cell (RBC)	4.1–5.3 million/mm³	4.2	4.0	3.8
	Hemoglobin (Hgb)	14–17.4 g/dL	15	13	11
	Hematocrit	42–52%	47%	40%	35%
	Platelets	140,000–400,000/µL	250	255	260
Arterial blood gas	PaO$_2$	80–95 mmHg	65	75	90
	PaCO$_2$	37–43 mmHg	47	50	45
	PH	7.35–7.45	7.4	7.32	7.36
	HCO$_3$	20–30 mmol/L	32	32	33
Basic metabolic panel	Glucose (fasting)	70–100 mg/dL	150	172	156
	Hgb A1C	<5.7%	6.7%	–	–
	Cholesterol	<200 mg/dL	210	–	–
	Low-density lipoprotein (LDL)	<70 mg/dL	130	–	–

(Continued)

(Continued)

Lab		Reference range	Hospital day 0: Emergency Department	Hospital day 1: ICU	Hospital day 2: ICU
	High-density lipoprotein (HDL)	>60 mg/dL	80	–	–
	Blood urea nitrogen (BUN)	6–25 mg/dL	25	28	30
	Creatinine	0.7–1.3 mg/dL	1.2	1.4	1.7
	Potassium	3.7–5.1 mEq/L	4	4.2	4.1
	Sodium	134–142 mEq/L	136	140	142
	Chloride	98–108 mEq/L	100	100	102
	Calcium	8.6–10.3 mg/dL	8.4	8.5	8.4
	Magnesium	1.2–1.9 mEq/L	1.4	1.3	1.4

Pause points

Based on the above information, what are the:
- Precautions for physical therapy?
- Examination priorities?
- Patient monitoring priorities?
- Potential reasons for abnormal laboratory values?

Hospital Day 2, ICU: Physical Therapy Examination

Subjective

"I can't look at my leg. When I do, I can't breathe."

Objective

Vital signs	Pre-treatment			Post-treatment
	Supine	Sitting	Standing	Sitting
Blood pressure (mmHg)	134/90	128/84	136/88	144/92
Heart rate (beats/min)	90	95	108	118
Respiratory rate (RR; breath/min)	24	28	32	34
Pulse oximetry on 2 L NC (SpO$_2$)	94%	93%	95%	92%
Borg scale	11/20	12/20	14/20	12/20
Pain	5/10 RLE 3/10 right side of thorax	5/10 RLE 3/10 right side of thorax	8/10 RLE 5/10 right side of thorax	6/10 RLE 5/10 right side of thorax
General	• Patient found supine in bed with head of bed (HOB) elevated 45 degrees. • RLE elevated with min serosanguineous drainage from incision. • Appears to be anxious, as shown by elevated respiratory rate upon introduction to patient. • Lines/equipment notable for telemetry, peripheral IV, right chest tube, 2 L O$_2$ by NC, CAM boot.			
Cardiovascular and pulmonary	• Inspection: shallow breathing, elevated RR, no accessory muscle use • Palpation: reduced expansion right middle and lower lobe. 2 + pedal pulses bilateral lower extremity (BLE) • Auscultation: diminished breath sounds bilateral lower lobes (BLL) R > L, occasional low-pitched expiratory wheeze right lower lobe (RLL), no crackles.			

(Continued)

(Continued)

Hospital Day 2, ICU: Physical Therapy Examination		
Gastrointestinal		• Mild abdominal distention
Genitourinary		• Voiding independently on bed pan, clear, yellow urine
Musculoskeletal	Range of motion (ROM)	• Bilateral upper extremity (BUE): within functional limit (WFL), except right shoulder flexion and abduction: 120 degrees, limited by right-sided pain • Left lower extremity (LLE): WFL • Right hip flexion: 90 degrees, limited by pain • Right knee flexion: 80 degrees, limited by pain • Right ankle: not tested due to CAM boot and precautions for no ROM at ankle
	Strength	• Left upper extremity (LUE): WFL • Right shoulder flexion: 3/5 • Right elbow flexion 4/5 • Right elbow extension: 4/5 • Right grip: 5/5 • LLE: WFL • Right hip flexion: 3-/5 • Right knee flexion: 2/5 • Right knee extension 2/5
	Aerobic	• Unable to perform standardized assessment at this time. • Refer to patient vital signs and signs and symptoms.
	Flexibility	• Not assessed at this time
	Other	• Not applicable
Neurological	Balance	• Static sitting: fair, able to maintain sitting with support of LUE × 60 seconds, then needing additional support secondary to fatigue. • Dynamic sitting: poor, requiring assistance to maintain sitting while reaching with either UE. • Static standing: poor requiring moderate to maximum assistance to maintain standing plus the assist of a second person to maintain NWB RLE.
	Cognition	• Alert and oriented (A&O) × 4
	Coordination	• Finger to nose: intact BUE • Toe tapping: LLE intact, unable to assess RLE
	Cranial nerves	• II–XII: intact
	Reflexes	• Not tested at this time
	Sensation	• Right plantar surface: decreased sensation to light touch
	Tone	• BUE: within normal limit (WNL) • BLE: WNL
	Other	• Not applicable
Functional status		
Bed mobility		• Scooting: moderate assistance × 1 • Bridge: unable to perform at this time • Left rolling: moderate assistance × 1, primarily to assist RLE • Supine to/from sit: maximal assistance × 1
Transfers		• Sit to/from stand: moderate to maximal assistance × 2 (1 person to assist at trunk, 1 person to assist RLE) with rolling walker (RW) • Bed to/from chair: moderate to maximal assistance × 2 using stand pivot technique

(Continued)

(Continued)

Hospital Day 2, ICU: Physical Therapy Examination	
Ambulation	• Hopped two steps with moderate to maximal assistance and an RW, however becoming very anxious, with elevated RR and increased pain.
Stairs	• Unsafe to trial at this time.

Assessment	
☑ Physical therapist's	*Assessment left blank for learner to develop.*

Goals	
Patient's	"I don't want to be in pain anymore."
Short term	1. *Goals left blank for learner to develop.* 2.
Long term	1. *Goals left blank for learner to develop.* 2.

Plan	
☐ Physician's ☑ Physical therapist's ☐ Other's	Patient will be seen for daily physical therapy including therapeutic exercise, bed mobility, transfer training, gait training and breathing exercises to improve strength, ROM, functional mobility, and endurance.

Bloom's Taxonomy Level	Case 12.A Questions
Create	1. Synthesizing the medical data and physical examination findings, develop an appropriate physical therapy assessment of the patient. 2. Develop two short-term physical therapy goals, including an appropriate timeframe. 3. Develop two long-term physical therapy goals, including an appropriate timeframe.
Evaluate	4. Discuss positive and negative prognostic indicators for this patient. 5. Describe how social history may impact discharge planning.
Analyze	6. Describe how this patient's rib fractures may affect ventilation. 7. Describe how this patient's weight-bearing status will affect endurance.
Apply	8. Discuss how to best perform gait training with this patient. 9. Implement strategies for energy conservation during gait training.
Understand	10. Interpret this patient's day 0 vital signs. 11. Does this patient have restrictive or obstructive lung disease or both? 12. What are the potential causes for impaired sensation of the RLE? 13. What is the relationship between rib fractures and a pneumothorax? 14. How can timing of medication administration assist with patient performance in physical therapy?
Remember	15. How will this patient's history of non–insulin-dependent diabetes mellitus (NIDDM) influence healing?

Bloom's Taxonomy Level	Case 12.A Answers
Create	1. The patient is a 62-year-old man admitted to the hospital s/p a 50-foot fall resulting in multiple rib fractures, right pneumothorax, and right open tibial/fibular fracture s/p ORIF. He presents with impaired strength, endurance, and functional mobility associated with the above injuries. His past medical history of COPD, obesity, NIDDM, and anxiety are also negative factors contributing to his functional status. He would benefit from skilled physical therapy services to improve strength, functional mobility, and endurance. 2. Short-term goals: • Patient will perform sit to/from stand transfers with moderate assistance × 1 to improve transfers out of bed within 1 week. • Patient will ambulate 10 feet with moderate assistance × 1 and RW while keeping O_2 saturation > 90% to ambulate to the bathroom. 3. Long-term goals: • Patient will perform sit to/from stand transfers with supervision to improve transfers out of bed within 2 weeks. • Patient will ambulate 25 feet with minimal assistance × 1 and RW keeping O_2 saturation > 90% to ambulate around his home.
Evaluate	4. Positive prognostic indicators include patient age, prior independent level of function. Negative prognostic indicators include comorbidities, sedentary lifestyle, lack of support at home. 5. This patient lives alone at home. Without help, he will need to be able to mobilize independently in order to get to the bathroom and take care of himself. Although it is a ranch-style home, there are two stairs to enter and laundry in the basement. This means the patient will need to be able to navigate some stairs to enter his home and will need someone to help with laundry. Given the extent of this patient's injuries, the change from his baseline functional level and the lack of help at home, it is recommended that this patient be discharged to an acute rehabilitation center.
Analyze	6. Rib fractures can make breathing very painful for this patient. This patient may frequently take short shallow breaths to reduce thoracic expansion and limit pain. This produces a restrictive lung condition, causing reduced inspiratory volumes, increased risk for pneumonia and potential respiratory failure. 7. Maintaining NWB of the RLE requires lifting the weight of this leg in addition to the weight of the CAM boot off the ground and maintaining this position during mobility. The increased muscle contraction for this task will increase metabolic demand and oxygen consumption. This will decrease the patient's endurance and increase fatigue.
Apply	8. Given the large amount of assistance this patient required to stand, gait training should begin in standing with assistance of two and an RW. First, the patient should focus on maintaining RLE NWB status in standing and performing weight shifts and mini-squats. After, the patient should progress to hopping in place with assistance and an RW, ensuring NWB is always maintained. Finally, the patient can progress to ambulating RLE NWB with assistance and an RW. Throughout gait training, caution should be taken with placement of a gait belt secondary to the chest tube. Having someone follow with a chair is also highly recommended due to patient fatigue. 9. Patient should self-monitor exertion using rate of Perceived Exertion (RPE) as well as dyspnea, using subjective rating of intensity or Borg Scale for rating breathlessness, as well as taking rest breaks as needed to assist in energy conservation and activity tolerance. Diaphragmatic and pursed lib breathing can be used to decrease respiratory rate, improve ventilation, and reduce dyspnea.
Understand	10. The patient's blood pressure is indicative of hypertension, which may be baseline for this patient, but is likely secondary to pain and anxiety. Heart rate is elevated, which may be secondary to pain, anxiety, blood loss, or a combination of these. Respiratory rate is elevated secondary to difficulty breathing and anxiety. Low oxygen saturation is consistent with hypoxic respiratory failure, which is likely resultant of rib fractures and pneumothorax. Temperature is normal. 11. This patient has both restrictive and obstructive lung disease. Restrictive lung disease is a result of recurrent rib fractures, where the obstructive disease is from his underlying COPD.

(Continued)

(Continued)

Bloom's Taxonomy Level	Case 12.A Answers
	12. Potential causes of impaired RLE sensation may be (a) secondary to neuropathy from diabetes or (b) peripheral nerve injury (tibial nerve) secondary to fracture. The patient should be asked if this is acute or chronic and exact distribution of sensory loss needs to be determined.
	13. Rib fractures can puncture the parietal pleura, causing increase air in the intrapleural space. This will increase the pressure in this space and can lead to atelectasis and lung collapse if left untreated.
	14. Providing physical therapy treatment soon after the administration of pain medication and nebulizer treatments will help control pain and improve ventilation. This will optimize the patient's ability to participate in therapy.
Remember	15. Diabetes will slow the healing process for the fracture and open areas of skin. This is secondary to impaired circulation and tissue damage associated with hyperglycemia. Up to 49% of individuals with DM present with arterial insufficiency causing impaired oxygen and nutrient supply to tissues.

Key points
1. Consider the complete patient picture including past medical history and history of present illness when prioritizing the components of the physical therapy examination.
2. Strategies to manage pain and anxiety will improve patient tolerance and outcomes.
3. Monitor the patient throughout the assessment and follow precautions to maintain patient safety.

General Information	
Case no.	12.B
Authors	Tracy Wall, PT, PhD
	Rachel Pata, PT, DPT, CI ISC, Board Certified Clinical Specialist in Cardiovascular & Pulmonary Physical Therapy
	Erin Lampron, PT, DPT, Board Certified Clinical Specialist in Neurologic Physical Therapy
Diagnosis	Multitrauma status post (s/p) 50-foot fall, multiple right (R) rib fractures, moderate R pneumothorax, open R tibial/fibular fracture with internal fixation.
Setting	Acute inpatient rehabilitation
Learner expectations	☐ Initial evaluation
	☑ Re-evaluation (2 weeks after admission to rehabilitation)
	☐ Treatment session
Learner objectives	1. Prioritize a comprehensive reexamination
	2. Prioritize a comprehensive plan of care
	3. Create an appropriate discharge plan

Medical	
Chief complaint	Rib and right lower extremity (RLE) pain
History of present illness	The patient is a 62-year-old man brought to hospital s/p a work-related fall 50 feet from a scaffold. He presented with acute shortness of breath, hypoxemia, and laceration of the RLE. He was diagnosed with multiple right-sided rib fractures, moderate right pneumothorax, and open right distal tibial/fibular fracture. The patient was stabilized with right chest tube placement and then underwent open reduction internal fixation (ORIF) of his RLE. He was at the acute care hospital × 14 days and has now been at inpatient rehabilitation × 2 weeks.
Past medical history (PMH)	Chronic obstructive pulmonary disease (COPD), obesity, non–insulin-dependent diabetes mellitus (DM), hypertension, anxiety
Past surgical history	s/p appendectomy 30 years ago

(Continued)

(Continued)

Medical	
Allergies	None.
Medications	Ambien, Lisinopril, Xanax, Albuterol, Metformin, Percocet, Lovenox, 1L O$_2$ by nasal cannula (NC)
Precautions/orders	Activity as tolerated Non–weight bearing (NWB) RLE Gentle active range of motion (AROM) of ankle to start at 4 weeks/Controlled Ankle Motion (CAM) boot at all times.

Social history	
Home setup	• Lives alone in a ranch-style home • Four steps to enter from the front door; two steps to enter from the garage. • Flight of steps to basement, where laundry is located.
Occupation	• Works full time as a commercial painter.
Prior level of function	• Independent in all functional mobility and activities of daily living (ADLs) without supplemental O$_2$. • Fatigue with prolonged community ambulation. • (+) Driving
Recreational activities	• Primarily sedentary during his time off, watches TV. • Meets up with friends at the bar twice a week. • Walks his dog around the block daily.

Lab		Reference range	Day 14: acute inpatient rehabilitation
Complete blood count (CBC)	White blood cell (WBC)	5.0–10.0 × 10^9/L	9.8
	Red blood cell (RBC)	4.1–5.3 million/mm^3	4.0
	Hemoglobin (Hgb)	14–17.4 g/dL	13
	Hematocrit	42–52%	42%
	Platelets	140,000–400,000/μL	255
Arterial blood gas (ABG)	PaO$_2$	80–95 mmHg	90
	PaCO$_2$	37–43 mmHg	45
	PH	7.35–7.45	7.4
	HCO$_3$	20–30 mmol/L	32
Basic metabolic panel (BMP)	Glucose (fast)	70–100 mg/dL	156
	Hgb A1C	<5.7%	–
	Cholesterol	<200 mg/dL	–
	Low-density lipoprotein (LDL)	<70 mg/dL	–
	High-density lipoprotein (HDL)	>60 mg/dL	–
	Blood urea nitrogen (BUN)	6–25 mg/dL	28
	Creatinine	0.7–1.3 mg/dL	1.4
	Potassium	3.7–5.1 mEq/L	4.2
	Sodium	134–142 mEq/L	140

(Continued)

(Continued)

Lab	Reference range	Day 14: acute inpatient rehabilitation
Chloride	98–108 mEq/L	100
Calcium	8.6–10.3 mg/dL	8.5
Magnesium	1.2–1.9 mEq/L	1.3

Pause points

Based on the above information, what are the priorities?
- Diagnostic tests and measures?
- Outcome measures?
- Treatment interventions?

Day 14, Acute Inpatient Rehabilitation: Physical Therapy Re-evaluation

Subjective

"I really want to go home but I am in so much pain."

Objective

Vital signs	Pre-treatment			Post-treatment
	Supine	Sitting	Standing	
Blood pressure (mmHg)	136/80	130/78	136/78	144/80
Heart rate (beats/min)	88	92	105	128
Respiratory rate (breaths/min)	24	24	26	35
Pulse oximetry on 1 L NC (SpO$_2$)	96%	96%	94%	93%
Borg scale	6/20	8/20	14/20	14/20
Pain	4/10 RLE 4/10 R side of thorax	5/10 RLE 4/10 R side of thorax	6/10 RLE 5/10 R side of thorax	6/10 RLE 5/10 R side of thorax
General	• Patient found supine in bed with head of bed (HOB) elevated 45 degrees. • RLE elevated with no drainage from incision • Notable anxiety and elevated respiratory rate (RR) when therapy arrives • Lines/equipment notable for 1L O$_2$ by NC, CAM boot			
Cardiovascular and pulmonary	• Inspection: shallow breathing, elevated RR, no accessory muscle use • Palpation: reduced expansion R middle and lower lobe • Pulses: 2 + pedal pulses bilaterally • Auscultation: diminished breath sounds bilateral lower lobes (BLL) R > L, occasional low-pitched expiratory wheeze right lower lobe (RLL), no crackles			
Gastrointestinal	• Reports normal bowel movement			
Genitourinary	• Voiding independently, urine clear			
Musculoskeletal	Range of motion	• Bilateral upper extremity (BUE): within functional limit (WFL) • Left lower extremity (LLE): WFL • RLE: WFL with the exception of R ankle, which is limited to ~5 degrees of dorsiflexion (DF) and plantar flexion (PF) with gentle AROM only		
	Strength	• BUE: WFL • LLE: 4/5 • R hip: 4/5 • R knee: 3/5 • R ankle: actively move ankle 5 degrees DF/PF		

(Continued)

(Continued)

Day 14, Acute Inpatient Rehabilitation: Physical Therapy Re-evaluation		
	Aerobic	• Patient ambulates 25 feet with minimal assistance and rolling walker (RW), maintaining RLE NWB, for 2-Minute Walk. • Postambulation vitals: heart rate: 115 beats per minute (beats/min); respiratory rate: 34 breaths/min, pulse oximetry = 93% on 1 L by NC, Rate of Perceived Exertion (RPE): 14/20, dyspnea: 2/4 ▶ Fig. 12.3
	Flexibility	• Not tested
	Other	• Not tested
Neurological	Balance	• Sitting balance: static and dynamic good • Static standing: contact guard assistance (CGA) with RW and RLE NWB • Dynamic standing: fair, as noted with gait
	Cognition	• Alert and oriented (A&O) × 4
	Coordination	• Finger to nose: intact BUE • Toe tapping: LLE intact, unable to assess RLE
	Cranial nerves	• II–XII: intact
	Reflexes	• Not tested
	Sensation	• Decreased light touch sensation on R plantar surface of foot
	Tone	• BUE: within normal limit (WNL) • BLE: WNL
	Other	• Patient has a follow-up appointment with ortho in 2 weeks
Functional status		
Bed mobility	• Rolling either direction: modified independent • Supine to/from sit: modified independent Requires increased time for all mobility	
Transfers	• Sit to/from stand: minimal assistance • Stand pivot transfer: CGA with RW, maintaining RLE NWB; verbal cues for pacing and pursed-lip breathing	
Ambulation	• Ambulated 50 feet with minimal assistance and RW, maintaining RLE NWB; verbal cues for pacing and pursed-lip breathing.	
Stairs	• Ascend/descend four steps with moderate assistance and bilateral handrails, maintaining RLE NWB; verbal cues for pacing and pursed-lip breathing.	
Other	• Patient has significant increase in anxiety with gait and especially stairs. He needs encouragement to continue along with cues to for breathing. He requires an occasional standing rest break during gait for encouragement to continue and to help him relax.	

Assessment	
☑ Physical therapist's	*Assessment left blank for learner to develop.*
Goals	
Patient's	"I want to walk by myself."
Short term	1. 　　　　　*Goals left blank for learner to develop.* 2.
Long term	1. 　　　　　*Goals left blank for learner to develop.* 2.

Rating of Perceived Exertion
Borg RPE Scale

6		How you feel when lying in bed or
7	Very, very light	sitting in a chair relaxed.
8		Little or no effort.
9	Very light	
10		
11	Fairly light	
12		Target range: How you should feel
13	Somewhat hard	with exercise or activity.
14		
15	Hard	
16		
17	Very hard	How you felt with the hardest
18		work you have ever done.
19	Very, very hard	
20	Maximum exertion	Don't work this hard!

Fig. 12.3 Radiologic evaluation of lower leg, ankle, and foot fracture fixation hardware.

Plan	
☐ Physician's ☑ Physical therapist's ☐ Other's	Patient will be seen for 1 to 2 hours a day × 5 to 7 days a week for physical therapy. Treatment will include bed mobility, transfer training, gait training, stair training, therapeutic exercises, breathing and pacing exercises, and energy conservation techniques.

Bloom's Taxonomy Level	Case 12.B Questions
Create	1. Synthesizing the medical data and physical examination findings, develop an appropriate physical therapy assessment of the patient. 2. Develop two short-term physical therapy goals, including an appropriate timeframe for the rest of his inpatient stay. 3. Develop two long-term physical therapy goals, including an appropriate timeframe for the rest of his inpatient stay.
Evaluate	4. Develop a discharge plan including prioritizing appropriate equipment needed to ensure safe return home. 5. Explain the impact of his contextual factors on his goals and outcomes.
Analyze	6. Describe how anxiety can change with the patient's given circumstances.
Apply	7. Design two appropriate interventions to improve gait. 8. Design two appropriate interventions to address anxiety and pain during mobility. 9. Design two appropriate interventions to improve transfers.
Understand	10. Describe the impact of bone healing and his PMH on his outcomes. 11. Describe the impact of his aerobic capacity on his outcomes.
Remember	12. What does normal bone healing look like (timeline)?

Bloom's Taxonomy Level	Case 12.B Answers
Create	1. The patient is a 62-year-old man with impaired mobility due to a recent fall from 50 feet resulting in multiple right rib fractures, right pneumothorax, and open right tibial/fibular fracture s/p ORIF. His functional mobility is limited due to not only impaired strength and endurance but also extensive PMH, current RLE NWB status, and anxiety. He would benefit from skilled physical therapy services to return to prior level of function. 2. Short-term goals: • Patient will ambulate 50 feet while maintaining NWB on RLE with CGA and RW to improve his ambulation within his home within 1 week. • Patient will ascend/descend a flight of stairs with bilateral handrails and minimal assistance to safely navigate between floors of his home within 1 week. 3. Long-term goals: • Patient will ambulate × 250 feet with modified independence using RW to navigate within his home within 2 weeks. • Patient will be independent with his home exercise program to improve BLE strength and muscle endurance within 2 weeks.
Evaluate	4. The patient will be discharged home with home health services (physical therapy, occupational therapy, nursing, home health aide). He will require an RW, rental wheelchair, and bedside commode. Depending on his functional progression and/or ability to obtain assistance, he may require a ramp for safe entry and exit of home. 5. The patient's past medical history of COPD and obesity, along with the current pain and anxiety, will increase the timeline needed for recovery. Additionally, acknowledgment should be given to the impact of DM on healing of the fracture and incision, which could prolong recovery.
Analyze	6. Pain and trauma from the fall have the potential to increase the patient's baseline anxiety, which could delay or limit progress and timeline.
Apply	7. Activities to improve balance and stability on one limb (LLE) must be considered. Two appropriate interventions would be (a) side-lying therapeutic exercise and (b) static standing with BUE support (i.e., RW) with RLE therapeutic exercise in all planes. Both of these interventions could focus on strengthening the gluteal muscles. 8. Appropriate interventions to address anxiety and pain during mobility are (a) imagery, (b) breathing exercises, and (c) meditation. If necessary, a referral to a psychologist may be necessary. 9. Two appropriate interventions to improve transfers are (a) single limb bridging and (b) practice of sit to stand transfers with RLE NWB starting with high surfaces to master the technique.
Understand	10. Due to PMH of DM, the patient may have a delay in healing of both incision site and bone. Consider nutritional support and patient education to maximize patient outcomes. 11. The patient's reduced aerobic capacity and deconditioning limit his functional mobility, thus increasing the time needed to reach his expected outcomes. Interventions to improve ventilation, energy conservation techniques, moderate-intensity aerobic exercise, and skeletal muscle conditioning can assist in improving his aerobic capacity.
Remember	12. Normal timeline for bone healing is 6 to 8 weeks. This can be delayed secondary to the patient's comorbidities.

Key points

1. The impact of prior level of function, PMH, and mental health should be considered when determining patient outcomes.

2. Patient education on current medical precautions on lifestyle choices should be incorporated into treatment.

3. For discharge planning, especially in a medically complex patient, consideration of equipment needs and home setup to maximize independence should be taken.

General Information

Case no.	12.C
Authors	Erin Lampron, PT, DPT, Board Certified Clinical Specialist in Neurologic Physical Therapy Tracy Wall, PT, PhD Rachel Pata, PT, DPT, CHSE, Board Certified Clinical Specialist in Cardiovascular & Pulmonary Physical Therapy
Diagnosis	Multitrauma status post (s/p) 50-foot fall, multiple right rib fractures, moderate right pneumothorax, open right tibial/fibular fracture s/p internal fixation.
Setting	Home
Learner expectations	☐ Initial evaluation ☑ Re-evaluation ☐ Treatment session
Learner objectives	1. Identify and interpret appropriate standardized tests and outcome measures based on client presentation and utility in the home care setting. 2. Describe the examination of the home environment including modification strategies to maximize safety and independence. 3. Develop an individualized, evidence informed physical therapy plan of care (POC).

Medical

Chief complaint	Right lower extremity pain
History of present Illness	The patient is a 62-year-old man currently participating in physical therapy in the home. He is now 8 weeks post open reduction internal fixation (ORIF) of right tibia/fibula. He was recently hospitalized × 14 days for acute shortness of breath and hypoxemia due multiple right-sided rib fractures and a moderate right pneumothorax, and a right distal tibial/fibular fracture s/p ORIF as a result of a fall. Prior to initiation of home health care services, he completed 4 weeks of inpatient rehabilitation. He is seen at visit 6 to complete a physical therapy reexamination due to a change in weight-bearing status.
Past medical history	Chronic obstructive pulmonary disease, obesity, non–insulin-dependent diabetes mellitus, hypertension, anxiety
Past surgical history	s/p appendectomy 30 years ago
Allergies	None
Medications	Ambien, Aspirin, Lisinopril, Xanax, Albuterol, Metformin, Ibuprofen
Precautions/orders	Activity as tolerated Weight bearing as tolerated (WBAT) right lower extremity (RLE) Controlled Ankle Motion (CAM) boot RLE when weight bearing

Social history

Home setup	• Lives alone in a ranch-style home. • Four steps to enter from the front door; two steps to enter from the garage. • Flight of steps + one handrail (part way) to basement, where laundry is located.
Occupation	• Works full time as a commercial painter.
Prior level of function	• Independent in all functional mobility and activities of daily living (ADLs) without supplemental O_2. • Fatigue with prolonged community ambulation • (+) Driving
Recreational activities	• Primarily sedentary during his time off, watches TV. • Meets up with friends at the bar twice a week. • Walks his dog around the block daily.
Home evaluation	• There is poor lighting in the bedroom and hallway. • Excess clutter within the main walking area is observed. • Throw rugs present in the bathroom.

Pause points

Based on the above information, what are the priorities?
- Diagnostic tests and measures?
- Outcome measures?
- Treatment interventions?

Physical Therapy Re-evaluation		
Subjective		
"I am very nervous about putting weight through this leg."		
Objective		

Vital signs	Pre-treatment	Post-treatment
	Sitting	Sitting
Blood pressure (mmHg)	136/74	144/80
Heart rate (beats/min)	88	126
Respiratory rate (breaths/min)	24	33
Pulse oximetry on room air (SpO$_2$)	96%	92%
Borg scale	8/20	13/20
Pain	2/10 RLE	5/10 RLE

General	• Patient seated in recliner chair upon start of visit with CAM boot on RLE. • Patient appears anxious with noted elevation in respiratory rate (RR).	
Cardiovascular and pulmonary	• Inspection: shallow breathing, elevated RR, no accessory muscle use • Palpation: 2 + pedal pulses bilateral lower extremity (BLE)	
Gastrointestinal	• Regular bowel movements	
Genitourinary	• Voiding independently, urine is clear	
Musculoskeletal	Range of motion (ROM)	• Bilateral upper extremity (BUE) active ROM (AROM): within normal limit (WNL). • BLE AROM: WNL, except right ankle, limited to 10-degree dorsiflexion (DF) and 12-degree plantar flexion (PF).
	Strength (tested sitting)	• BUE: within functional limit (WFL) • Left lower extremity (LLE): 4 + /5 throughout • Right hip flexion: 4/5 • Right knee extension: 4–/5 • Right knee flexion: 4/5 • Right DF: 3 + /5 within available ROM • Right PF: 3 + /5 within available ROM
	Aerobic	• 2-Minute Walk Test (2MWT) distance of 110 m (362 feet) with one standing rest break
	Flexibility	• Not tested
	Other	• Not applicable
Neurological	Balance	• Static sitting: good • Dynamic sitting: good • Static standing: supervision without BUE support • Dynamic standing: supervision without BUE when reaching minimally outside base of support, no loss of breath; minimal assistance without BUE support when reaching moderately outside base of support, delayed protective responses

(Continued)

(Continued)

Physical Therapy Re-evaluation		
	Cognition	• Alert and oriented (A&O) × 4
	Coordination	• Finger to nose: intact BUE • Heel to shin: intact BLE
	Cranial nerves	• I–XII: intact
	Reflexes	• Not tested
	Sensation	• BLE: intact to light touch with the exception of plantar surface of right foot, which is diminished
	Tone	• BUE: WNL • BLE: WNL
	Other	• 10 Meter Walk Test (10MWT) = 0.9 m/s (2.96 feet/s)
Functional status		
Bed mobility		• Rolling either direction: independent • Supine to/from sit: independent
Transfers		• Sit to/from stand: modified independent with use of rolling walker (RW)
Ambulation		• Ambulated household distances with modified independence and RW, demonstrating step-to gait pattern with increased time required. Gait deviations noted: short step length on the left, decreased right weight shift.
Stairs		• Ascend/descend four steps with supervision and bilateral handrails, demonstrating step-to pattern with rest at top.
Task specific		• Showering: home health aide provides assistance • Patient's sister lives nearby and has been assisting with laundry, cleaning, and cooking.
Sport specific		Not applicable
Other		• Patient demonstrates increase in anxiety with ambulation and stair negotiation. Patient exhibits reluctance to bear weight through RLE, requiring verbal and tactile cues for WBAT during mobility. Verbal cues required for pursed-lip breathing during activity.

Assessment	
☑ Physical therapist's	*Assessment left blank for learner to develop.*
Goals	
Patient's	"To walk normal"
Short term	1. *Goals left blank for learner to develop.* 2.
Long term	1. *Goals left blank for learner to develop.* 2.

Plan	
☐ Physician's ☑ Physical therapist's ☐ Other's	Patient will continue physical therapy in the home twice a week × 3 weeks. Treatment will include progressive gait training on level surfaces and elevations, therapeutic exercise (strengthening and aerobic conditioning), balance reeducation, energy conservation techniques, and patient education to reduce fall risk.

Bloom's Taxonomy Level	Case 12.C Questions
Create	1. Synthesizing the medical data and physical examination findings, develop an appropriate physical therapy assessment of the patient. 2. Develop two short-term physical therapy goals, including an appropriate timeframe for home care. 3. Develop two long-term physical therapy goals, including an appropriate timeframe for home care. 4. Design and implement a home exercise program (HEP), incorporating the frequency, intensity, time, type of exercise (FITT) principle
Evaluate	5. Describe the assessment of the environment, including assessment of fall risks within the home. 6. Identify modification strategies to reduce fall risk and improve overall safety for this patient.
Analyze	7. Interpret the patient's 2MWT and 10MWT scores 8. How can this information be used when creating the physical therapy POC (i.e., designing interventions, setting goals)?
Apply	9. Design and implement progressive gait training for this patient. 10. Design and implement two interventions to improve balance. 11. How should the physical therapist teach the patient to self-monitor? How should the physical therapist instruct this patient to progress activity/HEP?
Understand	12. How may the patient's medication for anxiety and pain influence the physical therapy POC?
Remember	13. Recall the role of the physical therapist in patient education. Identify appropriate education topics for this patient.

Bloom's Taxonomy Level	Case 12.C Answers

Create	1. The patient is a 62-year-old man who was recently hospitalized due to a fall resulting in multiple right rib fractures, right pneumothorax, and right tibial/fibular fracture s/p ORIF. He completed 4 weeks of inpatient rehabilitation and is currently participating in home physical therapy. New orders for WBAT RLE have been received. He demonstrates decreased strength and endurance, impaired balance, and hesitation to WB through RLE, all of which are contributing to limitations in functional mobility. He will benefit from continued skilled physical therapy services to include progressive gait training, therapeutic exercise, balance reeducation, and energy conservation techniques to maximize safety and independence in the home. To return to his work as a painter.
	2. Short-term goals:
	  • Patient will ambulate × 100 feet with supervision and single point cane to safely navigate around the first floor of his home within 1 week.
	  • Patient will ascend/descend flight of steps with supervision and a single point cane, demonstrating a step-to-step pattern, to safely navigate to basement within 1 week.
	3. Long-term goals:
	  • Patient will ambulate × 250 feet with modified independence using a single point cane to safely navigate to the mailbox and back within 3 weeks.
	  • Patient will ascend/descend a flight of stairs with modified independence and a single point cane, demonstrating a step-to-step pattern, to safely navigate to basement within 3 weeks.
	  • Patient will be independent with HEP for BLE ROM, strength, and muscle endurance using handout provided.
	4. A HEP should be individualized for each patient and include specific exercise instructions incorporating the FITT principle. This patient's HEP should include activities that target improving cardiovascular and pulmonary fitness, strength, and balance.
	Recommendations include performance of moderate-intensity aerobic activity (40–60% heart rate reserve [HRR]) at least 30 minutes a day × 5 days a week. For this patient, an appropriate recommendation would be to begin with 10 minutes of moderate-intensity walking thrice a day.
	Strength training at a moderate training intensity (50% of one repetition maximum [1RM]) is also recommended at least twice a week. This patient may benefit from LE strengthening exercises completed in standing with UE support (mini-squats, hip

(Continued)

(Continued)

Bloom's Taxonomy Level	Case 12.C Answers
	abduction/adduction, hip flexion/extension). Two to 3 sets of 10 to 15 repetitions at this moderate intensity would be recommended. The patient will also benefit from including activities aimed at improving balance as part of the prescribed HEP. Examples of standing balance activities that may be included: Romberg, sharpened Romberg, single leg stance activities, and braiding, all completed with UE support as needed for safety (use of the kitchen counter). A combination of two to five strength training/balance activities should be selected to maximize compliance with the HEP.
Evaluate	5. The assessment of the environment should include assessment of the accessibility and safety of the entrance/exit to the home (exterior accessibility) as well as all living, sleeping, and bathing space within the home (interior accessibility). The patient's activity and participation restrictions should be considered. For example, if the patient utilizes a laundry service and did not do his own laundry prior to injury, a focus need not be on access to the washer/dryer in the basement. The home assessment can be used to identify extrinsic risk factors for falls. Many environmental factors can be modified to reduce this risk. More specifically, the assessment of the home environment should include an evaluation of floors, furniture and durable medical equipment, lighting, stairways/steps, walkways, and thresholds within and outside of the home. There are several screening tools that may be used when completing the home assessment. Many of these include checklists that prompt the physical therapist to examine for the presence of clutter within main walking paths, narrow doorways, uneven flooring, loose mats or rugs, adequate lighting, stairs with sturdy railings, pets, and properly fitting nonslip footwear. In addition, the evaluation of safe mobility in and out of bed/chair/tub/toilet, the ability to reach frequently used items in the kitchen and prepare meals, and access to appropriate durable medical equipment should be included. The STEADI (Stopping Elderly Accidents, Deaths & Injuries) initiative, developed by the CDC, is considered a useful fall risk management tool for community-dwelling older adults. 6. Several extrinsic risk factors for falls can be identified for this patient based on findings from the home examination. These include poor lighting in the bedroom and hallway, clutter in main walking paths, inadequate railing to the basement, throw rugs in the bathroom, and the presence of a pet in the home. To reduce the risk of falls or potential for injury, recommendations should be provided to improve lighting within the home, declutter main walkways, install a sturdy rail running the entire length of the stairwell, and remove throw rugs.
Analyze	7. This patient's 2MWT distance (110 m) falls below the mean age-related value of 179.1 m for men. In addition, a walking speed of 0.9 m/s, as obtained by the 10MWT, falls below 1.34 m/s, the mean age-related walking speed value for men. 8. The 2MWT distance indicates decreased endurance and should prompt the therapist to design interventions to address this impairment. Implementing a walking program with the goal of increasing distance walked without rest breaks would be appropriate for this patient. The gait speed value acquired from the 10MWT indicates the patient may be at risk of falling. This finding should prompt the therapist to design a POC that includes a goal to decrease fall risk. Physical therapy intervention might include balance retraining, strengthening, and gait training activities, along with suggestions for home modification as appropriate. Age-/sex-related mean values for both the 2MWT and 10MWT should be utilized to establish objective and meaningful short- and long-term goals for this patient. An example of a long-term goal for this patient might be the following: In 3 weeks, the patient will ambulate at a modified independent level within the home using a straight cane with a walking speed of 1.34 m/s in order to reduce risk of falls.
Apply	9. Requirements for successful walking include LE support of body mass, production of locomotor rhythm, dynamic postural control of the moving body, propulsion in the intended direction, and adaptability to changing environment and task demands. Locomotor training should be task oriented, goal directed, and meaningful to the patient, progressed to maximally challenge the patient, and performed for a high number of repetitions.

(Continued)

(Continued)

Bloom's Taxonomy Level	Case 12.C Answers
	Gait training for this patient should include progression to the use of the least restrictive assistive device. Ambulation may be progressed from the use of an RW to a straight cane and ultimately no device. Gait training should minimize the use of compensatory strategies and optimize gait kinematics. For this patient, interventions that emphasize increased weight bearing on the RLE (i.e., step over obstacles with the left leg, use of verbal/tactile cueing for longer step length on the left) should be implemented to improve left step length and right weight shift during gait. An additional strategy for gait progression includes ambulation on a variety of surfaces (tile floor, carpet, outdoor terrain) and practice on elevations (stairs, curb).
	An emphasis on faster gait speed and increased ambulation distance (maximizing total number of steps) should also be included as part of this patient's progressive gait training.
	10. Balance retraining should include activities to improve dynamic postural control in standing, providing opportunities to improve efficiency and effectiveness of the patient's balance strategies. Activities should target the use of both equilibrium reactions (ankle and hip strategy) and protective responses (stepping strategy). For this patient, the physical therapist may consider performing balance activities that narrow the base of support (feet together, Romberg, sharpened Romberg, single leg stance) or change the standing surface (foam, wedge). These activities may be completed with eyes open or eyes closed. Ambulation with head turns, quick start/stops, changes in direction, and obstacle negotiation may be included to challenge the patient's postural control during gait. Side stepping, backward walking, and braiding may also be incorporated. Progression to performing balance activities without UE support should be considered.
	11. The patient should be instructed to use the tools selected for monitoring activity intensity in order to recognize when to take an activity break (self-pacing), as well as when progression is indicated.
	The Borg Rate of Perceived Exertion (RPE) Scale is a helpful tool when instructing a patient in self-monitoring activity intensity. Introducing the RPE, or modified RPE, with use of a visual aid is preferable. RPE should be monitored first at rest, to obtain a baseline value. Moderate intensity corresponds with RPE of 11 to 14 on a 6 to 20 scale. This patient should be instructed to take a break if the RPE exceeds 14, recovering long enough to reach his resting RPE value. In contrast, if the patient completes the prescribed activity at an intensity of less than 14, progression should be considered. The use of HRR is an additional method that may be employed for monitoring exercise intensity. A HRR of 40 to 60% corresponds with moderate-intensity exercise. This patient's HRR would be calculated between 116 and 130 beats/min. He would be instructed to monitor the HR at rest and during activity, with the goal of working within this target range. If the patient is able to complete an activity at a HR lower than this range, activity progression may be indicated. Using HRR as a measure of self-monitoring would require the patient to be able to take their own HR accurately. Progression of the HEP might include increasing the time spent during one bout of aerobic activity to 30 minutes (decrease rest time). Another strategy to progress the HEP would include completing strengthening and/or balance exercises with less UE support (one hand, then no hands with countertop close by). In addition, ankle weights can be added during strengthening exercises in order to maintain the moderate intensity required for maximal benefit.
Understand	12. It should be noted that individuals who take anti-anxiety medications may experience side effects such as drowsiness and decreased motor performance. Therefore, physical therapy should be scheduled accordingly to maximize the interventions and patient safety.
Remember	13. Patient education is a skilled intervention provided by physical therapists to improve compliance with the POC along with maximizing favorable outcomes. This patient would benefit from education addressing the change in weight-bearing status, energy conservation techniques, safety/fall risk reduction, general benefits of exercise, and anxiety management strategies.

Suggested Readings

2-minute walk test. Available at: https://www.srab.org/rehabilitation-measures/2 minute walk-test. Accessed March 1, 2020

10-meter walk test. Available at: Https//www.srab.org/rehabilitation-measures/10-meter walk-test. Accessed March 1, 2020

Academy of Acute Care Physical Therapy-APTA Taskforce on Lab Values. Laboratory Values Interpretation Resource. Pittsburgh, PA: APTA; 2017

Ahmad A, Abujbara M, Jaddou H, Younes NA, Ajlouni K. Anxiety and depression among adult patients with diabetic foot: prevalence and associated factors. J Clin Med Res. 2018; 10(5): 411–418

American College of Sports Medicine. ACSM's Guidelines for Exercise Testing and Prescription. 10th ed. Baltimore, MD: Lippincott, Williams and Wilkins; 2017

Anderson LW, Krathwohl DR. A Taxonomy for Learning, Teaching, and Assessing, Abridged Edition. Boston, MA: Allyn and Bacon; 2001

Armstrong P. Bloom's Taxonomy. https://cft.vanderbilt.edu/guides-sub-pages/blooms-taxonomy/. Accessed on April 1, 2018

Avin KG, Hanke TA, Kirk-Sanchez N, et al. Academy of Geriatric Physical Therapy of the American Physical Therapy Association. Management of falls in community-dwelling older adults: clinical guidance statement from the Academy of Geriatric Physical Therapy of the American Physical Therapy Association. Phys Ther. 2015; 95(6):815–834

Bohannon RW, Williams Andrews A. Normal walking speed: a descriptive meta-analysis. Physiotherapy. 2011; 97(3):182–189

Shirley Ryan AbilityLab. BORG Rating of Perceived Exertion. Available at: https://www.sralab.org/rehabilitation-measures/borg-rating-scale-perceived-exertion#older-adults-and-geriatric-care. Accessed March 11, 2020

Borg GA. Psychophysical bases of perceived exertion. Med Sci Sports Exerc. 1982; 14(5):377–381

Centers for Disease Control and Prevention. Stopping Elderly Accidents, Deaths & Injuries. Available at: Cdc.gov/steadi. Accessed March 1, 2020

Dechman G, Wilson CR. Evidence underlying breathing retraining in people with stable chronic obstructive pulmonary disease. Phys Ther. 2004; 84(12):1189–1197

Fruth SJ. Fundamentals of the Physical Therapy Examination: Patient Interviews and Tests & Measures. Burlington, MA: Jones & Bartlett Learning; 2014

Goodman CC, Fuller KS. Pathology: Implications for the Physical Therapist. 4th ed. St. Louis, MO: Saunders Elsevier; 2015

Hillegass E. Essentials of Cardiopulmonary Physical Therapy. 4th ed. St. Louis, MO: Elsevier; 2017

Jiao H, Xiao E, Graves DT. Diabetes and its effect on bone and fracture healing. Curr Osteoporos Rep. 2015; 13(5):327–335

Mackenzie L, Bates J, et al. Designing the Home Falls and Accidents Screening Tool (HOME FAST): selecting the items. Br J Occup Ther. 2000; 63:260–269

Marco CA, Sorensen D, Hardman C, Bowers B, Holmes J, McCarthy MC. Risk factors for pneumonia following rib fractures. Am J Emerg Med. 2019; 38(3):610–612

Middleton A, Fritz SL, Lusardi M. Walking speed: the functional vital sign. J Aging Phys Act. 2015; 23(2):314–322

Myers BA. Wound Management: Principles and Practice. 2nd ed. Upper Saddle River, NJ: Pearson Education, Inc.; 2008

O'Sullivan SB, Schmitz TJ, Fulk G. Physical Rehabilitation. Philadelphia, PA: F.A. Davis; 2019:400–433

Shumway Cook A, Woollacott MH. Motor Control: Translating Research into Clinical Practice. Philadelphia, PA: Lippincott Williams and Wilkins; 2017

Watchie J. Cardiovascular and Pulmonary Physical Therapy. 2nd ed. St. Louis, MO: Elsevier; 2010

Westerman RW, Hull P, Hendry RG, Cooper J. The physiological cost of restricted weight bearing. Injury. 2008; 39(7):725–727

Weinberger SE, Cockrill BA, Mandel J. Principles of Pulmonary Medicine. Philadelphia, PA: Saunders; 2008

13 Normal Pressure Hydrocephalus

General Information	
Case no.	13.A Normal-Pressure Hydrocephalus
Authors	Stephen J. Carp, PT, PhD, Board Certified Clinical Specialist in Geriatrics Physical Therapy
Diagnosis	Normal-pressure hydrocephalus
Setting	Neuro step-down unit in an acute care hospital
Learner expectations	☑ Initial evaluation ☐ Re-evaluation ☐ Treatment session
Learner objectives	1. List the common signs and symptoms of normal-pressure hydrocephalus pertinent to the physical therapist and discuss the rationale for the use of a ventriculoperitoneal (VP) shunt as a treatment option. 2. Interpret and incorporate into the plan of care the results of cognitive and fall-risk outcome measures. 3. Develop and defend the rationale for formulating an appropriate discharge plan for an acute care patient with multiple comorbidities and confounding social variables.

Medical	
Chief complaint	Unsteady gait, change in mental status
History of present illness	A 72-year-old man admitted to the acute care hospital through the emergency department with a chief complaint of progressive unsteadiness of gait and change in mental status over the past few weeks. He is not very verbal, and most information is provided by his wife. He was ambulating well up to 2 to 3 months ago when he began to complain of unsteadiness while walking and began to lose his balance. Wife states he had no history of falls up to 1 month ago but since that time she has witnessed a progressive increase in the frequency of his falls. She states the falls occur at all times during the day and at night, inside and outside the home. She cannot identify a pattern to the falls. The patient has grudgingly begun to use a cane at home. Over the past 2 weeks, the wife has noted that her husband has been increasingly confused especially with recent events. He can no longer balance the check book. Twice in the past month he has become lost while driving (she has since taken his car keys). She has also noted that he has been incontinent of urine a number of times over the past 2 weeks and was incontinent of stool once. He also experiences urgency, increased frequency, and nocturia. The patient confirms his wife's assessment about his mental status and loss of ambulatory balance but denies the urinary incontinence. They are both very worried that he has Alzheimer's disease.
Past medical history	Diabetic retinopathy, diabetes mellitus type II (DM2), elevated cholesterol and lipids, high blood pressure, cervical arthritis
Past surgical history	Cholecystectomy: 20 years ago; appendectomy: 35 years ago
Allergies	latex, penicillin, seasonal allergies
Medications	Atorvastatin (Lipitor), Glipizide, Metoprolol succinate, Flonase prn for seasonal allergies
Precautions/orders	Fall risk, VP shunt Activity as tolerated

Social history	
Home setup	• Two-story home with five steps to enter home with rail on the right. • Thirteen steps, rail on the left, to the second floor. • Bed and bath on the second floor. No bathroom on the first floor. • Has two married children residing within 30 minutes of home.
Occupation	• Retired from accounting 3 years ago due to an increased frequency in work mistakes. Has master's level education.

(Continued)

(Continued)

Social history	
Prior level of function	• Diminishment of function over past 3 months as evidenced by need to use walker or cane, frequent falls, decreased ability to perform hygiene, diminished social interaction. • Assistance to climb steps. • Independent with feeding, but requires assistance to bathe and occasionally to dress. • Stopped driving 3 months ago secondary to "memory issues."
Recreational activities	• Wife reports that immediately after retirement, he exercised regularly, traveled, gardened, and performed woodworking but over the past 6 months most of these activities have diminished or ended. • Over the past 3 months, his recreational activities have become limited to television watching.

Vital signs	Hospital day 0: neuro step-down unit
Blood pressure (mmHg)	130/90
Heart rate (beats/min)	82
Respiratory rate (breaths/min)	16
Pulse oximetry on room air (SpO$_2$)	97%
Temperature (°F)	98.7

Imaging/diagnostic test	Hospital day 0: Neuro step-down unit
Electrocardiogram (ECG)	1. Normal sinus rhythm. Rate 82. No ischemic changes
Magnetic resonance imaging (MRI)—brain	1. Mild cerebral and cerebellar atrophy, consistent with age, with otherwise normal-appearing gyri. 2. Dilated ventricles consistent with normal pressure hydrocephalus. 3. Otherwise, normal MRI of the brain ▶ Fig. 13.1

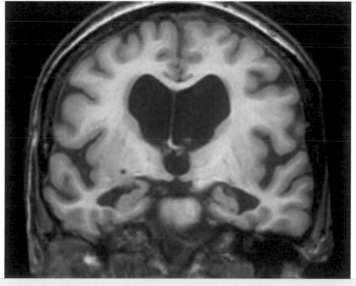

Fig. 13.1 The CT of the brain revealed mild cerebral atrophy and markedly dilated ventricles consistent with normal-pressure hydrocephalus. (Adapted from Kanekar S, ed. Neuroimaging. In: Imaging of Neurodegenerative Disorders. 1st ed. New York, NY: Thieme; 2015.)

(Continued)

Imaging/diagnostic test	Hospital day 0: Neuro step-down unit
MRI—cervical spine	1. Multilevel degenerative disk disease with degenerative joint disease at levels described above. 2. Posterior disk bulging with facet hypertrophy and uncovertebral joint spurring resulting in mild bilateral foraminal stenosis at C6–C7. 3. No significant cord impingement.

Medical management	Hospital day 0: Neuro step-down unit	Hospital day 1: Neuro intensive care unit	Hospital day 2: Neuro step-down unit
Medications	1. Atorvastatin (Lipitor) 2. Glipizide 3. Metoprolol succinate 4. Flonase prn for seasonal allergies	1. Atorvastatin (Lipitor) 2. Glipizide 3. Metoprolol succinate 4. Flonase prn for seasonal allergies	1. Atorvastatin (Lipitor) 2. Glipizide 3. Metoprolol succinate 4. Flonase prn for seasonal allergies
Procedures	1. Lumbar puncture (LP)	1. LP results: fluid clear 2. Left VP shunt 3. Endotracheal tube placed for procedure 4. Insert foley catheter	1. Successful extubation with transition to nasal cannula (NC) 2. Remove foley catheter

Lab		Reference range	Hospital day 0: Neuro step-down unit	Hospital day 1: Neuro intensive care unit	Hospital day 2: Neuro step-down unit
Complete blood count	White blood cell	$5.0–10.0 \times 10^9/L$	6.6	6.8	7.1
	Hemoglobin	14.0–17.4 g/dL	14.1	14.3	14.2
	Hematocrit	42–52%	42	42	42
	Red blood cell	4.5–5.5	5.1	5.2	5.2
	Platelet	140,000–400,000/μL	250	240	245
Metabolic Panel	Calcium	8.6–10.3 mg/dL	8.9		8.8
	Chloride	98–108 mEq/L	97		100
	Magnesium	1.2–1.9 mEq/L	1.8	Not reordered	1.8
	Phosphate	2.3–4.1 mg/dL	2.9		2.9
	Potassium	3.7–5.1 mEq/L	4.0		4.1
	Sodium	134–142 mEq/L	145		143
Other	Glucose	60–110 mg/dL	188	192	187
	Hemoglobin A1C	<6% of total hemoglobin	7.1	–	–
	Folate	3.6–20 ng/dL	10.0	10.0	9.8
	Ferritin	13–300 ng/mL	130	130	131

Pause points

Based on the above information, what are the priority:
- Diagnostic tests and measures?
- Outcome measures?
- Treatment interventions?

Hospital Day 2, Post-Op Day 1: Physical Therapy Examination				

Subjective

Patient: "I am not really sure why I was admitted to the hospital. I think they sent me here because I was falling. You best ask my wife. My neck and head hurt. Did I have an operation? Was something done to my neck??"

Wife: "I brought him here because I was very concerned that he has Alzheimer' disease or something similar. Over the past 3 months, he has been getting progressively confused and withdrawn. He has been falling and he can't control his urine. The neurologist here at the hospital ordered a lot of tests, which seemed to point toward a diagnosis of normal-pressure hydrocephalus. Yesterday morning, he had a shunt placed. The hope is the shunt decreases the amount of fluid in his brain, which hopefully will improve his symptoms."

Objective

Vital signs	Pre-treatment			Post-treatment
	Supine	Sitting	Standing	
Blood pressure (mmHg)	132/76	130/74	132/78	134/78
Heart rate (beats/min)	76	80	86	88
Respiratory rate (breaths/min)	14	16	26	28
Pulse oximetry on 2 L NC (SpO_2)	98%	97%	98%	98%
Borg scale	1	3	4	4
Pain	3/10 (incision at neck)	4/10 (incision at neck)	4/10 (incision at neck)	3/10 (incision at neck)

General	• Supine in bed, no acute distress • Wife present at bedside • Lines/equipment notable for peripheral intravenous (IV)
Head, ears, eyes, nose, and throat	• Emerging ecchymosis at the surgical site on the left neck. • Postoperative dressing clean/dry, intact
Cardiovascular and pulmonary	• Vital signs as above • No adventitious lung sounds • Calves are without edema, tenderness, or rubor, and without palpable cords. • Dorsalis pedis: 2 + bilaterally. Feet are warm
Gastrointestinal	• Denies diarrhea or constipation • Denies belly pain • Endorses good appetite
Genitourinary	• Endorses that he "wet the bed" this morning after foley catheter was removed. • Denies hematuria, pain with voiding, foul-smelling urine

Musculoskeletal	Range of motion (ROM)	• Cervical and lumbar spine ROM assessments deferred secondary to recent surgery. • All articular ROM assessments are full and painless. • No overt deformities noted.
	Strength	• Bilateral upper extremity (BUE): grossly 4/5 throughout • Bilateral lower extremity (BLE): grossly 4/5 throughout
	Aerobic	• Aerobic testing deferred secondary to postoperative day 1.
	Flexibility	• Articular ROM is normal and painless without deformity or pain. • Two-joint muscle length testing deferred at this time.
	Other	• No overt muscle wasting, or atrophy noted by visual inspection.

Neurological	Balance	Outcome measure	Presurgery	Postsurgery
		Montreal Cognitive Assessment (MoCA)	19/30	22/30
		Romberg—eyes open	12 seconds	14 seconds
		Romberg—eyes closed	8 seconds	12 seconds
		Timed Up and Go	16 seconds	13 seconds

(Continued)

(Continued)

Hospital Day 2, Post-Op Day 1: Physical Therapy Examination		
	Cognition	• See MoCA score above • Alert and oriented × 3: unsure of surgical procedure • Responds to questions but does not initiate conversation. • Able to follow simple one-step commands.
	Coordination	• Finger to nose: mild impairment in BUE • Heel to shin: mild impairment in BLE
	Cranial nerves	• I: intact olfactory sense bilateral via two stimuli. • II: visual acuity 20/20 with corrective lenses, visual fields intact via confrontation. • III, IV, VI: pupils equally reactive to light and accommodation. External ocular muscles intact. No ptosis noted. No twitches or flutters. No nystagmus noted. Pupils equal in size. Pupillary light reflex intact. • V: intact sensation both sides of face via cotton and pin. Masseter and pterygoid muscles intact. • VII: face symmetrical. Tongue sensation intact. • VIII: hearing intact bilaterally. Negative signs of vestibular nystagmus. • IX, X: palate elevates symmetrically. Gag reflex intact. Voice of normal amplitude. No hoarseness noted. • XI: sternocleidomastoid and upper trapezius muscles intact. • XII: tongue in midline. No atrophy or fasciculations noted.
	Reflexes	• Biceps: 1 + /4 bilaterally • Patellar: 1 + /4 bilaterally • Clonus: (–) bilaterally • Babinski: down-going bilaterally
	Sensation	• BUE: intact to light touch • BLE: intact to light touch, mild loss of vibratory sense from mid-calf to toe. • Upper extremity drift test is positive bilaterally.
	Tone	• BUE: rigid • BLE: rigid • Negative cogwheeling noted • No intentional or resting tremor noted. • No festination or difficulty initiating movement noted. • No "freezing" of gait noted.
	Other	• Dressing over left side of neck surgical site is clean, dry, and intact.
Functional status		
Bed mobility	• Rolling either direction: independent • Scooting up in bed: minimal assistance • Supine to/from sit: minimal assistance	
Transfers	• Sit to/from stand: minimal assistance • Bed to/from chair: moderate assistance using stand pivot transfer to bedside chair with rolling walker.	
Ambulation	• Ambulated 2 × 10 feet with moderate assistance and rolling walker; significant verbal and tactile cuing for gait sequencing with assistive device. • Gait deviations notable for mild LE ataxia, wide base of support, and multidirectional instability.	
Stairs	• Not applicable at this time.	

Assessment	
☑ Physical therapist's	*Assessment left blank for learner to develop.*
Goals	
Patient's	"I am really not sure why I am here. I want to go home with my wife and sleep in my own bed."
Short term	1.
	Goals left blank for learner to develop.
	2.
Long term	1.
	Goals left blank for learner to develop.
	2.

Plan	
☐ Physician's ☑ Physical therapist's ☐ Other's	Patient will be seen three to five times a week for therapeutic exercise, gait training, transfer training, endurance training, neuromuscular reeducation, patient and family education, and to facilitate discharge to appropriate care level.

Bloom's Taxonomy Level	Case 13.A Questions
Create	1. Synthesizing the medical data and physical examination findings, develop an appropriate physical therapy assessment of the patient. 2. Develop two short-term physical therapy goals, including an appropriate timeframe. 3. Develop two long-term physical therapy goals, including an appropriate timeframe.
Evaluate	4. Based on the physical therapy findings, determine and defend the discharge recommendation.
Analyze	5. Describe why removing cerebrospinal fluid via LP would decrease symptomology in a patient with normal-pressure hydrocephalus.
Apply	6. Design and implement two interventions for an ataxic gait pattern. 7. Design and implement two interventions for diminished standing balance.
Understand	8. What are the physical therapy implications for the home medications? 9. Why is it important to encourage cough and deep breathing in a postoperative patient?
Remember	10. What are the precautions of mobilizing someone day 1 post-VP shunt? 11. Define an ataxic gait pattern. 12. What are the symptoms of blood loss anemia? 13. Which of the three primary symptoms of normal-pressure hydrocephalus is often the least amenable for recovery by surgery?

Bloom's Taxonomy Level	Case 13.A Answers
Create	1. The patient is a 72-year-old, retired accountant, who resides in a two-story home with his wife. His children reside within 30 minutes. He was admitted to the hospital for surgical intervention (VP shunt) for symptomatic (urinary incontinence, gait dysfunction with falls, and confusion) normal-pressure hydrocephalus. Past medical history is significant for DM2, cervical arthritis, diabetic retinopathy, and elevated serum lipids and cholesterol. On day 2 of the admission, he underwent placement of a VP shunt. Postoperative course has been uneventful. Postoperative physical therapy consult revealed a 72-year-old man, looking his stated age, with a dressing on his neck. He is now alert and oriented × 3. From a system's viewpoint, he has musculoskeletal and neuromuscular deficits, leading to impairments with cognition, balance, bed mobility, transfers, and gait. His cardiovascular and pulmonary responses appear normal. He is at fall risk. Currently, he requires minimal to moderate assistance with most functional tasks including walking due to ataxia and diminished balance. Physical therapist's recommendation is to discharge to a skilled nursing facility for continued rehabilitation efforts prior to his returning home.

(Continued)

(Continued)

Bloom's Taxonomy Level	Case 13.A Answers
	2. Short-term goals: • The patient will be independent with all aspects of bed mobility within 5 days to be independent at home. • The patient will perform sit to/from stand transfers with supervision within 5 days to promote independence at home. 3. Long-term goals: • The patient will ambulate 50 feet with close supervision and least restrictive assistive device within 7 days to promote independence with home navigation. • The patient's wife will demonstrate proper body mechanics 100% of the time when assisting the patient within 7 days to prevent injury.
Evaluate	4. The discharge recommendation is to a skilled nursing facility. At the point of discharge from the acute care hospital, the patient was not sufficiently able to return home safely. He required additional rehabilitation efforts. With his age, comorbidities, and diminished functional status, acute medical rehabilitation was not an option; he could not tolerate 3 hours of intensive therapy per day. Therefore, he should receive graded physical/occupational therapy at a skilled nursing facility commensurate with his physical abilities prior to returning home.
Analyze	5. Removing a quantity of cerebrospinal fluid via LP temporarily lowers the volume and, hence, pressure within the cerebrospinal system. This temporarily decreases the patient's symptoms.
Apply	6. Interventions for gait ataxia include sitting on a Swedish ball and practicing anterior, posterior, and right and left weight shifts. This activity promotes core stability. Another intervention is performed in a pool—asking the patient to walk against the resistance of water—starting deep and moving to the shallow side. This activity will increase muscle strength, rhythmic activity, and dynamic balance in an arena of limited fear of falling. 7. Interventions for diminished standing balance include alternating one-leg stance (while guarded) and walking a supple surface (while guarded) such as a mat.
Understand	8. The physical therapy implications for the home medications are as follows: • Atorvastatin (Lipitor) 40 mg daily—the primary risk is rhabdomyolysis (muscle breakdown). This risk is amplified if the patient is older and/or taking medication for a hypothyroid. The physical therapist should monitor the patient for myalgia and refer the patient to the primary care practitioner (PCP) if this is noted. Hepatic issues have been noted in persons taking atorvastatin; therefore, the physical therapist should refer the patient to the PCP if signs/symptoms of liver disease occur. Atorvastatin may also increase blood sugar levels; therefore, individuals who have diabetes may need their blood sugar monitored pre- and postintervention. • Glipizide 10 mg daily: any therapist treating patients with diabetes should be aware of the signs of hypo-/hyperglycemia, risk of neuropathy, retinopathy, and renal failure, and integument precautions. • Metoprolol succinate 100 mg daily: this is a beta blocker medication, which decreases resting heart rate and heart rate with activity. Using the heart rate as a method of measuring workload is not valid. • Flonase prn for seasonal allergies has no physical therapy implications. 9. With anesthesia, there is the chance development of atelectasis, bronchitis, and pneumonia. Cough and deep breathing decrease this risk.
Remember	10. Patients and patient's families should be made aware of signs and symptoms of bleeding and infection. There is also the risk of shunt malfunction, which include behavioral changes, vomiting, or change in mental status or gait. Fall risk should be stressed to the patient and family. 11. Though there are many etiologies for ataxia, the gait pattern is relatively consistent: wide-based, shortened stride length, lack of heel strike at initial contact, slowed gait speed, and abducted arms. 12. The symptoms of blood loss anemia include a decrease in hemoglobin and hematocrit, paleness, shortness of breath, tachycardia, orthostatic hypotension, syncope, and diminished exercise endurance. Those patients with coronary artery disease may also experience anginal symptoms. 13. Research indicates that the ataxic gait pattern is often unaffected by the placement of a VP shunt.

Key points

1. Though the patient may have a primary diagnosis impacting one system, the physical therapist, as a PCP, must, at minimum, screen all systems. Pathologies may be primary to one system; however, the downstream effects and confounding variables often cross systems' boundaries.

2. When evaluating a patient with or with suspected dementia, a friend or relative with knowledge of the patient's behavior must be included, with permission of the patient, in the evaluation process.

3. The physical therapist is an important member of the acute care hospital health care team. The preferred term is to "consult" physical therapy rather than to "order" physical therapy. Consult implies interprofessional respect of the practitioner and the practitioner's unique knowledge content.

General Information

Case no.	13.B
Authors	Stephen J. Carp, PT, PhD, Board Certified Clinical Specialist in Geriatrics Physical Therapy
Diagnosis	Normal-pressure hydrocephalus
Setting	Skilled Nursing Facility (SNF)
Learner expectations	☑ Initial evaluation ☐ Re-evaluation ☐ Treatment session
Learner objectives	1. Translate and incorporate into the care plan data from one level of care (acute care hospital) to another level of care (skilled facility) to maximize patient outcomes. 2. Determine readiness to transfer from the skilled inpatient facility to home using evidence-based criteria. 3. Determine patient discharge needs to maximize patient's and his family's safety from skilled inpatient care to care at home.

Medical

Chief complaint	Status post implementation of a ventriculoperitoneal (VP) shunt for symptomatic normal-pressure hydrocephalus three days ago.
History of present illness	The patient is a 72-year-old man presents from an acute care hospital. Initially, he was admitted to the acute care hospital through the emergency department with a chief complaint of progressive unsteadiness of gait over the past few weeks, urinary incontinence, and change in mental status. He was ambulating well up to 2 to 3 months ago when he began to complain of unsteadiness while walking and loss of balance. Workup in the acute hospital: head computed tomography (CT), lumbar puncture, routine labs indicated a diagnosis of symptomatic normal-pressure hydrocephalus. A VP shunt was implanted 3 days ago. The post-op course was uneventful. The physical therapist at the hospital felt that he was not sufficiently functionally independent to return home. He was transferred to an SNF on hospital day 4, post-op day 3.
Past medical history	VP shunt 3 days ago, diabetic retinopathy, diabetes mellitus (DM) type II, elevated cholesterol and lipids, high blood pressure, cervical arthritis
Past surgical history	Cholecystectomy: 20 years ago; appendectomy: 35 years ago
Allergies	latex, PCN, seasonal allergies
Medications	Atorvastatin (Lipitor), Glipizide, Metoprolol succinate, Flonase prn for seasonal allergies
Precautions/orders	Fall risk, VP shunt Activity as tolerated

Social history

Home setup	• Two-story home with five steps to enter home with rail on right. • Thirteen steps, rail on left, to the second floor • Bed and bath on the second floor. No bathroom on the first floor • Has two married children residing within 30 minutes of home.

(Continued)

(Continued)

Social history	
Occupation	• Retired from accounting 3 years ago due to an increased frequency in work mistakes. Master's level education.
Prior level of function	• Diminishment of function over past 3 months as evidenced by need to use walker or cane, frequent falls, decreased ability to perform hygiene, diminished social interaction. • Assistance to climb steps. • Independent with feeding, but requires assistance to bathe and occasionally to dress. • Stopped driving 3 months ago secondary to "memory issues".
Recreational activities	• Wife reports that immediately after retirement, he exercised regularly, traveled, gardened, and performed woodworking but over the past 6 months most of this activity has diminished or ended. • Over the past 3 months, his recreational activities have become limited to television watching.

Vital signs	Day 2: SNF
Blood pressure (mmHg)	132/90
Heart rate (beats/min)	78
Respiratory rate (breaths/min)	17
Pulse oximetry on room air (SpO$_2$)	97%
Temperature (°F)	99.0

Day 2, SNF: Physical Therapy Examination
Subjective

Patient: "I had some type of head surgery. I can't remember why. Where is my wife? She knows the story. Is this a new hospital? I am confused. They ambulanced me from one hospital to another. I think they sent me here because I was falling".

Wife: "He was discharged from the acute care hospital to here for rehabilitation. He had a brain shunt placed due to hydrocephalus. The neurosurgeon said that he should improve over the next few weeks mentally, with his urine control and with his walking. He was too unsteady for me to bring him directly home from the acute care hospital. I am in my 70 s and he is a big man. I couldn't handle him."

Objective				
Vital signs	Pre-treatment			Post-treatment
	Supine	Sitting	Standing	
Blood pressure (mmHg)	130/70	132/68	126/68	130/74
Heart rate (beats/min)	78	82	86	84
Respiratory rate (breaths/min)	14	16	22	22
Pulse oximetry on room air (SpO$_2$)	98%	97%	98%	98%
Borg scale	1	3	5	2
Pain: posterior left side of neck	3/10	4/10	4/10	2/10
General	• Supine in bed, no acute distress • Appears tired but alert			
Head, ears, eyes, nose, and throat	• Emerging ecchymosis at surgical site left neck • No dressing • No drainage • Sutures intact			

(Continued)

(Continued)

Day 2, SNF: Physical Therapy Examination		
Cardiovascular and pulmonary	• Electrocardiography (during standing): ▶ Fig. 13.2 • No adventitious lung sounds • Calves are without edema, tenderness, or rubor • Dorsalis pedis: 2 + bilaterally. Feet are warm	
Gastrointestinal	• Denies diarrhea or constipation • Denies belly pain	
Genitourinary	• Wife endorses that he has not been incontinent for past 24 hours.	
Musculoskeletal	Range of motion (ROM)	• Cervical and lumbar spine ROM assessments deferred secondary to recent surgery. • All articular ROM assessments are full and painless. • No overt deformity
	Strength	• Bilateral upper extremity (BUE): grossly 4/5 throughout • Bilateral lower extremity (BLE): grossly 4/5 throughout
	Aerobic	• Aerobic testing deferred
	Flexibility	• Mild forward head deformity with accompanying thoracic kyphosis. • Articular ROM is normal and painless without deformity or pain. • Two-joint muscle length testing deferred at this time.
	Other	• No overt muscle wasting or atrophy noted by visual inspection.
Neurological	Balance	<table><tr><td>Outcome measure</td><td>Score</td></tr><tr><td>Montreal Cognitive Assessment (MoCA)</td><td>24</td></tr><tr><td>Romberg—eyes open</td><td>14</td></tr><tr><td>Romberg—eyes closed</td><td>11</td></tr><tr><td>Timed up and go</td><td>12</td></tr></table>
	Cognition	• See MoCA score above • Alert and oriented × 2 • Responds to questions but does not initiate conversation. • Able to follow simple one-step commands.
	Coordination	• Finger to nose: mild impairment in BUE • Heel to shin: mild impairment in BLE
	Cranial nerves	• I: intact olfactory sense bilateral via two stimuli. • II: visual acuity 20/20 with corrective lenses, visual fields intact via confrontation. • III, IV, VI: pupils equally reactive to light and accommodation. External ocular muscles intact. No ptosis noted. No twitches or flutters. No nystagmus noted. Pupils equal in size. Pupillary light reflex intact. • V: intact sensation both sides of face via cotton and pin. Masseter and pterygoid muscles intact. • VII: face symmetrical. Tongue sensation intact. • VIII: hearing intact bilaterally. Negative signs of vestibular nystagmus. • IX, X: palate elevates symmetrically. Gag reflex intact. Voice of normal amplitude. No hoarseness noted. The patient and his wife deny him having swallowing difficulties. • XI: sternocleidomastoid and upper trapezius muscles intact. • XII: tongue in midline. No atrophy or fasciculations noted.
	Reflexes	• Biceps: 1 + /4 bilaterally • Patellar: 1 + /4 bilaterally • Clonus: (−) bilaterally • Babinski: down-going bilaterally
	Sensation	• BUE: intact to light touch • BLE: intact to light touch, mild loss of vibratory sense from mid-calf to toe. • UE drift test is positive bilaterally.

(Continued)

(Continued)

Day 2, SNF: Physical Therapy Examination		
	Tone	• BUE: rigid • BLE: rigid • Negative cogwheeling noted • No intentional or resting tremor noted • No festination or difficulty initiating movement noted. • No "freezing" of gait noted
Functional status		
Bed mobility		• Rolling either direction: independent • Scooting up in bed: minimal assistance • Supine to/from sit: minimal assistance
Transfers		• Sit to/from stand: minimal assist. • Bed to/from chair: moderate assist using stand pivot transfer to bedside chair using rolling walker.
Ambulation		• Ambulated 2 × 25 feet with minimal to moderate assistance and rolling walker; required significant cueing for gait sequencing and attention to task, as he is easily distracted. • Gait is characterized by mild LE ataxia, wide base of support, and multidirectional instability.
Stairs		• Not applicable at this time.

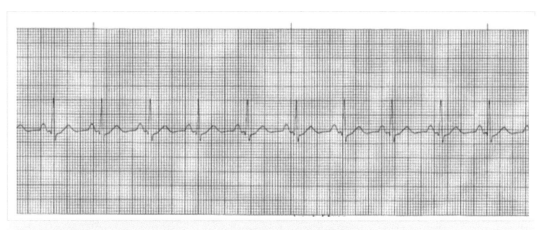

Fig. 13.2 The electrocardiogram indicated normal sinus rhythm at 78 beats per minute.

Assessment	
☑ Physical therapist's	*Assessment left blank for learner to develop.*
Goals	
Patient's	"They sent me here from the hospital after my brain surgery. I just want to go home with my wife and go out for breakfast with her."
Short term	1. *Goals left blank for learner to develop.* 2.
Long term	1. *Goals left blank for learner to develop.* 2.

	Plan
☐ Physician's ☑ Physical therapist's ☐ Other's	Will follow for 1 to 2 hours a day for bed mobility training, transfer training, gait training, static and dynamic balance activities, and cognitive activities (alone and in conjunction with balance activities).

Bloom's Taxonomy Level	Case 13.B Questions
Create	1. Synthesizing the medical data and physical examination findings, develop an appropriate physical therapy assessment of the patient. 2. Develop two short-term physical therapy goals, including an appropriate timeframe. 3. Develop two long-term physical therapy goals, including an appropriate timeframe.
Evaluate	4. Determine the proposed optimum discharge arena following the patient's skilled stay. 5. Based upon the arena of discharge chosen, consider necessary durable medical equipment (DME) and services required by the patient at that location.
Analyze	6. Why is the patient experiencing ataxia with UE and LE movement patterns?
Apply	7. Design and implement two interventions for an ataxic gait pattern. 8. Design and implement two interventions for diminished standing balance. 9. Since the patient has diabetes, the physical therapist must review diabetic foot precautions. List thee items you would teach the patient.
Understand	10. Briefly contrast services available at acute medical rehabilitation versus SNF. 11. What are the requirements for admission to an SNF? 12. What is the nurse staffing requirement for SNFs?
Remember	13. The patient has a fresh surgical wound. What are the systemic and local signs of a wound infection? 14. What are the Joint Commission's requirements for patient identification? 15. What is the Center for Disease Control and Prevention's handwashing guidelines for health care workers?

Bloom's Taxonomy Level	Case 13.B Answers
Create	1. This is a 72-year-old man admitted to the acute hospital due to progressive confusion, urinary incontinence, and gait dysfunction including falls. Workup was consistent with normal-pressure hydrocephalus and he underwent the placement of a VP shunt 4 days ago. Recovery was uneventful. His medical history includes diabetes (type II) with retinopathy. He also has elevated lipids and cholesterol and has been diagnosed in the past with cervical arthritis. He is retired and resides in a two-story home with his wife. Over the past few months, the wife has noted a marked decrease in his ability to ambulate safely. He has an increased frequency of falls. He is occasionally incontinent of urine and has shown a progressive cognitive decline. His physical examination here at the SNF is significant for mild generalized weakness. He has functional articular ROM albeit with mild neck stiffness. He has mild somatosensory loss in the stocking distribution. Distal pulses are palpable in his arms and legs. His feet are warm. Vital signs are blood pressure 132/70, respiratory rate 16, heart rate 76, and oxygen saturation 97% on room air. Functionally, he requires verbal cues for bed mobility, minimal assist with supine to sit to stand to sit to supine transfers, minimal assist on and off the toilet, and moderate assist in and out of the bathtub and car. He uses a walker to assist with transfers. He ambulates 35 feet with a rolling walker exhibiting moderate multidirectional instability. He is a fall risk as measured by his fall-risk measures. Fall-risk factors include history of falls, polypharmacy, diabetic retinopathy, diabetic sensory neuropathy, incontinence, and confusion. 2. Short-term goals: • Patient will be independent with supine to/from sit within 5 days to improve independence at home. • Patient will be independent with sit to/from stand transfers within 5 days to improve independence at home.

(Continued)

(Continued)

Bloom's Taxonomy Level	Case 13.B Answers
	3. Long-term goals: • Patient will ambulate × 100 feet with supervision and least restrictive assistive device within 10 days to safely navigate within home. • Patient will ascend/descend one flight of stairs with one railing and supervision within 10 days to get to second floor of home.
Evaluate	4. Based upon the physical findings, the expected prognosis based upon the primary diagnosis and comorbidities, premorbid functional status, and social situation, home with his wife appears to be the best discharge option at this time. 5. Once home, he should receive the optimum ambulatory aid (walker or cane) and commode, have shower/bath bars installed, and home care consultations for a home health aide, physical therapist, and nurse.
Analyze	6. Ataxia is a common sign associated with normal-pressure hydrocephalus (along with change in mental status and urinary incontinence). More often, it is seen in the LEs than the uppers but can be seen throughout the entire corpus.
Apply	7. Two interventions for an ataxic gait pattern are as follows: • Heel to toe walking, backward walking, side walking, braiding. • Ambulating on a variety of surfaces: floor, carpet, mat, grass. 8. Two interventions for diminished standing balance are as follows: • Unilateral leg standing, standing in place while tossing a ball or batting a balloon, tai chi, or yoga. 9. Three items you would teach the patient about diabetic foot precautions are as follows: • Check feet daily with a mirror for wounds, abrasions, blisters, redness, and dryness. • Contact the primary care practitioner (PCP) immediately if any of the above are noted. • Never walk barefoot or in socks. Always wear shoes.
Understand	10. Acute medical rehabilitation is the gold standard of rehabilitation. Services include rehabilitative nursing, medicine, physiatry, psychology, recreation therapy, occupational therapy, speech pathology, physical therapy, orthotics/prosthetics, wheelchair clinic, etc. Patients must be required to tolerate 3 hours of therapy care per day. Consideration must be given to the 65% rule for admission. 11. Skilled facilities typically support nursing, physician visits, physical therapy, occupational therapy, and speech pathology. For admission, the patient must have a skilled need. 12. Skilled facilities are required to have a registered professional nurse on premise 7 days per week.
Remember	13. Signs of a wound infection are as follows: Local: redness, warmth, exudate, cellulitis, pain, edema. Systemic: malaise, fever, change in mental status, elevated white blood cell count. 14. The Joint Commission requires two patient identifiers determined by the facility and utilized universally throughout the facility. These identifiers must be confirmed prior to any service provisions. 15. Hands must be washed prior to and after human and machine contacts. Hand sanitizer is sufficient for most encounters save when hands are visibly soiled or after use of the bathroom.

Key points

1. Regardless of the admitting diagnosis, if the patient has a risk factor for insensate feet, this must always be addressed via examination and teaching.

2. Limited rehabilitative and interventional services are available in an SNF. Advocate for a higher level of rehabilitation if the patient's rehabilitative, skilled, or medical needs exceed that provided by the skilled facility.

3. Gait dysfunction/gait ataxia is a common sign in patients with normal-pressure hydrocephalus. Interventions will always include balance/gait training. Ensure that at all times the patient is safely guarded. These patients are at a high risk of falls.

General Information	
Case no.	13.C
Authors	Stephen J. Carp, PT, PhD, Board Certified Clinical Specialist in Geriatrics Physical Therapy
Diagnosis	Normal-pressure hydrocephalus
Setting	Home
Learner expectations	☑ Initial evaluation ☐ Re-evaluation ☐ Treatment session
Learner objectives	1. List the common signs and symptoms of normal-pressure hydrocephalus pertinent to the physical therapist and discuss the rationale for the use of a ventriculoperitoneal shunt as a treatment option. 2. Interpret and incorporate into the plan of care the results of cognitive and fall-risk outcome measures. 3. Develop and defend the rationale for formulating an appropriate discharge plan for an acute care patient with multiple comorbidities and confounding social variables.

Medical	
Chief complaint	Unsteady gait, change in mental status
History of present illness	A 72-year-old man was admitted to home care from skilled nursing. He was originally admitted to the acute hospital through the emergency department with a chief complaint of progressive unsteadiness of gait, urinary incontinence, and change in mental status over the past few weeks. He underwent a ventriculoperitoneal shunt. The postoperative course was benign, and he was transferred to a skilled facility for further rehabilitation. He spent 9 days at a skilled facility where he received skilled physical therapy, occupational therapy, and nursing services. He was discharged to home yesterday. At home, he will receive physical therapy and occupational therapy three times per week. A nurse will visit once a day per week and a home health aide will assist 3 days per week.
Past medical history	Diabetic retinopathy, diabetes mellitus (DM) type II, elevated cholesterol and lipids, high blood pressure, cervical arthritis
Past surgical history	Cholecystectomy: 20 years ago; appendectomy: 35 years ago
Allergies	latex, PCN, seasonal allergies
Medications	Atorvastatin (Lipitor), Glipizide, Metoprolol succinate, Flonase prn for seasonal allergies
Precautions/orders	Fall risk

Social history	
Home setup	• Two-story home with five steps to enter home with rail on the right. The driveway is adjacent to the home. • Thirteen steps, rail on the left, to the second floor • Bed and bath on the second floor. No bathroom on the first floor • Has two married children residing within 30 minutes of home. • The wife is retired and is home all day.
Occupation	• Retired from accounting 3 years ago due to an increased frequency in work mistakes. Master's level education.
Prior level of function	• Diminishment of function over the past 3 months as evidenced by need to use walker or cane, frequent falls, decreased ability to perform hygiene, and diminished social interaction. In reviewing the notes from the acute hospital and skilled nursing facility (SNF), there appears to have been a gradual improvement in function. Gains appear to have been greater in cognition and urinary control more so than dynamic balance.

(Continued)

(Continued)

Social history

	• According to the SNF's discharge summary, the patient was independent with bed mobility. He required supervision for all transfers. He was walking 80 feet with a rolling walker with supervision and beginning to practice with a cane. He was able to ambulate up and down 13 steps with supervision and a handrail on the right. He could dress himself but required assistance with showering due to balance issues. He requires minimal assist in and out of the car. He is independent with toilet transfers. He has not had an episode of incontinence for 3 days.
Recreational activities	• The patient reports that immediately after retirement, he exercised regularly, traveled, gardened, and performed woodworking but over the past 6 months most of this activity has diminished or ended. • He states he enjoys television watching but wants to return to gardening and travel.

Pause points

Based on the above information, what are the priority:
• Diagnostic tests and measures?
• Outcome measures?
• Treatment interventions?

Physical Therapy Examination
Subjective

Patient: "Apparently I had something wrong with my brain... too much pressure. The surgeon placed a shunt from my brain to my belly to draw off the fluid. I really do not remember too much about the whole thing. After the surgery, they sent me to rehab to relearn how to walk. I think I am doing okay, but I do not want to use this walker anymore"

Wife: "It was something called normal-pressure hydrocephalus. The three symptoms are falling, inability to control urine, and confusion. He is much less confused now as compared with a week ago. He has not had any bathroom accidents for at least 3 days. I am still worried about his walking. He is still unsteady even with the walker."

Objective				
Vital signs	Pre-treatment			Post-treatment
	Supine	Sitting	Standing	
Blood pressure (mmHg)	130/72	130/68	132/70	134/70
Heart rate (beats/min)	78	82	84	84
Respiratory rate (breaths/min)	14	16	26	28
Pulse oximetry on room air (SpO_2)	98%	98%	98%	98%
Borg scale	1	2	4	3
Pain	0/10	1/10 (incision at neck)	1/10 (incision at neck)	1/10 (incision at neck)
General	• Sitting on a dining room chair, no acute distress. Wife present for interview • No lines or tubes			
Head, ears, eyes, nose, and throat	• Fading ecchymosis at surgical site on the left neck. No evidence of infection.			
Cardiovascular and pulmonary	• Vital signs as above • No adventitious lung sounds • Calves are without edema, tenderness, or rubor, and without palpable cords. • Dorsalis pedis: 2 + bilaterally. Feet are warm			
Gastrointestinal	• Denies diarrhea or constipation • Denies belly pain • Endorses good appetite			

(Continued)

(Continued)

Physical Therapy Examination		
Genitourinary		• Does remember that he was incontinent of urine a "few times" at rehab but not over the past few days. • Denies hematuria, pain with voiding, and foul-smelling urine
Musculoskeletal	Range of motion (ROM)	• Cervical ROM deferred. Lumbar ROM assessment deferred due to reported poor dynamic standing balance. • All articular ROM assessments are full and painless. • No overt deformities noted
	Strength	• Bilateral upper extremity (BUE): grossly 4/5 throughout • Bilateral lower extremity (BLE): grossly 4/5 throughout
	Aerobic	• Aerobic testing deferred
	Flexibility	• Articular ROM is normal and painless without deformity or pain. • Two-joint muscle length testing deferred at this time.
	Other	• No overt muscle wasting, or atrophy noted by visual inspection.
Neurological	Balance	

Outcome measure	Presurgery	Today
MoCA	19/30	24/30
Romberg—eyes open	12 seconds	14 seconds
Romberg—eyes closed	8 seconds	13 seconds
Timed up and go	16 seconds	13 seconds

	Cognition	• See MoCA score above. • Alert and oriented × 3; remains a bit unsure of reason for hospital course; events of past 2 weeks are not able to be recalled clearly. • Able to follow simple one- and two-step commands.
	Coordination	• Finger to nose: mild impairment in BUE • Heel to shin: mild impairment in BLE
	Cranial nerves	• I: intact olfactory sense bilateral via two stimuli. • II: visual acuity 20/20 with corrective lenses, visual fields intact via confrontation. • III, IV, VI: pupils equally reactive to light and accommodation. External ocular muscles intact. No ptosis noted. No twitches or flutters. No nystagmus noted. Pupils equal in size. Pupillary light reflex intact. • V: intact sensation both sides of face via cotton and pin. Masseter and pterygoid muscles intact. • VII: face symmetrical. Tongue sensation intact • VIII: hearing intact bilaterally. Negative signs of vestibular nystagmus • IX, X: palate elevates symmetrically. Gag reflex intact. Voice of normal amplitude. No hoarseness noted. • XI: sternocleidomastoid and upper trapezius muscles intact. • XII: tongue in midline. No atrophy or fasciculations noted.
	Reflexes	• Biceps: 1 + /4 bilaterally • Patellar: 1 + /4 bilaterally • Clonus: (−) bilaterally • Babinski: down-going bilaterally
	Sensation	• BUE: intact to light touch • BLE: intact to light touch, mild loss of vibratory sense from mid-calf to toe. • Upper extremity drift test negative bilaterally.

(Continued)

(Continued)

Physical Therapy Examination		
	Tone	• BUE: mildly rigid • BLE: mildly rigid • No cogwheeling noted • No intentional or resting tremor noted • No festination or difficulty initiating movement noted • No "freezing" of gait noted
Functional status		
Bed mobility		• Rolling either direction: independent • Scooting up in bed: independent • Supine to/from sit: independent
Transfers		• Sit to/from stand: independent • Bed to/from chair: independent using rolling walker
Ambulation		• Ambulated 2 × 80 feet with supervision and rolling walker; minimal tactile cues needed for gait pattern. Has mild multidirectional instability especially with turns and with uneven surfaces (tested on tile, carpet, and lawn). • Gait deviations notable wide base of support, and multidirectional instability.
Stairs		• Ascended and descended 13 steps with handrail with minimal assist and significant verbal cueing. Practiced with wife behind him for guarding. Once upstairs, patient sits in a chair at the top of steps until wife brings walker.

Assessment	
☑ Physical therapist's	*Assessment left blank for learner to develop.*
Goals	
Patient's	"I seem to be much clearer mentally and I can now, I hope, control my urine. Now I just need to walk better."
Short term	1. *Goals left blank for learner to develop.* 2.
Long term	1. *Goals left blank for learner to develop.* 2.

Plan	
☐ Physician's ☑ Physical therapist's ☐ Other's	Patient will be seen thrice a week for ambulation, dynamic and static balance activities, stair climbing, and transition from walker to cane. We will also discuss with the patient and his wife fall-risk mediation. We will also work with the wife on guarding techniques to be used with her husband when ambulating, using steps, bathing, and car transfers.

Bloom's Taxonomy Level	Case 13.C Questions
Create	1. Synthesizing the medical data and physical examination findings, develop an appropriate physical therapy assessment of the patient. 2. Develop two short-term physical therapy goals, including an appropriate timeframe. 3. Develop two long-term physical therapy goals, including an appropriate timeframe.
Evaluate	4. Determine the proposed optimum discharge plan following home physical therapy. 5. Why should a home health aide and nursing, who were also ordered along with a physical therapist and an occupational therapist, visit the patient? 6. What equipment should the physical therapist recommend for home, considering the only DME currently in the house are a walker and single point cane?

(Continued)

(Continued)

Bloom's Taxonomy Level	Case 13.C Questions
Analyze	7. How could the physical therapist incorporate the fact that the patient has diabetes into the evaluation, assessment, reassessments, and interventions?
Apply	8. Design and implement two interventions for an ataxic gait pattern that the patient could do at home 9. Design and implement two interventions for diminished standing balance that the patient could do at home.
Understand	10. At this point, can the patient be left home alone while the wife steps out of the house to shop?
Remember	11. What are signs and symptoms of hypoglycemia? Hyperglycemia?

Bloom's Taxonomy Level	Case 13.C Answers
Create	1. The patient is a 72-year-old, retired accountant, who resides in a two-story home with his retired wife. He was admitted to the hospital for surgical intervention (ventriculoperitoneal shunt) for symptomatic (urinary incontinence, gait dysfunction with falls, and confusion) normal-pressure hydrocephalus. He followed the acute say with a week at skilled. Past medical history is significant for diabetes mellitus type II, cervical arthritis, diabetic retinopathy, and elevated serum lipids and cholesterol. Postoperative course has been uneventful. He is now alert and oriented × 3 with mild forgetfulness about recent events. From a system's viewpoint, he has deficits in cognition, balance, bed mobility, transfers, and gait. His cardiovascular and pulmonary responses appear normal. He is at fall risk. Currently, he is independent with most basic activities of daily living (BADLs) but requires minimal assistance with higher-level transfers and ADLs. He is walking with supervision 80 feet with a walker. He can ascend/descend one flight of steps using two hands on the handrail and minimal assist of his wife. The plan is to treat him at home for 3 weeks and then discharge him to a local outpatient physical therapy facility for continued rehab. 2. Short-term goals: • The patient will ambulate around the backyard (× ~50 feet), which contains uneven terrain with supervision and rolling walker within 7 days to improve independence. • The patient will be independent with tub and toilet transfers within 7 days to improve independence. 3. Long-term goals:. • The patient will ambulate 200 feet independently on all surfaces with a cane within 3 weeks. • The patient will ascend/descend 13 steps with one rail and a cane independently within 3 weeks.
Evaluate	4. Following home physical therapy, the discharge recommendation is to an outpatient physical therapy clinic. It is anticipated that after 3 weeks of home therapy, the patient will be sufficiently safe to be driven to an outpatient physical therapy clinic to maximize his functional potential, including balance and endurance. Eventually, he will transition to a local fitness center to work with a certified trainer. 5. The home health aide was ordered because the patient continues to have difficulty with bath transfers and hygiene. The aide will assist him with these activities. The nurse was ordered due to the ongoing medical issues of the patient. He is diabetic and has hypercholesterolemia, hyperlipidemia, and diabetic retinopathy. The nurse will ensure, in the short term, that these medical conditions are appropriately assessed and addressed. The nurse can also check the surgical site for signs of infection. 6. Home DME for consideration may include a commode for downstairs, shower rails, and rails near the toilet. A second rail may be considered for the stairs to get into the house and the stairs to the second floor of the house.
Analyze	7. Since the patient has diabetes, it is important for the physical therapist to check his blood sugar prior to, during, and after intervention to garner information about his blood sugar control and his blood sugar response to activity. The physical therapist should encourage him to visit his ophthalmologist regularly, as well as encourage his wife to check his feet twice daily for ulceration or redness.

(Continued)

(Continued)

Bloom's Taxonomy Level	Case 13.C Answers
Apply	8. Interventions for gait ataxia, which can be done in the home, include sitting on a Swedish ball and practicing anterior, posterior, and right and left weight shifts, tossing a ball while standing with the physical therapist, walking on uneven surfaces, walking in the home, and stepping over objects strategically placed on the floor by the physical therapist. 9. Interventions for diminished standing balance, which can be performed at home, include alternating one-leg stance, walking a supple surface, such as a mat, reaching, step taps, and multidirectional stepping. The patient should perform the activities with proper guarding by the physical therapist ▶ Fig. 13.3
Understand	10. At this point, it is not advisable for the wife to leave the patient at home alone while she shops. Perhaps she can shop when the home health aide is present. The patient remains a bit confused over recent events and remains a fall risk.
Remember	11. Symptoms of hypoglycemia include sweating, tachycardia, change in mental status, and syncope. Symptoms of hyperglycemia include sweating, excessive thirst, tachycardia, and weight loss.

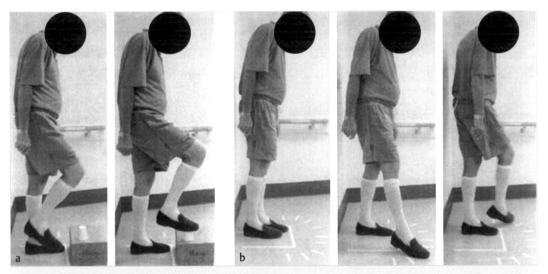

Fig. 13.3 (a,b) Examples of lower extremity coordination exercises which can be performed independently at home. (Adapted from Mehrholz J, ed. Maximizing muscle endurance and physical fitness. In: Physical Therapy for the Stroke Patient: Early Stage Rehabilitation. 1st ed. Stuttgart: Thieme; 2012.)

Key points
1. The physical therapist is the primary care practitioner when in the home. The physical therapist must consider all systems when evaluating the patient at home.
2. Outcome measures, especially with this patient, are extremely important as a guide to program advancement. These measures should be done at each visit.
3. In scenarios such as the one presented here, the therapist must remember that the primary caregiver, the wife, has needs and her needs must also be addressed.

Suggested Readings

Alamoudi NB, Alnajim RK, Alfaraj D. The typical triad of idiopathic normal pressure hydrocephalus in a 62-year-old male: a case report. Saudi J Emergency Med. 2020; 1(1):34–34

American College of Sports Medicine. ACSM's Guidelines for Exercise Testing and Prescription. 10th ed. Baltimore, MD: Lippincott, Williams and Wilkins; 2017

Bovonsunthonchai S, Witthiwej T, Ngamsombat C, Sathornsumetee S, Vachalathiti R. Gait alteration in patients with idiopathic normal pressure hydrocephalus after cerebral spinal fluid removal. Gait Posture. 2017; 57:256–257

Gallagher R, Marquez J, Osmotherly P. Gait and balance measures can identify change from a cerebrospinal fluid tap test in idiopathic normal pressure hydrocephalus. Arch Phys Med Rehabil. 2018; 99(11):2244–2250

Giordan E, Palandri G, Lanzino G, Murad MH, Elder BD. Outcomes and complications of different surgical treatments for idiopathic normal pressure hydrocephalus: a systematic review and meta-analysis. J Neurosurg. 2018; 131(4):1–13

Goodman CC, Fuller KS. Pathology: Implications for the Physical Therapist. 4th ed. St. Louis, MO: Saunders Elsevier; 2015

Griffa A, Van De Ville D, Herrmann FR, Allali G. Neural circuits of idiopathic normal pressure hydrocephalus: a perspective review of brain connectivity and symptoms meta-analysis. Neurosci Biobehav Rev. 2020; 112:452–471

Modesto PC, Pinto FCG. Home physical exercise program: analysis of the impact on the clinical evolution of patients with normal pressure hydrocephalus. Arq Neuropsiquiatr. 2019; 77(12):860–870

Montreal Cognitive Assessment. Available at: https://www.sralab.org/rehabilitation-measures/montreal-cognitive-assessment. Accessed May 1, 2020

Nassar BR, Lippa CF. Idiopathic normal pressure hydrocephalus: a review for general practitioners. Gerontol Geriatr Med. 2016; 2: 2333721416643702

Nikaido Y, Kajimoto Y, Akisue T, et al. Dynamic balance measurements can differentiate patients who fall from patients who do not fall in patients with idiopathic normal pressure hydrocephalus. Arch Phys Med Rehabil. 2019; 100(8):1458–1466

Oliveira LM, Nitrini R, Román GC. Normal-pressure hydrocephalus: a critical review. Dement Neuropsychol. 2019; 13(2):133–143

Peterson KA, Savulich G, Jackson D, Killikelly C, Pickard JD, Sahakian BJ. The effect of shunt surgery on neuropsychological performance in normal pressure hydrocephalus: a systematic review and meta-analysis. J Neurol. 2016; 263(8):1669–1677

Romberg Test. Available at: https://www.sralab.org/rehabilitation-measures/romberg-test. Accessed May 1, 2020

Sharpened Romberg Test. Available at: https://www.sralab.org/rehabilitation-measures/sharpened-romberg. Accessed May 1, 2020

Song M, Lieberman A, Fife T, et al. A prospective study on gait dominant normal pressure hydrocephalus. Acta Neurol Scand. 2019; 139(4):389–394

The Joint Commission. Standards. Available at: https://www.jointcommission.org/en/standards/. Accessed May 1, 2020

Timed Up and Go. Available at: https://www.sralab.org/rehabilitation-measures/timed-and-go. Accessed May 1, 2020

14 Osteoporosis

General Information	
Case no.	14.A Osteoporosis
Authors	Melissa Gilroy, DC, MSPAS, PA-C Sean Griech, PT, DPT, PhD, COMT, Board Certified Clinical Specialist in Orthopaedic Physical Therapy Julie M. Skrzat, PT, DPT, PhD, Board Certified Clinical Specialist in Cardiovascular & Pulmonary Physical Therapy
Diagnosis	Acute Compression Fracture of T12 Due to Osteoporosis
Setting	Emergency Department
Learner expectations	☑ Initial evaluation ☐ Re-evaluation ☐ Treatment session
Learner objectives	1. To understand the role of the physical therapist in the emergency department. 2. To consider differential diagnoses for a patient presenting with back pain. 3. To identify risk factors for vertebral compression fracture in the setting of osteoporosis.

Medical	
Chief complaint	Mid-back pain × 2 days
History of present illness	The patient is a 72-year-old woman with a history of osteoporosis presenting to the emergency department with mid-back pain that began acutely following a fall onto her backside 2 days prior. She fell while using the bathroom in the middle of the night. She states she used minimal lights to avoid waking her husband. The patient denies loss of consciousness or head trauma. No other injuries were reported. She denies numbness or paresthesia in the extremities. She reports one episode of urinary incontinence since the fall. Pain is described as sharp and rated as 8/10 since injury. It is localized to mid-back without radiation. There is minimal improvement of pain with acetaminophen 500 mg every 4 hours. It is worst with movement, particularly forward spinal flexion. She is able to sleep supine with knees bent.
Past medical history	Hypertension: diagnosed in her 40s; hyperlipidemia: diagnosed in her 40s; osteoporosis: diagnosed age 65 years; dual-energy X-ray absorptiometry (DEXA) scan (spine/hip) performed 7 years ago with a T-score of −2.5 and Z-score of −2; history of tobacco use: half pack per day since age 20 years; abstinent for 5 years; alcohol use: one to two glasses of wine each week.
Past surgical history	Total abdominal hysterectomy: age 45 years; no complications
Allergies	None
Medications	Lisinopril, Atorvastatin, Multivitamin, No herbals/supplements
Precautions/orders	Bedrest until cleared by neurosurgery Activity as tolerated Ambulate with assist

Social history	
Home setup	• Lives in a multilevel home with her husband who continues to work full-time. • Two steps without handrail to enter. • No bathroom on the first floor. • Bedroom and bathroom are located on the second floor. • Flight of stairs + one handrail to the second floor.
Occupation	• Elementary school teacher, retired 5 years ago.
Prior level of function	• Independent with functional mobility and activities of daily living (ADLs). • No regular exercise • (+) driver
Recreational activities	• Painting, sewing, scrapbooking • Enjoys visiting family and grandchildren.

Vital signs	Hospital day 0: emergency department
Blood pressure (mmHg)	134/88
Heart rate (beats/min)	102
Respiratory rate (breaths/min)	22
Pulse oximetry on room air (SpO$_2$)	98%
Temperature (°F)	98.6 (oral)

Imaging/diagnostic test	Hospital day 0: emergency department
Thoracic and lumbar spinal X-ray anteroposterior/lateral	1. X-ray shows presence of a moderate-grade anterior wedge fracture of T12 with approximately 30% degree of deformity. Cortical breaking and impaction of trabeculae are consistent with acute compression fracture. No other acute findings noted.
Thoracic and lumbar spinal magnetic resonance imaging (MRI)	▶ Fig. 14.1

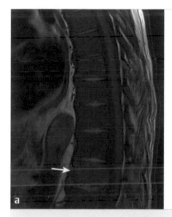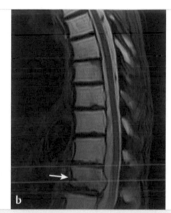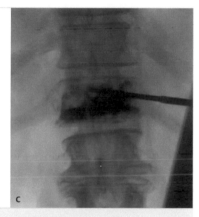

Fig. 14.1 (a) Sagittal T1-weighted sequence of the thoracic spine demonstrates diffuse metastatic infiltration of the bone marrow by a rectal mucinous adenocarcinoma (T1-weighted signal of the marrow significantly lower than the disk). (b) Sagittal T2-weighted sequence. *Arrows* in (a) and (b) show a T12 pathologic vertebral compression fracture. (c) Fluoroscopic image demonstrates adequate polymethyl methacrylate (PMMA) fill of the vertebral body from pedicle to pedicle and from end plate to end plate. (Adapted from 18.2 Current Information Based on Recent Literature and State-of-the-Art Practice. In: Beall D, ed. Vertebral Augmentation: The Comprehensive Guide to Vertebroplasty, Kyphoplasty, and Implant Augmentation. 1st ed. Stuttgart: Thieme; 2020.)

Medical management	Hospital day 0: emergency department
Medications	1. Lisinopril 2. Morphine PRN 3. Acetaminophen PRN 4. Colace PRN 5. Polyethylene glycol PRN
Consults	1. Neurosurgery: evaluate and treat for T12 compression fracture; nonoperative management recommended; stable fracture and cleared for physical therapy evaluation. 2. Geriatrics: evaluate and treat medical conditions of hypertension and untreated osteoporosis. 3. Physical therapy: evaluate and treat, disposition planning

Lab		Reference range	Hospital day 0: emergency department
Complete blood count	White blood cell	5.0–10.0 × 10^9/L	8.7
	Hemoglobin	12.0–16.0 g/dL	12.2
	Hematocrit	35.5–44.9%	37
	Red blood cell	4.5–5.5 million/mm^3	4.6
	Platelet	140,000–400,000/μL	250
Metabolic panel	Calcium	8.6–10.3 mg/dL	8.7
	Chloride	98–108 mEq/L	106
	Magnesium	1.2–1.9 mEq/L	1.2
	Phosphate	2.3–4.1 mg/dL	3.1
	Potassium	3.7–5.1 mEq/L	4.7
	Sodium	134–142 mEq/L	140
	Blood urea nitrogen	7–20 mg/dL	18
	Creatinine	0.7–1.3 mg/dL	1.02
	Anion gap	3–10 mEq/L	8
	CO$_2$	22–26 mEq/L	24

Pause points
Based on the above information, what are the priority: • Diagnostic tests and measures? • Outcome measures? • Treatment interventions?

Hospital Day 0, Emergency Department: Physical Therapy Examination		
Subjective		
"My back really hurts."		
Objective		
Vital signs	Pre-treatment	Post-treatment
Blood pressure (mmHg)	132/88	136/90
Heart rate (beats/min)	101	102
Respiratory rate (breaths/min)	20	22
Pulse oximetry on room air (SpO$_2$)	98%	96%
Pain	8/10 low back	8/10 low back
General	• Patient supine in bed. • Well developed, well nourished, awake/alert, appears stated age, in mild to moderate distress secondary to back pain. • Lines notable for peripheral intravenous (IV).	
Head, ears, eyes, nose, and throat	• Head normocephalic, atraumatic • Extraocular motion intact, pupils equal, round, and reactive to light and accommodation	
Cardiovascular and pulmonary	• Normal sinus rate and rhythm, no murmurs, rubs, gallops • S1 and S2 present, no S3 or S4 • Point of maximal impulse (PMI) is nondisplaced.	

(Continued)

(Continued)

Hospital Day 0, Emergency Department: Physical Therapy Examination		
Gastrointestinal	• Soft, nontender, nondistended • Positive bowel sound (BS) in all four quadrants. • No organomegaly	
Musculoskeletal	Range of motion	• Bilateral upper extremity (BUE): grossly within functional range • Bilateral lower extremity (BLE): grossly within functional range
	Strength	• BUE: grossly 4/5 • BLE: grossly 4/5 • Facial grimacing and subjective reports of low back pain with resisted shoulder flexion and hip flexion.
Neurological	Balance	• Static sitting, unsupported: supervision with BUE support • Dynamic sitting, unsupported: supervision with BUE support • Static standing, unsupported: minimal assistance • Dynamic standing, unsupported: minimal to moderate assistance • Dynamic standing, supported: minimal assistance with rolling walker
	Cognition	• Alert and oriented × 4
	Coordination	• Finger to nose: intact bilaterally
	Cranial nerves	• II–XII: intact
	Reflexes	• Patellar: 2 + bilaterally • Achilles: 2 + bilaterally • Babinski: negative bilaterally
	Sensation	• Intact and symmetric to light touch and deep pressure in BLE.
	Tone	• Normal throughout BUEs and BLEs
	Other	• No clonus in BLE
Functional status		
Bed mobility	• Rolling either direction: supervision. Patient educated on log roll technique. • Supine to/from sit: supervision with increased time, head of bed flat, no bedrails, used log roll technique ▶ Fig. 14.2a, b, c	
Transfers	• Sit to/from stand: contact guard assist • Stand pivot transfer: minimal assistance with no assistive device	
Ambulation	• Ambulated × 10 feet with minimal to moderate assistance and no assistive device. • Gait deviations notable for antalgic gait, flexed posture, decreased cadence, decreased bilateral (B/L) step length. • Ambulated × 25 feet with minimal assistance and rolling walker. • Gait deviations notable for above deficits, but to lesser degree. • Patient reports that while she does not like using a rolling walker, she feels more secure.	
Stairs	• Attempted to ascend/descend one step, but unable to complete due to pain.	

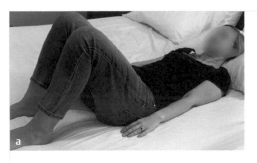
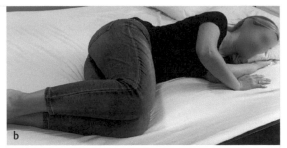
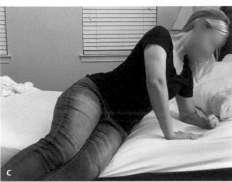

Fig. 14.2 (a-c) An example of the log roll technique to get in and out of bed.

Assessment	
☑ Physical therapist's	*Assessment left blank for learner to develop.*
Goals	
Patient's	"I want to get rid of this pain to go home."
Short term	1.
	Goals left blank for learner to develop.
	2.
Long term	1.
	Goals left blank for learner to develop.
	2.

Plan	
☐ Physician's ☑ Physical therapist's ☐ Other's	At this time, patient is not functioning at her baseline and, therefore, is not cleared to be discharged home. Patient would benefit from continued physical therapy to maximize functional mobility and safety.

Bloom's Taxonomy Level	Case 14.A Questions
Create	1. Synthesizing the medical data and physical examination findings, develop an appropriate physical therapy assessment of the patient. 2. Develop two short-term physical therapy goals, including an appropriate timeframe. 3. Develop two long-term physical therapy goals, including an appropriate timeframe. 4. Create a comprehensive home exercise program for this patient.
Evaluate	5. What are differential diagnoses for a patient presenting with back pain? How can they be ruled out?

(Continued)

(Continued)

Bloom's Taxonomy Level	Case 14.A Questions
Analyze	6. What components of the patient's history are important to consider in the evaluation of cauda equina syndrome?
Apply	7. How should the DEXA score be interpreted?
Understand	8. What risk factors are implicated in the development of osteoporosis?
	9. Why are the patient's blood pressure, heart rate, and respiratory rate elevated?
Remember	10. What is the definition of osteoporosis? How does it differ from osteopenia?

Bloom's Taxonomy Level	Case 14.A Answers
Create	1. The patient is a 72-year-old woman who presents to the emergency department status post fall with acute low back pain × 2 days. She was diagnosed with an acute compression fracture at T12 due to osteoporosis. Per neurosurgery, she is not a candidate for surgical interventions and, therefore, conservative management is recommended. She was previously independent with functional mobility and ADLs. Unfortunately, her primary limitation of pain warrants supervision—moderate assistance with/without an assistive device for functional mobility. Additionally, due to the pain, she is unable to successfully ascend/descend one step, impairing her ability to enter and exit her home and use bathroom, which is on the second floor. Finally, she has limited social support at home, since her husband continues to work full time. As a result of these, she is not safe to be discharged home. She would benefit from continued inpatient physical therapy for pain management and to maximize functional mobility and safety. Will continue to follow and progress as tolerated.
	2. Short-term goals:
	• Patient will independently perform bed mobility, utilizing logroll technique, within three visits to protect spine and promote independence.
	• Patient will independently perform all transfers with least restrictive assistive device within three visits to promote independence.
	3. Long-term goals:
	• Patient will be modified independent to ambulate a minimum of 50 feet, using the least restrictive assistive device, within seven visits to promote independence at home.
	• Patient will be modified independent to ascend/descend a flight of stairs, using one hand rail and a step-to pattern, within seven visits to be able to reach the second floor of home.
	• Patient will independently verbalize three ways to reduce fall risk within her home within 7 visits to maximize safety.
	4. The following is an example of a potential home exercise program for this patient. This exercise program should be prescribed to help prevent disease prevention. Only three to five exercises should be selected to ensure compliance.
	Strengthening:
	Frequency: 2 to 3 days a week
	Intensity: moderate, 60 to 80% 1 repetition maximum (RM)
	Time: 8 to 12 repetitions
	Type: mini-squats, standing hip abduction, bridges
	Aerobic training:
	Frequency: 3 to 5 days a week
	Intensity: moderate, 40 to < 60% heart rate reserve
	Time: 30 to 60 minutes a day
	Type: walking
Evaluate	5. The differential diagnoses for a patient with back pain can be broad, and many ruled out through an appropriate history and physical examination.
	Referred pain to the back from visceral complaints like pancreatitis (mid-back) or cholecystitis (right scapular) may be excluded in a patient who does not have associated abdominal pain, anorexia, and nausea/vomiting. Rupture of an abdominal aortic aneurysm may also cause referred back pain (mid to lower back). These patients may be identified by risk factors like older age, male sex, history of tobacco use,

(Continued)

(Continued)

Bloom's Taxonomy Level	Case 14.A Answers
	hypertension, hypercholesterolemia, known cardiovascular disease, etc. Any of these referred pain complaints can also be more definitively ruled out with appropriate imaging studies
	Other etiologies for consideration include malignancy or metastatic disease. The most common primary bone malignancy is multiple myeloma. Malignancies most likely to spread to the bone include prostate, thyroid, breast, lung, and renal cancers. These are typically identified on imaging studies but should be considered in patients with history of malignancy or based on other risk factors like advanced age, family history, hypercholesterolemia, and known cardiovascular disease.
	Various sources of infection like diskitis, osteomyelitis, or localized abscess may also present with back pain. These patients may have a history of immunosuppression, recent surgery or intervention, other infectious source (endocarditis, bacteremia), IV drug use, and may present with associated symptoms of fever and/or chills. A thorough history can help determine if an infectious etiology should be included on the differential and appropriate imaging can help identify the specific diagnosis
	Musculoskeletal considerations for back pain include herniated nucleus pulposus, spinal stenosis, muscular spasm/strain, spondylolisthesis, or bony fracture. A thorough history, physical examination, and appropriate imaging can be utilized to identify these conditions.
Analyze	6. Cauda equina syndrome is a condition in which the terminal nerve roots of the spinal cord are impinged, which can result in asymmetric multiradicular pain, leg weakness, and/or sensory loss in the lower extremities as well as bowel, bladder, or sexual dysfunction. Although not commonly caused by vertebral compression fractures, it is important to assess for these features in patients presenting with back pain. Failure to recognize and treat cauda equina syndrome in a timely fashion can result in permanent disability. This patient had one episode of urinary incontinence, which prompted the MRI evaluation to assess for integrity of the cord and nerve roots.
Apply	7. DEXA technology is used to measure bone mineral density (BMD), which is a reflection of bone strength. It is used to aid in the diagnosis of osteopenia and osteoporosis. The T-score is calculated by subtracting the mean BMD of a young adult reference population from the patient's BMD, then dividing by the standard deviation (SD) of young adult population. The Z-score is used to compare the patient's BMD to a population of peers. It is calculated by subtracting the mean BMD of an age, ethnicity, and sex-matched reference population from the patient's BMD, then dividing by the SD of the reference population.
	There are some discrepancies between medical organizations regarding what sites of BMD should be used to make the diagnosis of osteoporosis. The World Health Organization recommends using the T-score measured by DEXA at the femoral neck as the international standard for diagnosing osteoporosis. In contrast, the National Osteoporosis Foundation and the International Society for Clinical Densitometry suggest using the lowest T-score from the lumbar spine (L1–L4), total proximal femur, or femoral neck as determined by DEXA scanning in making the diagnosis of osteoporosis.
Understand	8. Risk factors for the development of osteoporosis include advanced age, history of previous fracture, long-term glucocorticoid therapy, low body weight (< 127 lb), parental history of hip fracture, cigarette smoking, excess alcohol use, and race/ethnicity (Caucasian with the highest risk). Of these, the greatest predictors for the development of osteoporosis are advanced age and history of previous fracture.
	9. The patient's blood pressure, heart rate, and respiratory rate are likely elevated due to the patient's reports of pain and anxiety.
Remember	10. Osteoporosis is a disease characterized by low bone mass. There are structural changes to the bone tissue, resulting in bone fragility. This puts an individual at risk of developing fractures, specifically at the hip, spine, and wrist. Osteoporosis, as defined by the World Health Organization, has a T-score less than −2.5. Osteopenia is a term used to describe a decrease in bone mineral density below normal reference values. Osteopenia, as defined by the World Health Organization, is a T-score between −1 and −2.5.

Key points
1. There is an increase in patients presenting at the emergency department with musculoskeletal complaints. Once acute pathology has been ruled out, physical therapists have the knowledge and abilities to implement therapeutic tests and measures to diagnosis and treat low back pain.
2. Physical therapists have the training and ability to integrate multiple date points to assist with disposition planning from the acute care setting.
3. Physical therapists can provide appropriate education on fall reduction techniques and proper body mechanics to assist in reducing incidence of vertebral compression fracture.

General Information	
Case no.	14.B
Authors	Melissa Gilroy, DC, MSPAS, PA-C Julie M. Skrzat, PT, DPT, PhD, Board Certified Clinical Specialist in Cardiovascular & Pulmonary Physical Therapy Sean Griech, PT, DPT, PhD, COMT, Board Certified Clinical Specialist in Orthopaedic Physical Therapy
Diagnosis	Acute compression fracture of T12 due to osteoporosis
Setting	Acute care hospital
Learner expectations	☐ Initial evaluation ☑ Re-evaluation ☐ Treatment session
Learner objectives	1. To understand the importance of an interdisciplinary team when treating an individual with acute low back pain. 2. To understand the importance of bracing for conservative management of low back pain. 3. To understand how health and wellness education begins in the acute care hospital.

Medical	
Chief complaint	Mid-back pain × 2 days
History of present illness	The patient is a 72-year-old woman presenting to the emergency department with mid-back pain that began acutely following a mechanical fall onto her backside 2 days prior. She was noted to have a T12 compression fracture on diagnostic imaging in the emergency department. Neurosurgery consulted and patient is not a surgical candidate. Instead, conservative management was recommended. Physical therapy was consulted for discharge planning and patient was deemed unsafe to be discharged home. As a result of inadequate pain management and being unsafe to be discharged home, patient was admitted to the neurosurgical/trauma service. Medical management to include thoracolumbosacral orthosis (TLSO) brace (▶ Fig. 14.3a, b) and pharmacological interventions. Pain, now managed medically, has improved to 4/10 from the previous 8/10. Gerontology consulted to assist in management of untreated osteoporosis and vitamin D deficiency.
Past medical history	Hypertension: diagnosed in her 40s; hyperlipidemia: diagnosed in her 40s; osteoporosis: diagnosed age 65 years; dual-energy X-ray absorptiometry (DEXA) scan (spine/hip) performed 7 years ago with a T-score of −2.5 and Z-score of −2; history of tobacco use: half pack per day since age 20 years; abstinent for 5 years; alcohol use: one to two glasses of wine each week.
Past surgical history	Total abdominal hysterectomy: age 45; no complications
Allergies	None
Medications	Lisinopril, Atorvastatin, Multivitamin, No herbals/supplements
Precautions/orders	Activity as tolerated TLSO brace when out of bed Fall risk

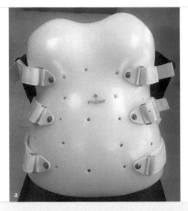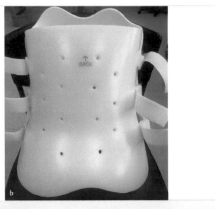

Fig. 14.3 (a,b) A thoracolumbosacral orthosis (TLSO) brace.

Social history	
Home setup	• Lives in a multilevel home with her husband who continues to work full time. • Two steps without handrail to enter. • No bathroom on the first floor. • Bedroom and bathroom are located on the second floor. • Flight of stairs + one handrail to the second floor.
Occupation	• Elementary school teacher, retired 5 years ago
Prior level of function	• Independent with functional mobility and activities of daily living (ADLs). • No regular exercise • (+) driver
Recreational activities	• Painting, sewing, scrapbooking • Enjoys visiting family and grandchildren.

Vital signs	Hospital day 0: emergency department	Hospital Day 1: ward
Blood pressure (mmHg)	134/88	120/82
Heart rate (beats/min)	102	88
Respiratory rate (breaths/min)	22	12
Pulse oximetry on room air (SpO₂)	98%	98%
Temperature (°F)	98.6 (oral)	98.6 (oral)

Lab		Reference range	Hospital day 0: emergency department	Hospital day 1: ward
Complete blood count	White blood cell	$5.0–10.0 \times 10^9$/L	8.7	8.5
	Hemoglobin	12.0–16.0 g/dL	12.2	12.1
	Hematocrit	35.5–44.9%	37	36.8
	Red blood cell	4.5–5.5 million/mm³	4.6	4.6
	Platelet	140,000–400,000/µL	250	251

(Continued)

(Continued)

Lab		Reference range	Hospital day 0: emergency department	Hospital day 1: ward
Metabolic panel	Calcium	8.6–10.3 mg/dL	8.7	8.7
	Chloride	98–108 mEq/L	106	105
	Magnesium	1.2–1.9 mEq/L	1.2	1.2
	Phosphate	2.3–4.1 mg/dL	3.1	3.2
	Potassium	3.7–5.1 mEq/L	4.7	4.7
	Sodium	134–142 mEq/L	140	139
	Blood urea nitrogen	7–20 mg/dL	18	18
	Creatinine	0.7–1.3 mg/dL	1.02	1.1
	Anion gap	3–10 mEq/L	8	8
	CO_2	22–26 mEq/L	24	24
Other	25-hydroxy vitamin D	25–80 ng/mL	–	12

Medical management	Hospital day 0: emergency department	Hospital day 1: ward
Medications	1. Lisinopril 2. Morphine PRN 3. Acetaminophen PRN 4. Colace PRN 5. Polyethylene Glycol PRN	1. Lisinopril 2. Morphine PRN 3. Acetaminophen PRN 4. Colace PRN 5. Polyethylene Glycol PRN 6. Calcium Carbonate 7. Vitamin D
Consults	1. Neurosurgery 2. Geriatrics 3. Physical therapy	1. Neurosurgery 2. Geriatrics 3. Physical therapy 4. Occupational therapy

Pause points
Based on the above information, what are the priority: • Diagnostic tests and measures? • Outcome measures? • Treatment interventions?

Hospital Day 1, Ward: Physical Therapy Re-evaluation				
Subjective				
"My pain is a little better. Can I try walking again?"				
Objective				
Vital signs	Pre-treatment			Post-treatment
	Supine	Sitting	Standing	
Blood pressure (mmHg)	128/88	129/89	124/88	125/80
Heart rate (beats/min)	87	89	91	95
Respiratory rate (breaths/min)	16	16	17	16
Pulse oximetry on room air (SpO_2)	98%	95%	96%	97%

(Continued)

(Continued)

Hospital Day 1, Ward: Physical Therapy Re-evaluation			
Pain	4/10 low back	5/10 low back	4/10 low back · 3/10 low back
General	• Patient seated in chair finishing breakfast, wearing TLSO. • Well developed, well nourished, awake/alert, appears stated age. • Lines notable for peripheral intravenous (IV), placed to saline lock (hep-lock).		
Head, ears, eyes, nose, and throat	• Head normocephalic, atraumatic • Extraocular motion intact (EOMI), pupils equal, round, and reactive to light and accommodation (PERRL).		
Cardiovascular and pulmonary	• Normal rate and rhythm, no murmurs, rubs, gallops • S1 and S2 present, no S3 or S4 • Point of maximal impulse (PMI) is nondisplaced.		
Gastrointestinal	• Soft, nontender, nondistended. • Positive bowel sound (BS) in all four quadrants. • No organomegaly.		
Musculoskeletal	Range of motion	• Bilateral upper extremity (BUE): grossly within functional range • Bilateral lower extremity (BLE): grossly within functional range	
	Strength	• BUE: grossly 4/5 • BLE: grossly 4/5	
	Aerobic	• Reported 10/20 on Rate of Perceived Exertion (RPE) Scale after ambulation trial.	
Neurological	Balance	• Static sitting, unsupported: independent • Dynamic sitting, unsupported: supervision with BUE support. Limited range due to TLSO brace. • Static standing, unsupported: supervision ▶ Fig. 14.4 • Dynamic standing, supported: supervision with rolling walker.	
	Cognition	• Alert and oriented × 4	
	Coordination	• Finger to nose: intact bilaterally	
	Cranial nerves	• II–XII: intact	
	Reflexes	• Patellar: 2 + bilaterally • Achilles: 2 + bilaterally • Babinski: negative bilaterally	
	Sensation	• Intact and symmetric to light touch and deep pressure in BLE	
	Tone	• Normal throughout BUEs and BLEs.	
	Other	• No clonus in BLE.	
Functional status			
Bed mobility	• Rolling either direction: supervision using logroll technique. • Supine to/from sit: supervision with increased time, head of bed flat, no bedrails, using logroll technique.		
Transfers	• Sit to/from stand: supervision. • Stand pivot transfer: supervision with rolling walker.		
Ambulation	• Ambulated × 50 feet with supervision and rolling walker. • Gait deviations notable for decreased cadence, decreased B/L step length, improved upright posture due to pain relief and use of TLSO brace.		
Stairs	• Ascend/descend one step × 2 trials with one handrail and minimal assistance.		
Other	• Required minimal assistance and verbal cues to don/doff TLSO brace.		

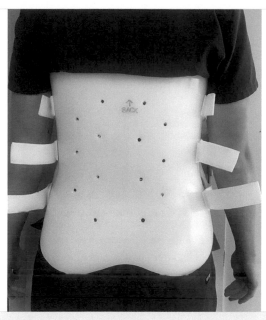

Fig. 14.4 An example of proper placement of the TLSO donned during static standing.

Assessment	
☑ Physical therapist's	*Assessment left blank for learner to develop.*
Goals	
Patient's	"To be able to walk again."
Short term	1.
	Goals left blank for learner to develop.
	2.
Long term	1.
	Goals left blank for learner to develop.
	2.

Plan	
☐ Physician's ☑ Physical therapist's ☐ Other's	Will continue to see patient two to four times a week for strength, balance, and functional mobility training. Safe to mobilize to bathroom and around unit with assistance.

Bloom's Taxonomy Level	Case 14.B Questions
Create	1. Synthesizing the medical data and physical examination findings, develop an appropriate physical therapy assessment of the patient. 2. Develop two short-term physical therapy goals, including an appropriate timeframe. 3. Develop two long-term physical therapy goals, including an appropriate timeframe.
Evaluate	4. What does the patient need to successfully complete to be discharged home?
Analyze	5. Without repeating a DEXA scan, how else can the patient be given a formal diagnosis of osteoporosis?
Apply	6. How does Vitamin D deficiency contribute to the development of osteoporosis?

(Continued)

(Continued)

Bloom's Taxonomy Level	Case 14.B Questions
Understand	7. What type of medication is the patient utilizing for management of moderate to severe pain and what are some potential side effects? 8. Explain what a vertebral compression fracture is. What are risk factors for the development of vertebral compression fractures?
Remember	9. What is the purpose of the TLSO brace? What risks are associated with its use and should be monitored in follow-up? 10. Name two balance assessments that would be appropriate to execute with this patient in this setting

Bloom's Taxonomy Level	Case 14.B Answers
Create	1. The patient is a 72-year-old woman who presented to the emergency department status post fall with acute low back pain × 2 days. Per neurosurgery, she is not a candidate for surgical interventions and conservative management is recommended. She was seen in the emergency department by a physical therapist and, due to increased pain and impaired functional level, was deemed unsafe to return home. She was admitted to Neurosurgery/Trauma service for conservative management, which includes use of TLSO brace. She was previously independent with functional mobility. With current medical management, her pain is better controlled, and she was able to progress functional mobility. She is, however, not at her functional baseline. She requires supervision—minimal assistance with rolling walker due to pain, decreased BLE strength, and impaired balance. She would benefit from continued physical therapy for pain management and to maximize functional mobility and safety. Will continue to follow and progress as tolerated. 2. Short-term goals: • Patient will independently demonstrate logroll technique 100% of the time when performing bed mobility within three visits to protect spine and decrease pain. • Patient will independently don/doff TLSO brace within three visits to protect spine and decrease pain. • Patient will participate in formal balance assessment next session to assess fall risk. 3. Long-term goals: • Patient will be modified independent to ambulate 100 feet, using least restrictive assistive device, within seven visits to independently mobilize within her home. • Patient will ascend/descend two steps with minimal assistance and no railings within seven visits to enter/exit home. • Patient will be modified independent to ascend/descend a flight of stairs, using one handrail and a step-to pattern, within seven visits to be able to reach the second floor of home.
Evaluate	4. In order to be successfully discharged home, the patient must be safe. Identification of initial cause of fall is essential. To follow up, understanding and implementation of education on fall prevention is also important. The patient's husband should also be present for the educational session for carryover at home. Education specific for the patient's husband should include information on proper body mechanics to assist the patient while also reducing his risk of injury. Functionally, the patient needs to be mobilizing at a modified independent to independent level and be able to don/doff the TLSO. The patient should be independent with bed mobility and transfers and modified independent for ambulation and stair negotiation. Two specific considerations need to be made around the patient's social support. Although the patient's husband is able to take 1 week off of work to assist the patient during her transition back to home, she will ultimately need to be self-sufficient. Planning needs to be given to (1) ascending/descending the two steps without a handrail to get in/out of the house and the flight of steps to the second floor where the bathroom is located and (2) consideration of getting rolling walker to/from the second floor. Depending on the patient's functional progress, it may be worthwhile to invest in a second rolling walker—one to keep on each floor—to maximize safety.

(Continued)

(Continued)

Bloom's Taxonomy Level	Case 14.B Answers
Analyze	5. A diagnosis of osteoporosis can be made based on bone mineral density (BMD) scoring from a DEXA scan or from the presence of a fragility fracture, defined as a fracture resulting from any fall from a standing height or less. The body should be able to sustain a fall from this height without fracture unless there is an underlying pathology decreasing the strength of the bone. The most common locations to see fragility fractures are the hip, spine, and the wrist.
Apply	6. Vitamin D helps stimulate the absorption of calcium from the gut. When this process is impaired, it can contribute to secondary hyperparathyroidism, drawing calcium from the bone and resulting in mineralization defects, and bone loss. Furthermore, patients with prolonged vitamin D deficiency can also experience muscle pain and weakness, contributing to falls and subsequent fragility fracture.
Understand	7. The patient is currently prescribed morphine for management of her back pain on an as-needed basis. Morphine is an opioid medication with potential side effects of nausea, vomiting, constipation, lightheadedness, dizziness, drowsiness, increased sweating, or dry mouth. Additionally, morphine is known to have addictive potential and should be used with caution. Consideration of risks and benefits to manage pain needs to be taken with this patient, as she is considered a fall risk. 8. A vertebral compression fracture occurs when significant compaction is placed on the weakened vertebral body causing a fracture and loss of height. Vertebral compression fractures can lead to severe and/or chronic pain, deformity, height loss, impaired ADLs, increased risk of pressure, pneumonia, and psychological distress. Although compression fractures are often the result of falls, they can happen with everyday activities such as twisting, bending, or sneezing. The cause of this patient's compression fracture was most likely her mechanical fall. Risk factors for the development of vertebral compression fractures include increased age, osteopenia, osteoporosis, a history of vertebral compression fractures, falls, inactivity, use of corticosteroids (or other medications), weight less than 117 lb, female sex, alcohol consumption, smoking, vitamin D deficiency, and depression. Based on this patient, her risk factors include increased age, osteoporosis, a history of falls, inactivity, being female, and vitamin D deficiency.
Remember	9. TLSO brace is a source of external support to protect the spine, limit spinal movements, and reduce pain. Use of a TLSO in nonoperative management of osteoporotic compression fracture can be controversial. Braces can contribute to the development of pressure injuries and subsequent soft-tissue infections. Use of bracing can also be associated with diminished pulmonary capacity and weakening of the axial musculature. Providers should consider the risks and benefits of bracing when developing a treatment plan for each individual patient. ▶ Fig. 14.5 10. Two balance assessments that would be appropriate to execute with this patient in the acute care setting are the Berg Balance Scale and Timed Up and Go (TUG). The Berg Balance Scale is a 14-item objective measure that assesses static balance and fall risk. The TUG assesses mobility, balance, walking ability, and fall risk in older adults. Both tests do not require an excessive amount of space, equipment, or time, and therefore are ideal to be implemented in the acute care setting. Upon completion of each test, the clinician can look at the total score to identify fall risk. Specific to the Berg Balance Scale, the clinician can look at individual item scores to identify specific tasks of concerns. Both components can guide physical therapy interventions.

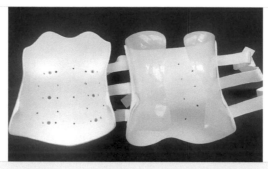

Fig. 14.5 The front and back of the TLSO.

Key points
1. Physical therapists, along with other members of the health care team (such as Gerontology), must work together to manage the patient's pain while also promoting function. It is imperative that this patient's function does not decline and that she does not develop hospital-acquired deconditioning. This could lead to further increase of health care resources (such as skilled nursing facility) and increased fall risk.
2. A TLSO brace is being used to protect the spine, limit spinal movements, and reduce pain. It is important for the patient and her husband to understand its value and how to properly don/doff it upon hospital discharge to prevent further spinal injury and an increase in pain.
3. Understanding what contributed to the initial fall and how to reduce fall risk begins in the acute care hospital. Additionally, because this patient has osteoporosis, physical therapists can also educate the patient and her husband on a home exercise program to help prevent disease progression.

General Information	
Case no.	14.C
Authors	Melissa Gilroy, DC, MSPAS, PA-C Sean Griech, PT, DPT, PhD, COMT, Board Certified Clinical Specialist in Orthopaedic Physical Therapy Julie M. Skrzat, PT, DPT, PhD, Board Certified Clinical Specialist in Cardiovascular & Pulmonary Physical Therapy
Diagnosis	Acute compression fracture of T12 due to osteoporosis
Setting	Home
Learner expectations	☑ Initial evaluation ☐ Re-evaluation ☐ Treatment session
Learner objectives	1. To understand that physical therapy treatment should be mindful of the whole patient, not just the chief complaint of back pain. 2. To understand the patient's risk of developing a subsequent vertebral fracture and how to prevent such from happening. 3. To perform a home evaluation that can help reduce fall risk and optimize safety.

Medical	
Chief complaint	Mid-back pain
History of present illness	The patient is a 72-year-old woman with history of osteoporosis who sustained a T12 compression fracture following a fall onto her backside 1 week ago. She presented to the hospital 2 days post fall and was admitted × 3 days for nonoperative management of her vertebral fracture. Pain was managed with oral medications and thoracolumbosacral orthosis (TLSO), and she was subsequently discharged home. Her osteoporosis and vitamin D deficiency are now being medically managed with daily vitamin D and calcium supplementation as well as alendronate, once weekly. She continues to use the TLSO brace for support and is tolerating this well. Physical Therapy consulted for fall risk assessment and safety.

(Continued)

(Continued)

Medical	
Past medical history	Hypertension: diagnosed in her 40s; hyperlipidemia: diagnosed in her 40s; osteoporosis: diagnosed age 65 years, DEXA scan (spine/hip) performed 7 years ago with a T-score of −2.5 and Z-score of −2; history of tobacco use: half pack per day since age 20 years; abstinent for 5 years; alcohol use: one to two glasses of wine each week.
Past surgical history	Total abdominal hysterectomy: age 45 years; no complications
Allergies	None
Medications	Lisinopril once daily, Atorvastatin once daily, Colace PRN, Acetaminophen PRN, Oxycodone/Acetaminophen PRN, Alendronate once weekly, Calcium carbonate daily, Vitamin D3 (cholecalciferol).
Precautions/orders	Activity as tolerated TLSO when out of bed

Social history	
Home setup	• Lives in a multilevel home with her husband who continues to work full time. • Two steps without handrail to enter. • No bathroom on the first floor. • Bedroom and bathroom are located on the second floor. • Flight of stairs + one handrail to the second floor.
Occupation	• Elementary school teacher, retired 5 years ago
Prior level of function	• Independent with functional mobility and activities of daily living (ADLs). • No regular exercise • (+) driver
Recreational activities	• Painting, sewing, scrapbooking • Enjoys visiting family and grandchildren

Pause points

Based on the above information, what are the priority:
• Diagnostic tests and measures?
• Outcome measures?
• Treatment interventions?

Physical Therapy Initial Examination		
Subjective		
"I don't want to fall again."		
Objective		
Vital signs	Pre-treatment	Post-treatment
Blood pressure (mmHg)	125/81	126/82
Heart rate (beats/min)	88	90
Respiratory rate (breaths/min)	14	14
Pulse oximetry on room air (SpO$_2$)	96	97
Pain	1/10 Low back	3/10 Low back
General	• Patient sitting in kitchen chair, wearing TLSO, rolling walker nearby. • Patient's husband present	

(Continued)

(Continued)

Physical Therapy Initial Examination		
Cardiovascular and pulmonary		• Normal rate • No adventitious heart or breath sounds
Gastrointestinal		• Opioid-related constipation, responding well to Colace, which she has been taking daily. She has also been weaning off opioid agents for pain management, taking only before bed.
Genitourinary		• Unremarkable
Musculoskeletal	Range of motion	• Bilateral upper extremity (BUE): grossly within functional range • Bilateral lower extremity (BLE): grossly within functional range
	Strength	• B shoulder flexion: 4/5 • B elbow flexion/extension: 4/5 • B wrist flexion/extension: 4/5 • B hip flexion: 4/5 • B knee flexion: 4/5 • B knee extension: 4/5 • B ankle dorsiflexion: 4/5 • Five Times Sit-to-Stand: 19 seconds
	Aerobic	• 2-Minute Walk Test: 140 m
Neurological	Balance	• Static sitting, unsupported: independent • Dynamic sitting, unsupported: modified independent with BUE support • Static standing, unsupported: independent • Dynamic standing, supported: supervision with rolling walker
	Cognition	• Alert and oriented × 4
	Coordination	• Finger to nose: intact bilaterally • Heel to shin: intact bilaterally
	Cranial nerves	• II–XII: intact
	Reflexes	• Patellar: 2 + bilaterally • Achilles: 2 + bilaterally • Babinski: negative bilaterally
	Sensation	• Intact and symmetric to light touch and deep pressure in BLE
	Tone	• Normal throughout BUEs and BLEs
	Other	• No clonus in BLE
Functional status		
Bed mobility		• Rolling either direction: independent using logroll technique. • Supine to/from sit: independent with increased time, head of bed flat, no bedrails, using logroll technique.
Transfers		• Sit to/from stand: independent • Stand pivot transfer: modified independent with rolling walker.
Ambulation		• Ambulated × 460 feet with supervision and rolling walker. • Gait deviations notable for decreased cadence, decreased B/L step length, improved upright posture due to pain relief and use of TLSO brace.
Stairs		• Ascend/descend flight of stairs + one rail with supervision, demonstrating step-to pattern.
Other		• Patient and her spouse bought a second rolling walker to allow one on each floor. • Patient is independent with donning/doffing TLSO brace.

(Continued)

(Continued)

Physical Therapy Initial Examination	
Abbreviated home evaluation	
Living room	• First floor • Carpeted floor • Sitting options include couch and recliner chair. • Coffee table creates narrow pathway. • TV has remote control access.
Kitchen	• First floor • Linoleum floor • One step between kitchen and living room. • Galley kitchen with high cabinets. • Mat by sink ▶ Fig. 14.6
Bedroom	• Second floor • Carpeted floor • Queen size bed • Narrow, dark hallway between bedroom and bathroom.
Bathroom	• Second floor • Tile floor • Vanity has two sinks. • Storage behind mirror and below vanity. • Tub shower • Bath mats by each sink and tub ▶ Fig. 14.7

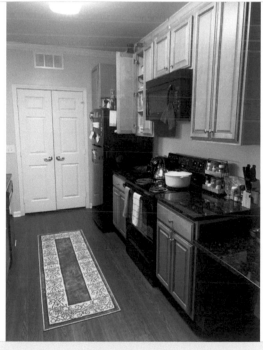

Fig. 14.6 The patient's kitchen, which was assessed during the home evaluation.

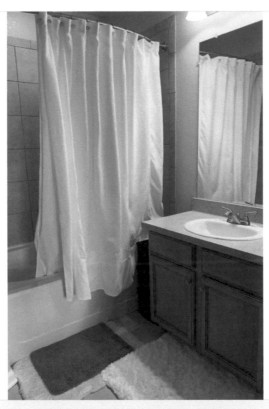

Fig. 14.7 The patient's bathroom, which was assessed during the home evaluation.

Assessment	
☑ Physical therapist's	*Assessment left blank for learner to develop.*
Goals	
Patient's	"To get back to how I was moving before."
Short term	1.
	Goals left blank for learner to develop.
	2.
Long term	1.
	Goals left blank for learner to develop.
	2.

Plan	
☐ Physician's ☑ Physical therapist's ☐ Other's	Will continue to see patient twice a week × 4 weeks. Treatment will include therapeutic exercise, gait training on level surfaces and stairs, balance interventions, and functional mobility training.

Bloom's Taxonomy Level	Case 14.C Questions
Create	1. Synthesizing the medical data and physical examination findings, develop an appropriate physical therapy assessment of the patient. 2. Develop two short-term physical therapy goals, including an appropriate timeframe. 3. Develop two long-term physical therapy goals, including an appropriate timeframe.

(Continued)

(Continued)

Bloom's Taxonomy Level	Case 14.C Questions
Evaluate	4. Based on the home evaluation, identify three modifications that can be made to reduce fall risk and improve safety. What further education can be provided?
Analyze	5. What class of medication is considered first line for managing the patient's osteoporosis in the long term and how does this medication work?
Apply	6. This patient is currently prescribed both acetaminophen and oxycodone/acetaminophen as needed, for management of her pain. What is a potential risk of combining these two medications?
Understand	7. What is the risk for this patient to develop a subsequent vertebral fracture?
	8. Interpret the patient's Five Times Sit-to-Stand results.
	9. Interpret the patient's 2-Minute Walk Test results.
Remember	10. State the purpose for the patient's home medications: lisinopril, atorvastatin, Colace, acetaminophen, oxycodone/acetaminophen, alendronate, calcium carbonate, vitamin D3 (cholecalciferol).

Bloom's Taxonomy Level	Case 14.C Answers
Create	1. The patient is a 72-year-old woman who is being evaluated in her home. She was recently admitted to the hospital for a T12 compression fracture, which was conservatively managed with pain medication and a TLSO brace. She presents with general deconditioning, as indicated by Vanual Muscle Test (MMT), Five Times Sit-to-Stand, and 2-Minute Walk Test. In addition, she has compromised balance, as she is currently using a rolling walker. She would benefit from continued physical therapy to improve strength, balance, and home safety. Will continue to follow and progress as tolerated.
	2. Short-term goals:
	• The patient will be independent with home exercise program within three visits to improve BLE muscular strength and endurance.
	• The patient will demonstrate two ways to modify her home within three visits to reduce fall risk.
	3. Long-term goals:
	• The patient will improve Five Times Sit-to-Stand to 12 seconds within seven visits to demonstrate an improvement in BLE strength.
	• The patient will improve 2-Minute Walk Test distance by 12 m within seven visits to demonstrate an improvement in endurance.
Evaluate	4. Three potential home modifications that can be made to reduce fall risk and improve safety are:
	• In the kitchen, move commonly used items to lower portion of shelves to reduce excessive neck extension (which could lead to posterior loss of balance) and need to use step stool.
	• In the upstairs hallway, place a night light in the hallway to illuminate the area in case the patient needs to use the bathroom in the middle of the night (as was the case of original injury).
	• In the kitchen and upstairs bathroom, either remove mats/rugs or ensure they are tacked down securely to prevent further tripping hazard.
Analyze	5. Oral bisphosphonates are generally considered first line for the management of osteoporosis in the postmenopausal woman and are effective in reducing risk of fragility fracture. Bisphosphonates work by inhibiting osteoclasts, cells that are responsible for bone resorption. They also appear to have effect in stimulating osteoblasts, cells responsible for the building up of bone.
Apply	6. Providing a patient with opioid and nonopioid options for pain management is a reasonable option to reduce the overall need for opioid use. Many agents will include a component of acetaminophen, which, when combined with over-the-counter acetaminophen-containing products, increases the risk of inadvertent acetaminophen overdose. Acetaminophen is one of the most common agents implicated in

(Continued)

(Continued)

Bloom's Taxonomy Level	Case 14.C Answers
	overdose and subsequent liver injury. It is important when prescribing these medications to discuss this risk with patients and assess their understanding. The recommended maximum daily dose of acetaminophen in the general population is 3 g, though some studies have shown safety up to 4 g daily.
Understand	7. Twenty percent (one in five) of women with a recent vertebral fracture in the setting of osteoporosis will sustain a new vertebral fracture within the next 12 months.
	8. The patient's current Five Times Sit-to-Stand time (19 seconds) is above the time for normal performance in community-dwelling older adults in her age group (12.6 seconds). Therefore, this patient is a fall risk.
	9. The patient's current 2-Minute Walk Test (140 m) is below the mean for retirement-dwelling older adults (150.4 m). This indicates that the patient has decreased endurance.
Remember	10. The purposes for the medications are as follows: • Lisinopril: angiotensin-converting enzyme (ACE) inhibitor, lowers blood pressure. • Atorvastatin: statin, treats hypercholesterolemia. • Colace: laxative, assists with opioid-related constipation. • Acetaminophen: analgesic, assists with pain control. • Oxycodone/acetaminophen: narcotic, assists with pain control. • Alendronate: treats and prevents osteoporosis. • Calcium carbonate: calcium dietary supplement. • Vitamin D3 (cholecalciferol): taken to increase intestinal absorption of calcium and phosphorous.

Key points
1. In addition to management of the patient's acute back pain, attention must be given to the initial cause of the back pain. In this case, it was the patient's fall. From there, the physical therapist must complete a comprehensive systems' review to best treat the patient.
2. It is important to acknowledge that 20% of women with a recent vertebral fracture in the setting of osteoporosis will sustain a new vertebral fracture within the next 12 months. Therefore, the physical therapist and the patient (and her family) should work together to optimize function and safety while reducing fall risk. An example of how this can be accomplished is through a comprehensive home exercise program.
3. Physical therapists are skilled in performing a thorough home evaluation to assist in reducing fall risk and optimizing safety. All rooms—internal and external—should be analyzed. Upon completion, suggestions and recommended modifications should be reviewed with the patient and her husband to understand what feasible changes are able to be implemented.

Suggested Readings

2-minute walk test. Available at: https://www.sralab.org/rehabilitation-measures/2-minute-walk-test. Accessed June 1, 2020

5 times sit to stand. Available at: https://www.sralab.org/rehabilitation-measures/five-times-sit-stand-test. Accessed June 1, 2020

American College of Neurological Surgeons. Vertebral compression fractures. Available at: https://www.aans.org/Patients/Neurosurgical-Conditions-and-Treatments/Vertebral-Compression-Fractures. Accessed June 1, 2020

American College of Sports Medicine. Available at: ACSM's Guidelines for Exercise Testing and Prescription. 10th ed. Baltimore, MD: Lippincott, Williams and Wilkins; 2017

Chang V, Holly LT. Bracing for thoracolumbar fractures. Neurosurg Focus. 2014; 37(1):E3

Cosman F, de Beur SJ, LeBoff MS, et al. Erratum to: Clinician's guide to prevention and treatment of osteoporosis. Osteoporos Int. 2015; 26(7):2045–2047

Crandall CJ, Newberry SJ, Diamant A, et al. Comparative effectiveness of pharmacologic treatments to prevent fractures: an updated systematic review. Ann Intern Med. 2014; 161(10):711–723

Goldstein CL, Chutkan NB, Choma TJ, Orr RD. Management of the elderly with vertebral compression fractures. Neurosurgery. 2015; 77 Suppl 4:S33–S45

Goodman CC, Fuller KS. Pathology: Implications for the Physical Therapist. 4th ed. St. Louis, MO: Saunders Elsevier; 2015

Johnell O, Oden A, Caulin F, Kanis JA. Acute and long-term increase in fracture risk after hospitalization for vertebral fracture. Osteoporos Int. 2001; 12(3):207–214

Kim HS, Strickland KJ, Mullen KA, Lebec MT. Physical therapy in the emergency department: a new opportunity for collaborative care. Am J Emerg Med. 2018; 36(8):1492–1496

Lebec MT, Jogodka CE. The physical therapist as a musculoskeletal specialist in the emergency department. J Orthop Sports Phys Ther. 2009; 39(3):221–229

Lips P, van Schoor NM. The effect of vitamin D on bone and osteoporosis. Best Pract Res Clin Endocrinol Metab. 2011; 25(4): 585–591

Longo UG, Loppini M, Denaro L, Maffulli N, Denaro V. Osteoporotic vertebral fractures: current concepts of conservative care. Br Med Bull. 2012; 102(1):171–189

McCarthy J, Davis A. Diagnosis and management of vertebral compression fractures. Am Fam Physician. 2016; 94(1):44–50

Newman M, Minns Lowe C, Barker K. Spinal orthoses for vertebral osteoporosis and osteoporotic vertebral fracture: a systematic review. Arch Phys Med Rehabil. 2016; 97(6):1013–1025

Plotkin LI, Lezcano V, Thostenson J, Weinstein RS, Manolagas SC, Bellido T. Connexin 43 is required for the anti-apoptotic effect of bisphosphonates on osteocytes and osteoblasts in vivo. J Bone Miner Res. 2008; 23(11):1712–1721

Prescott K, Stratton R, Freyer A, Hall I, Le Jeune I. Detailed analyses of self-poisoning episodes presenting to a large regional teaching hospital in the UK. Br J Clin Pharmacol. 2009; 68(2): 260–268

Rodan GA, Fleisch HA. Bisphosphonates: mechanisms of action. J Clin Invest. 1996; 97(12):2692–2696

Schumacher MA, Basbaum AI, Naidu RK. Opioid agonists & antagonists. In: Kertzung BG, ed. Basic and Clinical Pharmacology. 14th ed. New York, NY: McGraw Hill Education; 2018:559–565

Timed up and go. Available at: https://www.sralab.org/rehabilitation-measures/timed-and-go. Accessed June 1, 2020

Varacallo M, Seaman TJ, Jandu JS, Pizzutillo P. Osteopenia. Treasure Island, FL: StatPearls Publishing LLC; 2020

Wark JD, Westmore A. Studies of drugs and other measures to prevent and treat osteoporosis; a brief guide. Available at: https://www.who.int/ageing/publications/noncommunicable/alc_osteoporosis_brief.pdf?ua=1. Accessed June 1, 2020

Wood KB, Li W, Lebl DR, Ploumis A. Management of thoracolumbar spine fractures. Spine J. 2014; 14(1):145–164

15 Pneumonia

General Information	
Case no.	15.A Pneumonia
Author(s)	Julie M. Skrzat, PT, DPT, PhD, Board Certified Clinical Specialist in Cardiovascular & Pulmonary Physical Therapy Aaron S. Frey, DO
Diagnosis	Pneumonia with chronic obstructive pulmonary disease (COPD)
Setting	Emergency department, with transfer to the Intensive Care Unit
Learner expectations	☑ Initial evaluation ☐ Re-evaluation ☐ Treatment session
Learner objectives	1. Explain the pathophysiology of the patient's diagnosis. 2. Relate the pathophysiology and progression of pathology from chronic cardiovascular or pulmonary disorders to the clinical manifestations and activity/participation limitations seen in physical therapy practice. 3. Select, implement, and interpret physical therapy interventions based on the medical examination findings. 4. Develop an understanding of medical management and how it influences physical therapy plan of care.

Medical	
Chief complaint	Shortness of breath (SOB), productive cough
History of present illness	The patient is a 70-year-old man who presented to the emergency department yesterday with reports of a productive cough of thick yellow-greenish sputum and increasing dyspnea × 2 weeks. He denies nausea, vomiting, and diarrhea. He initially presented to the emergency department 1 week ago with similar complaints. He was diagnosed with a COPD exacerbation, prescribed azithromycin, and discharged home. However, after 3 days, his symptoms did not resolve, bringing him back to the emergency department today.
Past medical history	COPD on continuous 2L/min O_2 via nasal cannula at home, hypertension, hypercholesterolemia, atrial fibrillation, smoker × 50 years (1 pack/d)—quit 3 years ago
Past surgical history	Left knee replacement 3 years ago
Allergies	Latex
Medications	Lisinopril, Atorvastatin, Salmeterol, Albuterol inhaler, Warfarin, Metoprolol
Precautions/orders	Activity as tolerated

Social history	
Home setup	• Resides in a multilevel home with wife. • Three steps + one handrail to enter. • Half bath on the first floor. • Bedroom and bathroom are located on the second floor. • Flight of stairs + one handrail to the second floor.
Occupation	• Corporate lawyer for 42 years, retired 5 years ago.
Prior level of function	• Independent with functional mobility and activities of daily living (ADLs). • Modified independent for stairs, but required increased time. • (+) driver
Recreational activities	• Primarily watching TV and reading. • Used to enjoy gardening but now it requires too much energy, leaving him short of breath.

Hospital Day 0: Emergency Department		
Vital signs	Presentation	Corrected
Blood pressure (mmHg)	106/68	86/50
Heart rate (beats/min)	▶ Fig. 15.1	98
Respiratory rate (breaths/min)	36	22
Pulse oximetry (SpO$_2$)	84% 2L/min O$_2$ via nasal cannula	98% on BiPap
Temperature (°F)	101.2	100.1

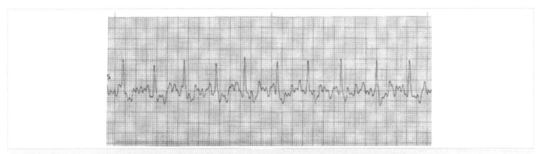

Fig. 15.1 The patient's electrocardiogram upon his arrival to the emergency department.

Imaging/diagnostic test	Hospital day 0: emergency department	Hospital day 1: intensive care unit
Chest X-ray	1. Flattening of diaphragm 2. Alveolar infiltrates in right lower lobe ▶ Fig. 15.2	1. Mild to moderate right pneumothorax with persistent right lower lobe infiltrates.
Ultrasound	1. No pericardial effusion	Not reordered
Sputum sample	1. Gram positive for *Streptococcus*	
Blood cultures	1. Negative	
Urine analysis	1. Negative	

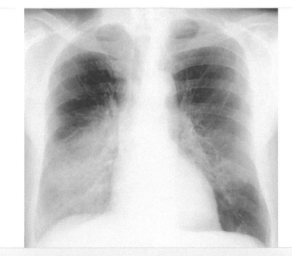

Fig. 15.2 The patient's chest x-ray upon his arrival to the emergency department. (Adapted from Krukemeyer M, ed. Cardiology, angiology, pulmonology. In: Introductory Guide to Medical Training: From Basic Sciences to Medical Specialties. 1st ed. New York, Thieme; 2015.)

Medical management	Hospital day 0: emergency department	Hospital day 1: intensive care unit
Medications	1. Intravenous (IV) fluids 2. Ceftriaxone IV 3. Methylprednisolone 60 mg IV 4. Duonebs, four times a day 5. Albuterol inhaler, every 2 hours PRN 6. Norepinephrine infusion to maintain mean arterial pressure (MAP) > 65 mmHg. 7. Acetaminophen 1,000 mg	1. Continued per medical plan of care
Respiratory	1. Placed on BiPap 2. Chest physical therapy/airway clearance techniques	1. Continued per medical plan of care
Procedures	1. Arterial line placed 2. Central line placed	1. Chest tube placed ▶ Fig. 15.3

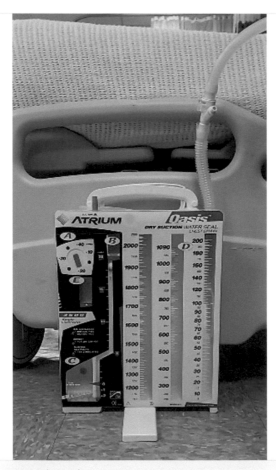

Fig. 15.3 An example of a patient's chest tube.

Lab		Reference range	Hospital day 0: emergency department	Hospital day 1: intensive care unit
Arterial blood gas	pH	7.35–7.45	7.32	7.37
	PaCO$_2$	37–43 mmHg	78	49
	PaO$_2$	80–95 mmHg	76	92
	HCO$_3^-$	20–30 mmol/L	23	25
Complete blood count	white blood cell	5.0–10.0 × 10^9/L	19.6	15.3
	Hemoglobin	14–17.4 g/dL	10.8	11.1
	Hematocrit	42–52%	36.5	38.2
	Red blood cell	4.1–5.3 million/mm^3	3.5	3.7
	Platelet	140,000–400,000/μL	115	240
Electrolytes	Calcium	8.6–10.3 mg/dL	8.9	9.1
	Chloride	98–108 mEq/L	98	100
	Magnesium	1.2–1.9 mEq/L	1.8	1.9
	Phosphate	2.3–4.1 mg/dL	2.9	2.8
	Potassium	3.7–5.1 mEq/L	4.2	4.5
	Sodium	134–142 mEq/L	141	140
Other	Cholesterol	<200 mg/dL	240	
	High-density lipoprotein (HDL)	≥35 mg/dL	67	
	Low-density lipoprotein (LDL)	65–180 mg/dL	198	Not reordered
	Triglycerides	<150 mg/dL	210	
	Blood urea nitrogen (BUN)	7–20 mg/dL	24	
	Creatinine	0.5–1.4 mg/dL	1.6	1.6
	Glucose	60–110 mg/dL	188	176
	brain natriuretic peptide (BNP)	<100 pg/mL	98	
	D-dimer	<400 ng/mL	58	Not reordered
	International normalized ratio (INR)	0.8–1.2	2.1	2.0
	Lactate	<2 mmol	3.0	1.2
	Troponin – 1	<0.03 ng/mL	0.02	
	Troponin – 2		0.01	Not reordered
	Troponin – 3		0.02	

Pause points

Based on the above information, what are the priorities?
- Diagnostic tests and measures?
- Outcome measures?
- Treatment interventions?

Hospital Day 2, Medical Ward: Physical Therapy Examination				
Subjective				
"It's so hard to breathe just sitting here, but I don't want to lose my ability to move."				
Objective				
Vital signs	Pre-treatment			Post-treatment
	Supine	Sitting	Standing	Sitting
Blood pressure (mmHg)	101/73	100/75	99/74	105/79
Heart rate (beats/min)	117	120	124	125
Respiratory rate (breaths/min)	27	30	32	31
Pulse oximetry on 4 L NC (SpO$_2$)	89%	90%	84%	91%
Borg scale	5/10 SOB			2/10 SOB, improved with upright posture
Pain	4/10, right flank			5/10, right flank
General	• Patient in bed, Fowler's position, (+) accessory muscle breathing • Lines notable for telemetry, NC, central line, arterial line, urinary catheter, chest tube			
Cardiovascular and pulmonary	• Auscultation: bilateral scattered rhonchi and bronchial breath sounds • Electrocardiography: atrial fibrillation with rapid ventricular response • Pulses: 2 + bilateral dorsalis pedis and posterior tibialis			
Gastrointestinal	• Abdomen slightly distended			
Genitourinary	• (+) urinary catheter			
Musculoskeletal	Range of motion	• Bilateral upper extremity (BUE): within functional range • Bilateral lower extremity (BLE): within functional range		
	Strength	• B shoulder flexion: 4/5 • B elbow flexion: 4/5 • B wrist extension: 4/5 • B hip flexion: 3 + /5 • B knee extension: 4/5 • B ankle dorsiflexion: 5/5 • Five Times Sit-to-Stand Test: 14.5 seconds		
	Aerobic	• Unable to perform standardized test at this time.		
	Flexibility	• Tight pectoralis major and minor, as demonstrated by rounded shoulder posture. • Suspect tight hip flexors due to reports of prolonged sitting at home: not tested due to inability to lie flat in side lying or prone.		
Neurological	Balance	• Static unsupported sitting: minimal assistance • Static standing: minimal assistance with rolling walker • Dynamic standing: minimal assistance with rolling walker		
	Cognition	• Alert and oriented × 4		
	Coordination	• Finger–to–nose: intact BUE		
	Cranial nerves	• Intact		
	Reflexes	• Patellar: 2 + bilaterally		
	Sensation	• Intact to light tough throughout BUE and BLE.		
	Tone	• Normal throughout BUE and BLE.		
	Other	• N/A		
Functional status				
Bed mobility	• Supine to sit: moderate assistance with head of bed elevated.			
Transfers	• Sit to/from stand: minimal assistance with rolling walker.			
Ambulation	• Ambulated 3 feet from bed to chair with minimal assistance and rolling walker.			
Stairs	• N/A			

Assessment	
☑ Physical therapist's	*Assessment left blank for learner to develop.*
Goals	
Patient's	"I want to get back home safely."
Short term	1. *Goals left blank for learner to develop.* 2.
Long term	1. *Goals left blank for learner to develop.* 2.

Plan	
☑ Physical therapist's	Will continue to see patient three to five times a week. Will continue to progress functional mobility as tolerated through strengthening and endurance interventions. Introduce various airway clearance techniques, including chest physical therapy, acapella, and huffing.

Bloom's Taxonomy Level	Case 15.A Questions
Create	1. Synthesizing the medical data and physical examination findings, develop an appropriate physical therapy assessment of the patient. 2. Develop two short-term physical therapy goals, including an appropriate timeframe. 3. Develop two long-term physical therapy goals, including an appropriate timeframe.
Evaluate	4. Explain the physical therapy findings and expected discharge disposition to the resident physician.
Analyze	5. Compare how pulmonary function tests would differentiate between a patient with obstructive lung disease and a patient with restrictive lung disease. 6. What is the rate and rhythm of the electrocardiogram (ECG) on the patient's day of admission?
Apply	7. Design and implement two interventions to improve energy conservation. 8. Design and implement two interventions—one stretching and one strengthening—to improve posture.
Understand	9. Interpret day 0's arterial blood gas. Based on the interpretation and assuming it is not compensated, what signs and symptoms would the physical therapist expect the patient to exhibit? 10. Does this patient have obstructive, restrictive, or both lung diseases?
Remember	11. What are precautions when mobilizing a patient with a chest tube? 12. What is the ratio for diaphragmatic breathing? 13. What is a pneumothorax? 14. Why does the patient's chest X-ray reveal a flattened diaphragm?

Bloom's Taxonomy Level	Case 15.A Answers
Create	1. The patient is a 70-year-old man who presented to the hospital with progressive SOB and productive cough. He was diagnosed with an acute exacerbation of COPD and pneumonia, with his course complicated by a right pneumothorax requiring insertion of a chest tube. From a mobility perspective, he demonstrates generalized deconditioning, with proximal muscle fatigue. This is likely due to decreased oxygenation (as shown through lower SpO_2 with movement) from pulmonary impairments and prolonged use of corticosteroids. As a result, he is unable to complete functional mobility independently. He would benefit from continued physical therapy to improve posture, endurance, strength, and airway clearance to maximize functional mobility and safety. Will continue to follow.

(Continued)

(Continued)

Bloom's Taxonomy Level	Case 15.A Answers
	2. Short-term goals: • Patient will perform supine to/from sit with head of bed flat and supervision to get in and out of bed at home within 4 days. • Patient will ambulate × 50 feet with rolling walker and supervision to navigate within home within 4 days. 3. Long-term goals: • Patient will ascend/descend 13 steps with a single handrail and supervision to get to the second floor bedroom within 7 days. • Patient will verbalize and implement two energy conservation techniques independently to assist in management of SOB within 7 days.
Evaluate	4. During the physical therapist's initial evaluation, the patient demonstrated a decrease in oxygenation with mobility. This is likely due prolonged supine position. Manual muscle testing revealed generalized weakness throughout all major muscle groups; however, it is particularly noticeable in bilateral hips. This is likely due to continued corticosteroid use. As a result of the patient's cardiac and pulmonary status, which is ultimately impairing circulation of oxygenated blood, the patient's muscles have decreased endurance and strength. Therefore, the patient requires minimal assistance for functional mobility. With improvement of pulmonary infections and continued inpatient physical therapy, it is anticipated that the patient will return to his baseline functional status (which was low functioning) and therefore will likely be able to return home with assistance and home physical therapy. This is, however, dependent on his ability to climb stairs since he has three steps to enter.
Analyze	5. Pulmonary Function Tests for obstructive and restrictive lung diseases differentiate as follows: Obstructive: decreased forced expiratory volume (FEV1), normal forced vital capacity (FVC). Restrictive: decreased FEV1, decreased FVC. 6. The ECG rate is ~100 beats per minute with a rhythm of atrial fibrillation.
Apply	7. Two interventions to improve energy conservation are: • The patient will use the Borg Dyspnea Scale to measure his SOB. When feeling SOB, the patient can implement diaphragmatic breathing. • The patient will plan his day's activities and incorporate rest break strategically. 8. Because this patient has COPD, he likely has a barrel chest, with tightened pectoralis major and pectoralis minor and elongated shoulder retractors. Therefore, two potential interventions are: • Stretching: roll a towel long way and place in the center of the bed. With the head of the bed flat, have the patient lie on the bed, with their spine parallel to towel. This should allow a stretch to the anterior chest. If the patient does not feel a stretch, build up the roll with more towels. • Strengthening: shoulder retractions. Depending on the patient's strength, this can be done with no weights (and ideally should be done first to ensure proper form), free weights, or theraband (tie to a stable surface).
Understand	9. On day 0, the patient demonstrates respiratory acidosis. This is shown by a decreased pH and increased carbon dioxide. It is not compensated for, as shown through a normal bicarb. Signs and symptoms the patient may display include restlessness, disorientation, confusion, headache, dyspnea, and/or cyanosis. 10. The patient has a combination of obstructive and restrictive diseases. COPD is obstructive diseases and the pneumonia and pneumothorax are restrictive diseases.
Remember	11. Precautions for mobilizing with the chest tube include keeping the chest tube below the level of insertion to prevent backflow into the patient's thorax cavity. 12. The ratio for diaphragmatic breathing is 1 second for inhalation and 2 seconds for exhalation. 13. A pneumothorax is an accumulation of air in the pleural cavity. It is caused by a defect in the visceral pleura or chest wall, and results in collapse of the lung on the affected side. As a result, it acts a restrictive disease. 14. The patient's diaphragm is flattened due to progressive COPD. With COPD, there is air trapping, causing the diaphragm to descend to accommodate the extra air in the lungs.

Key points
1. It is important for the physical therapist to synthesize all medical data (i.e., imaging, lab values, etc.) to understand how the patient's pathophysiology can affect functional status.
2. Consider the influence of long-term chronic disease management (i.e., corticosteroids) and how it can influence functional status.
3. Don't underestimate how what may seem like outpatient interventions can be incorporated into an inpatient environment.

General Information	
Case no.	15.B
Authors	Julie M. Skrzat, PT, DPT, PhD, Board Certified Clinical Specialist in Cardiovascular & Pulmonary Physical Therapy Sean F. Griech, PT, DPT, PhD, COMT, Board Certified Clinical Specialist in Orthopaedic Physical Therapy
Diagnosis	Generalized deconditioning
Setting	Home
Learner expectations	☑ Initial evaluation ☐ Re-evaluation ☐ Treatment session
Learner objectives	1. List potential environmental factors that may provide difficulty to the patient 2. Identify appropriate outcome measures based on the objective data provided for use in the home environment 3. Describe psychosocial implications of the patient's condition and implementation strategies for improving his quality of life 4. Develop a home exercise program for the home setting based on the patient's body structure and impairments to optimize his participation and quality of life

Medical	
Chief complaint	Generalized deconditioning, "easily short of breath."
History of present illness	Patient is a 70-year-old man who was recently hospitalized for 8 days with a diagnosis of right lower lobe pneumonia. Hospital course notable for a 5-day ICU stay. Medical management included intravenous (IV) antibiotics, IV corticosteroids, nebulizer treatments, BiPap, and right chest tube placement for pneumothorax. He was discharged home 3 days ago.
Past medical history	Chronic obstructive pulmonary disease (COPD) on 2L/min O_2 via nasal cannula at home, hypertension, hypercholesterolemia, atrial fibrillation, smoker × 50 years (1 pack/d)—quit 3 years ago.
Past surgical history	Left knee replacement 3 years ago
Allergies	Latex
Medications	Lisinopril, Atorvastatin, Salmeterol, Albuterol inhaler, Warfarin, Metoprolol
Precautions/orders	Activity as tolerated

Social history	
Home setup	• Resides in a multilevel home with wife. • Three steps + one handrail to enter. • Half bath is on the first floor. • Bedroom and bathroom are located on the second floor. • Flight of stairs + one handrail to the second floor.
Occupation	• Corporate lawyer for 42 years, retired 5 years ago.

(Continued)

(Continued)

Social history	
Prior level of function	• Prior to hospitalization: 　○ independent with ambulation. 　○ used to ambulate × 1 city block to church. 　○ modified independent for stairs, but required increased time. 　○ (+) driver
Recreational activities	• Primarily watching TV and reading. • Used to enjoy gardening but now it requires too much energy, causing him shortness of breath (SOB).

Pause points
Based on the above information, what are the priorities? • Diagnostic tests and measures? • Outcome measures? • Treatment interventions?

Physical Therapy Examination		
Subjective		
"That hospitalization took it out of me. I spent so much time in bed. I want to get stronger."		
Objective		
Vital signs	Pre-treatment	Post-treatment
Blood pressure (mmHg)	110/81	115/83
Heart rate (beats/min)	97	109
Respiratory rate (breaths/min)	15	21
Pulse oximetry on 2L/min O_2 via nasal cannula (SpO_2)	92%	90%
Borg scale	2/10 SOB	3/10 SOB
Pain	0–1/10, R flank where the chest tube was located	2/10, mid-thoracic region. Patient reports that this is due to deep breathing.
General	• Patient sitting with NC, portable oxygen tank, and rolling walker.	
Cardiovascular and pulmonary	• Breathing pattern: shallow, (+) accessory muscle breathing • Pulses: 2 + left radial: regularly irregular 2 + bilateral dorsalis pedis and posterior tibialis	
Gastrointestinal	• Reports constipation, but the patient attributes this to an increase in medication.	
Genitourinary	• Mild amounts of urinary leakage with coughing and sneezing, unable to quantify frequency. The patient attributes this to recent urinary catheter.	
Musculoskeletal	Range of motion	• bilateral upper extremity (BUE): within functional limits • bilateral lower extremity (BLE): within functional limits
	Strength	• B shoulder flexion: 4/5 • B elbow flexion: 4/5 • B wrist extension: 4/5 • B hip flexion: 3 + /5 • B knee extension: 3 + /5 • B ankle dorsiflexion: 5/5 • Five Times Sit-to-Stand Test: 12.0 seconds
	Aerobic	• 2-Minute Walk Test (2MWT): 350 feet. After completion, the patient reports increased SOB and demonstrates the following posture:

(Continued)

(Continued)

Physical Therapy Examination		
		▶ Fig. 15.4 Patient initially took NC off due to reports of "suffocating"; however, he was encouraged to put on and take deep, diaphragmatic breaths.
	Flexibility	• Trunk: tight pectoralis major and minor • BLE: tight hip flexors, hamstrings
	Other	• N/A
Neurological	Balance	• Timed Up and Go (TUG): 22 seconds
	Cognition	• Alert and oriented ×4
	Coordination	• Intact finger-to-nose bilaterally
	Cranial nerves	• Intact
	Reflexes	• Popliteal: 2+bilaterally
	Sensation	• Intact to light touch through BLUE
	Tone	• Normal
	Other	• N/A
Functional status		
Bed mobility	• Supine to sit: independent	
Transfers	• Sit to/from stand: independent	
Ambulation	• Ambulated household distances with rolling walker independently. Gait deviations notable for forward lead, decreased bilateral step length, decreased cadence.	
Stairs	• Ascend/descend flight of stairs + one rail with modified independence. • Stair deviations: placed bilateral hands on single handrail; occasionally "pulls" self up steps, especially toward top of flight; demonstrated step to pattern; required increased time.	

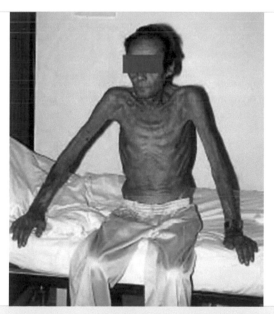

Fig. 15.4 An example of the tripod position the patient displayed upon completing the 2MWT (Adapted from Chronic obstructive pulmonary diseases. In: Steffers G, Credner S, ed. General Pathology and Internal Medicine for Physical Therapists. 1st ed. Stuttgart: Thieme; 2012.)

Assessment	
☑ Physical therapist's	*Assessment left blank for learner to develop*
Goals	
Patient's	"I want to be able to go up and down the steps without such difficulty."
Short term	1.
	Goals left blank for learner to develop.
	2.
Long term	1.
	Goals left blank for learner to develop.
	2.

Plan	
☑ Physical therapist's	Will continue to see the patient twice a week × 3 weeks. Treatment will include therapeutic exercise (lower extremity strengthening, aerobic conditioning), gait training on level surfaces and stairs, and energy conservation strategies.

Bloom's Taxonomy Level	Case 15.B Questions
Create	1. Synthesizing the medical data and physical examination findings, develop an appropriate assessment of the patient. 2. Develop two short-term physical therapy goals, including an appropriate timeframe. 3. Develop two long-term physical therapy goals, including an appropriate timeframe. 4. Develop a home exercise program, including interventions and exercise prescription, and identify how to hold the patient accountable.
Evaluate	5. Determine two referrals to other members of the health care team that this patient could potentially benefit from seeing.
Analyze	6. Based on the 2MWT results, is the patient above, at, or below the mean for individuals with COPD? 7. After completion of the 2MWT, why does the patient demonstrate a tripod position? 8. What is the appropriate interpretation of the TUG? Is the patient at risk of falling?
Apply	9. Design and implement two interventions to improve the patient's balance. 10. How should a physical therapist educate the patient to monitor his or her own vitals in the home environment?
Understand	11. Why does the patient report urinary incontinence with coughing and/or sneezing?
Remember	12. What are the potential side effects of prolonged corticosteroids? 13. What are clinical signs and symptoms to monitor for that would indicate a recurrent pulmonary infection?

Bloom's Taxonomy Level	Case 15.B Answers
Create	1. The patient is a 70-year-old man who was recently hospitalized × 8 days for an acute exacerbation of COPD and pneumonia. Hospital course was complicated by a pneumothorax requiring chest tube insertion. He has since been discharged home with home physical therapy. Upon initial evaluation, he demonstrates generalized decreased strength; however, it is most notable in bilateral hip flexors and knee extensors. He also demonstrates decreased endurance and fall risk, as shown through 2MWT and TUG, respectively. These deficits are further exemplified during gait and stair negotiation. He would benefit from continued physical therapy to improve strength, balance, and endurance, as well as posture to maximize functional mobility and safety. Will continue to follow. 2. Short-term goals: • The patient will ascend/descend flight of steps with a Borg score of < 2/10 within 4 days to be able to get to his second floor bedroom safely. • The patient will be independent with a BLE strength home exercise program within 4 days to maximize functional mobility.

(Continued)

(Continued)

Bloom's Taxonomy Level	Case 15.B Answers
	3. Long-term goals: • The patient will increase his 2MWT by 40 feet within 1 week to improve his endurance. • The patient will perform two bouts of 15 min/d on a restorator within 1 week to improve cardiovascular and BLE endurance. 4. The following is an example of a potential home exercise program for the home setting. Only three to five exercises should be selected to ensure compliance. *Strengthening*: > 2 d/week. Light intensity: 40–50% of one repetition maximum (1 RM). Moderate intensity: 60–70% of 1 RM (5–6 on a scale of 0–10). • Shoulder retractions, 3 × 10. • Mini-squats, hip abduction/adduction, hip flexion/extension with external support, 3 × 10. *Aerobic training*: ~3–5 times a week. Light intensity: 30 to < 40% of peak work rates. Vigorous intensity: 60–80% of peak work rates. • Walking, minimum of 10 minutes, at least 3 bouts a day. • Restorator, minimum of 10 minutes, at least 3 bouts a day. *Stretching*: • Anterior chest muscles with towel rolls, 30- to 60-second holds, × 3. To hold the patient accountable, a journal or tracking sheet can be developed. After meeting a standard, a reward of meaning to the patient can be provided.
Evaluate	5. Two referrals to other members of the health care team that this patient could potentially benefit from seeing are: • a physical therapist who specializes in pelvic floor, especially if his urinary incontinence continues. • an occupational therapist to assist with activities of daily living (ADLs) and instrumental ADLs (iADLs), being that he is deconditioned from hospitalization.
Analyze	6. The patient's current 2MWT (350 feet) is below the mean for individuals with COPD (492 feet or 150 meters). This indicates that the patient has decreased endurance. 7. After completing the 2MWT, the patient demonstrates a tripoding position due SOB. The patient's trunk musculature acts as trunk stabilizers and respiratory muscles. Because these muscles are working so hard to breath and ventilate, his posture is compromised, and he uses his upper extremities to stabilize his trunk. 8. The patient completed the TUG in 22 seconds. The cutoff score for community-dwelling adults is 13.5 seconds. This score indicates that the patient is at an increased risk for falls.
Apply	9. Two potential balance interventions include: • Using a countertop/kitchen table as external support, the patient can practice single-limb activities. This can assist with lower extremity strengthening, avoidance of obstacles around the home, and progressing functional mobility. • Walking while dual tasking. This would help improve his ability balance in various environments. 10. To measure the patient's heart rate, he can use his radial artery. Upon feeling the first pulsation, he should count beginning at zero. He should count the number of pulses for a minimum of 30 seconds and multiply × 2. However, because he does have a history of atrial fibrillation, it is advised he counts his pulse for the entire 60 seconds. To measure pulse oximetry, he can obtain a portable pulse oximetry monitor. To measure intensity of exercise, the patient should be using a Borg Scale.
Understand	11. The patient reports urinary incontinence with coughing and/or sneezing due to increased abdominal pressure, which is being exerted on the pelvic floor.
Remember	12. Potential side effects of corticosteroids include osteoporosis, osteonecrosis, increased risk of fractures, muscle weakness, and myopathy. It is important for physical therapists to keep these side effects in mind during interventions to prevent further damage. 13. Clinical signs and symptoms that could indicate a return of infection include (but are not limited to) fever, chills, fatigue, or malaise.

Key points	
1. When able, track patient's progression across settings with similar outcome measures.	
2. Develop an appropriate home exercise program—that has appropriate frequency, intensity, time, and type (FITT) parameters, targets long-term goals, and is specific to the setting—with a reward that is patient specific.	
3. Consider what airway clearance interventions can be implemented to optimize ventilation and, ultimately, improve oxygenation and activity tolerance.	

General Information	
Case no.	15.C
Authors	Julie M. Skrzat, PT, DPT, PhD, Board Certified Clinical Specialist in Cardiovascular & Pulmonary Physical Therapy Sean F. Griech, PT, DPT, PhD, COMT, Board Certified Clinical Specialist in Orthopaedic Physical Therapy
Diagnosis	Generalized deconditioning
Setting	Outpatient clinic
Learner expectations	☑ Initial evaluation ☐ Re-evaluation ☐ Treatment session
Learner objectives	1. Identify appropriate outcome measures based on the objective data provided for use in the outpatient clinic. 2. Correlate the impact of cardiovascular and pulmonary disorders and the effectiveness of pelvic floor functioning. 3. Develop a home exercise program for the outpatient setting based on the patient's body structure and impairments to optimize his participation and quality of life.

Medical	
Chief complaint	Generalized deconditioning, easily short of breath
History of present illness	The patient is a 70-year-old man who presents to an outpatient clinic with generalized deconditioning. Of note, he was recently hospitalized for right lower lobe pneumonia. The hospital course was notable for an 8-day stay, with 5 days spent in the ICU. Medical management included intravenous (IV) antibiotics, IV corticosteroids, nebulizer treatments, BiPap, and chest tube placement for pneumothorax. He was discharged home, where he received six home physical therapy sessions.
Past medical history	Chronic obstructive pulmonary disease (COPD) on 2L/min O_2 via nasal cannula at home, hypertension, hypercholesterolemia, atrial fibrillation, smoker×50 years (1 pack/d)—quit 3 years ago.
Past surgical history	Left knee replacement 3 years ago.
Allergies	Latex
Medications	Lisinopril, Atorvastatin, Salmeterol, Albuterol inhaler, Warfarin, Metoprolol
Precautions/orders	Activity as tolerated

Social history	
Home setup	• Resides in a multilevel home with wife. • Three steps + one handrail to enter. • Half bath is on the first floor. • Bedroom and bathroom are located on the second floor. • Flight of stairs + one handrail to the second floor.
Occupation	• Corporate lawyer for 42 years, retired 5 years ago.
Prior level of function	Currently: • independent with bed mobility, transfers, activities of daily living (ADLs). • modified independent for ambulation with use of rolling walker. • (–) driver

(Continued)

(Continued)

Social history	
	Prior to hospitalization: • independent with ambulation. • used to ambulate × 1 city block to church. • modified independent for stairs, but required increased time. • (+) driver
Recreational activities	• Primarily watching TV and reading. • Used to enjoy gardening, but now it requires too much energy, leaving him short of breath.

Pause points
Based on the above information, what are the priorities? • Diagnostic tests and measures? • Outcome measures? • Treatment interventions?

Physical Therapy Examination		
Subjective		
"The therapist at home really helped me so I can now go up and down steps without getting short of breath. I want to get continue to get strong."		
Objective		
Vital signs	Pre-treatment	Post-treatment
Blood pressure (mmHg)	110/81	115/83
Heart rate (beats/min)	97	109
Respiratory rate (breaths/min)	15	21
Pulse oximetry on 3 L NC (SpO_2)	92%	90%
Borg scale	2/10 shortness of breath (SOB)	3/10 SOB
Pain	0/10	2/10, mid-thoracic region. Patient reports this is due to deep breathing.
General	• Patient sitting in waiting room with NC, portable oxygen tank, and rolling walker Patient's wife accompanied him to visit.	
Cardiovascular and pulmonary	• Breathing pattern: shallow, (+) accessory muscle breathing • Pulses: 2 + left radial: regularly irregular 2 + bilateral dorsalis pedis and posterior tibialis	
Gastrointestinal	• Intermittent constipation with occasional strain and pain during defecation.	
Genitourinary	• Mild amounts of urinary leakage with coughing and sneezing, ~50% of the time.	
Musculoskeletal	Range of motion	• Bilateral upper extremity (BUE): ↓↓ shoulder flexion and abduction • Bilateral lower extremity (BLE): ↓↓ hip extension, knee extension
	Strength	• B shoulder flexion: 4/5 • B elbow flexion: 4/5 • B wrist extension: 4/5 • B hip flexion: 4/5 • B knee extension: 4/5 • B ankle dorsiflexion: 5/5

(Continued)

(Continued)

Physical Therapy Examination		
	Aerobic	• 6-Minute Walk Test: 1182 feet
	Flexibility	• Trunk: tight pectoralis major and minor • BLE: tight hip flexors, hamstrings
	Other	• N/A
Neurological	Balance	• Five Times Sit-to-Stand Test: 13.6 seconds • Gait speed assessment: 0.8 m/s
	Cognition	• Alert and oriented × 4
	Coordination	• Intact finger to nose bilaterally
	Cranial nerves	• Intact
	Reflexes	• Popliteal: normal bilaterally
	Sensation	• Intact to light touch
	Tone	• Normal
	Other	• N/A
Functional status		
Bed mobility	• Supine to sit: independent	
Transfers	• Sit to/from stand: independent	
Ambulation	• Ambulated 2 × 50 feet independently with rolling walker. • Gait deviations notable for decreased cadence.	
Stairs	• Ascend/descend flight of stairs + one rail • Stair deviations: step–to pattern	

Assessment	
☑ Physical therapist's	*Assessment left blank for learner to develop.*
Goals	
Patient's	"I want to be able to walk the block to church without getting short of breath."
Short term	1. *Goals left blank for learner to develop.* 2.
Long term	1. *Goals left blank for learner to develop.* 2.

Plan	
☐ Physician's ☑ Physical therapist's ☐ Other's	Will continue to see patient twice a week × 4 weeks. Treatment will include therapeutic exercise (proximal hip and pelvic floor strengthening, aerobic conditioning), gait training on level surfaces and stairs, and energy conservation strategies.

Bloom's Taxonomy Level	Case 15.C Questions
Create	1. Synthesizing the medical data and physical examination findings, develop an appropriate assessment of the patient. 2. Develop two short-term physical therapy goals, including an appropriate timeframe. 3. Develop two long-term physical therapy goals, including an appropriate timeframe. 4. Develop alternative strategies to intervention if patient expresses health insurance and/or financial limitations, affording him a total of four physical therapy sessions.
Evaluate	5. Determine potential referral sources to other health care providers.
Analyze	6. Analyze the relationship between the primary diagnosis of COPD and reports of pelvic floor dysfunction. 7. Based on the 6-Minute Walk Test, is the patient above, at, or below the mean for individuals with COPD? What is the minimally detectable change that needs to be achieved to show improvement in endurance?
Apply	8. Design and implement two interventions to improve the patient's aerobic capacity. 9. Design and implement two interventions to improve the patient's balance. 10. Design and implement two interventions to improve energy conservation.
Understand	11. Based on the patient's medications, what outcome measure should the physical therapist use to accurately measure exercise intensity?
Remember	12. How much fraction of inspired oxygen is the patient receiving if he is on 2 L of oxygen via NC?

Bloom's Taxonomy Level	Case 15.C Answers
Create	1. The patient is a 70-year-old man who had an acute exacerbation of COPD and pneumonia. He was hospitalized for 8 days followed by a course of home physical therapy, and now presents for outpatient physical therapy. Upon initial evaluation, he presents with generalized deconditioning, muscular weakness (primarily hip strength and pelvic floor), and endurance, which contribute to limited stair climbing and an increased fall risk. His limited gait speed is also a significant contributor to these deficits. He is a good candidate for skilled physical therapy services. 2. Short-term goals: • The patient will improve gait speed on level surface by 0.1 m/s within 2 weeks to improve independence with community ambulation. • The patient will improve hip flexion strength by 1 manual muscle testing (MMT) grade in 2 weeks to allow improved ability to climb stairs. 3. Long-term goals: • The patient will improve Five Times Sit to Stand to < 12 seconds within 4 weeks to show improved endurance and decreased fall risk. • The patient will tolerate walking one block with a Borg score of < 3/10 within 4 weeks to be able to walk to church. 4. If the patient expresses health insurance and/or financial limitations, a comprehensive home exercise program with strengthening, balance, and endurance interventions and education on how to monitor vitals and signs and symptoms could be provided. Follow-up visits could be scheduled ad lib to assess tolerance and progress interventions. Additionally, the physical therapist could write an advocacy letter to the insurance company requesting more visits. If this is unsuccessful, community resources/grants could be investigated. Finally, pro bono physical therapy services could be provided.
Evaluate	5. The patient could benefit from referrals to outpatient pulmonary rehabilitation, and pelvic floor physical therapist. The patient should also continue regular follow-ups with his pulmonologist.

(Continued)

(Continued)

Bloom's Taxonomy Level	Case 15.C Answers
Analyze	6. The trunk can be viewed as a soda can. With optimal internal pressures, as regulated by the trunk's muscles, skeletal system, vocal cords, diaphragm, and pelvic floor, the trunk remains stable and has proper posture. However, in the patient with COPD, he has a chronic cough. Coughing opens the vocal cords, and therefore requires contraction of the pelvic floor to stabilize the trunk. However, with repetitive coughing, there becomes an increase in abdominal cavity pressures. This may lead to the pelvic floor weakening, leading to urinary incontinence. ▶ Fig. 15.5a, b 7.7. Based on the 6-Minute Walk Test, the patient's ambulation distance (1,182 feet) is below the mean for individuals with COPD (1,247 feet). The minimally detectable change that needs to be achieved to show improvement in endurance is 54 meters, or 177 feet.
Apply	8. To improve the patient's aerobic capacity, the patient could walk on the treadmill for a minimum of 10 minutes, × 3 bouts at a light (30% to <40% of peak work rates). The patient should ambulate approximately three to five times a week. To progress, the patient should increase time. This would also assist the patient with proximal hip strengthening. The patient could also use the arm ergometer for a minimum of 10 minutes, × 3 bouts. Strength and endurance of upper extremity muscles is important for functional tasks (i.e., carrying grocery bags). 9. Considering improving the patient's independence with community ambulation, two potential balance interventions include: • Treadmill ambulation with gradual increases in speed to work on improving patient confidence and improving gait speed. • Toe tapping on cones—this will help work on both stepping up on to a curb and progressing toward single-limb stance. 10. To assist the patient with energy conversation, the patient could monitor his signs and symptoms using the Borg Scale or Medical Research Council (MRC) Dyspnea Scale. The patient could also benefit from learning diaphragmatic breathing to control breathing pattern.
Understand	11. The physical therapist should use the Borg Scale to accurately measure the patient's exercise intensity. This is because the patient is taking metoprolol, a beta-blocker. Metoprolol lowers the patient's heart rate and, therefore, it will not increase with exercise intensity.
Remember	12. The patient is receiving 28% fraction of inspired oxygenation through 2L/min O_2 via nasal cannula.

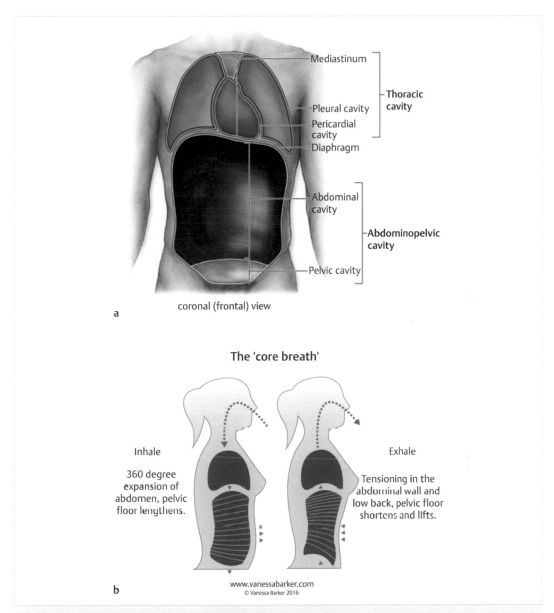

coronal (frontal) view

a

The 'core breath'

Inhale

360 degree
expansion of
abdomen, pelvic
floor lengthens.

Exhale

Tensioning in the
abdominal wall and
low back, pelvic floor
shortens and lifts.

www.vanessabarker.com
© Vanessa Barker 2016

b

Fig. 15.5 (a, b) The respiratory and pelvic diaphragm work together to control internal pressures to maintain posture and breathing. During inspiration, both diaphragms descend. During exhalation, both diaphragms ascend. **(a)** (Adapted from https://quizlet.com/210876730/ap-body-cavities-and-serous-membranes-flash-cards.) **(b)** (Adapted from https://mongoosebodyworks.com/breathing-for-core-optimization-and-wellbeing/.)

Key points
1. Be conscious of the patient's overall situation, including financial. The patient and the physical therapist should work as a team to develop an efficient, effective plan of care.
2. Consider addressing signs and symptoms outside of the primary system impaired. This includes the genitourinary system. Refer out if necessary.
3. Especially as the patient works at higher intensities, select an appropriate outcome measure to assess exertion, as heart rate may not always be appropriate.

Suggested Readings

2-Minute Walk Test. Available at: https://www.sralab.org/rehabilitation-measures/2-minute-walk-test. Accessed April 1, 2018

6-Minute Walk Test. Available at: https://www.sralab.org/rehabilitation-measures/6-minute-walk-test. Accessed April 1, 2018

American College of Sports Medicine. ACSM's Guidelines for Exercise Testing and Prescription. 10th ed. Baltimore, MD: Lippincott, Williams and Wilkins; 2017

ATS Committee on Proficiency Standards for Clinical Pulmonary Function Laboratories. ATS statement: guidelines for the six-minute walk test. Am J Respir Crit Care Med. 2002; 166(1): 111–117

Bohannon RW. Normative reference values for the two-minute walk test derived by meta-analysis. J Phys Ther Sci. 2017; 29 (12):2224–2227

Buatois S, Miljkovic D, Manckoundia P, et al. Five times sit to stand test is a predictor of recurrent falls in healthy community-living subjects aged 65 and older. J Am Geriatr Soc. 2008; 56(8): 1575–1577

Bui KL, Nyberg A, Maltais F, Saey D. Functional tests in chronic obstructive pulmonary disease, part 1: clinical relevance and links to the international classification of functioning, disability, and health. Ann Am Thorac Soc. 2017; 14(5):778–784

Bui KL, Nyberg A, Maltais F, Saey D. Functional tests in chronic obstructive pulmonary disease, part 2: measurement properties. Ann Am Thorac Soc. 2017; 14(5):785–794

Chui KK, Hood E, Klima DW. Meaningful change in walking speed. Top Geriatr Rehabil. 2012; 28(2):97–103

Crisafulli E, Torres A. COPD 2017: a year in review. COPD. 2018; 15 (2):118–122

Daabis R, Hassan MM, Zidan M. Endurance and strength training in pulmonary rehabilitation for COPD patients. Egypt J Chest Dis Tuberc. 2016; 66:231–236

Martinez-Garcia M Del M, Ruiz-Cardenas JD, Rabinovich RA. Effectiveness of smartphone devices in promoting physical activity and exercise in patients with chronic obstructive pulmonary disease: a systematic review. COPD. 2017; 14(5):543–551

Five times Sit to Stand. Available at: https://www.sralab.org/rehabilitation-measures/five-times-sit-stand-test. Accessed April 1, 2018

Frownfelter D, Dean E. Cardiovascular and Pulmonary Physical Therapy: Evidence to Practice. St. Louis, MO: Saunders Elsevier; 2012

Gloeckl R, Teschler S, Jarosch I, Christle JW, Hitzl W, Kenn K. Comparison of two- and six-minute walk tests in detecting oxygen desaturation in patients with severe chronic obstructive pulmonary disease: a randomized crossover trial. Chron Respir Dis. 2016; 13(3):256–263

Goodman CC, Fuller KS. Pathology: Implications for the Physical Therapist. 4th ed. St. Louis, MO: Saunders Elsevier; 2015

Hillegass E. Essentials of Cardiopulmonary Physical Therapy. 4th ed. St. Louis, MO: Elsevier; 2017

Holland AE, Spruit MA, Troosters T, et al. An official European Respiratory Society/American Thoracic Society technical standard: field walking tests in chronic respiratory disease. Eur Respir J. 2014; 44(6):1428–1446

Jácome C, Cruz J, Oliveira A, Marques A. Validity, reliability, and ability to identify fall status of the Berg balance scale, BESTest, Mini-BESTest, and Brief-BESTest in patients with COPD. Phys Ther. 2016; 96(11):1807–1815

Kennedy CC. Handgrip strength in chronic obstructive pulmonary disease: ready for prime time or frailty research tool? Ann Am Thorac Soc. 2017; 14(11):1630–1631

Maltais F, Decramer M, Casaburi R, et al. ATS/ERS Ad Hoc Committee on Limb Muscle Dysfunction in COPD. An official American Thoracic Society/European Respiratory Society statement: update on limb muscle dysfunction in chronic obstructive pulmonary disease. Am J Respir Crit Care Med. 2014; 189(9):e15–e62

Mandell LA, Wunderink RG, Anzueto A, et al. Infectious Diseases Society of America, American Thoracic Society. Infectious Diseases Society of America/American Thoracic Society consensus guidelines on the management of community-acquired pneumonia in adults. Clin Infect Dis. 2007; 44 Suppl 2:S27–S72

Massery M. Musculoskeletal and neuromuscular interventions: a physical approach to cystic fibrosis. J R Soc Med. 2005; 98 Suppl 45:55–66

McCarthy B, Casey D, Devane D, Murphy K, Murphy E, Lacasse Y. Pulmonary rehabilitation for chronic obstructive pulmonary disease. Cochrane Database Syst Rev. 2015(2):CD003793

McNamara RJ, McKeough ZJ, McKenzie DK, Alison JA. Water-based exercise training for chronic obstructive pulmonary disease. Cochrane Database Syst Rev. 2013(12):CD008290

Menadue C, Piper AJ, van 't Hul AJ, Wong KK. Non-invasive ventilation during exercise training for people with chronic obstructive pulmonary disease. Cochrane Database Syst Rev. 2014(5): CD007714

Ngai SPC, Jones AYM, Tam WWS. Tai Chi for chronic obstructive pulmonary disease (COPD). Cochrane Database Syst Rev. 2016 (6):CD009953

Pierobon A, Sini Bottelli E, Ranzini L, et al. COPD patients' self-reported adherence, psychosocial factors and mild cognitive impairment in pulmonary rehabilitation. Int J Chron Obstruct Pulmon Dis. 2017; 12:2059–2067

Puhan MA, Gimeno-Santos E, Cates CJ, Troosters T. Pulmonary rehabilitation following exacerbations of chronic obstructive pulmonary disease. Cochrane Database Syst Rev. 2016; 12(12): CD005305

Reid WD, Yamabayashi C, Goodridge D, et al. Exercise prescription for hospitalized people with chronic obstructive pulmonary disease and comorbidities: a synthesis of systematic reviews. Int J Chron Obstruct Pulmon Dis. 2012; 7:297–320

Rochester CL, Vogiatzis I, Holland AE, et al. ATS/ERS Task Force on Policy in Pulmonary Rehabilitation. An official American Thoracic Society/European Respiratory Society Policy Statement: Enhancing implementation, use, and delivery of pulmonary rehabilitation. Am J Respir Crit Care Med. 2015; 192(11):1373–1386

Shumway-Cook A, Brauer S, Woollacott M. Predicting the probability for falls in community-dwelling older adults using the timed up & go test. Phys Ther. 2000; 80(9):896–903

van Dort MJ, Geusens P, Driessen JHM, et al. High imminent vertebral fracture risk in subjects with COPD with a prevalent or incident vertebral fracture. J Bone Miner Res. 2018; 33(7): 1233–1241

Vincent EE, Chaplin EJ, Williams JEA, et al. Experiences of patients undergoing pulmonary rehabilitation during an exacerbation of chronic respiratory disease. Chron Respir Dis. 2017; 14(3):298–308

Wedzicha JA, Miravitlles M, Hurst JR, et al. Management of COPD exacerbations: a European Respiratory Society/American Thoracic Society guideline. Eur Respir J. 2017; 49(3):1600791

Yasir M, Sonthalia S. Corticosteroid Adverse Effects. Treasure Island, FL: StatPearls Publishing; 2019

16 Women's Health

General Information	
Case no.	16.A Women's Health
Authors	Karen Snowden, PT, DPT, Board Certified Clinical Specialist in Women's Health Physical Therapy Kathleen Ehrhardt, MMS, PA-C, DFAAPA Rebecca Maidansky, PT, DPT
Diagnosis	Twin pregnancy complicated by low back pain
Setting	Outpatient clinic
Learner expectations	☑ Initial evaluation ☐ Re-evaluation ☐ Treatment session
Learner objectives	1. Explain the pathophysiology of the patient's diagnosis. 2. Relate the pathophysiology and progression of pathology to clinical manifestations and activity/participation limitations seen in physical therapy practice. 3. Select, implement, and interpret physical therapy interventions based on the medical examination findings. 4. Identify special considerations when treating a pregnant patient.

Medical	
Chief complaint	Low back pain, 28-week twin pregnancy
History of present illness	The patient is a 32-year-old woman G2P1001 who is 28 weeks pregnant with twins. She was seen yesterday by her obstetrician and cleared of any pregnancy-related complications. She reports babies have been actively moving. She denies contractions, vaginal bleeding, or loss of vaginal fluid. She complains of new-onset left-sided lumbar pain and intermittent sharp, shooting pain left buttock and posterior left thigh; rated 6/10. The pain started 1 week ago after lifting her 2-year-old toddler. Pain worsens with activities requiring forward bending, transfers in/out of bed, and rolling in bed. Denies bowel or bladder dysfunction. She tried acetaminophen and warm compresses, which provided mild relief. States she tripped on sidewalk when she was 12 weeks pregnant but caught herself and didn't fall to the ground; no residual pain from this incident.
Past medical history	L5/S1 disk herniation 5 years ago treated with physical therapy. Term pregnancy delivered vaginally 2 years ago.
Past surgical history	Right anterior cruciate ligament (ACL) repair age 18 years.
Allergies	None
Medications	Prenatal vitamins, Folic acid, Iron
Precautions/orders	Activity as tolerated

Social history	
Home setup	• Resides in a multilevel home with husband and 2-year-old son. • Two steps + two handrails to enter. • Master bedroom and bathroom is on the first floor. • Half bath is on the first floor. • Son's bedroom and nursery is on the second floor. • Flight of stairs + one handrail to the second floor.
Occupation	• Elementary school teacher
Prior level of function	• Independent with ambulation • Drives
Recreational activities	• Enjoys swimming and spending time with husband and son.

Imaging/diagnostic tests	
Prenatal labs (obtained at 8 weeks' gestation)	Blood type: AB+, no antibodies Complete blood count—hematocrit: 21.2%; hemoglobin: 6.7 g/dL; mean corpuscular volume (MCV): 44.3 fL; platelets: 181,000 µL; white blood cells: 7,000 µL venereal disease research laboratory (VDRL)/rapid plasma reagin (RPR): negative. Urine culture/screen: negative Hepatitis B virus surface antigen (HBsAg): negative Human immunodeficiency virus (HIV) testing: negative Chlamydia: negative Gonorrhea: negative Pap Test: negative Purified protein derivative (PPD): negative
12-week dating ultrasound	Gestational age: 12 weeks and 1 day Obstetric ultrasound revealed diamniotic/dichorionic twin pregnancy Twin 1, right: normal first trimester scan. Nuchal translucency of 1.4 mm. Posterior placenta. Normal amount of amniotic fluid. Fetal heart action at 150 beats/min. Appropriate growth. Normal fetal anatomy Twin 2, left: normal first trimester scan. Nuchal translucency of 1.2 mm. Posterior placenta. Normal amount of amniotic fluid. Fetal heart action at 156 beats/min. Normal fetal anatomy
20-week prenatal ultrasound	Gestational age: 20 weeks and 3 days Shows appropriate growth of both twins. Twin 1, right: 298 g Twin 2, left: 300 g No fetal anomalies of either twin. Both placentae appear normal and posterior.
24- to 28-week labs	Complete blood count: 1-hour glucose level: 125 mg/dL
24-week prenatal ultrasound	Gestational age: 28 weeks and 1 day Shows appropriate growth of both twins. Twin 1, right: 1,000 g Twin 2, left: 1,005 g No fetal anomalies of either twin. Both placentae appear normal and posterior.

Pause points
Based on the above information, what are the priorities? • Diagnostic tests and measures? • Outcome measures? • Treatment interventions?

Physical Therapy Examination			
Subjective			
"Can you help with my back pain? I am also worried about it affecting the pregnancy."			
Objective			

Vital signs	Pre-treatment			Post-treatment
	Supine	Sitting	Standing	Sitting
Blood pressure (mmHg)	90/60	110/70	98/64	112/68
Heart rate (beats/min)	66	60	62	62
Respiratory rate (breaths/min)	14	12	12	14
Pulse oximetry on room air (SpO$_2$)	100%	100%	100%	100%

(Continued)

(Continued)

Physical Therapy Examination				
Pain	5/10 L lumbar	6/10 L lumbar; L buttock and posterior L thigh	6/10 L lumbar	4/10 L lumbar
General	• Patient is sitting, leaning to the right; appears uncomfortable. • Patient's husband has accompanied her to visit.			
Cardiovascular and pulmonary	• Auscultation: 2/6 mid-systolic murmur without radiation. • Lungs clear to auscultation bilaterally. • Pulses: 2 + bilateral dorsalis pedis and posterior tibialis; 1 + pitting edema to anterior shin bilaterally.			
Gastrointestinal	• Gravid, nontender, no palpable contractions			
Musculoskeletal	Range of motion	• Bilateral upper extremity (BUE): within functional limit (WFL) • Lumbar spine: flexion: 49 degrees; end range pain extension: 23 degrees right lateral flexion: 23 degrees left lateral flexion: 15 degrees; end range pain • B hip flexion: 118 degrees • B hip extension: 10 degrees • B knee flexion: 128 degrees • B knee extension: 0 degrees		
	Strength	• BUE: WFL • L hip flexion: 4–/5 • R hip flexion: 4/5 • L hip extension: 4–/5 • R hip extension: 4 + /5 • L hip abduction: 3 + /5 • R hip abduction: 4/5 • B knee extension: 4/5 • B knee flexion: 4/5 • B ankle dorsiflexion: 4 + /5 • B ankle plantar flexion: 4 + /5		
	Aerobic	• Borg Rate of Preceived Exertion (RPE) while ascending/descending 1 flight of stairs: 12/20		
	Flexibility	• Pectoralis major and minor: shortened as demonstrated by posture • B hamstring: decreased L > R; passive straight leg raise (SLR): L 76 degrees; R 85 degrees • B quadriceps: within normal limit (WNL) tested in standing • B adductors: WNL tested in standing		
	Posture	• B rounded shoulders		
Neurological	Balance	• Tandem stance, eyes open: 30 seconds B • Tandem stance, eyes closed: 30 seconds B, increased sway • Single-limb stance, left, eyes open: 18 seconds • Single-limb stance, right, eyes open: 30 seconds • Single-limb stance, left, eyes closed: 8 seconds • Single-limb stance, right, eyes closed: 19 seconds		

(Continued)

(Continued)

Physical Therapy Examination		
	Cognition	• Alert and oriented × 4
	Coordination	• Finger-to-nose: intact bilaterally
	Cranial nerves	• II–XII: intact
	Reflexes	• Patellar: 2 + bilaterally • Achilles: 2 + bilaterally
	Sensation	• Bilateral lower extremity (BLE): intact to light touch • Denies saddle anesthesia
	Tone	• BUE and BLE: normal
	Other	• (+) slump L • (–) supine sacroiliac joint (SIJ) compression • (–) side-lying SIJ distraction • (–) thigh thrust • (–) Flexion, abduction, and external rotation (FABER) • (+) L straight leg raise • (+) Trendelenburg in L single-leg stance. • (+) Centralization of leg pain with repeated lumbar extension, standing.
Functional status		
Bed mobility		• Rolling right and left: independent • Supine to/from sit: independent, but moves slowly
Transfers		• Sit to/from stand: modified independent using BUEs
Ambulation		• Ambulated 90 feet independently. • Gait deviations notable for wide base of support, decreased L stance time, and L Trendelenburg during R stance phase.
Stairs		• Ascend/descend flight of stairs: modified independent with handrail for UE weight-bearing assist, demonstrates step-to pattern.
Task Specific		• Patient reports unable to lift 2-year-old son from floor due to pain. • Patient reports decreased pain with extension-biased exercises, and increased pain with flexion-biased exercises.

Assessment	
☑ Physical therapist's	*Assessment left blank for learner to develop.*
Goals	
Patient's	"I want relief from my back pain."
Short term	1. *Goals left blank for learner to develop.* 2
Long term	1. *Goals left blank for learner to develop.* 2.

Plan	
□ Physician's ☑ Physical therapist's □ Other's	Plan to treat two times per week × 6 weeks with lumbosacral and LE therapeutic exercise, balance training, pain management, and education in proper body mechanics and posture.

Bloom's Taxonomy Level	Case 16.A Questions
Create	1. Synthesizing the medical data and physical examination findings, develop an appropriate physical therapy assessment of the patient. 2. Develop two short-term physical therapy goals, including an appropriate timeframe. 3. Develop two long-term physical therapy goals, including an appropriate timeframe.
Evaluate	4. Differential diagnosis would involve ruling out what medical red flags when evaluating this patient?
Analyze	5. List four musculoskeletal causes or classifications to consider when determining the source/cause of this patient's back pain.
Apply	6. Describe appropriate education to empower this patient in actively managing her pain. 7. When administering exercise interventions, what precautions must be considered with this patient?
Understand	8. Discuss factors associated with this patient's edema. 9. Discuss at least three reasons why pregnant women are at increased risk for back pain. 10. List other potential physical therapy options if this patient does not make progress after two to three physical therapy treatments?
Remember	11. Explain "term pregnancy." 12. What does the "G2P1" in G2P1001 mean?

Bloom's Taxonomy Level	Case 16.A Answers
Create	1. The patient is a 32-year-old woman, 28 weeks pregnant with twins, presenting to physical therapy with a 1-week history of left lumbar pain and intermittent posterior radicular left thigh pain. She states it began after lifting her 2-year-old toddler; one week ago. The pain remains unchanged over the past week and she rates it 6/10 on the numeric pain scale. Physical examination reveals limited forward and lateral left lumbar flexion, left hip weakness, decreased flexibility left hamstrings, decreased balance in left single-leg stance, and altered gait pattern. She is independent in all functional mobility. Her goal is to be able to lift her toddler. She would benefit from physical therapy to address above deficits to maximize pain-free mobility and ability to lift and care for her toddler. Will continue to follow. 2. Short-term goals: • Patient will be able to independently roll in bed with < 2/10 pain within 2 weeks for improved sleep and increased independence at home. • Patient will be able to ascend and descend a flight of stairs independently with < 2/10 pain within 2 weeks in order to obtain access to the second-floor bedrooms. 3. Long-term goals: • Patient will be able to transfer from sit to stand while holding toddler with < 2/10 pain in 6 weeks to improve functional mobility in caring for her toddler. • Patient will be able to lift her toddler from the floor with proper body mechanics and < 2/10 pain in 6 weeks to improve functional mobility in caring for her child.
Evaluate	4. Possible red flags to consider when evaluating a patient with back pain include cancer, infection, fracture, and cauda equina syndrome. Cancer is unlikely in this patient due to age, no prior history, and she denies being awakened with night time pain except with rolling. Fracture is unlikely due to no recent trauma. She does not have a fever or general malaise, which rules out infection. The patient does not report saddle anesthesia, incontinence, or progressive neurologic deficits, which rules out cauda equina syndrome. When treating a pregnant woman with back pain, one must also consider possible labor contractions as a cause of back pain. Labor contractions may are rhythmical and not

(Continued)

(Continued)

Bloom's Taxonomy Level	Case 16.A Answers
	alleviated by rest or position changes. This patient was able to reduce her pain with repeated lumbar extension, thereby indicating a high likelihood of a musculoskeletal cause being the source of her back pain. Additionally, physical therapists must observe for elevated blood pressure each session, especially in a woman pregnant at 20 weeks or beyond. Although unrelated to back pain, this could be a sign of preeclampsia (diastolic pressure > 90 mmHg) or eclampsia (140/90 mmHg after 20 weeks gestation). If ignored, it could be life-threatening for both the mother and baby. Other symptoms of preeclampsia may include headache, nontransient edema (hands, animals, feet, face), visual changes, severe heartburn, and change in reflexes.
Analyze	5. Potential musculoskeletal causes of back pain may include mechanical, muscular, neurogenic, pelvic girdle, and/or left hip. Classification of lumbar pain into intervention groups would also be an acceptable answer: mobilization, specific exercise, immobilization, traction.
Apply	6. Aside from instruction in home exercise intervention, education in proper posture and body mechanics would help this patient in understanding how to avoid worsening her back pain and how to alleviate it. Special attention should be given to activities requiring forward trunk flexion, as this exacerbated her back and leg pain during the examination. She should be advised to keep her spine upright while bending and using her legs to lift her child; if lifting off the floor, assuming a half-kneeling position when lifting the child may prevent the onset of back pain. When carrying her child, she should hold the child against her torso and avoid resting the toddler on one hip. When lifting household items such as a laundry basket from the floor, a half-kneeling position allows for independence with ADLs while reducing the risk of injury. ▶ Fig. 16.1 When sitting she can utilize a small towel or lumbar roll to support her natural lordosis, and should avoid slouching. In bed, she may benefit from positioning a pillow between her knees and placing a small folded towel under her growing uterus to alleviate added strain to her low back while sleeping. Utilization of a heating pad or cold pack to the low back for short periods may also be considered, with the same skin precautions considered in all patients. 7. Women are encouraged to maintain their fitness level during uncomplicated pregnancies. Exercise has many physical and emotional benefits, and can reduce pregnancy-related hypertension, gestational diabetes, and excessive gestational weight gain. Women who exercise during pregnancy are more likely to exercise postpartum, and exercise can be performed safely without adverse complications to babies. Pregnant women are encouraged to maintain adequate hydration during exercise, and avoid overheating and exercising beyond fatigue, and to perform exercise or activities that are unlikely to cause a fall. Exercises in prone lying position should be avoided after the first trimester (3 months).
Understand	8. Edema in pregnancy is very common due to increased water retention. It can also develop as a result of pressure of the uterus on the inferior vena cava and iliac veins. Edema is usually in the distal extremities, such as ankles and wrists. Edema in pregnancy can be concerning if associated with preeclampsia. Usually with preeclampsia, patients often have peripheral and facial edema. 9. Three reasons that patients who are pregnant are at an increased risk for back pain are (1) ligamentous and joint laxity, (2) increased weight gain, and (3) changes in posture resulting in a shift in center of gravity. All of these alter the patient's body mechanics. This patient's history of previous back pain puts her at greater risk for back pain during pregnancy. 10. If this patient is not seeing improvements in her symptoms after two to three visits, consider (1) altering treatment, for example, adjust exercise, reinforce home strategies, lumbar orthosis, initiate safe modalities; (2) confer with another physical therapist; and/or (3) refer to an obstetric-trained physical therapist. If lack of progress continues, the patient may need to be referred back to doctor for further evaluation.
Remember	11. "Term pregnancy" refers to childbirth between 37 and 42 weeks of the pregnancy. On average, singleton pregnancies last 39 to 40 weeks and twin pregnancies last 36 weeks. 12. The G stands for gravida, or number of pregnancies. The P stands for parity, or number of births carried beyond 20 weeks (live births and stillbirths). G2P1 describes this patient who has been pregnant twice (G2), had one childbirth (P1), and is currently pregnant.

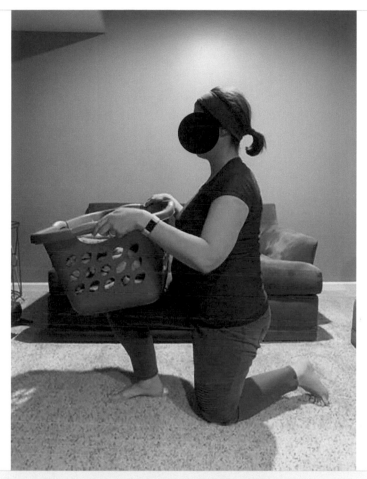

Fig. 16.1 Half-kneeling allows for upright posture and reduced strain when performing activities of daily living. The patient is encouraged to use her legs when moving up and down, and to avoid forward bending of the spine.

Key points
1. Pregnancy-related low back pain is common. As experts in musculoskeletal function, physical therapists play an important role in helping reduce pain and optimize function during the perinatal period.
2. Physical therapists must perform a comprehensive musculoskeletal examination to determine the cause of a patient's back pain while screening for potential medical complications. Differential diagnosis along with careful monitoring of vital signs will ensure a pregnant woman's safety during physical therapy intervention.
3. Exercise is safe and encouraged with women having an uncomplicated pregnancy. Precautions are taken for women carrying multiples (more than one baby). Pregnant women should not exercise beyond the point of fatigue. If a woman is experiencing a complicated or high-risk pregnancy (including pregnancy with multiples), she must be closely monitored for safety and may benefit from the care of an obstetric-trained physical therapist.

General Information	
Case no.	16.B
Authors	Kathleen Ehrhardt, MMS, PA-C, DFAAPA Karen Snowden, PT, DPT, Board Certified Clinical Specialist in Women's Health Physical Therapy
Diagnosis	Twin pregnancy complicated by low back pain
Setting	Acute care hospital

(Continued)

(Continued)

General Information	
Learner expectations	☑ Initial evaluation ☐ Re-evaluation ☐ Treatment session
Learner objectives	1. Explain the pathophysiology of the patient's diagnosis. 2. Understand that "bedrest" is defined in various ways depending on the facility and medical providers. 3. Select, and implement physical therapy interventions based on the medical condition and musculoskeletal examination findings. 4. Develop a physical therapy plan of care that safely contributes to the medical management of a high-risk patient on bedrest.

Medical	
Chief complaint	Low back pain, 33-week twin pregnancy, in preterm labor
History of present illness	The patient is a 32-year-old woman G2P1001 who is 33 weeks pregnant with twins and admitted to the labor and delivery unit with increasing back pain and regular contractions. Patient with a naturally occurring dichorionic/diamniotic twin pregnancy that has been complicated by low back pain and left lower extremity (LLE) sciatica. She participated in outpatient physical therapy and had significant improvement of her back pain. Yesterday the patient's back pain worsened and she noticed regular contractions every 6 to 8 minutes starting early this morning. She reports that the babies were moving well prior to the start of the contractions, but the movement has subsequently decreased. She is very anxious. She denies any fluid or vaginal bleeding.
Past medical history	L5/S1 disk herniation 5 years ago; treated with physical therapy Term pregnancy delivered vaginally 2 years ago.
Past surgical history	Right anterior cruciate ligament (ACL) repair age 18 years
Allergies	None
Medications	Prenatal vitamins, Folic acid, Iron, Acetaminophen PRN for back pain
Precautions/orders	Bedrest due to preterm labor; physical therapy evaluate and treat

Social history	
Home setup	• Resides in a multilevel home with husband and 2-year-old son. • Two steps + two handrails to enter. • Master bedroom and bathroom are on the first floor. • Half bath is on the first floor. • Son's bedroom and nursery are on the second floor. • Flight of stairs + one handrail to the second floor.
Occupation	• Elementary school teacher
Prior level of function	• Independent with ambulation • Drives
Recreational activities	• Enjoys swimming and spending time with husband and son.

Vital signs	Hospital day 0: labor and delivery	Hospital day 1: labor and delivery
Blood pressure (mmHg)	110/62 supine, left arm	111/65
Heart rate (beats/min)	68	70
Respiratory rate (breaths/min)	14	13
Pulse oximetry on room air (SpO$_2$)	100%	98%
Temperature (°F)	98.6	98.4

Imaging/diagnostic test	Hospital day 0: labor and delivery
External fetal monitoring	• Twin A fetal heart rate (FHR) in 120 s with good variability and accelerations. • Twin B FHR in 120 s with good variability and accelerations. • No decelerations noted. Regular contractions every 6 minutes. • Category I FHR pattern in both fetuses.
Fetal ultrasound	• Twin A and Twin B both in vertex presentation. • Twin A female, estimate fetal weight = 2,350 g. • Twin B male, estimated fetal weight = 2,245 g. • Two fundal placentas grade 2. Estimated gestational age = 34 weeks
Transvaginal ultrasound	• Cervical length is 30 mm.
Urine analysis and culture	• Negative
Sterile speculum examination	• Cervix appears dilated to 2 cm. • Ferning: negative
Fetal fibronectin (fFN)	• Positive
Rectovaginal group B streptococcal culture	• Positive

Medical management	Hospital day 0: labor and delivery	Hospital day 1: labor and delivery
Medications	1. Intravenous (IV) fluids 2. Betamethasone 3. Penicillin G 4. Nifedipine	Continued per medical plan of care.
Continuous external fetal monitoring	Continued per medical plan of care.	Continued per medical plan of care.
Compression stockings	Continued per medical plan of care.	Continued per medical plan of care.
Bedrest with left-sided wedge	Continued per medical plan of care.	Continued per medical plan of care.
Indwelling urinary catheter	Continued per medical plan of care.	Continued per medical plan of care.

Lab		Reference range	Hospital day 0: labor and delivery	Hospital day 1: labor and delivery
Complete blood count	White blood cell	$5.0–10.0 \times 10^9$/L	16.7	17.8
	Hemoglobin	14.0–17.4 g/dL	11.2	11.4
	Hematocrit	42–52%	33.6	34.2
	Red blood cell	4.5–5.5 million/mm^3	4.6	4.8
	Platelet	140,000–400,000/µL	250	300
Metabolic panel	Calcium	8.6–10.3 mg/dL	9.8	10
	Chloride	98–108 mEq/L	106	104
	Magnesium	1.2–1.9 mEq/L	1.7	1.7
	Phosphate	2.3–4.1 mg/dL	3.1	3.3
	Potassium	3.7–5.1 mEq/L	4.7	4.8
	Sodium	134–142 mEq/L	140	138
	Blood urea nitrogen	7–20 mg/dL	16	17
	Creatinine	0.7–1.3 mg/dL	1.00	1.12
	Anion gap	3–10 mEq/L	4	5
	CO_2	22–26 mEq/L	23	22
Other	Glucose	60–110 mg/dL	102	98
Type and screen	–	–	AB +, antibody negative	–

Based on the above information, what are the priorities?
- Diagnostic tests and measures?
- Outcome measures?
- Treatment interventions?

Hospital Day 2, Labor and Delivery:
Physical Therapy Examination

"Prior to the initial evaluation, the physical therapist sought clarification regarding the patient's activity restriction. It was confirmed the patient is able to ambulate to and from the bathroom and perform active range of motion (AROM) exercises in bed with proper monitoring for safety."

Subjective

"I'm having back pain, but thankfully my preterm labor has stopped."

Objective

Vital signs	Pre-treatment	Post-treatment
Blood pressure (mmHg)	98/60	112/70
Heart rate (beats/min)	68	62
Respiratory rate (breaths/min)	14	14
Pulse oximetry on room air (SpO$_2$)	100%	100%
Pain	5/10 B lumbar	5/10 B lumbar

General		• Patient left side-lying in bed. • Thrombo-Embolus Deterrent (TED) stockings to knees bilaterally. • Lines notable for IV in left hand, indwelling catheter in bladder.
Cardiovascular and pulmonary		• Auscultation: 2/6 mid-systolic murmur without radiation • Lungs clear to auscultation bilaterally. • Pulses: 2 + bilateral dorsalis pedis and posterior tibialis. 1 + pitting edema to anterior shin bilaterally.
Gastrointestinal		• Gravid, nontender, no palpable contractions
Posture		• Mild cervical protraction • Rounded shoulders • Excessive lumbar lordosis ▶ Fig. 16.2
Musculoskeletal	Range of motion (ROM)	• Bilateral upper extremity (BUE): within functional limits (WFL) • Bilateral lower extremity (BLE): WFL with the exception of left hip, which actively externally rotates ~20 degrees. • Lumbar spine: WFL with the exception of flexion, which is limited ~75% due to body habitus; pain with end range flexion.
	Strength	• BUE: 5/5 • BLE: > 3 + /5 as demonstrated through functional mobility
	Aerobic	• Not tested
	Flexibility	• Pectoralis major and minor: shortened bilaterally, as demonstrated by posture. • Hamstrings: shortened bilaterally; straight leg raise (SLR), passively: 30 degrees. • Piriformis: tightness in left
Neurological	Balance	• Unable to achieve single leg stance bilaterally.
	Cognition	• Alert and oriented × 4
	Coordination	• Finger to nose: intact bilaterally • Heel to shin: intact bilaterally
	Cranial nerves	• II–XII: intact
	Reflexes	• Patellar: 2 + bilaterally • Achilles: 2 + bilaterally

(Continued)

(Continued)

Hospital Day 2, Labor and Delivery: Physical Therapy Examination		
	Sensation	• BUE and BLE: intact to light touch, deep pressure
	Tone	• BUE and BLE: normal
Functional status		
Bed mobility	• Rolling either direction: independent, central lumbar pain. • Supine to/from sit: modified independent with the head of the bed elevated ~35 degrees and use of bed rails, (+) central lumbar pain.	
Transfers	• Sit to/from stand: modified independent with use of BUEs, (+) central lumbar pain.	
Ambulation	• Ambulated × 15 feet independently. • Gait deviations notable for wide base of support, reduced pelvic rotation, and decreased cadence.	

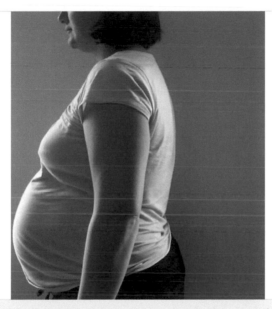

Fig. 16.2 Posture is assessed from the anterior, posterior, and lateral views. Observation of this lateral view reveals the patient has cervical protraction, rounded shoulders, and excessive lumbar lordosis. (Source: Graham and Sheila, CC BY 2.0, via Wikimedia Commons.)

Assessment	
☑ Physical therapist's	*Assessment left blank for learner to develop*
Goals	
Patient's	"Reduce back pain" "Care for my child and do household chores without starting pre-term labor"
Short term	1. *Goals left blank for learner to develop* 2.
Long term	1. *Goals left blank for learner to develop* 2.

Plan	
☐ Physician's ☑ Physical therapist's ☐ Other's	Plan to treat once daily with education in body mechanics and transfer training, breathing exercises using incentive spirometry, therapeutic exercise in supine/side-lying to maintain ROM and strength and prevent thromboembolism, and pain reduction techniques × 7 days.

Bloom's Taxonomy Level	Case 16.B Questions
Create	1. Synthesizing the medical data and physical examination findings, develop an appropriate physical therapy assessment of the patient. 2. Develop two short-term physical therapy goals, including an appropriate time frame. 3. Develop two long-term physical therapy goals, including an appropriate time frame.
Evaluate	4. Explain the physical therapy findings and expected discharge disposition. 5. Assess the woman's emotional and psychological disposition. 6. Explain how the patient and physical therapist can differentiate labor contractions from musculoskeletal back pain beyond the use of electronic monitoring.
Analyze	7. What adverse medical condition must a clinician monitor for when a patient is on bedrest?
Apply	8. Describe and implement patient safety education for this pregnant woman who desires to sometimes lay supine. 9. Describe and implement three physical therapy interventions to reduce this patient's pain and improve function.
Understand	10. Describe why patients who are pregnant develop physiologic anemia. 11. Explain why a calcium channel blocker is used for the treatment of preterm labor. 12. Describe why patients with multifetal gestation have a higher risk for preterm labor. 13. Describe signs and symptoms of preterm labor.
Remember	14. What are the benefits of physical therapy for a pregnant woman on bedrest? 15. Why must physician orders for "bedrest" be verified prior to working with high-risk pregnant patients in physical therapy?

Bloom's Taxonomy Level	Case 16.B Answers

Create	1. The patient is a 32-year-old woman, 33 weeks pregnant with twins, who was admitted to the inpatient labor and delivery unit with preterm labor and back pain. Her physical therapy examination reveals difficulty and pain with bed mobility and transfers. She reports back pain during bed mobility, transfers, and activities requiring lumbar flexion (i.e., lifting an object off the ground). She states "I'm so scared. My doctor wants me to stay pregnant for at least another week, and any day beyond that would be even better for the babies' development." Patient would benefit from physical therapy improve body mechanics and posture, perform safe therapeutic exercise to for education in safe mobility and avoidance of eliciting labor contractions, prevent deconditioning and blood clots, transfer training to reduce excessive use of abdominals and energy conservation and education in positioning strategies for reduced pain during labor and delivery. Will continue to follow.
	2. Short-term goals:
	  • Patient will be able to self-determine the difference between labor contractions and back spasms within three visits to reduce risk of preterm birth.
	  • Patient will be able to perform bed mobility and transfers with < 3/10 back pain within three visits to improve functional mobility.
	  • Patient will be independent with home exercise program within three visits to maintain BUE and BLE ROM and strength for independent functioning.
	3. Long-term goals:
	  • Patient will demonstrate increased awareness of good posture and body mechanics within seven visits to reduce back pain.
	  • Patient will report two ways to reduce back pain during labor in seven visits to ease pain during childbirth.

(Continued)

(Continued)

Bloom's Taxonomy Level	Case 16.B Answers
Evaluate	4. Patient is on bedrest to reduce risk of preterm labor. It is essential the physical therapist verify the restrictions associated with this medical order (see "Remember" below) and educate the patient to abide by the restrictions for safety of herself and unborn babies. Blood pressure, heart rate, pulse oximetry, and uterine activity should be monitored during physical therapy sessions. Physical therapists must understand how to monitor for labor contractions with and without electronic monitoring in order to assist in the goal of avoiding the onset of labor. It was determined this patient was cleared to perform physical therapist-prescribed AROM exercises, bed mobility, transfers, and ambulation to/from her bathroom with appropriate monitoring. Formal manual muscle testing is not necessary for patients on bedrest; the evaluation should focus on functional ability. During the modified physical therapy evaluation, the patient reported back pain and demonstrated difficulty and poor quality of movement with bed mobility, transfers, and ambulation. She verbalized little knowledge in understanding how her breath, posture and body mechanics could assist in reducing her back pain and potentially influence eliciting uterine contractions. It is anticipated this patient will do well in physical therapy for reduced back pain while on modified bedrest to reduce the risk of preterm birth prior to 35 weeks' gestation as desired by her medical team. Anticipate patient will return home before or following childbirth, and follow up with outpatient physical therapy for postpartum rehabilitation. 5. Patient expressed anxiety and fear related to activity bringing on the onset of labor, risking preterm childbirth. Anxiety and fear associated with high-risk pregnancies is common. Childbirth prior to 35 weeks' gestation can impact fetal outcomes and result in a newborn spending greater time in the neonatal intensive care unit (NICU). 6. Electronic fetal monitoring and uterine activity monitoring can be utilized to reassure a woman if her activity is "safe," meaning activity is not inducing uterine contractions, which could put her babies at risk of preterm birth. Uterine contractions and back spasms can both be experienced as back pain. Educating this pregnant woman in the difference between uterine and musculoskeletal contractions may help reduce the patent's anxiety and empower her to understand how she can move and function while keeping her and her babies safe. Positional changes can elicit and reduce her back pain. She can monitor if changes in position reduce her back pain or if the pain is a more rhythmical pattern (indicating greater likelihood of uterine or labor contractions). Nonrhythmical pain that can be started and stopped based on position would more likely occur with back spasms. Teaching the patient how to differentiate the cause of her back pain is particularly helpful if she is discharged home while still pregnant, where she would not have electronic uterine monitoring.
Analyze	7. Clinicians must monitor for signs and symptoms related to thromboembolisms, whether deep vein thrombosis (DVT) or pulmonary embolus (PE), when a patient is on bedrest.
Apply	8. Laying supine during the third trimester can result in supine hypotensive syndrome (also referred to as vena cava syndrome). The inferior vena cava lies anterior to the lumbar vertebrae and can be occluded by an enlarged uterus when a pregnant woman lays supine. This inferior vena cava compression can result in hypotensive syndrome. Signs and symptoms of hypotensive syndrome include shortness of breath, dizziness, pallor, restlessness, nausea, LE paresthesia, cold/clammy skin, visual disturbances, reduced blood pressure (systolic), and increased maternal heart rate. Semi-supine or side-lying positioning can improve blood flow and alleviate these symptoms. 9. Physical therapy interventions to reduce the patient's pain and improve function include the following: **Positioning/posture:** education in use of pillows and towel rolls for positioning and pain control. Patient is educated to avoid supine positioning for more than 3 minutes. Patient and caregivers are advised to monitor bony prominences for signs of skin breakdown. Additional education for positioning strategies to reduce back pain during labor and delivery may involve support for lumbar extension and avoiding excessive lumbar flexion. The patient practices these postures during treatment **Mobility training:** patient is educated in and practices rolling and transitional movements with proper breathing to avoid increased intra-abdominal pressure and Valsalva maneuver. Breathing and "exhale during effort" is reinforced with ambulation and

(Continued)

(Continued)

Bloom's Taxonomy Level	Case 16.B Answers
	transfers on/off the toilet as well as in/out of bed. Education is provided to utilize the controls on the hospital bed for raising and lowering the head to assist with bed mobility and transfers and to monitor for uterine contractions during transfers and ambulation. **Therapeutic exercise:** AROM exercises are initiated slowly while observing equipment monitoring uterine contractions. One to two exercises for each body part is initiated, for 5 to 10 repetitions each. Proper breathing is reinforced. Exercises may be increased or decreased during future treatments depending on the patient's response. Examples: AROM of all joints of extremities and neck, small-range lower trunk rotation, pelvic tilts, side-lying hip external rotation (clamshells), diaphragmatic breathing, stretching of the pectoral, hamstring, and piriformis muscles unilaterally in side-lying position. Relaxation techniques such as visual imagery and deep breathing can be beneficial in alleviating stress, anxiety, and fear associated with high-risk pregnancies. **Modalities:** consider heating pad/cold pack and massage for reducing back pain.
Understand	10. Pregnant women have physiologic anemia in pregnancy due to hemodilution. There is an increase in plasma volume but not an increase in red cell mass.
	11. Calcium channel blockers are used in the treatment of preterm labor to block calcium ions through the cell membrane and cause relaxation of the myometrium, or uterine muscle.
	12. Preterm labor and delivery are more common in women with multiple gestation because of the increased distention of the uterus from more than one fetus. The distension causes increase in oxytocin receptors and increases the manufacturing of prostaglandins, which cause contraction and subsequent dilation of the cervix.
	13. Signs and symptoms of preterm labor include bloody show (pink or red vaginal bleeding), menstrual-like cramps, abdominal or intestinal cramps without diarrhea, suprapubic pressure, and/or backache unresponsive to postural changes.
Remember	14. Physical therapy aims to minimize the negative effects of bedrest without increasing the risk of complications for the mother and fetus(es). If cleared by the physician, physical therapy helps maximize mobility, maintain ROM and functional strength, promote circulation, and assist in respiratory mechanics. There are also psychological benefits. The physical therapist can help the patient identify safe activity and exercise while reducing fear.
	15. "Bedrest" is analogous to "activity restriction" and may be prescribed for pregnant women despite lacking evidence of its effectiveness. Clarification of bedrest restrictions may be necessary prior to treating the patient in order to ensure safety. Examples of bedrest: strict bedrest (no upright activity or bathroom privileges), bedrest in Trendelenburg, bedrest with bathroom privileges, and activity limited but not necessarily to bed. Levels of activity restriction vary among facilities and providers and may change during the pregnancy from one day to the next day.

Key points
1. Proactively communicate with nursing and medical staff prior to each physical therapy treatment, as a patient's status can change quickly.
2. Bedrest and activity restriction are often prescribed for women with high-risk pregnancies in an attempt to improve pregnancy outcomes. Verify patient's restrictions prior to initiating physical therapy.
3. Recognize safety precautions specific to treating pregnant women.
4. Focus physical therapy interventions on promoting patient's safe mobility and function.

General Information	
Case no.	16.C
Authors	Kathleen Ehrhardt, MMS, PA-C, DFAAPA Karen Snowden, PT, DPT, Board Certified Clinical Specialist in Women's Health Physical Therapy
Diagnosis	Postpartum urinary incontinence (UI)

(Continued)

(Continued)

General Information	
Setting	Outpatient clinic
Learner expectations	☑ Initial evaluation ☐ Re-evaluation ☐ Treatment session
Learner objectives	1. Explain the pathophysiology of the patient's diagnosis. 2. Relate the pathophysiology and progression of pathology to clinical manifestations and activity/participation limitations seen in obstetric physical therapy practice. 3. Select, implement, and interpret physical therapy interventions based on the medical examination findings. 4. Develop an understanding of medical management and how it influences physical therapy plan of care.

Medical	
Chief complaint	Postpartum UI
History of present illness	The patient is a 32-year-old G2P1203 woman who presents to the office for evaluation of postpartum UI. She describes her symptoms as loss of a small amount of urine with cough, laugh, and sneeze. She denies fever, hematuria, and dysuria. She delivered twins vaginally 5 weeks ago at 35.5 weeks' gestation. Both infants were born without forceps or vacuum assistance; there was no associated vaginal tear or episiotomy. Both son and daughter are doing well and growing appropriately. She is currently breastfeeding. She was seen by her obstetrician 2 days ago and told she has a stage 1 uterine prolapse and urethral hypermobility. Ob-gyn reassured her that UI should improve postpartum. Urine dip was negative in the office; it was sent to lab for urine analysis. She is healing appropriately from childbirth and referred to pelvic floor physical therapy for evaluation and treatment. Postpartum depression screen was negative.
Past medical history	L5/S1 disk herniation 5 years ago treated with physical therapy. Recurring back pain in recent twin pregnancy; received physical therapy antepartum. Term pregnancy delivered vaginally 2 years ago (son). Preterm twin pregnancy delivered vaginally 5 weeks ago (son and daughter).
Past surgical history	Right anterior cruciate ligament (ACL) repair age 18 years, postpartum tubal ligation.
Allergies	None
Medications	Prenatal vitamins
Precautions/orders	Activity as tolerated

Social history	
Home setup	• Resides in a multilevel home with husband, 2-year-old son and 5-week old twins. • Two steps + two handrails to enter. • Master bedroom and bathroom on the first floor. • Half bath on the first floor. • Children's bedrooms on the second floor. • Flight of stairs + one handrail to the second floor.
Occupation	• Elementary school teacher, currently on maternity leave.
Prior level of function	• Independent with ambulation. • Drives
Recreational activities	• Enjoys swimming and spending time with husband and son.

Imaging/diagnostic tests	Results (from test 2 days prior)
Urine analysis	• Negative

Pause points
Based on the above information, what are the priorities?
• Diagnostic tests and measures?
• Outcome measures?
• Treatment interventions?

Physical Therapy Examination		
Subjective		
"I lose my urine when I cough or sneeze."		
Objective		
Vital signs	Pre-treatment	Post-treatment
Blood pressure (mmHg)	108/68	112/70
Heart rate (beats/min)	62	62
Respiratory rate (breaths/min)	14	14
Pulse oximetry on room air (SpO$_2$)	100%	100%
Borg scale	2/10	2/10
Pain	0/10	0/10
General	• Patient is sitting in chair and appears comfortable.	
Cardiovascular and pulmonary	• Auscultation: regular rate and rhythm without murmur. • Lungs clear to auscultation bilaterally. • Pulses: 2+ bilateral dorsalis pedis and posterior tibialis. • No peripheral edema	
Gastrointestinal	• Abdomen is soft, nontender, without organomegaly.	
Genitourinary	• External genitalia without lesion, cervix is 1.2 cm superior to introitus, urethral hypermobility.	
Musculoskeletal	Diastasis rectus abdominis (DRA): positive • 4.5 cm superior to umbilicus: 4 cm. • Umbilicus: 5.5 cm • 4.5 cm inferior to umbilicus: 7 cm. Doming is present with active contraction of rectus abdominis ▸ Fig. 16.3	
Pelvic function	Bladder	• Voids every 60 minutes • UI with laugh, cough, sneeze; denies urgency • Uses liner pad protection (one daily) daytime only.
	Bowels	• Denies dysfunction
	Sexual	• Not yet attempted intercourse postpartum.
	Pain	• None reported
Pelvic floor Internal vaginal examination	External integument	• Within normal limits (WNLs)
	Manual Muscle Test (MMT)/strength	• R: 2/5 • L: 2/5
	Endurance	• Maximum hold 2 seconds × 5 repetitions.
	Quality of contraction	• Uses accessory abdominal muscles during pelvic floor muscle (PFM) contraction.
	Sensation	• Intact to light touch.
	Pain	• Mild tenderness L levator ani.
	Urethral mobility	• Hypermobile
	Tone	• WNLs

(Continued)

(Continued)

Physical Therapy Examination	
Functional status	
Bed mobility	• Rolling right and left independent • Supine to/from sit: independent
Transfers	• Sit to/from stand: independent
Ambulation	• Ambulate > 500 feet independently
Stairs	• Ascend/descend a flight of stairs independently.
Sport specific	• Has not yet returned to exercise.

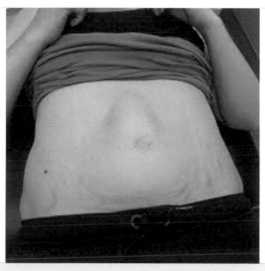

Fig. 16.3 Diastasis rectus abdominis is a separation of the rectus abdominis muscle bellies during pregnancy. This may result in doming (or bulging) of the abdomen along the linea alba postpartum

Assessment	
☑ Physical therapist's	*Assessment left blank for learner to develop.*
Goals	
Patient's	"Eliminate UI"
Short term	1. *Goals left blank for learner to develop* 2.
Long term	1. *Goals left blank for learner to develop* 2.

Plan	
☐ Physician's ☑ Physical therapist's ☐ Other's	Treat patient once every 3 weeks × 4 visits within 12 weeks. Treatment to consist of pelvic floor and abdominal strengthening exercise, education on pelvic floor protection strategies, posture, and body mechanics.

Bloom's Taxonomy Level	Case 16.C Questions
Create	1. Synthesizing the medical data and physical examination findings, develop an appropriate physical therapy assessment of the patient. 2. Develop two short-term physical therapy goals, including an appropriate timeframe. 3. Develop two long-term physical therapy goals, including an appropriate timeframe.
Evaluate	4. Explain the physical therapy findings and expected discharge disposition.
Analyze	5. Describe how to assess for a diastasis rectus abdominis (DRA). 6. Explain how this woman's symptoms could put her at greater risk of low back pain.
Apply	7. Design and implement two physical therapy interventions to improve this patient's bladder control. 8. Discuss two reasons why education in posture and biomechanics is an appropriate intervention in this patient's physical therapy plan of care.
Understand	9. Describe how to instruct a woman to properly perform an isolated PFM contraction. 10. Based on this patient's symptoms, name four muscles requiring strengthening. 11. Describe a precaution to consider with this patient when implementing abdominal muscle strengthening.
Remember	12. Describe the structures that make up the pelvic floor. 13. Describe how pelvic floor muscle strength is determined. 14. Explain why a urinalysis is ordered in the evaluation of a female with UI.

Bloom's Taxonomy Level	Case 16.C Answers
Create	1. The patient is a 32-year-old postpartum female status post spontaneous vaginal delivery of twins 5 weeks ago. She is breastfeeding. She presents with stress urinary incontinence (SUI), stage 1 uterine prolapse, bladder frequency, pelvic floor muscle (PFM) weakness, and DRA. She would benefit from pelvic physical therapy. Will continue to follow. 2. Short-term goals: • Patient will demonstrate improved sitting posture when nursing within 6 weeks to reduce risk of back pain. • Patient will demonstrate improved body mechanics with bending, lifting, carrying, and caring for her children within 6 weeks to reduce risk of back pain reoccurrence. 3. Long-term goals: • Patient will demonstrate improved PFM strength of at least 3/5 within 12 weeks for reduction in episodes of UI and reduced pad protection. • Patient will demonstrate improved abdominal strength as evidenced by reduction of DRA in 12 weeks for safe return to recreation and exercise.
Evaluate	4. SUI is a loss of urine during exertion, such as laughing, coughing, and sneezing. Pregnancy and vaginal birth are associated risk factors for the development of pelvic organ prolapse (POP), SUI, and urethral hypermobility. A stage 1 uterine prolapse is "mild," but indicative of laxity of the pelvic structures. Postpartum urethral hypermobility, SUI, and bladder frequency may result from the inability of the striated PFMs to sufficiently contract and produce closure of the urethra. Physical therapists are musculoskeletal experts qualified to evaluate and treat pelvic floor musculature. External palpation of the levator ani muscles determines if a patient has the ability to contract these muscles. Formal PFM strength testing requires an internal MMT, vaginally or rectally, by a pelvic floor–trained (PF) physical therapist. This patient's pelvic floor strength was therefore assessed by a PF physical therapist and rated 2/5 bilaterally, which is "poor"; this describes a weak squeeze of the muscles and no muscle elevation or lift during the contraction. The muscles also lacked endurance or ability to hold the contraction for more than 2 seconds. Diastasis rectus abdominis (DRA) is a separation of the rectus abdominis muscles, causing an increase in the width of the linea alba or inter-recti distance (IRD). A DRA may spontaneously resolve shortly after childbirth but must be assessed in all postpartum women. Impairments left untreated may result in reduced functional abdominal strength, pelvic floor dysfunction, posture and respiratory abnormalities, lumbopelvic pain, and cosmetic disfigurement, and could increase the risk for lumbopelvic issues later in life.

(Continued)

(Continued)

Bloom's Taxonomy Level	Case 16.C Answers
	Assessment of posture and body mechanics postpartum is necessary to determine if intervention is required to mitigate back pain. Postpartum body changes along with a history of back pain and lifestyle changes postpartum such as breastfeeding and childcare, increase this woman's risk for back pain.
Analyze	5. The size and location of a DRA is determined by measuring the IRD typically at the level of the umbilicus and superior and inferior to the umbilicus. Measuring methods utilized in physical therapy include real-time ultrasound, calipers, tape measure, and finger width method. ▶ Fig. 16.4 The patient is positioned in supine or hooklying, and the IRD is measured during active truck flexion (curl-up) as the patient exhales.
	6. The pelvic floor muscles, multifidus, transversus abdominis (TrA), and respiratory diaphragm make up the body's deep "core" muscles. Weakness in any of these muscle groups interferes with lumbopelvic stability and function. This can lead to altered biomechanical function and back pain.
Apply	7. Physical therapy interventions to improve this patient's bladder control and prevent back pain are implemented as follows:
	a) **Therapeutic exercise for PFM strength training:** The patient is instructed in the proper technique for performing an isolated PFM contraction and prescribed a home exercise program (HEP): Perform a PFM contraction for 2- to 3-second hold × 8 repetitions, two times a day in gravity-eliminated position (supine or side-lying), 5 days weekly. Patient is educated that performing the exercises for a minimum of 6 weeks offers best results. Progression of the program would involve advancing the HEP each session as appropriate, including performance of exercises in antigravity positions (e.g., sitting, standing) and during functional tasks (e.g., lifting child).
	b) **Education in behavior modification:** The patient is taught strategies such as performing a PFM contraction prior to a cough or sneeze to reduce SUI, bladder retraining to reduce voiding frequency, and pelvic floor protection strategies to manage intra-abdominal pressures to reduce excessive downward force on the pelvic organs and muscles. Learning to manage intra-abdominal pressures during lifting and childcare is important to reduce the risk of worsening this woman's uterine prolapse.
	c) **Posture and body mechanics education:** The patient's history of back pain during pregnancy is a risk factor for postpartum back pain. Childcare tasks and postpartum weak core muscles can also increase this patient's risk for back pain. The patient is educated in and practices upright sitting posture with the lumbar spine well supported while breastfeeding, and utilization of good body mechanics when performing childcare and activities of daily living. Supervised PFM training and behavioral techniques should be offered as a first-line treatment to women with urinary incontinence (UI).
	8. Two reasons why education in posture and body mechanics are appropriate for this patient are:
	a) Reducing strain and risk of injury is important due to this patient's history of back pain and dysfunction.
	b) Poor posture and body mechanics while performing new activities such as childcare and breastfeeding can bring on strain and pain of the spine and surrounding muscles which may be weakened postpartum.
Understand	9. Effective verbal cueing encourages proper technique for an isolated PFM contraction by using words similar to:
	• "Take a breath in and as you exhale, lift and squeeze the PFMs."
	• "Tighten the anus as if stopping the passing of gas."
	• "Lift the vagina up and in."
	• "Pull the tailbone toward the pubic bone, etc."
	Instruction to use submaximal effort helps isolate deep, local PFM activation from the global activity of the abdominal, gluteal, and hip adductor accessory muscles.
	10. Four core muscles that may require strengthening include any of the following: pelvic floor, transverse abdominis (TrA), rectus abdominis, respiratory diaphragm, and multifidus.
	11. The bladder base depresses during an abdominal curl, putting women at risk of pelvic floor dysfunction and pelvic organ prolapse (POP) when performing abdominal curl

(Continued)

(Continued)

Bloom's Taxonomy Level	Case 16.C Answers
	activities. The patient was instructed on how to perform a TrA contraction and then progressed to performing this along with mini-abdominal curls, with a focus on lifting the shoulder blades off the mat while exhaling. She was instructed to pre-activate the TrA and avoid breath holding with each repetition. She was also advised to approximate and manually support the rectus abdominis muscle bellies to reduce the IRD and facilitate neuromotor retraining of the muscles. Enforcing proper technique is necessary to safely and effectively strengthen the abdominal muscles while reducing adverse effects. This technique was carried over into instruction during functional activities that require trunk flexion during times of increased abdominal pressure, such as when transferring supine to/from sit.
Remember	12. The pelvic floor consists of various visceral and neurovascular structures in addition to the superficial genital and deep levator ani muscles, and anal sphincter. The levator ani muscles form a sling laterally between the ischial tuberosities and from the pubis anteriorly to the coccyx posteriorly, to support the pelvic viscera. 13. Screening a patient to determine if she has the ability to contract and relax the PFMs can be achieved with external palpation medial to the ischial tuberosities. A MMT of the PFMs requires an internal digital vaginal or rectal examination. 14. A urinalysis is ordered in the evaluation of a female patient with incontinence to rule out infection as the etiology. A symptom of urinary tract infection (UTI) is loss of urine.

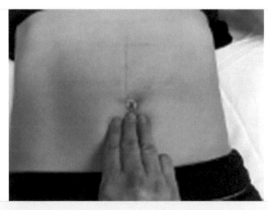

Fig. 16.4 The finger-width method is commonly used to screen for a DRA, by assessing the inter-recti distance superiorly, inferiorly, and at the level of the umbilicus.

Key points
1. Physical therapy for women postpartum is effective in reducing pain and disability and has lifelong implications by reducing the risks for issues later in life.
2. Physical therapy implementation of abdominal, pelvic floor, and "core" strengthening exercises is effective in reducing DRA and SUI in women postpartum.
3. Consider the psychosocial status of postpartum patients and routinely screen for postpartum depression.

Suggested Readings

Birsner ML, Gyamfi-Bannerman C. Physical Activity and Exercise During Pregnancy and the Postpartum Period ACOG Committee Opinion Summary, Number 804. Obstetrics and Gynecology. 2020 Apr 1;135(4):E178-88

America College of Obstetricians and Gynecologists' Committee on Practice Bulletins—Obstetrics. Practice bulletin no. 171: management of preterm labor. Obstet Gynecol. 2016; 128(4): e155–e164

Bo K, Frawley HC, Haylen BT, et al. An International Urogynecological Association (IUGA)/International Continence Society (ICS) joint report on the terminology for the conservative and nonpharmacological management of female pelvic floor dysfunction. Int Urogynecol J Pelvic Floor Dysfunct. 2017; 28(2): 191–213

Boyle R, Hay-Smith EJC, Cody JD, Mørkved S. Pelvic floor muscle training for prevention and treatment of urinary and fecal incontinence in antenatal and postnatal women: a short version Cochrane review. Neurourol Urodyn. 2014; 33(3):269–276

Brown S, Gartland D, Perlen S, McDonald E, MacArthur C. Consultation about urinary and faecal incontinence in the year after childbirth: a cohort study. BJOG. 2015; 122(7):954–962

Burgio KL. Update on behavioral and physical therapies for incontinence and overactive bladder: the role of pelvic floor muscle training. Curr Urol Rep. 2013; 14(5):457–464

Carrera Pérez C, Da Cuña Carrera I, González González Y. What is the best exercise for rehabilitation of abdominal diastasis rehabilitation? Rehabilitacion (Madr). 2019; 53(3):198–210

Casanova R, Chuang A, Goepfert AR, Hueppchen NA, Weiss PM. Beckmann and Ling's Obstetrics and Gynecology. 8th ed. Philadelphia, PA: Wolters Kluwer; 2019

Chiarello CM, McAuley JA, Hartigan EH. Immediate effect of active abdominal contraction on inter-recti distance. J Orthop Sports Phys Ther. 2016; 40(3):177–183

Cunningham FG, Leveno KJ, Bloom SL, et al. Williams Obstetrics. 25th ed. New York, NY: McGraw Hill; 2018

Fernandes da Mota PG, Pascoal AGBA, Carita AIAD, Bø K. Prevalence and risk factors of diastasis recti abdominis from late pregnancy to 6 months postpartum, and relationship with lumbo-pelvic pain. Man Ther. 2015; 20(1):200–205

Flenady V, Wojcieszek AM, Papatsonis DN, et al. Calcium channel blockers for inhibiting preterm labour and birth. Cochrane Database Syst Rev. 2014(6):CD002255

Fox NS, Saltzman DH, Fishman A, Klauser CK, Gupta S, Rebarber A. Gestational age at cervical length and fetal fibronectin assessment and the incidence of spontaneous preterm birth in twins. J Ultrasound Med. 2015; 34(6):977–984

García-Sánchez E, Ávila-Gandía V, López-Román J, Martínez-Rodríguez A, Rubio-Arias JÁ. What pelvic floor muscle training load is optimal in minimizing urine loss in women with stress urinary incontinence? A systematic review and meta-analysis. Int J Environ Res Public Health. 2019; 16(22):4358

Gleason JL, Richter HE, Redden DT, Goode PS, Burgio KL, Markland AD. Caffeine and urinary incontinence in US women. Int Urogynecol J Pelvic Floor Dysfunct. 2013; 24(2):295–302

Heenan AP, Wolfe LA, Davies GA, McGrath MJ. Effects of human pregnancy on fluid regulation responses to short-term exercise. J Appl Physiol (1985). 2003; 95(6):2321–2327

Irion JM, Irion GL, Lewis K, Giglio M. Current trends of physical therapy interventions for high-risk pregnancies. J Womens Health Phys Therap. 2012; 36(3):143–157

Joueidi Y, Vieillefosse S, Cardaillac C, et al. Impact of the diastasis of the rectus abdominis muscles on the pelvic-perineal symptoms: review of the literature. Prog Urol. 2019; 29(11):544–559

Kanayama N, Fukamizu H. Mechanical stretching increases prostaglandin E2 in cultured human amnion cells. Gynecol Obstet Invest. 1989; 28(3):123–126

Keskin EA, Onur O, Keskin HL, Gumus II, Kafali H, Turhan N. Transcutaneous electrical nerve stimulation improves low back pain during pregnancy. Gynecol Obstet Invest. 2012; 74(1):76–83

Laycock J, Jerwood D. Pelvic floor muscle assessment: the PERFECT scheme. Physiotherapy. 2001; 87(12):631–642

Lee D, Hodges PW. Behavior of the linea alba during a curl-up task in diastasis rectus abdominis: an observational study. J Orthop Sports Phys Ther. 2016; 46(7):580–589

Lee SW, Khaw KS, Ngan Kee WD, Leung TY, Critchley LA. Haemodynamic effects from aortocaval compression at different angles of lateral tilt in non-labouring term pregnant women. Br J Anaesth. 2012; 109(6):950–956

Massery M. The Linda Crane Memorial Lecture: The patient puzzle: piecing it together. Cardiopulm Phys Ther J. 2009; 20(2):19–27

Massery M. Musculoskeletal and neuromuscular interventions: a physical approach to cystic fibrosis. J R Soc Med. 2005; 98 Suppl 45:55–66

McCarty-Singleton S, Sciscione AC. Maternal activity restriction in pregnancy and the prevention of preterm birth: an evidence-based review. Clin Obstet Gynecol. 2014; 57(3):616–627

Memon H, Handa VL. Pelvic floor disorders following vaginal or cesarean delivery. Curr Opin Obstet Gynecol. 2012; 24(5): 349–354

Middlekauff ML, Egger MJ, Nygaard IE, Shaw JM. The impact of acute and chronic strenuous exercise on pelvic floor muscle strength and support in nulliparous healthy women. Am J Obstet Gynecol. 2016; 215(3):316.e1–316.e7

Moore KL, Agur AMR, Dalley AF. Essential Clinical Anatomy. 4th ed. Philadelphia, PA: Wolters Kluwer/Lippincott Williams and Wilkins; 2011

Okido MM, Valeri FL, Martins WP, Ferreira CHJ, Duarte G, Cavalli RC. Assessment of foetal wellbeing in pregnant women subjected to pelvic floor muscle training: a controlled randomised study. Int Urogynecol J Pelvic Floor Dysfunct. 2015; 26(10):1475–1481

Park H, Han D. The effect of the correlation between the contraction of the pelvic floor muscles and diaphragmatic motion during breathing. J Phys Ther Sci. 2015; 27(7):2113–2115

Serrao C, Barton A, Thompson J, Briffa NK. Real time transabdominal ultrasound to assess bladder base position during pelvic floor contraction and abdominal curl up in exercising women. Physiotherapy. 2015; 101:e1517

Townsend MK, Devore EE, Resnick NM, Grodstein F. Acidic fruit intake in relation to incidence and progression of urinary incontinence. Int Urogynecol J Pelvic Floor Dysfunct. 2013; 24 (4):605–612

van Benten E, Pool J, Mens J, Pool-Goudzwaard A. Recommendations for physical therapists on the treatment of lumbopelvic pain during pregnancy: a systematic review. J Orthop Sports Phys Ther. 2014; 44(7):464–473, A1–A15

van de Water ATM, Benjamin DR. Measurement methods to assess diastasis of the rectus abdominis muscle (DRAM): a systematic review of their measurement properties and meta-analytic reliability generalisation. Man Ther. 2016; 21:41–53

van Wingerden JP, Ronchetti I, Sneiders D, Lange JF, Kleinrensink GJ. Anterior and posterior rectus abdominis sheath stiffness in relation to diastasis recti: abdominal wall training or not? J Bodyw Mov Ther. 2020; 24(1):147–153

Wood LN, Anger JT. Urinary incontinence in women. BMJ. 2014; 349:g4531

Zeleke BM, Bell RJ, Billah B, Davis SR. Symptomatic pelvic floor disorders in community-dwelling older Australian women. Maturitas. 2016; 85:34–41

17 Total Knee Replacement

General Information	
Case no.	17.A Total Knee Replacement
Authors	Melissa Brown, MSPAS, PA-C
	Julie M. Skrzat, PT, DPT, PhD, Board Certified Clinical Specialist in Cardiovascular & Pulmonary Physical Therapy
Diagnosis	Periprosthetic infection of total knee replacement (TKR)
Setting	Medical-surgical floor in an acute care hospital
Learner expectations	☑ Initial evaluation
	☐ Re-evaluation
	☐ Treatment session
Learner objectives	1. Explain the pathophysiology of the patient's diagnosis.
	2. Recognition and integration of medical precautions/orders into physical therapy plan of care.
	3. Identify signs and symptoms of disease progression.

Medical	
Chief complaint	Right knee pain and fever
History of present illness	The patient is a 73-year-old man with a past medical history of a right TKR 3 months ago. He presented to the emergency department yesterday with sudden-onset right knee pain, swelling, and fever of 101.2 °F. The pain started upon awakening 2 days ago and has progressed to a now constant 10/10 sharp, aching pain. He noted swelling and redness of the knee, along with an inability to bear weight on the right leg for the past 24 hours. He also endorsed severe pain with movement of his knee in all planes of motion. Initial evaluation in the emergency department revealed a leukocytosis of 16.7×10^9/L, and erythrocyte sedimentation rate (ESR) of 85 mm/h, and C-reactive protein (CRP) of 115 mg/L. Arthrocentesis was performed, which yielded 25 mL of turbid yellow fluid. He has been started on intravenous (IV) vancomycin and cefepime.
Past medical history	Hypertension, hyperlipidemia, type 2 diabetes mellitus
Past surgical history	Right knee replacement at age 72 years without complications.
	Appendectomy at age 24 years without complications.
Allergies	None
Medications	Lisinopril, Atorvastatin, Metformin
Precautions/orders	Activity as tolerated
	Non–weight-bearing (NWB) on right lower extremity (RLE).

Social history	
Home setup	• Resides in a two-story home with his wife.
	• One step without handrail to enter.
	• No bathroom on the main level.
	• Bedroom and bathroom are located on the second floor.
	• Flight of stairs + one handrail to the second floor.
Occupation	• Police officer, retired 7 years ago.
Prior level of function	• Independent with functional mobility and activities of daily living (ADLs).
	• Very active; gym 3 × week participated in cardio and strength training.
	• (+) driver
Recreational activities	• Fishing and hiking

Vital signs	Hospital day 0: emergency department	Hospital day 1: ward
Blood pressure (mmHg)	122/74	132/68
Heart rate (beats/min)	108	104
Respiratory rate (breaths/min)	24	21
Pulse oximetry on room air (SpO$_2$)	99%	98%
Temperature (°F)	101.8 (oral)	100.8 (oral)

Imaging/diagnostic test	Hospital day 0: emergency department	Hospital day 1: ward
Right knee X-ray	1. Well-fixed and cemented components of TKR with good alignment ▶ Fig. 17.1	1. Not reordered.
Synovial fluid analysis and culture	1. Viscosity: low 2. White blood cell (WBC) count: 113,000 3. Polymorphonuclear cell count: 86% 4. Gram stain: positive 5. Crystals: negative	1. Culture: positive for gram + cocci in clusters.
Blood cultures	1. No growth to date.	1. No growth to date.

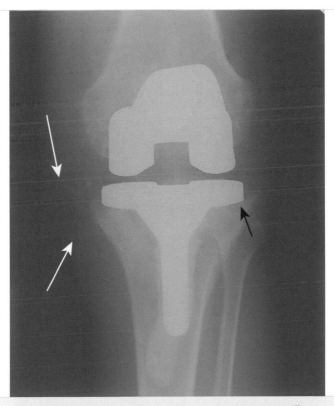

Fig. 17.1 Radiographs of the knee demonstrate changes of total knee arthroplasty. A joint effusion is present, with surrounding soft-tissue swelling. Bone loss and lucency outline portions of the femoral and tibial components (*black arrows*). Soft-tissue gas (*white arrows*) is seen along the medial joint line. (Adapted from Garcia G, ed. Case 167. A 51-year-old man presents with redness and swelling of the knee. In: RadCases: Musculoskeletal Radiology. 1st ed. New York, NY: Thieme; 2010.)

Medical management	Hospital day 0: emergency department	Hospital day 1: ward
Medications	1. Vancomycin IV 2. Cefepime IV 3. Lisinopril 4. Atorvastatin 5. Insulin glargine 6. Insulin lispro 7. Heparin SQ 8. Oxycodone PO prn 9. Morphine IV prn 10. Colace PO prn 11. Acetaminophen prn 12. Ketorolac prn	Continued per medical plan of care.
Procedures	1. Right knee arthrocentesis	1. Arthroscopic irrigation and debridement of right knee.

Lab		Reference range	Hospital day 0: emergency department	Hospital day 1: ward
Complete blood count	WBC	$5.0-10.0 \times 10^9/L$	16.7	17.8
	Hemoglobin	14.0–17.4 g/dL	14.1	14.6
	Hematocrit	42–52%	42.5	43.2
	Red blood cell	4.5–5.5 million/mm³	4.6	4.8
	Platelet	140,000–400,000/μL	399	401
Metabolic Panel	Calcium	8.6–10.3 mg/dL	9.2	9.4
	Chloride	98–108 mEq/L	106	104
	Magnesium	1.2–1.9 mEq/L	1.7	1.7
	Phosphate	2.3–4.1 mg/dL	3.1	3.3
	Potassium	3.7–5.1 mEq/L	4.7	4.8
	Sodium	134–142 mEq/L	140	138
	Blood urea nitrogen	7–20 mg/dL	18	17
	Creatinine	0.7–1.3 mg/dL	1.02	1.12
	Anion gap	3–10 mEq/L	8	10
	CO_2	22–26 mEq/L	24	22
Other	Glucose	60–110 mg/dL	168	187
	CRP	<3.0	115	
	Uric acid	3.4–7.0 mg/dL	3.6	
	International normalized ratio	0.8–1.2	0.9	Not reordered
	Lactate	<2 mmol	1.8	

Pause points

Based on the above information, what are the priorities?
- Diagnostic tests and measures?
- Outcome measures?
- Treatment interventions?

	Hospital Day 1, Ward: Physical Therapy Examination			
	Subjective			
	"I am anxious to move, but want to get back to my routine."			
	Objective			
Vital signs	Pre-treatment			Post-treatment
	Supine	Sitting	Standing	Sitting
Blood pressure (mmHg)	130/80	128/80	132/82	128/78
Heart rate (beats/min)	104	107	110	110
Respiratory rate (breaths/min)	17	20	22	18
Pulse oximetry on room air (SpO_2)	96%	99%	97%	98%
Pain	10/10, right knee			8/10, right knee
General	• Patient supine in bed, awake but fatigued, R knee Immobilizer present. • Lines notable for telemetry, hep-lock IV.			
Cardiovascular and pulmonary	• Auscultation: normal rate. No murmurs, rubs, or gallops. Lungs clear to auscultation. • Rhythm strip ▶ Fig. 17.2 • Pulses: 2 + bilateral dorsalis pedis and posterior tibialis.			
Musculoskeletal	Inspection	• R knee erythematous, swollen, and warm to palpation. Three arthroscopic incisions well-approximated without discharge.		
	Range of motion (ROM)	• Bilateral upper extremity (BUE): within functional range. • R hip and ankle: within functional range. • R knee: not tested due to knee immobilizer. • Left lower extremity (LLE): within functional range.		
	Strength	• B shoulder flexion: 5/5 • B elbow flexion: 5/5 • B wrist extension: 5/5 • B hip flexion: 4/5 • R knee: not tested due to knee immobilizer. • L knee extension: 4/5 • R ankle dorsiflexion: 3/5 (resistance not applied due to WB status). • L ankle dorsiflexion: 4/5		
	Aerobic	• Reported 14/20 on Rate of Perceived Exertion (RPE) Scale during transfers.		
	Flexibility	• Not tested		
Neurological	Balance	• Static sitting, unsupported: close supervision • Dynamic sitting, unsupported: contact guard assistant • Static standing: contact guard assistance with rolling walker. • Dynamic standing: minimal assistance with rolling walker.		
	Cognition	• Alert and oriented × 4		
	Coordination	• Finger to nose: intact bilaterally		
	Cranial nerves	• II–XII: intact		
	Reflexes	• L patellar: 2 + • Achilles: 1 + bilaterally		
	Sensation	• Intact to light touch.		
	Tone	• Normal throughout BUEs and bilateral lower extremities (BLEs).		
	Other	• N/A		

(Continued)

(Continued)

Hospital Day 1, Ward: Physical Therapy Examination	
Functional status	
Bed mobility	• Rolling right: supervision with head of the bed (HOB) flat, no bed rails.
	• Rolling left: minimal assistance to move right lower extremity (RLE), with HOB flat, no bedrails.
	• Supine to sit: supervision at trunk, minimal assistance for RLE; HOB flat.
Transfers	• Sit to/from stand: minimal assistance with rolling walker.
Ambulation	• Ambulated 20 feet with minimal assistance and rolling walker; demonstrated 3-point, step-to gait pattern.
	• Gait deviations notable for increased WB through BUE with bilateral scapular elevation.
	• Verbal cues provided throughout for maintenance of WB precautions.
Stairs	• Not tested
Other	• Activity Measure for Post-Acute Care (AM-PAC) score: 18/24.

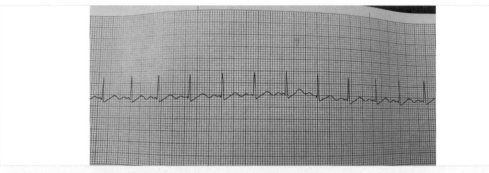

Fig. 17.2 Rhythm strip.

Assessment	
☑ Physical therapist's	*Assessment left blank for learner to develop*
Goals	
Patient's	"I want to get back to doing what I did before."
Short term	1.
	Goals left blank for learner to develop
	2.
Long term	1.
	Goals left blank for learner to develop
	2.

Plan	
☑ Physical therapist's	Will continue to see patient three to five times a week for strength and endurance interventions to maximize functional mobility and safety.

Bloom's Taxonomy Level	Case 17.A Questions
Create	1. Synthesizing the medical data and physical examination findings, develop an appropriate physical therapy assessment of the patient. 2. Develop two short-term physical therapy goals, including an appropriate timeframe. 3. Develop two long-term physical therapy goals, including an appropriate timeframe.
Evaluate	4. If the patient is to remain NWB on RLE at hospital discharge, how could the physical therapist educate the patient on ascending the stairs to get to his bathroom?
Analyze	5. What is the rate and rhythm of the rhythm strip on the patient's day of admission? Identify three reasons why the patient may have this rate and rhythm.
Apply	6. Design and implement two interventions to decrease the risk of developing a deep vein thrombosis.
Understand	7. Discuss classification of periprosthetic infection and at what timeframe is a patient at most risk for developing a periprosthetic infection. 8. Why was a uric acid level and crystals ordered. 9. Interpret the patient's AM-PAC score. 10. Why is the patient's blood glucose elevated.
Remember	11. What do WBCs and CRP measure? Why are they elevated.

Bloom's Taxonomy Level	Case 17.A Answers
Create	1. The patient is a 73-year-old man who presents with sudden onset of right knee pain, swelling, and fever. Medical workup included arthrocentesis, which revealed septic arthritis. Physical therapy evaluation showed decreased RLE strength, specifically right quadriceps, and decreased aerobic capacity as shown by sinus tachycardia and 14/20 RPE on Borg Scale during transfers. As a result of these physical findings and medical precautions of NWB, he required use of rolling walker and minimal assistance to complete all functional mobility. He would benefit from continued physical therapy to improve above deficits through ROM, strengthening, endurance, and functional training to maximize functional mobility and safety. Will continue to follow thrice a week and progress as tolerated. 2. Short-term goals: • Patient will perform supine to/from sit independently with HOB flat within 4 days to be independent at home. • Patient will be independent with home exercise program for BLE muscle strengthening and endurance within 4 days to optimize functional mobility. 3. Long-term goals: • Patient will ambulate 100 feet with rolling walker and supervision, demonstrating reciprocal gait pattern, within 7 days to be able to mobilize around home. • Patient will ascend/descend a flight of stairs + one rail with supervision within 7 days to get in and out of home.
Evaluate	4. If the patient were to remain NWB on RLE at hospital discharge, the patient could demonstrate a hop-to pattern with LLE on the steps while placing bilateral hands on the single handrail. Assuming the patient is not ascending the flight of stairs multiple times a day, the patient's wife could assist by placing the rolling walker on the second floor to use after successful stair negotiation. The patient and his wife could also have a chair set up for the patient to rest, since hopping on one leg is more metabolically demanding, especially considering physiological changes that occur with aging and hospitalization.
Analyze	5. The patient's rhythm strip reads a rate of 110 beats/min and a rhythm of sinus tachycardia. Explanations for this patient's rate and rhythm include pain (10/10), anxiety (as reported by subjective), and/or in response to metabolic demand.
Apply	6. Two interventions to decrease the risk of developing a deep vein thrombosis are ankle pumps (in any position) or active mobility. Other interventions may include leg exercises, proper hydration, mechanism compression, and assessment regarding the need for referral to a physician. By having the patient perform active movements, facilitation of venous return is occurring.
Understand	7. Timeframe of periprosthetic infection is often divided into three categories: early, delayed, and late. Early is defined as infection that occurs within the first 3 months after

(Continued)

(Continued)

Bloom's Taxonomy Level	Case 17.A Answers
	implantation. Delayed is the period between 3 and 24 months, and late is more than 2 years after implantation. Patients are at greatest risk during the early timeframe.
	8. Serum uric acid level and evaluation of arthrocentesis fluid for crystals evaluate the etiology of the presenting complaint. Gout and pseudogout present with similar symptoms to an acute septic arthritis, which include a painful, erythematous, hot, swollen joint. Gout results from an accumulation of monosodium urate crystals within a joint space. Gout is often diagnosed with elevated serum uric acid levels and negatively birefringent crystals in arthrocentesis fluid. Pseudogout results from the accumulation of calcium pyrophosphate dehydrate crystals within the joint space. Pseudogout will have positive birefringent crystals on arthrocentesis evaluation. Proper evaluation determines proper diagnosis, which guides appropriate treatment.
	9. AM-PAC "6-clicks" is a functional assessment instrument used in the acute care setting. The AM-PAC measures three domains: basic mobility, daily activities, and applied cognition. Physical therapists use the basic mobility domain, which includes the following components: rolling, sitting down on and standing up from a chair, moving from lying on back to sitting on the side of the bed, moving to/from bed to chair, walking in the hospital room, and climbing three to five stairs with a railing. It is ranked on a 4-point scale with 1 being dependent and 4 being independent. The patient's AM-PAC score is 18/24 because he scored a 3 on all functional components, which is based on his functional performance during his initial evaluation.
	10. The body will respond to a stressful experience, such as a significant infectious process, by triggering several hormones in order to maintain energy stores. Blood glucose will be elevated due to elevations in counter-regulatory hormones. Increased secretion of catecholamines and glucagon initially raise glucose where increased secretion of cortisol and growth hormone leads to prolonged hyperglycemia in stress states.
Remember	11. The patient's WBCs are elevated, which is also known as leukocytosis. The increase in WBCs is likely due to an infection, as found in the patient's arthrocentesis performed on hospital day 1. The infection supports the patient's clinical manifestations of fever and inflammation and pain at the knee joint. CRP is a protein made by the liver. It is an inflammatory biomarker. It is elevated as a result of the bacterial infection found in the patient's arthrocentesis.

Key points
1. It is important for the physical therapist to synthesize all medical data (i.e., imaging, lab values, etc.) to understand how the patient's pathophysiology can affect functional status and to assess for red flags at every session.
2. It is important to identify medical precautions/orders prior to treating the patient, as they have the ability to change physical therapy management and potentially discharge planning.
3. Considering the length of time physical therapists spend with patients during evaluations and subsequent treatment sessions, they are in prime positions to monitor for signs and symptoms that could be indicative of disease progression, both within a session and over time.

General Information	
Case no.	17.B
Authors	Melissa Brown, MSPAS, PA-C
	Julie M. Skrzat, PT, DPT, PhD, Board Certified Clinical Specialist in Cardiovascular & Pulmonary Physical Therapy
Diagnosis	History of total knee replacement (TKR) with periprosthetic infection, endocarditis, and sepsis
Setting	Medical intensive care unit (ICU) in an acute care hospital
Learner expectations	☑ Initial evaluation
	☐ Re-evaluation
	☐ Treatment session

(Continued)

(Continued)

General Information	
Learner objectives	1. Explain the pathophysiology of acute respiratory distress syndrome. 2. Relate the pathophysiology and progression of pathology to clinical manifestations and activity/participation limitations seen in physical therapy practice. 3. Differentiate how physical therapy plans of care differ between patients who are intubated and patients who are not intubated. 4. Develop an understanding of ICU acquired weakness and the ICU triad and how it can impact physical therapy's plan of care.

Medical	
Chief complaint	Endocarditis and sepsis
History of present illness	The patient is a 73-year-old man with a past medical history of a right TKR 3 months ago. He presented to the emergency department 3 days ago with sudden-onset right knee pain, swelling, and fever of 101.2 °F. Arthrocentesis was performed and he was started on intravenous (IV) vancomycin and cefepime. The following day, he was taken to the operating room (OR) for arthroscopic irrigation and debridement. Final cultures grew methicillin-resistant *Staphylococcus aureus* from the right knee as well as blood cultures. On hospital day 2, he developed chest pain, shortness of breath, worsening fever, and a new-onset heart murmur. A transthoracic echocardiogram was performed and confirmed the finding of a vegetation on the tricuspid valve. A diagnosis of acute bacterial endocarditis was made. On hospital day 3, he was transferred to the ICU after becoming hypotensive and tachypneic. He was intubated on hospital day 4.
Past medical history	Hypertension, hyperlipidemia, and type 2 diabetes mellitus
Past surgical history	Arthroscopic irrigation and debridement 2 days ago. Right knee replacement at age 72 without complications initially. Appendectomy at age 24 without complications.
Allergies	None
Home Medications	Lisinopril, Atorvastatin, Metformin
Precautions/orders	Contact precautions Non–weight-bearing (NWB) on right lower extremity (RLE). Bedrest on hospital day 3, ICU day 1. Activity as tolerated on hospital day 5, ICU day 3.

Social history	
Home setup	• Resides in a two-story home with his wife. • One step without handrail to enter. • No bathroom on the main level. • Bedroom and bathroom are located on the second floor. • Flight of stairs + one handrail to the second floor.
Occupation	• Police officer, retired 7 years ago.
Prior level of function	• Independent with functional mobility and activities of daily living (ADLs). • Very active; gym thrice a week, participated in cardio and strength training. • (+) driver
Recreational activities	• Fishing and hiking

Vital signs	Hospital day 0: emergency department	Hospital day 2: ward	Hospital day 4: ICU day 2
Blood pressure (mmHg)	122/74	118/68	108/66 (on vasopressors)
Heart rate (beats/min)	108	112	104
Respiratory rate (breaths/min)	24	21	18

(Continued)

(Continued)

Vital signs	Hospital day 0: emergency department	Hospital day 2: ward	Hospital day 4: ICU day 2
Pulse oximetry (SpO$_2$)	99% room air	94% on 2 L/min O$_2$ via nasal cannula	100% On mechanical ventilation via endotracheal tube (ETT) FiO$_2$: 60% Tidal volume: 6 mL/kg ideal body weight (IBW) Positive end expiratory pressure (PEEP): 5 cm H$_2$O
Temperature (°F)	101.8 (tympanic)	100.8 (tympanic)	102.6 (tympanic)

Imaging/diagnostic test	Hospital day 0: emergency department	Hospital day 2: ward	Hospital day 4: ICU day 2
Right knee X-ray	1. Well-fixed and cemented components of TKR with good alignment	N/A	N/A
Chest X-ray	N/A	1. Bilateral lung fields clear without infiltrates. Heart size normal. Impression: no acute cardiopulmonary findings.	1. Diffuse bilateral nodular densities in early stages of cavitation ▶ Fig. 17.3
Chest computed tomography (CT)	N/A	1. No evidence of infiltrate, effusion, or infarction. cardiovascular and pulmonary silhouette appears normal.	1. Subpleural nodular lesions without necrosis suspicious for septic emboli ▶ Fig. 17.4
Arthrocentesis, synovial fluid analysis and culture	1. 25-mL turbid yellow fluid, cultures pending	1. Methicillin-resistant *S. aureus*	1. Methicillin-resistant *S. aureus*, sensitive to van-comycin, linezolid, dapsone.
Blood cultures	1. Negative	1. Methicillin-resistant *S. aureus*	1. Methicillin-resistant *S. aureus*, sensitive to van-comycin, linezolid, dapsone.

Medical management	Hospital day 0: emergency department	Hospital day 2: ward	Hospital day 4: ICU day 2
Medications	1. Lisinopril 2. Insulin glargine 3. Insulin lispro 4. Vancomycin 5. Cefepime	1. Vancomycin IV 2. Cefepime IV 3. Oxycodone PO prn 4. Morphine IV prn 5. Colace PO prn 6. Acetaminophen 1,000 mg 7. Ketorolac prn 8. Lisinopril 9. Atorvastatin 10. Insulin glargine 11. Insulin lispro 12. Heparin SQ	1. Vancomycin IV 2. Cefepime IV 3. Norepine phrine 4. Propofol 5. Insulin drip 6. Heparin SQ 7. Protonix IV 8. Fentanyl IV prn
Procedures	1. Right knee arthrocentesis	1. Arthroscopic irrigation and debridement of right knee in the OR.	1. Insertion of arterial line, central line, endotracheal tube, foley catheter, orogastric (OG) tube.

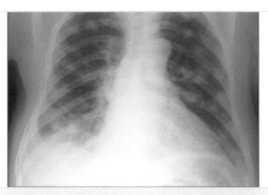

Fig. 17.3 The patient's chest X-ray on hospital day 4, ICU day 2. (Adapted from Gunderman R, ed. Lung. In: Essential Radiology. Clinical Presentation, Pathophysiology, Imaging. 3rd ed. New York, NY: Thieme; 2014.)

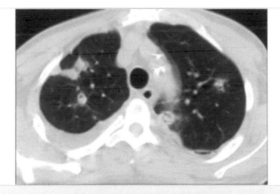

Fig. 17.4 The patient's chest CT on hospital day 4, ICU day 2. (Adapted from Gunderman R, ed. Lung. In: Essential Radiology. Clinical Presentation, Pathophysiology, Imaging. 3rd ed. New York, NY: Thieme; 2014.)

Lab values		Reference range	Hospital day 0: emergency department	Hospital day 2: ward	Hospital day 4: ICU day 2
Complete blood count	White blood cell (WBC)	$5.0–10.0 \times 10^9$/L	16.7	18.0	24.2
	Hemoglobin	14.0–17.4 g/dL	14.1	13.8	13.6
	Hematocrit	42–52%	42.5	42.0	41.4
	Red blood cell	4.5–5.5 million/mm³	4.6	4.8	4.7
	Platelet	140,000–400,000/μL	399	401	566
Metabolic panel	Calcium	8.6–10.3 mg/dL	9.2	9.4	9.1
	Chloride	98–108 mEq/L	106	104	100
	HCO_3^-	22–26 mEq/L	24	25	18
	Magnesium	1.2–1.9 mEq/L	1.7	1.5	1.2
	Phosphate	2.3–4.1 mg/dL	3.1	3.0	2.8
	Potassium	3.7–5.1 mEq/L	4.7	4.9	5.1
	Sodium	134–142 mEq/L	140	138	132
	Blood urea nitrogen	7–20 mg/dL	18	16	22

(Continued)

(Continued)

Lab values		Reference range	Hospital day 0: emergency department	Hospital day 2: ward	Hospital day 4: ICU day 2
Other	Creatinine	0.7–1.3 mg/dL	1.02	1.21	2.52
	Glucose	60–110 mg/dL	168	180	202
	C-reactive protein	<3.0	115		Not reordered
	Uric acid	3.4–7.0 mg/dL	3.6	Not reordered	Not re-ordered
	International normalized ratio	0.8–1.2	0.9		1.0
	Lactate	<2 mmol	1.8	2.1	4.2
	Troponin 1	<0.03 ng/mL	Not ordered	0.01	0.03
	Troponin 2		Not ordered	0.01	0.03
	Troponin 3		Not ordered	0.02	0.02
Arterial blood gas	pH	7.35–7.45		7.31	7.12
	$PaCO_2$ (mmHg)	37–43	Not ordered	43	60.4
	PaO_2 (mmHg)	80–95		85	34
	HCO_3^-	20–30		21	18

Pause points

Based on the above information, what are the priorities?
• Diagnostic tests and measures?
• Outcome measures?
• Treatment interventions?

Hospital Day 5, ICU Day 3: Physical Therapy Examination

Subjective

Patient nonverbal due to endotracheal tube, however nodding appropriately to questions.

Objective

Vital signs	Pre-treatment			Post-treatment
	Supine	Sitting	Standing	Sitting
Blood pressure (mmHg)	132/78	130/80	123/72	135/85
Heart rate (beats/min)	126	135	140	127
Respiratory rate (breaths/min)	25	25	27	24
Oxygen saturation (mechanically ventilated via endotracheal tube; assist control, 40% FiO_2, PEEP 5)	94	95	96	95
Pain	2/10, throat due to endotracheal tube. 3/10, right knee			2/10, right knee
General	• Patient supine in bed, sedated but arousable, no acute distress. • Lines notable for telemetry, central line, arterial line, endotracheal tube, urinary catheter, OG tube.			
Cardiovascular and pulmonary	• Auscultation: tachycardia, 2/6 diastolic murmur heard best at the left fourth intercostal space. Lungs scattered rhonchi throughout. • Pulses: 1+ bilateral dorsalis pedis and posterior tibialis.			

(Continued)

(Continued)

Hospital Day 5, ICU Day 3: Physical Therapy Examination		
Gastrointestinal		• Soft, nontender, nondistended • No hepatosplenomegaly
Musculoskeletal	Inspection	• R knee mild erythema and swelling. 3 arthroscopic incisions well approximated without drainage.
	Range of motion (ROM)	• Bilateral upper extremity (BUE): within functional range • R hip and ankle: within functional range • R knee: not tested due to knee immobilizer • Left lower extremity (LLE): within functional range
	Strength	• B shoulder flexion: 3+/5 • B elbow flexion: 4/5 • B wrist extension: 4/5 • B hip flexion: 3+/5 • R knee: not tested due to knee immobilizer. • L knee: 3+/5 • R ankle dorsiflexion: 3/5 • L ankle dorsiflexion: 3/5
	Aerobic	• Reported 16/20 on Rate of Perceived Exertion (RPE) Scale during transfers.
	Flexibility	• Not tested
Neurological	Balance	• Static sitting, unsupported: minimal assistance • Dynamic sitting, unsupported: moderate assistance • Static standing: minimal assistance with rolling walker. • Dynamic standing: moderate assistance with rolling walker.
	Cognition	• Richmond Agitation–Sedation Scale (RASS): (–1) • Confusion Assessment Method for the Intensive Care Unit (CAM-ICU): (+).
	Coordination	• Not tested due to inability to follow one-step commands consistently.
	Cranial nerves	• Optic, oculomotor, trochlear, abducens, and spinal accessory intact. • Others not tested.
	Reflexes	• L patellar: 2+ • Achilles: 1+ bilaterally
	Sensation	• Not tested
	Tone	• Normal throughout BUEs and BLEs
	Other	• N/A
Functional status		
Bed mobility		• Rolling right: moderate assistance • Rolling left: maximal assistance at trunk and to move right lower extremity. • Supine to sit: moderate assistance, head of bed flat, use of bedrails.
Transfers		• Sit to stand: moderate assistance with rolling walker. • Stand to sit: minimal assistance with rolling walker.
Ambulation		• Ambulated 3 feet from bed to chair with moderate assistance and rolling walker, demonstrated NWB status with verbal cues.
Other		• Activity Measure for Post-Acute Care (AM-PAC): 11/24. • Functional Status Scale for the Intensive Care Unit (FSS-ICU): 13/35.

Assessment	
☑ Physical therapist's	*Assessment left blank for learner to develop.*
Goals	
Patient's	Patient writing "I want the tube [ETT] out."
Short term	1.
	Goals left blank for learner to develop.
	2.
Long term	1.
	Goals left blank for learner to develop.
	2.

Plan	
☑ Physical therapist's	Will continue to see patient three to five times a week for ROM, strength, endurance, airway clearance, and positioning interventions to maximize functional mobility and safety.

Bloom's Taxonomy Level	Case 17.B Questions
Create	1. Synthesizing the medical data and physical examination findings, develop an appropriate assessment of the patient.
	2. Develop two short-term physical therapy goals, including an appropriate timeframe.
	3. Develop two long-term physical therapy goals, including an appropriate timeframe.
Evaluate	4. What is the relationship between periprosthetic infection and the development of endocarditis?
Analyze	5. A murmur is heard at the left fourth intercostal space. What valve is likely affected? How does this impact the physical therapy plan of care?
Apply	6. Name three interventions—one for strengthening, one for endurance, and one for function—that can be implemented in the ICU.
Understand	7. What laboratory values indicate the patient has a bacterial infection?
	8. Why would a patient with endocarditis present with low back pain?
	9. Interpret the patient's RASS and CAM-ICU scores.
	10. Interpret the patient's FSS-ICU score.
	11. What precautions are necessary when mobilizing a patient with an endotracheal tube?
	12. What are two reasons for the vent to trigger a high-pressure alarm? What are two reasons for the vent to trigger a low-pressure alarm?
Remember	13. What are the criteria for systemic inflammatory response syndrome (SIRS)? Based on these data, does this patient have SIRS?

Bloom's Taxonomy Level	Case 17.B Answers
Create	1. The patient is a 73-year-old man who initially presented to the hospital with septic arthritis. He subsequently developed acute bacterial endocarditis, acute hypoxic respiratory failure, and septic shock with multiple septic emboli to the lungs. On ICU day 2, vasopressors weaned and physical therapy consult was placed. During physical therapy evaluation, lines were notable for endotracheal tube, arterial line, central line, telemetry, foley catheter, and OG tube. Physical examination revealed altered cognition as shown through RASS and CAM-ICU and diffuse weakness in BUE and bilateral lower extremity, which is likely attributed to ICU-acquired weakness. He was able to participate in mobility trial, requiring moderate assistance with rolling walker to complete. Primary limitations include decreased aerobic capacity and muscle weakness. He would benefit from continued physical therapy to improve above deficits to maximize functional mobility and safety. Will continue to follow five times a week and progress as tolerated.

(Continued)

(Continued)

Bloom's Taxonomy Level	Case 17.B Answers
	2. Short-term goals: • Patient will tolerate supported sitting out of bed×2 hours every day in 5 days to improve hemodynamic stability, ventilation, and oxygenation. • Patient will perform stand pivot transfers with rolling walker and minimal assistance within 5 days to improve functional independence. 3. Long-term goals: • Patient will demonstrate diaphragmatic breathing independently within 10 days to maximize ventilation and oxygenation and decrease shortness of breath. • Patient will improve his FSS-ICU score by 5 points in 10 days to demonstrate an improvement in functional mobility.
Evaluate	4. Periprosthetic infection can lead to endocarditis from bacteria spreading through the blood stream and seeding on a heart valve. The joint space is very vascular and the infection can enter the blood stream easily.
Analyze	5. A murmur at the left fourth intercostal space is likely indicative of a pathology at the tricuspid valve, which separates the right atrium and right ventricle.

Apply	6. Three interventions that can be implemented in the ICU are as follows:
	• Strengthening:
	  ○ Bilateral upper extremities: With the patient in supine, theraband (of appropriate resistance) can be attached to the patient's bedrails. From there, the patient can complete upper extremity therapeutic exercise (i.e., bicep curls, triceps extensions, proprioceptive neuromuscular facilitation proprioceptive neuromuscular facilitation (PNF) patterns, etc.).
	  ○ Bilateral uppers and lower extremities: Therapeutic exercise will be dependent on the patient's position. Such exercises can include quad sets, glut sets, and ankle pumps for supine and seated marching and long arc quads (as able) in sitting.
	• Endurance: The patient can complete cycling—whether via an in-bed cycle or restorator—to improve cardiovascular and muscle endurance.
	• Functional: The patient should progress from unsupported sitting activities (i.e., static sitting with breathing) to standing activities (walking).

Understand	7. Laboratory values associated with bacterial infection include elevation of WBCs, erythrocyte sedimentation rate, C-reactive protein, and lactate levels. Increase in WBCs, specifically neutrophils is an immune response to fight the bacterial infection. Erythrocyte sedimentation rate and C-reactive protein levels are inflammatory markers. Serum lactate is a marker of hypoperfusion which can indicate sepsis 8. Infective endocarditis is a bacterial infection of the endocardium. The inner lining also covers the heart valves. The bacteria may form into a thrombus, which can be dislodged and become an embolus, traveling to various parts of the body. This includes the back, which could present as acute low back pain. 9. An interpretation of the patient's RASS and CAM-ICU scores are as follows: • RASS: The RASS is an instrument to assess level of alertness in a patient in the ICU. It is scored on a 10-level scale. The patient's score of (−1) indicates that the patient is drowsy, but has sustained awakening to voice (eye opening and contact>10 seconds). ▶ Fig. 17.5 • CAM-ICU: The CAM-ICU is an instrument to assess delirium in a patient in the ICU. By having a positive CAM-ICU, the patient is experiencing delirium. ▶ Fig. 17.6. 10. FSS-ICU is a functional assessment used in the ICU. The test measures rolling, supine to sit, unsupported static sitting, sit to stand transfer, and ambulation. It is ranked on a 7-point scale, with 1 being complete dependence and 7 being complete independence. The patient's FSS-ICU score is 13/35 based on the following scores: • Rolling: 2—maximal assistance to roll. • Supine to sit: 3—moderate assistance • Unsupported static sitting: 4—minimal assistance • Sit to stand: 3—moderate assistance • Ambulation: 1—ambulated<50 feet

(Continued)

(Continued)

Bloom's Taxonomy Level	Case 17.B Answers

	11. When mobilizing a patient with an endotracheal tube, the following precautions should be taken:
	• discussion with the medical team regarding risk–benefit of physical therapy during acute medical conditions.
	• observation of the location of the endotracheal tube before and after physical therapy interventions.
	• observation of the location of the ventilator prior, during, and after mobilization.
	• anticipation of the patient's movements and how that impacts patient's proximity to the ventilator.
	• understanding the meaning of high- and low-pressure ventilator alarms.
	12. In regard to ventilator alarms:
	• Two reasons for high-pressure ventilator alarms include:
	  ○ Coughing, increase in secretions.
	• Two reasons for low-pressure ventilator alarms include:
	  ○ Disconnection between tubing and ventilator, leak in ventilator circuitry.

Remember	13. To be diagnosed with SIRS, the patient must have two or more of the following variables: fever > 38 °C (100.4 °F) or < 36 °C (96.8 °F), heart rate > 90 beats/min, respiratory rate > 20 breaths/min or arterial carbon dioxide tension < 32 mmHg, and abnormal WBC count (> 12,000/ μL or < 4,000/ μL or > 10% immature [band] forms). The patient meets all four of the SIRS criteria: temperature (102.6 °F), heart rate (124 beats/min), respiratory rate (20 breaths/min), and elevated WBC count (24,200/μL).

Score	Classification	(RASS)
+4	Combative	Overtly combative or violent; immediate danger to staff
+3	Very agitated	Pulls on or removes tube(s) or catheter(s) or has aggressive behavior toward staff
+2	Agitated	Frequent non-purposeful movement or patient–ventilator dyssynchrony
+1	Restless	Anxious or apprehensive but movements not aggressive or vigorous
0	Alert and calm	Spontaneously pays attention to caregiver
−1	Drowsy	Not fully alert, but has sustained (more than 10 seconds) awakening, with eye contact, to voice
−2	Light sedation	Briefly (less than 10 seconds) awakens with eye contact to voice
−3	Moderate sedation	Any movement (but no eye contact) to voice
−4	Deep sedation	No response to voice, but any movement to physical stimulation
−5	Unarousable	No response to voice or physical stimulation

https://doi.org/10.1371/journal.pone.0207174.t001

Fig. 17.5 Richmond Agitation Sedation Scale (Adapted from https://www.researchgate.net/figure/Richmond-agitation-sedation-scale-RASS-score_tbl1_328945668.)

Key points
1. Acute hypoxic respiratory failure can be caused by multiple conditions, all of which ultimately result in decreased oxygen content of the arterial blood. In this patient's case, it was due to multiple septic pulmonary emboli that originated from the bacterial vegetation on the tricuspid valve.
2. Medical management of acute hypoxic respiratory failure (i.e., intubation, anti-inflammatories, medications, etc.) may alter the patient's physical and cognitive status. Therefore, physical therapy plans of care should begin with low levels of activity to monitor for tolerance before progressing to greater functional activities.

(Continued)

(Continued)

Key points

3. Physical therapy may be implemented with patients who are intubated; however, it may require greater communication and coordination of care among other health care providers (i.e., nursing, respiratory therapists, physicians, etc.) compared to patients who are not intubated.

4. ICU-acquired weakness and the ICU triad of delirium, pain, and agitation may limit a patient's ability to physically and cognitively participate in physical therapy. Plans of care must be modified to accommodate both while keeping the patient safe.

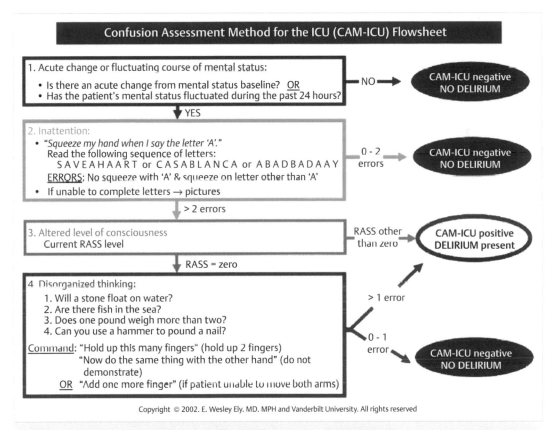

Fig. 17.6 Confusion Assessment Method for the Intensive Care Unit. (Adapted from https://uploadsssl.webflow.com/5b0849daec50243a0a1e5e0c/5bad3d0db04 cd51ee28f45c3_CAM-ICU-flowsheet.pdf.)

General Information	
Case no.	17.C
Authors	Melissa Brown, MSPAS, PA-C Julie M. Skrzat, PT, DPT, PhD, Board Certified Clinical Specialist in Cardiovascular & Pulmonary Physical Therapy
Diagnosis	Intensive care unit (ICU) weakness after hospitalization for right knee periprosthetic infection, endocarditis, acute hypoxic respiratory failure, and sepsis
Setting	Acute inpatient rehabilitation

(Continued)

(Continued)

General Information	
Learner expectations	☑ Initial evaluation ☐ Re-evaluation ☐ Treatment session
Learner objectives	1. Understand complications of a prolonged hospitalization stay and how to monitor for them in an inpatient rehabilitation setting. 2. Develop a comprehensive physical therapy plan of care for a patient who is medically complex. 3. Identify and implement appropriate outcome measures.

Medical	
Chief complaint	"Will I ever get back to how I was before this happened?"
History of present illness	The patient is a 73-year-old man with a past medical history of a right total knee replacement 3 months ago who presented to the emergency department 2 weeks ago with a right periprosthetic infection secondary to methicillin-resistant *Staphylococcus aureus*. He had arthroscopic irrigation and debridement of the right knee on hospital day 1. He subsequently developed endocarditis with vegetation of the tricuspid valve on hospital day 2. His conditioned worsened as he developed hypotension, tachypnea, and leukocytosis. He was transferred to the ICU on hospital day 3, and intubated on ICU day 2, hospital day 4 due to acute hypoxic respiratory failure and septic shock. He was intubated × 5 days and required vasopressor support with norepinephrine, and an insulin drip to control serum glucose level. The infection was initially treated with intravenous (IV) vancomycin and cefepime. He was discharged to inpatient rehabilitation center after a 14-day hospital stay. He is receiving 6 weeks of IV vancomycin for treatment of endocarditis.
Past medical history	Hypertension, hyperlipidemia, type 2 diabetes mellitus
Past surgical history	Arthroscopic irrigation and debridement of right knee 13 days ago. Right knee replacement at age 72 years initially without complications. Appendectomy at age 24 years without complications.
Allergies	None
Home Medications	Lisinopril, Atorvastatin, Metformin
Precautions/orders	Activity as tolerated Partial weight bearing (WB) on right lower extremity (RLE).

Social history	
Home setup	• Resides in a two-story home with his wife • One step without handrail to enter • No bathroom on the main level • Bedroom and bathroom are located on the second floor • Flight of stairs + one handrail to the second floor
Occupation	• Police officer, retired 7 years ago
Prior level of function	• Independent with functional mobility and activities of daily living (ADLs) • Very active; gym 3 × week participated in cardio and strength training • (+) driver
Recreational activities	• Fishing and hiking

Vital signs	Hospital day 0: emergency department	Hospital day 14: step-down unit	Day 1: acute inpatient rehabilitation
Blood pressure (mmHg)	122/74	124/80	128/82
Heart rate (beats/min)	108	84	80
Respiratory rate (breaths/min)	16	14	14
Pulse oximetry on room air (SpO$_2$)	99%	95%	96%
Temperature (°F)	101.8 (oral)	98.2 (oral)	97.8 (oral)

Medical management	Hospital day 0: emergency department	Hospital day 14: step-down unit	Day 1: acute inpatient rehabilitation
Medications	1. Lisinopril 2. Insulin glargine 3. Insulin lispro 4. Vancomycin 5. Cefepime	1. Lisinopril 2. Insulin glargine 3. Insulin lispro 4. Heparin 5. Protonix 6. Vancomycin	1. Lisinopril 2. Atorvastatin 3. Insulin glargine 4. Insulin lispro 5. Vancomycin

Lab		Reference range	Hospital day 14: step-down unit	Day 1: acute inpatient rehabilitation
Complete blood count	White blood cell	5.0–10.0 × 10^9/L	14.4	14.2
	Hemoglobin	14.0–17.4 g/dL	14.1	14.2
	Hematocrit	42–52%	42.6	42.8
	Red blood cell	4.5–5.5 million/mm^3	4.7	4.8
	Platelet	140,000–400,000/μL	336	340
Metabolic panel	Calcium	8.6–10.3 mg/dL	9.8	9.7
	Chloride	98–108 mEq/L	104	106
	HCO$_3^-$	23–30 mEq/L	26	27
	Magnesium	1.2–1.9 mEq/L	1.7	1.7
	Potassium	3.7–5.1 mEq/L	4.9	4.8
	Sodium	134–142 mEq/L	139	138
	Blood urea nitrogen	7–20 mg/dL	17	18
	Creatinine	0.7–1.3 mg/dL	1.52	1.48
Other	Glucose	60–110 mg/dL	146	138
	C-reactive protein	<3.0	35	Not reordered
	Lactate	<2 mmol	1.4	
	Procalcitonin	<1.5 ng/mL	1.0	
	Vancomycin	15–20 mcg/mL	17	

Pause points

Based on the above information, what are the priorities?
- Diagnostic tests and measures?
- Outcome measures?
- Treatment interventions?

Day 1, Acute Inpatient Rehabilitation: Physical Therapy Examination				
Subjective				
"I've had enough of the hospital. I want to go home to my dog."				
Objective				
Vital signs	Pre-treatment			Post-treatment
	Supine	Sitting	Standing	Sitting
Blood pressure (mmHg)	134/82	132/80	130/78	136/82
Heart rate (beats/min)	78	80	82	80
Respiratory rate (breaths/min)	14	16	15	14
Pulse oximetry on room air (SpO$_2$)	97%	99%	95%	96%
Pain	2/10, right knee			3/10, right knee
General	• Patient sitting up in bed, appears tired. • Lines notable for peripherally inserted central catheter (PICC) right basilic vein.			
Cardiovascular and pulmonary	• Auscultation: normal rate. 2/6 diastolic murmur heard best at the left fourth intercostal space. Lungs clear with decreased breath sounds at bases. • Pulses: 2 + bilateral dorsalis pedis and posterior tibialis.			
Musculoskeletal	Inspection	• R knee: mild swelling, no erythema. 3 arthroscopic incisions well approximated.		
	Range of motion (ROM)	• Bilateral upper extremity (BUE): within functional range. • Left lower extremity (LLE): within functional range. • R hip and ankle: within functional range. • R knee: lacks terminal knee extension.		
	Strength	• B shoulder flexion: 3 + /5 • B elbow flexion: 4/5 • B wrist extension: 4/5 • B hip flexion: 3 + /5 • R knee extension: 3-/5 • L knee extension: 3 + /5 • R ankle dorsiflexion: 3 + /5 • L ankle dorsiflexion: 3 + /5 • Five Times Sit-to-Stand: 75 seconds		
	Aerobic	• Patient performed recumbent elliptical bike × 6 minutes on level 1. Rate of perceived exertion (RPE) 16/20.		
	Flexibility	• Not tested		
Neurological	Balance	• Static sitting, unsupported: minimal assistance • Dynamic sitting, unsupported: moderate assistance • Static standing: moderate assistance with rolling walker. • Dynamic standing: maximal assistance with rolling walker.		
	Cognition	• Orientated to person, place, and time. Patient is unsure of situation. • Montreal Cognitive Assessment (MoCA): 23/30.		
	Coordination	• Finger to nose: intact bilaterally • Heel to shin: attempted bilaterally, however had difficulty completing due to bilateral lower extremity (BLE) weakness.		
	Cranial nerves	• I–XII: intact		
	Reflexes	• L patellar: 2 + • Achilles: 1 + bilaterally		
	Sensation	• Intact to light touch but diminished with 5.07/10-g monofilament testing on plantar aspects of feet. • Vibratory sensation: 20-second bilateral great toes and 10-second lateral malleoli.		
	Tone	• Low muscle tone		

(Continued)

(Continued)

	Day 1, Acute Inpatient Rehabilitation: Physical Therapy Examination	
	Other	• Respiratory function: Incentive spirometer: able to achieve 1,000 mL × 5 with proper form. Additional trials demonstrate compromise of posture and integrity of breathing (▶ Fig. 17.7). Productive cough of thin white secretions after use of recumbent elliptical trainer.
	Functional status	
Bed mobility		• Rolling right: moderate assistance • Rolling left: moderate assistance • Supine to sit: maximal assistance, head of bed flat, use of bedrails. • Sit to supine: moderate assistance, head of bed flat, use of bedrails.
Transfers		• Sit to stand: maximal assistance with rolling walker. • Stand to sit: moderate assistance with rolling walker.
Ambulation		• Ambulated 2 × 10 feet with moderate assistance and rolling walker; demonstrated partial WB RLE within moderate verbal and tactile cues.
Stairs		• N/A due to safety concerns.

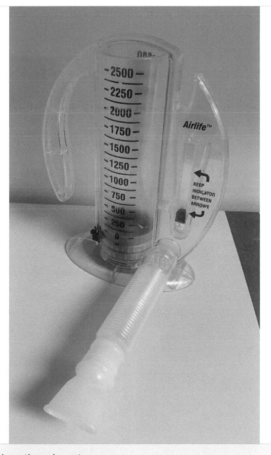

Fig. 17.7 An example of an incentive spirometer.

Assessment	
☑ Physical therapist's	*Assessment left blank for learner to develop.*

Goals	
Patient's	"To get back home."
Short term	1.
	Goals left blank for learner to develop.
	2.
Long term	1.
	Goals left blank for learner to develop.
	2.

Plan	
☑ Physical therapist's	Will continue to see patient 30 to 90 minutes a day for 1 to 2 weeks for ROM, strength, endurance, balance, motor control, airway clearance, and mobility training to maximize function and safety.

Bloom's Taxonomy Level	Case 17.C Questions
Create	1. Synthesizing the medical data and physical examination findings, develop an appropriate assessment of the patient.
	2. Develop two short-term physical therapy goals, including an appropriate timeframe.
	3. Develop two long-term physical therapy goals, including an appropriate timeframe.
Evaluate	4. Explain why the patient is on insulin for management of type 2 diabetes mellitus and why he is not back on metformin.
Analyze	5. Interpret the patient's spirometry results. What physiological changes have occurred that produce these results?
	6. Interpret the 5 x Sit to Stand.
	7. Interpret the patient's MoCA.
	8. Interpret the patient's sensory findings.
Apply	9. What are three interventions—one for strengthening, one for aerobic, and one for stretching—that can be implemented in this setting? Be sure to include frequency, intensity, time, and type (FITT) principles.
Understand	10. Explain the importance of infusing vancomycin at a slow rate.
Remember	11. What precautions are necessary when mobilizing a PICC line?

Bloom's Taxonomy Level	Case 17.C Answers
Create	1. The patient is a 73-year-old man with a past medical history of a right total knee replacement 3 months ago who initially presented to the emergency department with a right periprosthetic infection secondary to methicillin-resistant *S. aureus*. Hospital stay was complicated by endocarditis, acute hypoxic respiratory failure, and sepsis, which required a 5-day ICU stay with intubation, pressor support, and antibiotics. He has since stabilized, but due to prolonged hospitalization and subsequent sequelae, he has been admitted to acute inpatient rehabilitation. Physical therapy initial evaluation showed global BUE, BLE, and trunk musculature strength deficits; decreased cardiovascular and pulmonary capacity as demonstrated by incentive spirometer, productive cough, and decreased breath sounds; and impaired balance due to decreased muscle strength and decreased sensation. As a result of these, he requires minimal to maximal assistance with rolling walker to complete all functional mobility. He would benefit from continued physical therapy to improve above deficits to maximize functional mobility and safety. Will continue to follow and progress as tolerated. Will discuss and work with occupational therapist (OT) and speech-language pathologist (SLP) to maximize outcomes. Physical therapist to see 1 to 2 hours a day×5 to 7 days a week.
	2. Short-term goals:
	• Patient will perform 15 minutes on a recumbent elliptical trainer at level 1 within 7 days to improve his aerobic capacity.
	• Patient will perform sit to/from stand with minimal assistance and rolling walker, demonstrating good quadriceps control by not "plopping" onto chair when sitting, within 7 days to become more independent with functional mobility.

(Continued)

(Continued)

Bloom's Taxonomy Level	Case 17.C Answers
	3. Long-term goals: • Patient will perform incentive spirometer to 2,000 mL × 10 repetitions independently within 14 days to demonstrate improved respiratory capacity. • Patient will verbalize two energy conservation techniques independently within 14 days to be independent with functional tasks at home and prevent shortness of breath.
Evaluate	4. Patients who are hospitalized are often transitioned from oral diabetic medication to insulin to obtain better glucose control. Glucose will often be elevated due to an acute stress response and insulin allows for tighter control. Metformin increases the risk of lactic acidosis and is often held during hospitalizations.
Analyze	5. An incentive spirometer is a used to promote lung expansion after surgery or lung pathology by having the patient inhale slowly and deeply into the device. Since the patient was on a ventilator and immobile for an extended period of time, (a) his trunk muscles, including diaphragm, are weak, which prevent a mechanical disadvantage to breathing at ideal total lung capacity and (b) he needs to improve oxygenation through expansion of alveoli. An incentive spirometer can assist with both of these goals. The patient's volume of 1,000 mL is below normal average lung volumes. Ideally, a patient should be inspiring between 2,000 and 3,000 mL. Additionally, it is encouraged to perform 10 repetitions before resting. The fact that the patient has a decreased inspiratory volume and can only perform five times with proper form gives an indication of muscle weakness and ongoing recovery of his underlying pulmonary condition. 6. The Five Times Sit-to-Stand Test is an objective measurement to quantify functional lower extremity strength and fall risk. Normative cutoff is at 12 seconds. Since the patient took 75 seconds to complete Five Times Sit-to-Stand, he has lower extremity weakness and is at a fall risk. 7. The MoCA is a 30-question test that assesses for mild cognitive impairments. It assesses cognition in the visuospatial and executive functions, naming, memory, attention, language, abstraction, and orientation domains. A score of ≥ 26 is considered normal. 8. On the planter aspects of the patient's feet, sensation is intact to light touch but diminished with 5.07/10-g monofilament testing and vibration. The patient's diminished sensation to monofilament testing and vibration is indicative of a loss of protective sensation, likely due to the patient's past medical history of diabetes mellitus. This makes the patient susceptible to the development of diabetic ulcers.

Apply	9. Three interventions that can be included in this setting's rehabilitation program include:
	 • Strengthening:
	   ○ Frequency: minimum of 2 days a week.
	     Intensity: 60 to 80% of 1 rep max, RPE = 5 to 6/10.
	     Time: minimum of one set of 10 to 15 reps.
	     Type: 8 to 10 exercises involving major muscle groups using theraband or free weights.
	     Upper extremities: shoulder girdle, retractors
	     - Lower extremities: pelvic and hip muscles, eccentric quadriceps.
	 • Aerobic:
	   ○ Frequency: minimum of 3 days a week.
	     Intensity: 40 to 80% of heart rate reserve, RPE = 11 to 16/20.
	     Time: minimum of 10 minutes × 3 trials a day, with goal of 20 to 60 minutes per session.
	     Type: ambulation
	 • Flexibility
	   ○ Frequency: minimum of 2 days a week.
	     Intensity: stretch to the point of feeling tightness.
	     Time: 30 to 60 seconds
	     Type: any activity that maintains or increases flexibility using slow movements.

Understand	10. Rapid infusion of vancomycin can lead to "red man" syndrome. Vancomycin is also ototoxic and nephrotoxic and proper dosing is imperative.
Remember	11. A PICC is used for long-term nutrition, medications, and in this patient's case, antibiotics. This patient's PICC is placed in the right upper arm into the basilic vein. Because of the placement PICC, physical therapists should be mindful not to take blood pressures over the line and should have the patient avoid heavy lifting. Additionally, the patient should cover the PICC line with an appropriate dressing

(Continued)

Bloom's Taxonomy Level	Case 17.C Answers
	during shower or bathing. Finally, the physical therapist should monitor for signs and symptoms of infection, bleeding, blood clots, pulmonary embolus, and allergies to local anesthetic, latex, sterile preparation solutions, or flushing solutions.

Key points

1. Complications of a prolonged hospital stay may arise in a multitude of systems, including but not limited to musculoskeletal, neurological (including cognition), integumentary, cardiovascular, and pulmonary. It is imperative that a comprehensive evaluation be performed and monitored for adverse signs and symptoms throughout the rehabilitation stay.

2. The physical therapy plan of care should include interventions to target the musculoskeletal, neurological, integumentary, cardiovascular, and pulmonary system. The latter is especially relevant when one considers that the patient had a prolonged hospitalization due to respiratory failure and, therefore, oxygenation throughout the body was impaired.

3. Selected outcome measures should cover identified deficits. However, they should also be selected to see a noticeable change during the rehabilitation stay.

Suggested Readings

Academy of Acute Care Physical Therapy. Laboratory Values Interpretation Resource. Available at: http://c.ymcdn.com/sites/www.acutept.org/resource/resmgr/docs/2017-Lab-Values-Resource.pdf. Accessed January 8, 2017

AM-PAC. Available at: http://am-pac.com/category/home/. Accessed July 1, 2019

Melo TA, Duarte ACM, Bezerra TS, França F, Soares NS, Brito D. The five times sit-to-stand test: safety and reliability with older intensive care unit patients at discharge. Rev Bras Ter Intensiva. 2019; 31(1):27–33

Bencardino JT, Hassankhani A. Calcium pyrophosphate dihydrate crystal deposition disease. Semin Musculoskelet Radiol. 2003; 7(3):175–185

Brower RG. Consequences of bed rest. Crit Care Med. 2009; 37(10) Suppl:S422–S428

Ciccone CD. Pharmacology in Rehabilitation. 5th ed. Philadelphia, PA: F.A. Davis Company; 2015

Falvey JR, Mangione KK, Stevens-Lapsley JE. Rethinking hospital-associated deconditioning: proposed paradigm shift. Phys Ther. 2015; 95(9):1307–1315

Five Times Sit to Stand Test. Available at: https://www.sralab.org/rehabilitation-measures/five-times-sit-stand-test#pulmonary-diseases. Accessed March 8, 2020

Frownfelter D, Dean E. Cardiovascular and Pulmonary Physical Therapy: Evidence to Practice. St. Louis, MO: Saunders Elsevier; 2012

Hammer GD, McPhee SJ. Pathophysiology of Disease: An Introduction to Clinical Medicine. 8th ed. New York, NY: McGraw-Hill Education; 2019

Hillegass E, Puthoff M, Frese EM, Thigpen M, Sobush DC, Auten B, Guideline Development Group. Role of physical therapists in the management of individuals at risk for or diagnosed with venous thromboembolism: evidence-based clinical practice guideline. Phys Ther. 2016; 96(2):143–166

Hillegass E. Essentials of Cardiopulmonary Physical Therapy. 4th ed. St. Louis, MO: Elsevier; 2017

Huang M, Chan KS, Zanni JM, et al. Functional status score for the ICU: an international clinimetric analysis of validity, responsiveness, and minimal important difference. Crit Care Med. 2016; 44(12): e1155–e1164

Jameson JL, Fauci AS, Kasper DL, Hauser SL, Longo DL, Loscalzo J. Harrison's Principles of Internal Medicine. 20th ed. New York, NY: McGraw-Hill Education; 2018

Jette DU, Brown R, Collette N, Friant W, Graves L. Physical therapists' management of patients in the acute care setting: an observational study. Phys Ther. 2009; 89(11):1158–1181

Jette DU, Stilphen M, Ranganathan VK, Passek SD, Frost FS, Jette AM. Validity of the AM-PAC "6-clicks" inpatient daily activity and basic mobility short forms. Phys Ther. 2014; 94(3):379–391

Jette DU, Stilphen M, Ranganathan VK, Passek SD, Frost FS, Jette AM. AM-PAC "6-clicks" functional assessment scores predict acute care hospital discharge destination. Phys Ther. 2014; 94(9):1252–1261

Katzung BG. Basic & Clinical Pharmacology. 14th ed. New York, NY: McGraw-Hill Education; 2018

Kaukonen KM, Bailey M, Pilcher D, Cooper DJ, Bellomo R. Systemic inflammatory response syndrome criteria in defining severe sepsis. N Engl J Med. 2015; 372(17):1629–1638

Montreal Cognitive Assessment. Available at: https://www.mocatest.org/about/. Accessed March 6, 2020

Morris PE, Goad A, Thompson C, et al. Early intensive care unit mobility therapy in the treatment of acute respiratory failure. Crit Care Med. 2008; 36(8):2238–2243

Nordon-Craft A, Moss M, Quan D, Schenkman M. Intensive care unit-acquired weakness: implications for physical therapist management. Phys Ther. 2012; 92(12):1494–1506

Osmon DR, Berbari EF, Berendt AR, et al. Infectious Diseases Society of America. Diagnosis and management of prosthetic joint infection: clinical practice guidelines by the Infectious Diseases Society of America. Clin Infect Dis. 2013; 56(1):e1–e25

Parry SM, Denehy L, Beach LJ, Berney S, Williamson HC, Granger CL. Functional outcomes in ICU—what should we be using?: an observational study. Crit Care. 2015; 19:127

Pescatello L Sr, ed. ACSM Guidelines for Exercise Testing and Prescription. 10th ed. Baltimore, MD: Lippincott, Williams and Wilkins; 2017

Peterson ML, Lukens K, Fulk G. Physical function measures used in the intensive care unit: a systematic review. J Acute Care Phys Ther. 2018; 9(2):78–90

Ragavan VK, Greenwood KC, Bibi K. The Functional Status Score for the Intensive Care Unit Scale - is it reliable in the intensive care unit? Can it be used to determine discharge placement? JACPT.

Sessler CN, Gosnell MS, Grap MJ, et al. The Richmond agitation-sedation scale: validity and reliability in adult intensive care unit patients. Am J Respir Crit Care Med. 2002; 166(10):1338–1344

Thrush A, Rozek M, Dekerlegand JL. The clinical utility of the functional status score for the intensive care unit (FSS-ICU) at a long-term acute care hospital: a prospective cohort study. Phys Ther. 2012; 92(12):1536–1545

Tortora GJ, Derrickson BH. Principles of Anatomy & Physiology. 15th ed. Hoboken, NJ: 2016

18 Spinal Cord Injury

General Information	
Case no.	18.A Spinal Cord Injury
Authors	Pamela Bartlo, PT, DPT, Board Certified Clinical Specialist in Cardiovascular & Pulmonary Physical Therapy Kevin Jenney, PT, DPT Board Certified Clinical Specialist in Neurologic Physical Therapy
Diagnosis	Spinal cord injury (SCI)
Setting	Acute care hospital
Learner expectations	☑ Initial evaluation ☐ Re-evaluation ☑ Treatment session
Learner objectives	1. Describe at least three important aspects of physical therapy evaluation for this patient. 2. Explain the primary goals of physical therapy in the acute management of this patient. 3. Detail the components and parameters for physical therapy interventions for this patient.

Medical	
Chief complaint	Back pain, numbness in bilateral lower extremities (BLEs).
History of present illness	The patient is a 25-year-old man admitted to the emergency department status post motor vehicle accident. His car rolled over and he was trapped inside. Emergency Medical Services (EMS) arrived at the scene within 15 minutes and extrication took approximately 30 minutes. In the field, the patient was placed on a long board with a cervical collar. He reported no feeling in his lower back, abdomen, or legs. He reported pain in mid-back and left chest (Glasgow Coma Scale [GCS] = 14). Transportation time from the scene to the emergency department was 10 minutes.
Past medical history	None
Past surgical history	Tonsillectomy at age 8 years.
Allergies	Seasonal allergies to pollen.
Medications	None

Social history	
Home setup	• Resides in a third -floor apartment alone. • Two steps into building—no railings. • Three flights of stairs to apartment with left railing for ascension (no elevator in building). • Parents live in a two-story house in the area.
Occupation	• Full-time manager of a corporate pharmacy store.
Prior level of function	• Independent with functional mobility and activities of daily living (ADLs). • (+) driver
Recreational activities	• Played recreational sports and exercised at least 3 days per week for at least 30 to 60 minutes.

Vital signs	Hospital day 0: emergency department
Blood pressure (mmHg)	112/70
Heart rate (beats/min)	69
Respiratory rate (breaths/min)	12
Pulse oximetry on 2 L nasal cannula (NC; SpO$_2$)	97%
Temperature (°F)	98.9 °F

Diagnostic test	Hospital day 0: emergency department	Hospital day 2: surgical intensive care unit (SICU)
Chest X-ray	(+) posterior fractures at ribs 5 and 6 (–) for signs of pleural effusion, pneumothorax, or internal hemorrhage in thoracic cavity.	• Not reordered
Spine computed tomography (CT) scan	(+) fractures at the vertebral body and right pedicle of T7 (+) fractures at the transverse processes of T5 and T6. (+) Diffuse edema noted at T5–T8 region of spine.	• Post-op day 1: (+) surgical fusion of T6–T8. Good fixation of plates and screws.
Magnetic resonance imaging (MRI)	(+) spinal compression and ischemia at T7.	• Not reordered

▶ Fig. 18.1

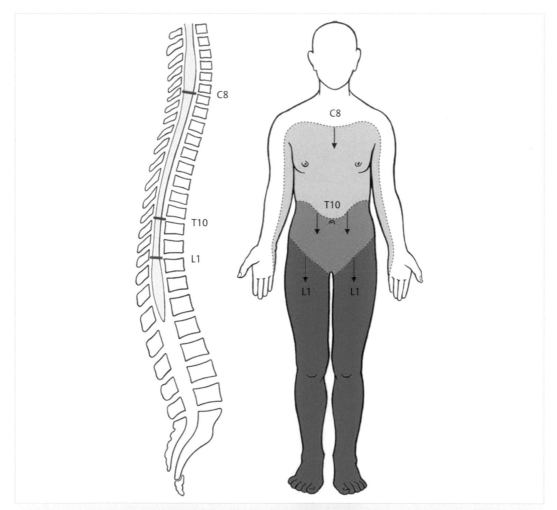

Fig. 18.1 A visual representation of levels of potential spinal cord injuries and associated areas of the body affected. (Adapted from Bähr M, Frotscher M, eds. Spinal Cord Syndromes. In: Topical Diagnosis in Neurology: Anatomy, Physiology, Signs, Symptoms. 6th ed. New York, NY: Thieme; 2019.)

Medical management	Hospital day 0: emergency department	Hospital day 2: SICU
Medications	1. Intravenous (IV) fluids. 2. Oxycodone 5 mg every 4 hours. 3. Norepinephrine 1 mcg/kg/min.	1. Continued per medical plan of care. 2. Oxycodone 5 mg every 4 to 6 hours until hospital day 5, then change to acetaminophen 325 mg every 6 hours. 3. Metoclopramide (Reglan) 1 mg/kg.
Respiratory	1. Placed on 2 L O_2 NC.	1. Continue per medical plan of care.
Procedures	1. Spine stabilization until surgery. 2. Foley catheter placed.	1. Continue per medical plan of care.
Precautions/Orders	1. Bed rest 2. Telemetry	1. Out of bed as tolerated. 2. Telemetry 3. Spinal fusion surgery precautions (no bending forward past 90 degrees, no twisting/rotation through thoracic spine, no lifting > 5 lbs). 4. Physical therapy consultation

Lab		Reference range	Hospital day 0: emergency department	Hospital day 2: SICU
Arterial blood gas	pH	7.35–7.45	7.42	7.38
	$PaCO_2$	35–45	36	45
	PaO_2	75–95	77	94
	HCO_3^-	23–29	25	26
Complete blood count	White blood cell	5.0–10.0 × 10^9/L	8.1	8.8
	Hemoglobin	14.0–17.4 g/dL	15.1	15.8
	Hematocrit	42–52%	43.7	44.2
	Red blood cell	4.5–5.5 million/mm^3	4.6	4.9
	Platelet	140,000–400,000/μL	152	162
Electrolytes	Calcium	8.6–10.3 mg/dL	8.9	9.7
	Chloride	98–108 mEq/L	101	98
	Magnesium	1.2–1.9 mEq/L	1.3	1.4
	Phosphate	2.3–4.1 mg/dL	3.4	3.2
	Potassium	3.7–5.1 mEq/L	4.2	4.2
	Sodium	134–142 mEq/L	135	137
Other	Blood urea nitrogen	7–20 mg/d	18.2	Not reordered
	Creatinine	0.5–1.4 mg/dL	1.1	Not reordered
	Glucose	60–10 mg/dL	201	116
Coagulation	Prothrombin time	10–14 seconds	10.1	10.8
	Partial thromboplastin time	25–35 seconds	25.2	26.4
	International normalized ratio	2.0–3.0	1.8	2.1

Pause points
Based on the above information, what are the priorities?
• Examination tests?
• Outcome measures?
• Treatment interventions?

Hospital Day 3, SICU: Physical Therapy Examination		
Subjective		
"My back hurts right where they did the surgery" Patient with complaints of left posterior rib pain from fractures as well. Patient reports that he hasn't been out of bed yet but has sat up with the head of the bed raised.		
Objective		

Vital signs	Pre-treatment	During treatment	Post-treatment
	Supine	Sitting	Sitting
Blood pressure (mmHg)	118/70	98/65	108/65
Heart rate (beats/min)	72	90	76
Respiratory rate (breaths/min)	12	16	12
Pulse oximetry on 2 L NC (SpO_2)	96%	94%	97%
Borg scale	6/20	15/20	11/20
Pain	6/10 at back 4/10 at ribs	8/10 at back 5/10 at ribs	5–6/10 at back 4/10 at ribs

General	• Patient supine in bed. • Lines/equipment notable for telemetry, urinary catheter, 2 L O_2 via NC, BLE compression stockings, and bilateral sequential compression devices ▶ Fig. 18.2.	
Head, ears, eyes, nose, and throat (HEENT)	• No discernable abnormalities present.	
Cardiovascular and pulmonary	• Heart sounds: normal S1 and S2 with no murmurs or abnormal sounds noted. • Breathing pattern: notable for diaphragmatic breathing. • Breath sounds: slight decrease in inspiratory sounds in bilateral basilar lung segments anteriorly and posteriorly. No other adventitious sounds noted. • Pedal pulses: 2 + bilateral dorsalis pedis and posterior tibialis.	
Gastrointestinal	• No discernable issues	
Genitourinary	• (+) foley catheter	
Musculoskeletal	Range of motion (ROM)	• Bilateral upper extremity (BUE): within functional range. • Bilateral lower extremity (BLE): passive ROM (PROM)—within functional limit (WFL); no active ROM noted.
	Strength	• B shoulder flexors and abductors: 4/5 due to pain in back. • B shoulder extensors, adductors, internal rotators, and external rotators: 5/5. • B elbow flexors, extensors, supinator, and pronator: 5/5. • B wrist and hand: 5/5 • BLE: 0/5 throughout all muscle groups. • Abdominals: 0/5
	Aerobic	• Unable to perform standardized test at this time. • Able to complete bed mobility and transfers with minimal to moderate shortness of breath.

(Continued)

(Continued)

		Hospital Day 3, SICU: Physical Therapy Examination
	Flexibility	• No abnormal issues found with flexibility at this time. • Spinal motion not tested due to postsurgical restrictions.
Neurological	Balance	• Static unsupported sitting: minimal assistance with BUE support. • Dynamic unsupported sitting: minimal assistance with BUE support. • Standing balance: not appropriate at this time.
	Cognition	• Alert and oriented × 4
	Coordination	• Finger to nose: intact bilaterally • Heel to shin: unable to perform bilaterally.
	Cranial nerves	• I–XII: intact
	Reflexes	• Babinski's reflex: (+) bilaterally • No other reflexes present below T7 level.
	Sensation	• BUE: intact to light touch, pain, temperature, and proprioception. • BLE: absent for light touch, pain, temperature, and proprioception. • Trunk: sensation intact until about T6–T7 level, absent distally.
	Tone	• BUE: normal • BLE: hypotonic/flaccid throughout • No clonus elicited during PROM assessment.
		Functional status
Bed mobility		• Rolling either direction: contact guard assistance with LE preparation and management; using BUEs, bedside rails, and momentum. • Supine to/from sit: moderate assistance with LE management and trunk.
Transfers		• Bed to/from chair: moderate assistance with slide board.
Ambulation		• Not applicable
Stairs		• Not applicable
Task specific		• Wheelchair mobility: patient unable to propel wheelchair at this time. Will assess after discharge from ICU.
Sport specific		• N/A

	Assessment
☑ Physical therapist's	*Assessment left blank for learner to develop*
	Goals
Patient's	"I want to get out of here." "I'd love to walk again."
Short term	1. *Goals left blank for learner to develop* 2.
Long term	1. *Goals left blank for learner to develop* 2.

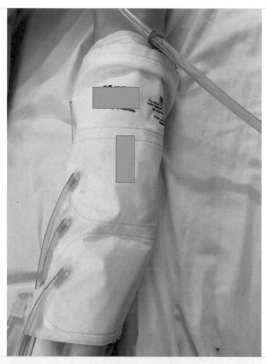

Fig. 18.2 Lower extremity intermittent pneumatic compression device.

	Plan
☐ Physician's ☑ Physical therapist's ☐ Other's	Will continue to see patient five to seven times a week to progress functional mobility. Will continue to progress balance, bed mobility, transfers, wheelchair mobility, and safety through strengthening and endurance interventions and education on respiratory mechanics, airway clearance, and positioning. Will coordinate functional plan with occupational therapy and rehabilitation plan with physician and discharge planner.

Bloom's Taxonomy Level	Case 18.A Questions
Create	1. Synthesizing the medical data and physical examination findings, develop an appropriate physical therapy assessment of the patient. 2. Develop two short-term physical therapy goals, including an appropriate timeframe. 3. Develop two long-term physical therapy goals, including an appropriate timeframe.
Evaluate	4. Discuss the physical therapist's evaluation findings with occupational therapist in order to devise an interprofessional plan of care.
Analyze	5. Explain concern about pH, $PaCO_2$, and PaO_2 levels in a person with acute SCI and why it is important to follow those blood values. 6. Why is it important to track the patient's electrolytes?
Apply	7. Describe at least two functional mobility interventions for the initial treatment sessions in acute care with physical therapist. Be specific as to the parameters and position of interventional techniques. 8. Design and implement two interventions to improve respiratory capacity and airway clearance. 9. What interventions could the physical therapist provide if the patient became symptomatic due to a decrease in blood pressure and a recovery was not seen within 3 to 5 minutes?

(Continued)

(Continued)

Bloom's Taxonomy Level	Case 18.A Questions
Understand	10. Did the patient's vital signs respond appropriately to the physical therapy interventions performed on day 3? Why is it important to monitor vital signs before, during, and after physical therapy sessions with this patient?
Remember	11. What are the implications of the spinal surgery precautions to mobility in the physical therapy sessions? 12. What are the two pulmonary complications that are most likely to occur at this point in the patient's care?

Bloom's Taxonomy Level	Case 18.A Answers
Create	1. The patient is a 25-year-old man who presented to the hospital status post motor vehicle accident. The patient was diagnosed with an incomplete SCI at the T7 level—American Spinal Injury Association (ASIA) classification B—and posterior rib fractures of ribs 5 and 6. The patient underwent T6–T8 spinal fusion and will follow post-op spinal fusion precautions of forward flexion, lifting, and spinal rotation. As a result of his spinal injury, the patient presents with lack of motor and sensory nerve function below T7 at this time. He is using 2 L O_2 via NC to maintain proper oxygen saturations. All other lab findings are appropriate at this time. He would benefit from continued physical therapy to improve above deficits to maximize functional mobility and safety. Will continue to follow and progress as tolerated. 2. Short-term goals: • Patient will perform rolling in either direction without use of bed rails with contact guard assistance within 3 days to promote independence with bed mobility. • Patient will perform slide board transfer from bed to/from chair with minimal assistance within 3 days to promote independence with transfers. 3. Long-term goals: • Patient will perform slide board transfer bed to/from chair with contact guard assistance within 7 days to promote independence with transfers. • Patient will independently propel wheelchair a minimum of 100 feet on level surface, avoiding 100% of obstacles, to promote independence.
Evaluate	4. The physical therapist should discuss the findings regarding UE strength, lack of LE motor and sensory function, and mobility. The physical therapist and occupational therapist should develop a plan to optimize the patient's skills for bed mobility, endurance, transfers, wheelchair mobility, wheelchair prescription, pulmonary education and interventions, and education regarding other ancillary complications (bowel and bladder, etc.). At a minimum, the physical therapist should take the lead on pulmonary interventions, wheelchair prescription, wheelchair mobility, endurance, and flexibility/maintaining ROM.
Analyze	5. The patient is likely to have a decrease in inspiratory volumes. The thoracic cage muscles are involved although most are intact. This will lead to some decrease in inspiratory volumes, at least early on in the rehab process. All mobility will also take more effort for the patient placing even more demand on the pulmonary system. Therefore, it is important to monitor vital signs to make sure that the patient is still getting enough PaO_2 volumes to sustain the body's demand and that the lack of inspiration isn't leading to decrease volumes, hence increase $PaCO_2$, which could cause problems with the body's pH. 6. An SCI can impact the patient's sympathetic nervous system, which in turn can impact organ function, including production and regulation of fluid electrolyte levels. Since the electrolytes can impact the patient's cardiovascular system, renal system, and liver, it is important for the medical team to monitor these lab values, and for the physical therapist to watch for any adverse signs and symptoms pre-, peri-, or postrehabilitation.
Apply	7. Two functional mobility interventions for the initiation of physical therapy include: • Bed mobility: The physical therapist should be specific about teaching the patient how to position LEs, how to use UEs to develop momentum, and, of course, safety

(Continued)

(Continued)

Bloom's Taxonomy Level	Case 18.A Answers
	precautions, especially within the confines of the spinal precautions. Anecdotally, the patient should practice these techniques at least three times to each side during each session. Supine to sit should also be practiced at least three to four times per session. • Transfers: the physical therapist should work with the patient on sliding board transfers. Education and practice on the placement of the board, positioning of LEs and UEs, safety issues, and strategies should be implemented. These should be practiced at least three to four times during each session. 8. The patient should be educated on the need to maintain or improve inspiratory volumes. Interventions to promote this include deep breathing, diaphragmatic breathing, inspiratory hold, breath stacking, or other inspiratory breathing techniques. Again, anecdotally, these should be performed for at least 1 to 3 minutes each session and the patient should be educated to perform them at least once or twice a day. For airway clearance, the patient should be educated on how to produce an effective and efficient cough and why maintaining an upright posture is important. For coughing, splinting technique or other self-assisted cough techniques may need to be implemented if the patient is unable to generate a strong enough cough independently. This should only need to be taught once and then have the patient demonstrate them once or twice over the first few physical therapy sessions to ensure they are being performed accurately and effectively. 9. In the short term, the physical therapist should elevate the patient's LEs, but for a more long-term solution, an abdominal binder, and/or compression stockings may be added to assist with blood pressure regulation. Initially, generic off-the-shelf stockings can be used. However, if it is determined that the patient will need them long term to maintain venous return, then custom progressive resistance stockings should be prescribed and obtained for the patient.
Understand	10. The patient's vital signs did respond appropriately to the physical therapy interventions performed on day 3. It is important to watch heart rate due to increased physical demand on the patient since he is unable to use his LEs. The physical therapist needs to ensure that motion and mobility aren't placing too high of a demand on the patient's cardiac system. Blood pressure is also important to monitor to assess for tolerance to physical demands. However, it is important to be mindful that the patient has lost muscle contractions to assist with venous return, and therefore he is at risk of developing postural hypotension. Respiratory rate and O_2 saturations give the physical therapist the ability to monitor that physical activity isn't placing too high of a pulmonary demand on the patient either.
Remember	11. The physical therapist will need to educate the patient on the spinal surgery precautions and evaluate that the patient understands them. During interventions, the physical therapist must make sure that the patient is not flexing or rotating the spine. 12. The patient is at risk of developing a pulmonary embolism, atelectasis, or pulmonary infection (most likely pneumonia). The patient is at a lower risk of developing a pneumothorax, pleural effusion, or pulmonary edema.

Key points

1. It is important for the physical therapist to evaluate motor and sensory nerve function regularly for this patient as there may be some improvement with time, to fully evaluate patient's mobility, and to assess how other body systems are being impacted by the SCI and how those reactions may impact the patient's rehab with physical therapy.

2. Primary goals for physical therapy management of this patient in the acute care setting are to stabilize his pulmonary system and prevent complications, encourage mobility and upright activities, and prepare the patient for the next phase of rehabilitation.

3. Program parameters should include mobility, functional movements, and pulmonary training as the main types of rehab. Duration should be about 15 to 20 minute in total with multiple rests for the patient. Intensity will be determined based on patient's subjective complaints and vital sign responses. Frequency should be most days of the week to prepare for the next phase of rehab.

General Information	
Case no.	18.B
Authors	Pamela Bartlo, PT, DPT, Board Certified Clinical Specialist in Cardiovascular & Pulmonary Physical Therapy Kevin Jenney, PT, DPT Board Certified Clinical Specialist in Neurologic Physical Therapy
Diagnosis	Thoracic spinal cord injury (SCI)
Setting	Subacute rehabilitation
Learner expectations	□ Initial evaluation □ Re-evaluation ☑ Treatment session
Learner objectives	1. Describe important intervention techniques and strategies for this patient at this level of care. 2. Differentiate primary intervention focus and secondary interventions. 3. Explain the interaction between patient's current functional status and his cardiorespiratory endurance.

Medical	
Chief complaint	Lack of mobility and strength.
History of present illness	The patient is a 25-year-old man who was admitted to the hospital after a motor vehicle accident. He sustained an incomplete SCI at the T7 level and posterior fractures at ribs 5 and 6. The patient underwent spinal fusion of T6–T8 on hospital day 1. He spent 2 days in intensive care unit (ICU) and 6 days on the ward. Upon medical stabilization, the patient was transferred to subacute rehabilitation yesterday.
Past medical history	None
Past surgical history	Tonsillectomy at age 8 years.
Allergies	Seasonal allergies to pollen.
Medications	Acetaminophen prn
Precautions/orders	• Out of bed as tolerated. • Spinal fusion surgery precautions (no bending forward past 90 degrees, no twisting/rotation through thoracic spine, no lifting greater than 10 lbs) for another 5 weeks.

Social history	
Home setup	• Resided in a third-floor apartment alone. • Two steps into building—no railings. • Three flights of stairs to apartment with left railing for ascension (no elevator in the building). • Parents live in a two-story house in the area. For discharge planning: • Patient will be going to parents' house. His parents' house has two steps to enter; however, they are in the process of installing a ramp. He will have a bedroom and a half bath on the first floor. Full bath is on the second floor and family is still figuring out ways to get the patient there for bathing. • Long term, the patient will be looking into changing his apartment to a first-floor unit in the future.
Occupation	• Full-time manager of a corporate pharmacy store. For discharge planning: • The patient will remain out of work on short-term disability for the time being, but he would like to return to his job as soon as he can.
Prior level of function	• Independent with functional mobility and activities of daily living (ADLs). • (+) driver For discharge planning: • The patient would like to get back to being independent including driving himself as soon as he can.
Recreational activities	• Played recreational sports and exercised at least 3 days per week for at least 30 to 60 minutes. For discharge planning: • Long term, the patient would like to get active again in the future.

Medical management	
Supplemental O_2	Prescribed up to 2 L O_2 via nasal cannula (NC) only if needed to maintain O_2 saturations > 90%.
Compression stockings	Calf length compression stockings to be worn when patient out of bed.

Pause points
Based on the above information, what are the priorities? • Physical therapy tests and measures? • Standardized endurance measures? • Treatment interventions?

Day 2, Subacute Rehab: Physical Therapy Treatment Session
(Patient did participate in bed-level physical therapy evaluation yesterday, however, was tired from the transfer between facilities. Therefore, he did not complete a functional assessment or outcome measures. The first half of the documentation is from yesterday's initial evaluation, whereas the functional assessment and outcome measures are from today's session)

Subjective
"I just want to get home again and be able to do things myself. I don't want to rely on my parents for very long."

Objective			
Vital signs	Pre-treatment	During treatment	Post-treatment
	Sitting	Sitting	Sitting
Blood pressure (mmHg)	116/74	142/78	n/a
Heart rate (beats/min)	68	115	75
Respiratory rate (breaths/min)	N/A	N/A	N/A
Pulse oximetry on room air (SpO_2)	96%	92%	95%
Borg scale	N/A	14/20	N/A
Pain	2/10 posterior spine	4/10 site of rib fractures	3/10 posterior spine and site of rib fractures
General	• Patient presents to physical therapy rehab gym in standard wheelchair with foley catheter and compression stockings on bilateral LEs.		
Head, ears, eyes, nose, and throat (HEENT)	• No discernable abnormalities present.		
Cardiovascular and pulmonary	• Heart sounds: normal S1 and S2 sounds. No murmurs or abnormal sounds noted. • Breath sounds: slight decrease in breath sounds in bilateral bases, posterior > anterior. No adventitious sounds noted.		
Gastrointestinal	• No discernable issues.		
Genitourinary	• (+) foley catheter. • Physical Therapist noted in medical plan of care that patient will gradually be transitioned to intermittent catheter training.		
Musculoskeletal	Range of motion (ROM)	• Bilateral upper extremity (BUE): within normal range. • Bilateral lower extremity (BLE): passive ROM (PROM)—within functional limit (WFL); no active ROM noted.	
	Strength	• BUE: grossly 5/5 throughout. • BLE: 0/5 throughout all muscle groups. • Abdominals: 0/5	

(Continued)

(Continued)

	Day 2, Subacute Rehab: Physical Therapy Treatment Session	
	Aerobic	• Not assessed at this time.
	Flexibility	• BUE: no limitations at this time. • BLE: no limitations at this time. • Spinal motion not tested due to postsurgical restrictions.
	Other	• Will assess patient's tolerance to use of static standing frame as able and as appropriate based on patient's blood pressure responses.
Neurological	Balance	• Static unsupported sitting: minimal assistance without BUE support. • Dynamic unsupported sitting: supervision with BUE support. • Long sit balance on mat table: supervision without BUE support. • Dynamic long sitting on mat table: Supervision with BUE support on side of weight shift; minimal assistance without BUE support.
	Cognition	• Alert and oriented × 4
	Coordination	• Finger to nose: intact bilaterally • Heel to shin: unable to perform bilaterally.
	Cranial nerves	• I–XII: intact
	Reflexes	• Babinski reflex (+) B feet. • No other reflexes present below T7 level.
	Sensation	• BUE: intact to light touch, pain, temperature, and proprioception throughout. • BLE: slight sensation to deep pressure on lateral, proximal right thigh—3/5 trials; absent for light touch, pain, temperature, and proprioception. • Thoracic cage: sensations intact until about T6–T7 level and then absent below.
	Tone	• BUE: normal • BLE: hypotonic/flaccid throughout. No signs of hypertonicity developing at this time.
	Functional status	
Bed mobility		*All bed mobility done on therapy mat table without use of any bed rails or other assistive devices* • Rolling either direction: minimal assistance. Patient needs occasional verbal cues for LE preparation and management. • Rolling prone to supine: supervision assistance with occasional verbal cues for LE management. • Supine to sit: minimal assistance for trunk control and LE management. Occasionally, during the last portion of the movement, the patient requires maximal assistance to prevent from shifting his trunk too far in the opposite direction and losing his balance.
Transfers		• Chair to mat: contact guard assistance with sliding board; occasional minimal assistance for sliding board placement and wheelchair part management. • Mat to chair: minimal assistance due to slight incline in height differential between surfaces with sliding board; also occasional minimal assistance for sliding board placement and wheelchair part management.
Wheelchair propulsion		• Propels standard frame wheelchair × 300 feet with BUE. • 14/20 on Borg Scale and shortness of breath 3/10 on modified Borg Scale.
Stairs/ramp negotiation		• Ascend/descend 10-feet ramp using standard frame wheelchair with supervision: minimal assistance.

(Continued)

(Continued)

Day 2, Subacute Rehab: Physical Therapy Treatment Session	
Task specific	• Per patient's medical chart, he is independent to wash UEs and trunk, however, requires minimal assistance for LEs, and will begin bowel and bladder program with nursing over the next week.
Sport specific	• Not assessed at this time. • Patient would like to return to sports or activities at some point but is focusing on function to go home at this time.

Physical therapy endurance tests/measure	
6-Minute Push Test (6 MPT) with wheelchair	• 6 MPT is the wheelchair propulsion equivalent of the 6-Minute Walk Test for ambulation. • This patient was able to perform 6 MPT. See case-specific questions.
General endurance measure	• Patient can perform approximately 6 to 8 minutes of aerobic UE exercise prior to rest needed with dyspnea 3–4/10 on modified Borg Scale.

Assessment	
☑ Physical therapist's	*Assessment left blank for learner to develop*
Goals	
Patient's	"I want to get out of rehab and not depend on my parent's so much."
Short term	1. *Goals left blank for learner to develop* 2.
Long term	1. *Goals left blank for learner to develop* 2.

Plan	
☐ Physician's ☑ Physical therapist's ☐ Other's	Physical therapist will see patient five to seven times a week to progress functional mobility and promote independence with wheelchair management. Therapeutic interventions to include UE endurance and strengthening, endurance training, bed mobility training, transfer training, wheelchair training on even and uneven surfaces, airway clearance, standing tolerance, and patient education.

Bloom's Taxonomy Level	Case 18.B Questions
Create	1. Synthesizing the medical data and physical examination findings, develop an appropriate physical therapy assessment of the patient. 2. Develop two short-term physical therapy goals, including an appropriate timeframe. 3. Develop two long-term physical therapy goals, including an appropriate timeframe.
Evaluate	4. Describe the most likely outcome for patient on the 6 MPT wheelchair propulsion test. Be specific about distance, Borg rating, vital sign response, and possible patient symptom report.
Analyze	5. Why is it important to watch vital signs with regard to positioning and exercise with this patient? 6. How could use of an inspiratory muscle training device assist with this patient's overall rehab?
Apply	7. Explain two methods to incorporate pulmonary interventions into the physical therapy rehab session. Be specific with regard to positioning, parameters, and cueing. 8. Discuss how to progress patient's endurance. Be specific with regard to frequency, intensity, time, and mode(s).

(Continued)

(Continued)

Bloom's Taxonomy Level	Case 18.B Questions
	9. Describe how the patient's sitting balance and pulmonary status impact each other. How can improving one alter the patient's ability with the other?
Understand	10. When working toward independent mobility, why is it important to emphasize positioning, technique, and safety in addition to independence?
	11. Explain the primary neuro goals, secondary pulmonary goals, other system goals (i.e., genitourinary, integumentary, etc.) of physical therapy interventions at this time. Do not need to be written as goals, but as the overall goals of this level of care on these systems.
Remember	12. What is the importance of positioning, use of stander, or abdominal binder for this patient in the subacute rehab setting?

Bloom's Taxonomy Level	Case 18.B Answers
Create	1. The patient is a 25-year-old man who presented to subacute rehab after 8 days in the acute care hospital following a motor vehicle accident. He sustained an incomplete SCI at T7 level and posterior fractures of ribs 5 and 6. He underwent spinal fusion at levels T6–T8 and has spinal fusion precautions. As a result of his injury, he presents with lack of motor and sensory nerve function below T7 at this time, impairing respiratory mechanics, balance, and mobility. He continues to require assistance for all functional mobility and ADLs, and therefore was transferred to subacute rehab. Will continue to follow and progress as tolerated.
	2. Short-term goals:
	• Patient will independently use the inspiratory muscle trainer for 5 to 10 breaths/trial, twice a day at the prescribed level within 2 weeks to improve respiratory mechanics.
	• Patient will independently propel wheelchair × 800 feet on level surface, avoiding 100% of obstacles, within 2 weeks to promote independence.
	• Patient will tolerate upright positioning in the standing frame for 10 minutes while performing upper body weight shifts without adverse signs and symptoms within 2 weeks to promote BLE extension ROM and blood pressure responses to upright.
	3. Long-term goals:
	• Patient will perform 6 MPT for 1,600 feet without rest needed and Borg rating < 14 within 4 weeks to improve functional mobility and endurance.
	• Patient will independently perform bed to/from chair transfers using sliding board within 4 weeks to improve independence.
	• Patient will independently ascend/descend ramp within 4 weeks to enter/exit home.
Evaluate	4. Patient should propel at least 1,000 feet with BUE without rest needed. In this case, the patient probably propelled slightly less than that and needed some rest due to the rib fractures and new injury causing some decrease in endurance.
	• Borg Scale will probably be at least 14 to 15 due to new injury.
	• Vitals will see blood pressure, heart rate, and respiratory rate increase.
	• Should have no adverse symptoms. However, if he does, it is likely to be shortness of breath and fatigue. This could be due to impaired gas exchange due to weakened inspiratory muscle strength. Another adverse sign or symptom may be upper body soreness due to new overuse.
Analyze	5. It is important to monitor the patient's vital signs due to the patient using his BUEs more frequently. This will require increased oxygen consumption and may result in decreased BUE muscle endurance. As a result, frequent rests may be needed. The patient's rib fractures and decreased muscle strength throughout thoracic cage and its impact on posture (and ultimately respiratory mechanics) must also be considered. The physical therapist will want to focus on upright positioning and vital sign response.
	6. Utilization of the inspiratory muscle-training device is important to strengthen the patient's diaphragm and accessory muscles, which have become weak due to the loss of motor function of the lower thoracic muscles. Use of an inspiratory muscle trainer will also maintain inspiratory capacity to help prevent fluid buildup or other pulmonary complications.

(Continued)

(Continued)

Bloom's Taxonomy Level	Case 18.B Answers
Apply	7. Any therapeutic interventions that directly or indirectly improve inspiratory capacity, muscle strength, or endurance are appropriate. Some examples include: • The incorporation of deep breathing or breath stacking while working on sitting balance or standing in standing frame. • Working on upright posture positioning to strengthen thoracic muscles during rest from other exercise. • Education on airway clearance/coughing techniques. The patient should perform such interventions as needed. Prone on elbows position should be encouraged for coughing since patient is still unable to flex his trunk. • Progressing aerobic endurance exercises. Any aerobic exercise will help improve his endurance, which in turn will improve pulmonary status (i.e., wheelchair propulsion, UE ergometer, pushups, etc.) • Providing the patient with an inspiratory muscle trainer and having them perform it outside of physical therapy as part of a home exercise program to strengthen muscles while not using physical therapy time for it. 8. To progress the patient's endurance, the physical therapist should focus on aerobic and strengthen training. Wheelchair propulsion is an appropriate functional activity that promotes aerobic endurance training. The patient can perform the activity for as long as possible, with the goal for a minimum of 6 to 8 minutes. The patient's Borg score should be ~12 to 13/20. To progress the patient, duration should be increased first, followed by a reduction in the number of rest breaks. Finally, intensity can be increased. The patient's goal should be at least 12 minutes of aerobic exercise and/or wheelchair propulsion by discharge to allow functional tasks to be completed without rest needed. 9. Due to the lack of muscle control below T7, the thoracic cage muscles will be impacted too. He will not have low back extensors nor all of his abdominal muscles. Sitting posture will be flexed, thus decreasing anterior thoracic cage expansion. This will likely decrease inspiratory volumes, thus limiting the amount of oxygen being inhaled and thus available for delivery to muscles. The muscles will have decreased endurance due to less oxygen delivery and therefore the patient will fatigue quicker and feel more shortness of breath due to less inspiratory volumes. The more upright posture we can get the patient into, the more "normal" the inspiratory volumes will be, thus allowing endurance to improve more because oxygen will be inhaled more and then delivered more to the muscles.
Understand	10. It is important to make sure the patient uses safe body mechanics, positioning, and techniques during transfers to reduce long-term complications. The patient should focus on performing the appropriate techniques for carryover to different surfaces. Propelling his wheelchair using correct body mechanics and proper positioning will help avoid overuse injuries at the shoulder or further spinal issues in the upper back. These same factors apply to positioning for bed mobility, ramp negotiation, dressing, etc. Again, it is the physical therapist's responsibility to ensure mobility is being performed correctly, not just independently, to prevent adverse consequences. 11. At this stage of rehabilitation, the primary goals are related to neurological system. Rehabilitation should focus on maximizing muscle strength and endurance, transfers, mobility, and functional movements. Primary goals: • Bed mobility should move toward independence. Focus on patient managing setup of LEs. • Transfer training with and without the slide board. Vary the surface level type and heights. Focus on management of board and wheelchair equipment, as well as safety during the transfer. • Wheelchair propulsion should be focused on endurance, and also on UE positioning and strengthening. It is important at this stage to start patient propelling in correct positions and postures to try to prevent rotator cuff or other shoulder overuse injuries later on. • Wheelchair propulsion should include even and uneven surfaces, such as ramps. Emphasis should be on safety and control. • Resistance exercise for UEs and trunk is important. Start with moderate weight and repetitions. Progress to higher weight and lower reps for greater strength gains for mobility needs.

(Continued)

(Continued)

Bloom's Taxonomy Level	Case 18.B Answers
	• Get the patient set up with a loaner wheelchair that is more appropriate for someone with an SCI: keep in mind seat cushion, back, axle position, footrest/plate decisions, etc. Final wheelchair prescription can occur in outpatient therapy, but the patient should be sent home in one similar to what he will get in the end ▶ Fig. 18.3. Secondary goals by system: • Cardiovascular and pulmonary system: It is important to increase endurance, improve inspiratory capacity, and maximize strength of diaphragm and accessory muscles as much as possible; ensure venous return is sufficient and educate on effective and efficient coughing and airway clearance. It is important that the patient is educated on why pulmonary complications are important. Pulmonary complications are the leading cause of death in people with SCI, so the patient needs to be aware of why and how to change positions, perform an effective and efficient cough, and proper positioning to assist with airway clearance. Patient may need to continue wearing compressing stockings (custom vs. off the shelf?) and/or abdominal binder if blood pressure consistently drops in upright. They may also assist with deep vein thrombosis prevention. An abdominal binder may assist in maintaining abdominal integrity during inspiration. Most likely due to his thoracic level injury, he won't need long-term compression stockings or abdominal binder, but it is important to keep them in mind in case. Education regarding pulmonary embolism and other secondary conditions is important too. • Integumentary system: Assess skin integrity daily (especially pressure points and where spinal incision is located). Educate patient on consistent pressure-relief movements. Prescribe appropriate wheelchair seat cushion and back to assist with appropriate support with least amount of pressure. • Genitourinary: Physical therapists should work with medical and nursing staff to assist with bowel and bladder training. Discuss sexual functioning with patient and provide education, referrals, and resources as needed. • Orthopaedic: Physical therapists should discuss the possibility of shoulder injury due to overuse and poor positioning. The patient should be prescribed strengthening exercises and educated on positioning and strategies to help prevent injury. • Other system interventions and education as needed and appropriate.
Remember	12. The importance of the various pieces of equipment are as follows: • Abdominal binder: An abdominal binder can primarily assist with stabilization of abdominal contents and pressure regulation. By maintaining abdominal position and not allowing the abdomen to distend anteriorly during inspiration, it allows the intrathoracic pressure to become negative, thus allowing gas to enter the lungs at optimal levels. This will maintain oxygen inspiration and ultimately diffusion into the blood and delivery to the tissues. • Upright positioning: Upright positioning is important to place the diaphragm in as close to optimal length tension relationship as possible, thus allowing greater excursion and optimal inspiratory ability. It also assists in decreasing fluid buildup, as fluid will be pulled toward the lower lobes of the lung where it is typically easier for the patient to clear via coughing. • Use of a stander: Use of a stander can have many positive implications. From the cardiovascular and pulmonary standpoint, it can help with building tolerance to upright position and stabilizing venous return. Upright standing promotes improved gastrointestinal motility and slows the process of long bone demineralization, which can lead to osteoporosis. It is similar to upright sitting posture in relation to diaphragm excursion and fluid movement for airway clearance ▶ Fig. 18.4.

Key points

1. It is important for the physical therapist to work endurance and pulmonary treatments into the main rehab goals at this time. The main goals will need to be mobility, function, and safety so there won't always be time dedicated specifically to pulmonary interventions. Including them as part of the overall physical therapy plan of care will allow the therapist to address function and pulmonary system.

(Continued)

(Continued)

Key points

2. Some patients may really struggle with inspiratory capacity and venous return early on in their recovery. The subacute rehab stage becomes integral in maximizing the patient's pulmonary strength and ability through specific pulmonary muscle strengthening (inspiratory muscle training) and overall endurance training. The physical therapist should pay close attention to blood pressure responses in upright and assist with stabilization of venous return as needed to allow the patient to safely maintain upright positioning for most of the day.

3. Education becomes more important in subacute rehab. It is important for the physical therapist to provide education for all the systems (neurologic, orthopaedic, etc.). Special time and education should be given regarding education of possible pulmonary complications. The patient must begin to understand the importance of positioning, movement, etc., to prevent possibly pulmonary complications such as pulmonary embolism, pulmonary infection, atelectasis, etc.

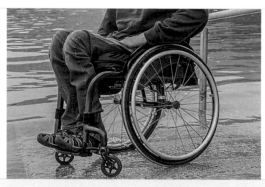

Fig. 18.3 Wheelchair positioning is important for function, prevention of pressure ulcers, and for optimal pulmonary function. (Adapted from https://www.wallpaperflare.com/black-wheelchair-near-gray-concrete-wall-disability-accident-wallpaper-wxjec.)

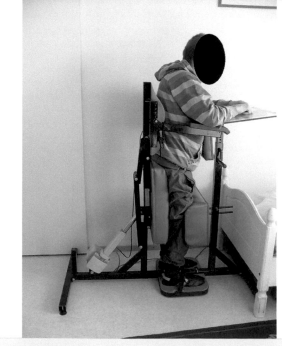

Fig. 18.4 Upright standing frame for optimal cardiovascular and pulmonary function and upper extremity activities. (Source: Memasa, CC BY-SA 3.0, via Wikimedia Commons.)

General Information

Case no.	18.C
Authors	Pamela Bartlo, PT, DPT, Board Certified Clinical Specialist in Cardiovascular & Pulmonary Physical Therapy Kevin Jenney, PT, DPT Board Certified Clinical Specialist in Neurologic Physical Therapy
Diagnosis	Spinal cord injury (SCI)
Setting	Outpatient clinic
Learner expectations	☐ Initial evaluation ☐ Re-evaluation ☑ Treatment session
Learner objectives	1. Describe important intervention techniques and strategies for this patient at this level of care. 2. Apply strategies to maximize function while also developing planning for discharge from physical therapy restorative services. 3. Explain importance of prevention of pulmonary complications.

Medical

Chief complaint	Recovering from a thoracic SCI.
History of present illness	The patient is a 25-year-old man who was admitted to the hospital after a motor vehicle accident. He sustained a T7 incomplete SCI and fractures at posterior ribs 5 and 6. He underwent spinal fusion of T6–T8. He spent 2 days in intensive care unit (ICU), another 6 days in acute neurorehabilitation, and then 3 weeks at subacute neuro rehab. He has been living at his parent's house for 1 week.
Past medical history	None
Past surgical history	Tonsillectomy at age 8 years.
Allergies	Seasonal allergies to pollen.
Medications	Ibuprofen prn
Precautions/orders	Activity as tolerated Spinal fusion surgery precautions (no bending forward past 90 degrees, no twisting/rotation through thoracic spine, no lifting greater than 10 lbs) for another 2 weeks.

Social history

Home setup	• Resided in a third-floor apartment alone. • Two steps into building—no railings. • Three flights of stairs to apartment with left railing for ascension (no elevator in building). • Parents live in a two-story house in the area. Currently: The patient resides at his parents' home. It has a ramp to enter. He is primarily staying on the first floor, which has a bedroom and half bathroom. The full bath is on the second floor and his family helps him get onto steps, after which he lifts himself up steps backward on his buttocks. Family carries the wheelchair up to the top of the stairs and help him transfer back into it. He has a shower chair and equipment from occupational therapy (OT) to assist with his bathing in the full bath. Future planning: The patient and his parents are looking into securing him a first-floor apartment that should be ready in about 4 weeks. At that time, he will have a ramp to enter the apartment. They are currently unsure if doorways will be wide enough for the wheelchair, so that is still being explored.
Occupation	• Full-time manager of a corporate pharmacy store. Future planning: The patient would like to return to work in about 4 to 6 weeks once he is able to function on his own.

(Continued)

(Continued)

Social history	
Prior level of function	• Independent with functional mobility and activities of daily living (ADLs). • (+) driver Currently: The patient is able to perform bed mobility and most of transfers with supervision, however does require contact guard—minimal assistance sporadically. He is able to propel his wheelchair on even surfaces × 1,000 feet and ascend/descend a ramp independently. He is modified independent for dressing with use of equipment provided by occupational therapist. Future planning: The patient would like to get back to being independent including driving himself. The family is looking into a driver evaluation and subsequent modifications to his car to allow him to drive independently. The evaluation is scheduled for next week and modifications to the car should take approximately 2 weeks according to the patient's report.
Recreational activities	• Played recreational sports and exercised at least 3 days per week for at least 30 to 60 minutes. Future planning: The patient wants to start getting active again. He would like weightlifting exercises he can do at home and is interested in knowing the kind of wheelchair sports available in his area.

Medical management	
Compression stockings	Calf length compression stockings to be worn when the patient is out of bed as needed.

Pause points
Based on the above information, what are the priority: • Physical therapy tests and measures? • Standardized endurance measures? • Treatment interventions?

Physical Therapy Treatment Session
Subjective
"I want to do everything myself, get back to work, and start working out some. I don't want to feel like I can't do anything."

Objective

Vital signs	Pre-treatment	During treatment	Post-treatment
	Sitting	Sitting	Sitting
Blood pressure (mmHg)	122/81	147/82	n/a
Heart rate (beats/min)	70	135	67
Respiratory rate (breaths/min)	n/a	n/a	n/a
Pulse oximetry on room air (SpO$_2$)	98%	94%	n/a
Borg scale	n/a	15/20	n/a
Pain	0/10	1/10 posterior spine	0–1/10 posterior spine
General	• Patient has had an outpatient physical therapy evaluation and has begun with interventions to address functional mobility, safety, endurance, and education for prevention of secondary complications.		

(Continued)

(Continued)

	Physical Therapy Treatment Session	
	• The patient is using a wheelchair on loan and is awaiting the permanent wheelchair prescription that the outpatient Physical therapy is scheduled to do with a wheelchair vendor on his fourth physical therapy treatment session. • Patient reports that he isn't wearing the compression stockings anymore as "they are too hard to wear". • Patient reports that his ribs don't usually bother him unless he is really breathing heavy and then he may feel slight pain.	
Head, ears, eyes, nose, and throat (HEENT)	• No discernable abnormalities present.	
Cardiovascular and pulmonary	• Cardiac auscultation: normal S1 and S2 sounds. No murmurs or abnormal sounds noted. • Breath sounds: slight decrease in breath sounds in bilateral bases posterior > anterior. No adventitious sounds noted.	
Gastrointestinal	• No discernable issues except patient reports occasional constipation that is resolved with over-the-counter stool softener.	
Genitourinary	• Independent with his bowel and bladder management.	
Musculoskeletal	Range of motion (ROM)	• Bilateral upper extremity (BUE): within normal range. • Bilateral lower extremity (BLE): no active ROM noted throughout. • Passive ROM (PROM): BLE hip extension is to neutral only. B knee extension is to full neutral. B plantar flexion is still full range.
	Strength	• BUE: 5/5 throughout all major muscle groups. • BLE: 0/5 throughout all muscle groups. • Abdominal muscles: 1/5 in rectus abdominis and external intercostals.
	Aerobic	• Patient will be evaluated on wheelchair propulsion endurance. • Overall endurance will also be assessed.
	Flexibility	• BUE: no abnormal issues noted. • BLE: bilateral tight hip flexors noted, as bilateral hip extension to neutral only. The Physical therapy will need to address with the patient for the future. • Spinal motion not tested due to postsurgical restrictions.
	Other	• Patient had been tolerating exercise in static standing frame for 10 to 12 minutes as per the Physical therapy notes from subacute rehab. Patient's tolerance was limited by hypotensive response to upright.
Neurological	Balance	• Static unsupported sitting: independent without UE support. • Dynamic unsupported sitting: independent without UE support for minimal bilateral weight shifting outside of base of support; required UE support for greater weight shifting outside of base of support. • Long sit balance on mat table: independent without UE support. • Dynamic long sitting on mat table: independent with UE support on side of weight shift for minimal to moderate range weight shifts. Still requires CG assistance for maximal range weight shifting, even with UE support.

(Continued)

(Continued)

Physical Therapy Treatment Session		
	Cognition	• Alert and oriented × 4
	Coordination	• Finger to nose: intact bilaterally • Heel to shin: unable to perform bilaterally
	Cranial nerves	• I–XII: intact
	Reflexes	• Babinski's reflex (+) B feet • No other reflexes present below T7 level
	Sensation	• BUE: intact for all sensation and proprioception • BLE: slight sensation to deep pressure on lateral, proximal thighs bilaterally—L 1–L 2 dermatomes. No other sensation noted throughout LEs for any level of sensation or proprioception • Trunk: sensations intact until T6–T7 level and then absent below
	Tone	• BUE: normal • BLE: bilateral hip flexion has slight hypertonicity noted. All other hip muscles with hypotonicity or flaccidity noted
Functional status		
Bed mobility	*All bed mobility done on therapy mat table* • Rolling either direction: independent; occasional verbal cues for LE preparation and management • Rolling prone to/from supine: supervision; occasional cues for LE management. • Supine to sit: contact guard assistance—supervision with LE management and trunk. Patient with good control but occasionally requires assistance at the last range of transfer to sitting to ensure he doesn't weight shift too far and lose balance • Sit to supine: contact guard assistance—supervision. Similar to supine to sit, patient requires assistance for last quarter range of transfer for controlled descent at trunk	
Transfers	• Chair to/from mat with slide board: supervision; occasional verbal cues for safety	
Wheelchair propulsion	• Propel lightweight frame wheelchair × 1,000 feet • Afterward, patient reports moderate fatigue and mild shortness of breath	
Stairs/ramp negotiation	• Ascend/descend 10-feet ramp using lightweight frame wheelchair independently • Patient did however require assistance at the top of the ramp to manage opening/closing of a door without safety concerns of rolling down the ramp • Patient can perform and maintain a wheelie position for 30 seconds with minimal assistance	
Task specific	• Car transfers: minimal to moderate assistance; unable to get wheelchair into and out of the car independently • Floor transfers: not assessed as this time	
Sport specific	• Physical therapy gave patient information on local wheelchair leagues for basketball, sled hockey, skiing, and racing (wheelchair road races). Physical therapy will check in with patient in a couple of weeks to see if there are sport-specific tasks he'd like to work on • Patient stated that he wants to begin lifting weights again at the gym, so the physical therapy will work with him to develop a modified lifting plan over the next couple of weeks	
Other	• Patient had been tolerating exercise in static standing frame for 10 to 12 minutes as per physical therapy notes from subacute rehab. Patient's tolerance was limited by hypotensive response to upright. Will assess standing tolerance in outpatient physical therapy within a few visits	

Physical therapy endurance tests/measure	
6-Minute Push Test (6 MPT) with wheelchair	• Patient able to perform 6 MPT for 1,300 feet with heart rate 137 and O_2 saturations 95% right atrial (RA). Patient's Borg response was 14/20 or "somewhat hard." Modified Borg Dyspnea Scale response was 3/10 or "moderate shortness of breath."
General endurance measure	• Patient can perform approximately 15 to 20 minutes of aerobic UE exercise prior to rest needed

Assessment	
☑ Physical therapist's	*Assessment left blank for learner to develop*
Goals	
Patient's	"I want to get out of rehab and not depend on my parents so much."
Short term	1. *Goals left blank for learner to develop* 2.
Long term	1. *Goals left blank for learner to develop* 2.

Plan	
☐ Physician's ☑ Physical therapist's ☐ Other's	Physical therapy will see patient twice to thrice a week to progress mobility, independence, safety, and aerobic capacity. Plan of care will incorporate transfers, balance, resistance and aerobic exercise, and education for prevention of postinjury complications

Bloom's Taxonomy Level	Case 18.C Questions
Create	1. Synthesizing the medical data and physical examination findings, develop an appropriate physical therapy assessment of the patient 2. Develop two short-term physical therapy goals, including an appropriate timeframe. 3. Develop two long-term physical therapy goals, including an appropriate timeframe.
Evaluate	4. Describe the current barriers to independence with all bed mobility and transfers. Explain possible interventions to overcome those barriers and achieve independence.
Analyze	5. Why is the hip, knee, and ankle PROM important? What should the physical therapy do with the patient to maintain/improve this? 6. What barriers are present that prevent the patient from living on his own and returning to work? What other resources, health care professionals, or other people can assist with achieving the level of independence needed?
Apply	7. Discuss at least two interventions to improve the patient's strength to allow for independence and return to leisure activities that he wants to pursue. 8. Why is periodic and consistent pressure relief important for this patient and what techniques/strategies would the physical therapy teach him to perform this consistently? 9. Describe at least two topics (not from questions 10 and 11) the physical therapy would educate the patient on related to his injury and possible complications. Make sure to include how to assess the patient's learning.
Understand	10. What is autonomic dysreflexia (AD) and what signs or symptoms would the physical therapy educate the patient to watch for with this complication? 11. What is heterotopic ossification (HO) and why is it important for this patient to know about?
Remember	12. What are Americans with Disabilities Act (ADA) guidelines for door width, maximum rise of a ramp, and recommended turning space in a kitchen? 13. What are the components to consider when prescribing a wheelchair for this patient?

Bloom's Taxonomy Level	Case 18.C Questions
Create	1. The patient is a 25-year-old man who presented to outpatient physical therapy after 3 weeks in a subacute rehab facility following a motor vehicle accident. He sustained an incomplete SCI at the T7 level and posterior rib fractures of ribs 5 and 6. He underwent spinal fusion at T6–T8 and currently has spinal precautions. He currently requires contact guard—supervision for most of mobility, but higher-level tasks such as floor to/from chair and car transfers require greater assistance due to decreased endurance, decreased flexibility, and impaired balance. He would benefit from continued physical therapy to improve above deficits. Will continue to follow 2. Short-term goals: • Patient will independently perform supine to/from sit, demonstrating controlled ascent and descent, within 3 weeks to be independent at home. • Patient will independently perform sliding board transfers within 3 weeks to get to/off of stairs, which he needs to do to get to the second floor of home. • Patient will perform UE ergometer exercise × 18 minutes at moderate intensity with Borg Scale rating of 13/20 within 3 weeks to improve cardiovascular endurance. (Intensity would be set based on what level allowed the patient to complete the exercise, but at a level of somewhat hard to really improve endurance.). • Patient will independently manage opening/closing door at the top of a ramp 3/5 trials within 3 weeks to be independent at home. 3. Long-term goals: • Patient will independently perform 6 MPT for 2,000 feet with Borg for perceived exertion rating of 12/20, modified Borg of 2 to 3, and O_2 saturations at least 94% RA within 5 weeks to improve cardiovascular endurance. • Patient will independently perform passive hip extension stretching 3 days a week within 5 weeks to improve hip ROM. • Patient will independently perform floor to/from chair transfer within 5 weeks to get to/off of stairs, which he needs to do to get to the second floor of home. • Patient will independently perform car transfer while managing his wheelchair within 5 weeks to promote independence.
Evaluate	4. The largest barriers for bed mobility and transfers at this time are the patient's strength—both UE and core—and balance. The physical therapy and patient should work on task training directly to allow the patient to successfully master bed mobility and transfers. Interventions should be strengthening exercise for UEs and balance activities in short sit, long sit, and in his wheelchair. For crossover of task and increased confidence, environmental conditions can be modified.
Analyze	5. Since this patient will be sitting for long periods of time, he is susceptible to losing BLE ROM, specifically hip and knee extension and ankle plantar flexion. Therefore, if stretching and positioning is not performed, the patient could quickly lose range and potentially develop fixed contractures. That could lead to problems with skin integrity, joint integrity, and muscle/ligament/tendon integrity. The Physical therapy should teach the patient prone stretching and positioning and develop a home exercise program to be implemented outside of the clinic. For plantar flexion, positioning and education may be facilitated in the wheelchair or stretching using a towel in long sit 6. Barriers for living alone and return to work are bed mobility, all transfers (including floor to/from chair and car), managing doors at top of ramps, and cardiovascular endurance. Physical therapy, occupational therapist (OT), and a vocational training professional may be able to assist with these barriers. Equipment and modifications to the car and/or home may assist. Consideration of work modifications may also be warranted. To identify the challenges, it is best to have the patient and employer go through normal daily tasks and see what may be difficult for the patient. Afterward, the rehab team can work with the patient to see what barriers can be addressed in therapy and what may need equipment of workplace modification
Apply	7. Potential interventions to address the patient's strength and allow for independence and return to leisure activities that he wants to pursue are UE ergometer, weightlifting with weights/dumbbells, weightlifting with circuit training, weight training with body weight resistance, and wheelchair propulsion without or with resistance. Exercise prescription should be based on American College of Sports Medicine (ACSM) guidelines. 8. A major complication for people with SCI is skin breakdown. The patient should be educated on how lack of sensation can impact skin integrity, and the importance of

(Continued)

(Continued)

Bloom's Taxonomy Level	Case 18.C Questions
	frequent position changes in bed and while using the wheelchair. The physical therapist should educate the patient on dips, lateral leaning, and other techniques for pressure relief. The education should focus on how to do the technique(s) for pressure relief, how often to perform them, and for how long. The physical therapist should also make sure to educate the patient on the other impacts to skin integrity: nutrition, body weight, shear, friction, moisture, and, of course, his sensation. ▶ Fig. 18.5.
	9. There are a variety of topics to educate the patient on, including, but not limited to, the risk of developing pulmonary complications such as pneumonia, urinary tract infections, skin breakdown, diabetes mellitus, obesity, spasticity, mental health issues such as depression or anxiety, loss of bone density, and loss of ROM and joint integrity. The Physical therapist can use a variety of methods to educate the patient: handouts, videos, support groups, etc. It is very important to assess the patient's understanding. It isn't enough to just ask if he has any questions. The Physical therapist could have him repeat back to the information provided or have him explain it to a family member or other patient. Additionally, the Physical therapist could ask him questions about the information. Any other methods of assessment would be fine too. It is important to verify that he learned the information and didn't just listen to it.
Understand	10. AD happens in around 40% of people with SCI at T6 or above. This patient's SCI is just below T6, so he is still at a moderate risk of developing AD at some point in his life. The patient should be aware that it will be a fairly rapid rise in blood pressure with lower heart rate. The Physical therapist should educate the patient that the symptoms he may feel are feeling flush or pink in the cheeks, a pounding headache, heavy sweating, anxiety, blurry vision, and possibly trouble breathing. This is a medical emergency and the patient should call 911 immediately. In the meantime, he should sit up immediately to help reduce the elevated blood pressure and look for potential causes for the AD such as tight clothing or a pressure injury. The patient could try inserting a urinary catheter in case there is a urinary tract blockage triggering the AD. Otherwise, the patient should wait for medical assistance. Most incidences of AD are not fatal since they are caught early.
	11. HO is the formation of bone in the soft tissue and/or muscle. It occurs in up to 50% of people with SCI. For people with SCI, it can occur in almost any soft-tissue area, but it is frequently in the LEs around or near joints. One of the main signs of HO is localized pain, but in this case, the patient may not feel it due to loss of sensation from the SCI, so the patient must keep an eye out for localized swelling that will begin to look similar to a tumor or growth. As the HO grows, it may impact motion in the nearest joint too, so the patient should make note of any loss of motion not connected with stretching. Conservative treatment interventions include nonsteroidal anti-inflammatory drugs and radiation. Surgery to remove the calcification can be done if conservative methods fail.
Remember	12. Door width must be a minimum of 32 inches, maximum ramp rise must be 30 inches, recommended kitchen measurements for wheelchair negotiation are 40 to 60 inches depending on the layout of the kitchen.
	13. See Table 18.1 for considerations with wheelchair prescription. This patient should be more mobile, able to perform pressure relief on his own, and be active. The Physical therapy would want to look for a more agile axle and seat setup, antitippers, and good-quality seat and back, but there is no need for a wheelchair with power, maximum pressure relief, recline, or tilt-in-space.

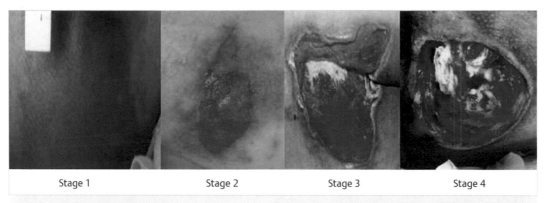

| Stage 1 | Stage 2 | Stage 3 | Stage 4 |

Fig. 18.5 Progression of pressure ulcer.

Table 18.1 Wheelchair design considerations

Component	Explanation	Options
Type of propulsion	• Consider whether the patient can propel the chair on their own for extended periods or if power is needed for mobility.	• Power • Manual
Frame	• Rigid frames: better for individuals who are larger, have multiple medical and/or physical impairments, or more sedentary; more energy efficient so may be better for active users and wheelchair sports, etc. They tend to be lighter so this model is easier for a driver to transfer the frame in/out of the car. • Folding: better for individuals who are more mobile, have less medical and/or physical impairments, or more active in the community.	• Rigid • Folding

Wheel type	• Consider weight, durability, and ease of propulsion:
	  ○ Spoke wheels: aid shock absorption, lighter, easier to propel, but require more maintenance.
	  ○ Mag wheels: durable, less maintenance, but less shock absorption, and heavier so more difficult to propel.
		• Spoke
		• Mag

Wheel locks	• Type of brake needed is usually based on the patient's balance, reaching ability, strength, and hand function.	• Pull to lock • Push to lock • Retractable • Need for break extension.
Seat	• Used for positioning and to assist with pressure control. • Should be fitted well to the patient so as not to increase pressure especially on bony prominences.	• Generic foam • Custom foam • Foam and gel • Gel • Air cells
Back rest	• Used for proper positioning to maintain neutral spine position as much as possible and to distribute weight onto ischial tuberosities and posterior legs.	• Firm, minimum contour • Custom contour back—covered in foam, with gel inserts, or with air cells.
Back height		• High profile • Low profile • Custom measurement

(Continued)

(Continued)

Component	Explanation	Options
Antitippers	• Important accessory for safety to prevent backward tipping of the wheelchair. • Can inhibit curb negotiation or wheelies needed for other functional mobility.	• Wheeled antitippers • Padded antitippers
Recline	• Ability for the seat back angle to increase beyond 90 degrees. • The purpose of recline is to allow pressure relief off the ischial tuberosities by shifting weight more toward the sacrum and spine. There are some shearing forces that may occur as the patient moves into/out of the reclined position.	• Yes/no
Tilt-in-space	• "Tilt-in-space" refers to the seating area to tilt as one piece on top of the wheelchair frame. • The purpose of tilt is to allow pressure relief without changing the overall seating position of the patient and limiting shearing forces. The chair moves in the sagittal plane to take pressure off the ischial tuberosities and place it on the spine for a short period of time. It may be more expensive, add weight to the chair, and need mechanical power to perform the tilt.	• Yes/no
Other	• Other features including, but not limited to, foot plates, arm rests, head rests, alternate power sources, tire type, and quick release wheels are not covered here, but would be considerations in full wheelchair prescription.	

Note: This is meant to cover basic considerations. Proficiency with wheelchair prescription requires further knowledge beyond this table.

Key points
1. This is the last stage of rehab, so it is important to help the patient become as functionally independent as he can while maintaining safety too.
2. Building endurance is still crucial at this point. Strength and endurance will be the two main factors impacting function and quality of life. Work with the patient to find which activities and exercises will improve his endurance and strength the most and that he will continue with after he is discharged from Physical therapy.
3. Education is paramount at this point. Mortality rates for people with SCI are due mostly to secondary complications, the most common of those being pulmonary complications. It is of utmost importance at this stage of rehab to educate the patient on all the possible complications related to SCI and what he should do if he experiences any of them. Written resources are especially valued since these may happen months or years in the future after physical therapy has been completed.

Suggested Readings

Curt A, Van Hedel HJ, Klaus D, Dietz V, EM-SCI Study Group. Recovery from a spinal cord injury: significance of compensation, neural plasticity, and repair. J Neurotrauma. 2008; 25(6):677–685

Berlowitz DJ, Wadsworth B, Ross J. Respiratory problems and management in people with spinal cord injury. Breathe (Sheff). 2016; 12(4):328–340

Boninger ML, Waters RL, Chase T, et al; Consortium for Spinal Cord Medicine. Preservation of Upper Limb Function Following Spinal Cord Injury: A Clinical Practice Guideline for Health-Care Professionals. Washington, DC: Paralyzed Veterans of America; 2005

Cardozo CP. Respiratory complications of spinal cord injury. J Spinal Cord Med. 2007; 30(4):307–308

Dietz V, Fouad K. Restoration of sensorimotor functions after spinal cord injury. Brain. 2014; 137(Pt 3):654–667

Goodman CC, Heick J, Lazaro RT. Differential Diagnosis for Physical Therapists: Screening for Referral. 6th ed. St Louis, MO: Elsevier; 2018

O'Sullivan SB, Schmitz TJ, Fulk G. Physical Rehabilitation. 7th ed. Philadelphia, PA: F.A. Davis Company; 2019

Sheel AW, Reid WD, Townson AF, Ayas NT, Konnyu KJ, Spinal Cord Rehabilitation Evidence Research Team. Effects of exercise training and inspiratory muscle training in spinal cord injury: a systematic review. J Spinal Cord Med. 2008; 31(5):500–508

Soumyashree S, Kaur J. Effect of inspiratory muscle training (IMT) on aerobic capacity, respiratory muscle strength and rate of perceived exertion in paraplegics. J Spinal Cord Med. 2020; 43 (1):53–59

Wing PC, Dalsey WC, Alvarez E, et al.; Consortium for Spinal Cord Medicine. Early Acute Management in Adults with Spinal Cord Injury: A Clinical Practice Guideline for Health-Care Providers. Washington, DC: Paralyzed Veterans of America; 2008

Torres-Castro R, Vilaró J, Vera-Uribe R, Monge G, Avilés P, Suranyi C. Use of air stacking and abdominal compression for cough assistance in people with complete tetraplegia. Spinal Cord. 2014; 52(5):354–357

Aslan SC, Randall DC, Krassioukov AV, Phillips A, Ovechkin AV. Respiratory training improves blood pressure regulation in individuals with chronic spinal cord injury. Arch Phys Med Rehabil. 2016; 97(6):964–973

Zbogar D, Eng JJ, Noble JW, Miller WC, Krassioukov AV, Verrier MC. Cardiovascular stress during inpatient spinal cord injury rehabilitation. Arch Phys Med Rehabil. 2017; 98(12):2449–2456

Goldman JM, Rose LS, Williams SJ, Silver JR, Denison DM. Effect of abdominal binders on breathing in tetraplegic patients. Thorax. 1986; 41(12):940–945

Wadsworth BM, Haines TP, Cornwell PL, Paratz JD. Abdominal binder use in people with spinal cord injuries: a systematic review and meta-analysis. Spinal Cord. 2009; 47(4):274–285

Askari S, Kirby RL, Parker K, Thompson K, O'Neill J. Wheelchair propulsion test: development and measurement properties of a new test for manual wheelchair users. Arch Phys Med Rehabil. 2013; 94(9):1690–1698

6 minute arm test. Rehab Measures Database. Available at: https://www.sralab.org/rehabilitation-measures/six-minute-arm-test. Accessed May 1, 2020

Bhise AR, Solanki R, Shukla YU, Prabhakar MM. Using six-minute-push-test to measure cardiovascular fitness in spinal cord injury patients in Indian hospital setting. Arch Phys Med Rehabil. 2015; 96(10):e75

Cowan RE, Callahan MK, Nash MS. The 6-min push test is reliable and predicts low fitness in spinal cord injury. Med Sci Sports Exerc. 2012; 44(10):1993–2000

Gauthier C, Grangeon M, Ananos L, Brosseau R, Gagnon DH. Quantifying cardiorespiratory responses resulting from speed and slope increments during motorized treadmill propulsion among manual wheelchair users. Ann Phys Rehabil Med. 2017; 60(5):281–288

Jacobs PL, Nash MS. Exercise recommendations for individuals with spinal cord injury. Sports Med. 2004; 34(11):727–751

Bochkezanian V, Raymond J, de Oliveira CQ, Davis GM. Can combined aerobic and muscle strength training improve aerobic fitness, muscle strength, function and quality of life in people with spinal cord injury? A systematic review. Spinal Cord. 2015; 53(6):418–431

Hsieh JTC, Connolly SJ, McIntyre A, et al. Spasticity following spinal cord injury. In: Eng JJ, Teasell RW, Miller WC, et al. eds. Spinal Cord Injury Rehabilitation Evidence. Version 6.0. 2016

Riebe D, Ehrman JK, Liguori G, Magal M. ACSM's Guidelines for Exercise Testing and Prescription. 10th ed. Philadelphia, PA: Wolters Kluwer; 2018

Garber SL, Bryce TN, Gregorio-Torres TL. Pressure Ulcer Prevention and Treatment Following Injury: A Clinical Practice Guideline for Health-Care Providers. 2nd ed. Washington, DC: Consortium for Spinal Cord Medicine; 2014

Lindan R, Joiner E, Freehafer AA, Hazel C. Incidence and clinical features of autonomic dysreflexia in patients with spinal cord injury. Paraplegia. 1980; 18(5):285–292

Meyers C, Lisiecki J, Miller S, et al. Heterotopic ossification: a comprehensive review. JBMR Plus. 2019; 3(4):e10172

Teasell RW, Mehta S, Aubut JL, et al. SCIRE Research Team. A systematic review of the therapeutic interventions for heterotopic ossification after spinal cord injury. Spinal Cord. 2010; 48(7):512–521

Americans with Disabilities Act. Compliance Directory. Available at https://www.ada-compliance.com/. Accessed May 2020

Ciccone C. Pharmacology in Rehabilitation. 5th ed. Philadelphia, PA: F.A. Davis Company; 2016

Ko HY. Revisit spinal shock: pattern of reflex evolution during spinal shock. Korean J Neurotrauma. 2018; 14(2):47–54

Batavia M. The Wheelchair Evaluation: A Clinician's Guide. 2nd ed. Sudbury, MA: Jones and Bartlett Publishers; 2010

Susiwala S. Wheelchair Prescription. Available at: https://www.slideshare.net/sharminsusiwala22/wheelchair-prescription. Accessed May 2020

EnableNSW and Lifetime Care & Support Authority. Guidelines for the prescription of a seated wheelchair or mobility scooter for people with a traumatic brain injury or spinal cord injury. EnableNSW and Lifetime Care & Support Authority; Sydney; 2011

19 Back Surgery

General Information	
Case no.	19.A Back Surgery
Authors	Josh Fede, PT, DPT, MTC, CSCS, USATF-L1 Brian Goonan, PT, DPT, Board Certified Clinical Specialist in Orthopaedic Physical Therapy Scott Siverling, PT, DPT, Board Certified Clinical Specialist in Orthopaedic Physical Therapy, Fellow of the American Academy of Orthopedic Physical Therapy
Diagnosis	Lower back, right lateral hip, and right foot pain
Setting	Acute care hospital
Learner expectations	☑ Initial evaluation ☐ Re-evaluation ☐ Treatment session
Learner objectives	1. Understand any postoperative complications and when you refer back to physician. 2. Understand postoperative restrictions for this particular surgery and be able to provide education to the patient. 3. Identify goals, provide education, discuss support and home setup, and prepare for discharge.

Medical	
Chief complaint	Chronic right-sided lower back pain, lateral hip pain, and foot pain
History of present illness	The patient is a 51-year-old man who reports approximately 2.5-year history of progressive lower back pain with right lower extremity (RLE) pain and weakness. As his sensation diminished in the right lower leg, his gait was adversely affected, and ultimately, he underwent an L5–S1 lumbar microdiscectomy 1 year ago. He recently went back to his surgeon for 1-year follow-up. Currently, he continues to have radicular symptoms down his RLE, including "shooting" pain down into the heel of his foot, numbness along the lateral and posterior aspects of the RLE, and gross weakness. He feels that he has exhausted conservative management with previous physical therapy and pain management. He discussed surgical options with his physician, and his physician recommended a multilevel fusion (L4–L5/L5–S1) in order to relieve his radicular symptoms. Benefits and risks of the surgery were discussed with the patient and he agreed to move forward with the elective procedure.
Past medical history	Hypertension, hypercholesterolemia, gastroesophageal reflux disease (GERD)
Past surgical history	L5–S1 discectomy, cholecystectomy, appendectomy
Allergies	None
Medications	Lisinopril, Lipitor, Omeprazole
Precautions/orders	Activity as tolerated

Social history	
Home setup	• Lives in a two-story home with his wife and three children. • Bedroom is on the second floor. • Has a guest bedroom and half bath on the first floor.
Occupation	• Financial advisor
Prior level of function	• Independent with functional mobility and activities of daily living (ADLs). • Married father of three children. • (+) driver
Recreational activities	• Occasionally plays basketball in the summer. • Works out at the gym once or twice times a week but has not exercised in over 1 year.

Vital signs	Hospital day 1, postoperative, ward
Blood pressure (mmHg)	135/84
Heart rate (beats/min)	85
Respiratory rate (breaths/min)	20
Pulse oximetry on room air (SpO$_2$)	98%

Medical management	Hospital day 1: postoperative, ward
Medications	1. Acetaminophen prn pain 2. Ibuprofen prn pain 3. Oxycodone prn pain
Neurosurgery team	1. Monitor hemoglobin (Hgb) and hematocrit (Hct) with complete blood count (CBC). 2. Monitor for signs and symptoms related to deep vein thromboses (DVTs). 3. Manage pain, continue current regimen. 4. Incision clear/dry/intact

Precautions	• Activity as tolerated
	• Fall risk
	• Spinal precautions:
	  ○ Avoid bending and twisting.
	  ○ Avoid lifting, pushing, and/or pulling > 20 lb for 2 weeks
	  ○ Avoid prolonged sitting > 30 min
	• Brace (▶ Fig. 19.1)
	• Full weight bearing (FWB) bilateral lower extremity (BLE).
	• Telemetry

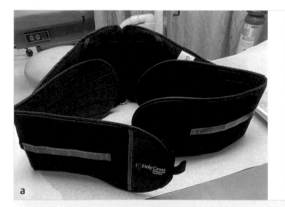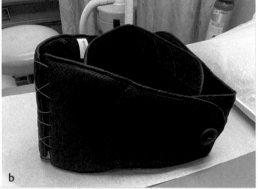

Fig. 19.1 (a,b) Back brace typically used postoperatively for a spinal fusion surgery. The brace helps act as a reminder through proprioceptive feedback to limit bending and rotation immediately after surgery. Additionally, the brace offers compression, which can help with post-op pain and soreness.

Lab		Reference range	Hospital day 1: postoperative, ward
CBC	White blood cell	$5.0–10.0 \times 10^9$/L	6.4
	Red blood cell	4.1–5.3 million/mm^3	4.7
	Hgb	14–17.4 g/dL	15
	Hct	42–52%	47%
	Platelets	140,000–400,000/μL	250
Basic metabolic panel	Glucose	70–100 mg/dL	90
	Hgb A1C	<5.7%	6.7%
	Cholesterol	<200 mg/dL	210
	low-density lipoprotein	<100 mg/dL	130
	High-density lipoprotein	>40 mg/dL	80
	Blood urea nitrogen	6–25 mg/dL	25
	Creatinine	0.7–1.3 mg/dL	1.2
	Potassium	3.7–5.1 mEq/L	4
	Sodium	134–142 mEq/L	136
	Chloride	98–108 mEq/L	100
	Calcium	8.6–10.3 mg/dL	8.4
	Magnesium	1.2–1.9 mEq/L	1.4

Pause points

Based on the above Information, what are the priorities:
• Diagnostic tests and measures?
• Outcome measures?
• Treatment Interventions?

Hospital Day 2, Post-Op Day 1, Ward: Physical Therapy Examination
Subjective

Patient reports that he is "sore" along the lumbopelvic hip complex and bilateral sacroiliac joint regions. Additionally, he reports that he still feels "numbness" along the shin and dorsum of the foot, with occasional "shooting" pains along the same distribution.
"My surgeon said this is normal, and it will return."

Objective		
Vital signs	Pre-treatment	Post-treatment
Blood pressure (mmHg)	130/82	132/84
Heart rate (beats/min)	75	77
Respiratory rate (breaths/min)	18	21
Pulse oximetry on room air (SpO$_2$)	98%	96%
Pain	2/10 along spinal incision	5/10 along spinal incision
General	• Patient supine in bed, no apparent distress. • Patient's wife at bedside. • Lines notable for intravenous line access. • Dressing over the incision clean, dry, and intact.	
Head, ears, eyes, nose, and throat	• (–) congestion, sore throat, or otalgia	

(Continued)

(Continued)

		Hospital Day 2, Post-Op Day 1, Ward: Physical Therapy Examination	
Cardiovascular and pulmonary		• (–) chest pain, palpitations, edema, aspiration, shortness of breath, orthopnea. • (–) cough, congestion, wheezing, or sputum production.	
Gastrointestinal		• Unremarkable	
Genitourinary		• (–) dysuria, frequency, urgency, blood in urine	
Musculoskeletal	Range of motion (ROM)	Right	Left
		• Upper extremity (UE): within functional limit (WFL). • Hip flexion: 0–90 degrees • Hip abduction: 0–26 degrees • Hip external rotation: 0–25 degrees • Hip internal rotation: 0–15 degrees • Knee flexion: WFL • Knee extension: WFL • Ankle dorsiflexion: WFL • Ankle plantar flexion: WFL	• UE: WFL • Hip flexion: 0–105 degrees • Hip abduction: 0–35 degrees • Hip external rotation: 0–30 degrees • Hip internal rotation: 0–23 degrees • Knee flexion: WFL • Knee extension: WFL • Ankle dorsiflexion: WFL • Ankle plantar flexion: WFL
		Lumbar ROM limited by postoperative restrictions.	
	Strength	• UE: WFL • Hip flexion: > 3 + /5 as demonstrated by functional mobility. • Hip abduction: > 3 + /5 as demonstrated by functional mobility. • Knee extension: 3 + /5 • Knee flexion: 4/5 • Ankle dorsiflexion: 3/5 • Ankle eversion: 3 + /5 • Ankle plantar flexion: 4/5 • Great toe extension: 4/5	• UE: WFL • Hip flexion: > 3 + /5 as demonstrated by functional mobility. • Hip abduction: > 3 + /5 as demonstrated by functional mobility. • Knee extension: 5/5 • Knee flexion: 5/5 • Ankle dorsiflexion: 5/5 • Ankle eversion: 5/5 • Ankle plantar flexion: 5/5 • Great toe extension: 5/5
	Special tests	• (+) Flexion, abduction, and external rotation (FABER). • (+) Active Straight Leg Raise (SLR) Test. • Five Times Sit-to-Stand: 3 with rolling walker assist (untimed due to patient not completing 5 repetitions).	
	Flexibility	• (+) Tibial and dorsal foot pain with passive SLR at approximately 30 degrees.	
Neurological	Balance	• Sitting, static: supervision • Sitting, dynamic: contact guard assistance. Limited range due to brace. • Standing, static: supervision with rolling walker. • Standing, dynamic: contact guard assistance with rolling walker. • Single limb stance: unable to stand on RLE > 1 second due to decreased strength and increased pain.	
	Cognition	• Alert and oriented × 4	
	Coordination	• Finger to nose: intact bilaterally	
	Cranial nerves	• II–XII: intact	

(Continued)

(Continued)

	Hospital Day 2, Post-Op Day 1, Ward: Physical Therapy Examination	
	Reflexes	• Patellar: 2 + bilaterally • Achilles: 1 + on right, 2 + on left
	Sensation	• Left lower extremity (LLE): intact to light touch. • RLE: diminished light touch and pinprick at L5 and S1 dermatome levels.
	Functional status	
Bed mobility	• Rolling either direction: minimal assistance • Supine to/from sit: minimal assistance	
Transfers	• Sit to/from stand: contact guard assistance with rolling walker.	
Ambulation	• Ambulated × 50 feet with contact guard assistance and rolling walker, verbal cues provided for upright posture. • Gait deviations notable for decreased cadence.	
Stairs	• Ascend/descend five steps with contact guard assistance and minimal assist. • Demonstrated step-to pattern	

Assessment	
☑ Physical therapist's	*Assessment left blank for learner to develop.*
Goals	
Patient's	"I want to go home. I want to walk without a walker."
Short term	1. 　　　*Goals left blank for learner to develop.* 2.
Long term	1. 　　　*Goals left blank for learner to develop.* 2.

Plan	
☑ Physical therapist's	Will continue to follow daily for functional mobility training within the confines of spinal precautions and newly implemented brace. Throughout, will educate and reinforce postsurgical precautions, importance of brace. Prior to discharge, will institute a walking program and provide a home exercise program.

Bloom's Taxonomy Level	Case 19.A Questions
Create	1. Synthesizing the medical data and physical examination findings, develop an appropriate physical therapy assessment of the patient. 2. Develop two short-term physical therapy goals, including an appropriate timeframe. 3. Develop two long-term physical therapy goals, including an appropriate timeframe.
Evaluate	4. What education should the physical therapist provide to the patient regarding his diminished sensation? 5. What strategies can be provided for the patient in order to follow his post-op precautions and mobilize safely once he has been discharged to his home?
Analyze	6. How is BLE sensation tested to definitively determine the area of diminished sensation? 7. Considering this patient has restrictions with spinal flexion and rotations, what would be an appropriate technique for supine to sit transfer?
Apply	8. What functional tasks should be addressed in daily physical therapy until the patient's discharge? 9. How should functional progression be measured?

(Continued)

(Continued)

Bloom's Taxonomy Level	Case 19.A Questions
Understand	10. What therapeutic exercise would be appropriate to prescribe on this patient's initial evaluation? 11. What education can be provided to the patient to help diminish the risk of DVT and pulmonary embolism?
Remember	12. If the patient were to complain of mid-thoracic pain, especially after meals, what might be suspected? 13. Besides difficulty with gait and lower extremity weakness, what complaints/signs might the patient have if there is cauda equina involvement?

Bloom's Taxonomy Level	Case 19.A Answers
Create	1. The patient is a 51-year-old man status post surgical lumbar fusion. He was previously independent with functional mobility and ADLs. He currently exhibits decreased BLE ROM, RLE strength, RLE sensation, and impaired balance. This, in combination with his newly implemented spinal precautions, brace, and pain, is contributing to his limitations in mobility. He currently requires contact guard—minimal assistance and use of rolling walker to mobilize. He will benefit from continued therapeutic interventions with integration of spinal precautions and brace; also, specific education on an exercise regimen will maximize functional mobility and safety. Will continue to follow. 2. Short-term goals: • Patient will perform Five Times Sit-to-Stand in < 15 seconds within 3 days to improve BLE strength. • Patient will independently perform supine to/from sit within 3 days to improve functional mobility for home. • Patient will independently verbalize and implement 3/3 spinal precautions 100% of the time within 3 days to protect his spine. 3. Long-term goals: • Patient will ambulate 150 feet with distance supervision and rolling walker within 7 days to improve functional mobility at home. • Patient will ascend/descend 12 steps with supervision and a single handrail within 7 days to improve functional mobility at home. • Patient will independently don/doff brace within 7 days to protect his spine and promote independence at home.
Evaluate	4. The physical therapist should educate the patient that a temporary alteration in sensation following surgery is normal. The patient should be educated that nerve regeneration can be slow and unpredictable and that pain may accompany nerve regeneration. Sensation should be reassessed periodically. 5. To mobilize safely while maintaining spinal precautions, the patient should: • change position once every 30 minutes to prevent pressure injuries. • ambulate frequently to decrease the risk of DVTs. • be educated on how to assess his home living situation—remove objects and/or throw rugs from floor to decrease fall risk, ask for assistance from family/caregiver to pick up/carry larger objects. • practice activity pacing and modification.
Analyze	6. To test lower extremity sensation, sensation should be tested on the UEs to ensure that the patient knows what to expect. The patient should close his eyes and respond "yes" when he feels the physical therapist's touch. The physical therapist should lightly touch the skin in varying patterns to assess dermatome levels. The physical therapist can use Q-tip, tissue, or finger as light touch instrument. The Semmes-Weinstein filaments can also be used. 7. The appropriate technique for the supine to sit transfer would be the "log roll" technique, where the patient rolls toward his side, and proceeds to use his arms and legs to rise (like a seesaw) from side-lying to sitting at the edge of the bed.

(Continued)

(Continued)

Bloom's Taxonomy Level	Case 19.A Answers
Apply	8. Functional tasks such as bed mobility, transfers, and gait training on even and uneven surfaces should be addressed in daily physical therapy sessions.
	9. Ways to objectively track functional progression include noting the amount of assistance needed, utilization of assistive devices, gait speed, gait distance, mobility deviations, or outcome measures such as the Activity Measure for Post-Acute Care (AMPAC) 6-Clicks or Five Times Sit-to-Stand.
Understand	10. Therapeutic exercises that would be appropriate to prescribe at this patient's initial evaluation include ankle pumps, long arc quads, heel slides, and sit to stands with assistance. Acknowledgement should also be given to the UEs; therefore, light UE motions without resistance can also be prescribed.
	11. To help diminish the risk of developing a DVT and/or pulmonary embolism, the patient should first be educated on signs and symptoms and why he is at risk. Further, the patient can be educated on the importance of ankle pumps, frequent mobility throughout the day, the use of an incentive spirometer, and diaphragmatic breathing.
Remember	12. If the patient were to complain of mid-thoracic pain, especially after meals, GERD "flare" (gallbladder has been removed) or stomach ulcer may be suspected.
	13. Complaints/signs that could indicate cauda equina involvement include difficulty with urination, especially initiating and saddle anesthesia. Urinary retention is the most common initial (and persistent) symptom in cauda equine syndrome; however, saddle anesthesia is the most common symptom of post-op acquired cauda equine syndrome.

Key points
1. Red flags need to be constantly monitored. Such red flags for this case include DVT, pulmonary embolism, and cauda equina syndrome.
2. Assessment of myotome and dermatome needs to be consistent and reassessed, especially because of the patient's recent spinal surgery.
3. Progressing functional tasks, while maintaining precautions and other restrictions, and maximizing safety are priorities during the acute phase of recovery.

General Information	
Case no.	19.B
Authors	Josh Fede, PT, DPT, MTC, CSCS, USATF-L1
	Brian Goonan, PT, DPT, Board Certified Clinical Specialist in Orthopaedic Physical Therapy
	Scott Siverling, PT, DPT, Board Certified Clinical Specialist in Orthopaedic Physical Therapy, Fellow of the American Academy of Orthopedic Physical Therapy
Diagnosis	Lower back, right lateral hip and foot pain
Setting	Outpatient clinic
Learner expectations	☑ Initial evaluation
	☐ Re-evaluation
	☐ Treatment session
Learner objectives	1. To stress the importance of recognizing possible red flags.
	2. Appreciate the importance of testing peripheral neurological structures.
	3. Discuss the differential diagnosis of lateral hip pain in a patient with primary lumbar spine issues.

Medical	
Chief complaint	Right-sided lower back pain, lateral hip pain, and foot pain
History of present illness	The patient is a 51-year-old man who reports approximately 2.5-year history of progressive lower back pain and right-sided radiculopathy. He underwent an L5–S1 microdiscectomy approximately 1 year ago; however, during recovery, he began to have

(Continued)

(Continued)

Medical	
	difficulty lifting his R foot while walking. Additionally, his dorsal foot pain advanced to an "unbearable" level. At this point, he elected to have a lumbar spinal fusion (L4–L5/L5–S1). Following 6 weeks of postoperative recovery, he is presenting for outpatient physical therapy evaluation.
Past medical history	Hypertension, hypercholesterolemia, gastroesophageal reflux disease.
Past surgical history	L5–S1 discectomy, cholecystectomy, appendectomy, L4–L5/L5–S1 fusion (6 weeks ago).
Allergies	None
Medications	Lisinopril, Lipitor, Omeprazole
Precautions/orders	Spinal precautions Activity as tolerated

Social history	
Home setup	• Lives in a two-story home with his wife and three children. • Bedroom is on the second floor. • Has a guest bedroom and half bath on the first floor.
Occupation	• Financial advisor
Prior level of function	• Currently using a rolling walker for static and dynamic standing mobility, uses adaptive equipment for bathing. • Married father of three children. • (+) driver (currently not driving)
Recreational activities	Prior to surgery: • Occasionally plays basketball in the summer. • Works out at the gym once or twice a week but has not exercised in over 1 year.

Medical management	Surgeon's office, 1 week ago
Follow-up	• Review of the patient's postoperative computed tomography (CT) scan shows that he underwent an L4–L5/L5–S1 fusion, posterior approach 5 weeks ago. • Fusion healing well, all hardware intact, satisfactory alignment maintained. • Incision healed • Post-op brace discontinued.

Pause points
Based on the above information, what are the priorities: • Diagnostic tests and measures? • Outcome measures? • Treatment interventions? Based on the above information: • What red flags are important to look for? • What is the hypothesis for the ongoing leg pain?

Physical Therapy Examination	
Subjective	

"It feels like my right foot is on fire sometimes and it feels really swollen"
The patient reports some difficulty with sleeping due to foot pain. Additionally, he states: "my back aches if I'm doing too much or just at the end of the day." "my hip hurts the most, especially when I'm just trying to walk a few blocks" (about 10 min). He reports decreased lower back and buttock pain but complains of a lower back ache with prolonged sitting or standing (> 10–15 minutes).
"I can feel more of my leg than before surgery, it just kind of gets itchy sometimes, but that's no big deal"

Objective		
Vital signs	**Pre-treatment**	
Blood pressure (mmHg)	128/88	
Heart rate (beats/min)	71	
Respiratory rate (breaths/min)	22	
Pulse oximetry on room air (SpO$_2$)	99%	
Pain	0–1/10, low back, at rest 5/10, low back, at worst, occurs with prolonged standing/walking, > 15 minutes	
General	Observation	Patient is ambulating with a rolling walker.
Musculoskeletal	Range of motion (ROM)	• Bilateral upper extremity (BUE): within functional limit (WFL). • Lumbar ROM: limited by postoperative precautions. • Left lower extremity (LLE): WFL • Right lower extremity (RLE): WFL with the exception of external rotation (ER): 0 to 15 degrees, limited by lateral hip pain at end range.
	Strength	**Right** / **Left**
		• UE: WFL • UE: WFL • Hip extension: 3 + /5 • Hip extension: 5/5 • Hip abduction: 3 + /5 • Hip abduction: 5/5 • Knee extension: 4 + /5 • Knee extension: 5/5 • Knee flexion: 4/5 • Knee flexion: 5/5 • Ankle dorsiflexion: 3/5 • Ankle dorsiflexion: 5/5 • Ankle eversion: 3 + /5 • Ankle eversion: 5/5 • Ankle plantar flexion: 4/5 (6 single leg heel raises) • Ankle plantar flexion: 5/5 • Great toe extension: 4/5 • Great toe extension: 5/5 • 30-Second Sit to Stand = 9 repetitions
	Flexibility	• (+) Tibial and dorsal foot pain with passive straight leg raise (SLR) at approximately 48 degrees
Neurological	Balance	• Sitting, static: independent • Sitting, dynamic: independent • Standing, static: modified independent with rolling walker • Standing, dynamic: modified independent with rolling walker. • Single limb stance: unable to stand on right LE > 1 second; complains of lateral R hip pain with single limb stance; evidence of Trendelenburg motion in single limb attempts. • Timed Up and Go (TUG) Test = 19.1 seconds.
	Cognition	• Alert and oriented × 4.
	Coordination	• Finger to nose: intact bilaterally • Heel to shin: intact bilaterally

(Continued)

(Continued)

Physical Therapy Examination		
	Cranial nerves	• II–XII: intact
	Reflexes (deep tendon reflexes)	• Patellar: 2 + bilaterally • Achilles: 2 + bilaterally
	Sensation	• LLE: intact to light touch • RLE: diminished to light touch and pinprick at L5 and S1 dermatome levels
Integumentary	Skin integrity	• Unremarkable, incisions well healed
Functional status		
Bed mobility		• Rolling either direction: independent • Supine to/from sit: independent
Transfers		• Sit to/from stand: modified independent with rolling walker.
Ambulation		• Ambulated × 250 feet with modified independence using rolling walker. • Gait deviations notable for decreased cadence, decreased right hip extension, and (+) right Trendelenburg gait. • After ambulation trial, patient reported pain at the lateral right hip and general LE fatigue.
Stairs		• Ascend/descend 12 steps with modified independence using single handrail. • Demonstrated step-to pattern. • After ambulation trial, patient reported lateral right hip pain, particularly when ascending steps.
Other		• 40-Meter Fast-Paced Walk Test = 25.5 seconds • Oswestry Disability Index (ODI) score = 46% (► Fig. 19.2)

ODI Score Interpretation	Disability
0–20%	Minimal disability
21–40%	Moderate disability
41–60%	Severe disability
61–80%	Crippling back pain
81–100%	Bed bound

Source: Fairbank JC, Pynsent PB. The Oswestry disability index. Spine 2000;.25(22):2940–2953.

Assessment	
☑ Physical therapist's	*Assessment left blank for learner to develop*
Goals	
Patient's	"I really want to start walking more for exercise."
Short term	1. *Goals left blank for learner to develop* 2.
Long term	1. *Goals left blank for learner to develop* 2.

Plan	
☑ Physical therapist's	Plan of care should include education, exercise prescription to address strength and motion deficits meant to improve function, manual therapy for joint/soft-tissue restrictions and/or pain modulation, and functional training to meet the demands on performing transfers, ambulation, and stairs regularly.

Modified Oswestry Low Back Pain Disability Questionnaire

Name:_____ Date: ____/____/_____

Please Read:

This questionnaire has been designed to give your doctor/therapist information as to how your back pain has affected your ability to manage everyday life. Please answer every section, and mark in each section only the **one** box that best describes your condition today.

We realize you may feel that two of the statements in any one section relate to you, but please just mark the box which most closely describes your current condition

Section 1 – Pain Intensity	Section 6 – Standing
☐ I can tolerate the pain I have without having to use pain medication.	☐ I can stand as long as I want without increased pain.
☐ The pain is bad but I manage without having to take pain medication.	☐ I can stand as long as I want but increases my pain.
☐ Pain medication provides me complete relief from pain.	☐ Pain prevents me from standing for more than 1 hour.
☒ Pain medication provides me moderate relief from pain.	☒ Pain prevents me from standing for more than ½ hour.
☐ Pain medication provides me little relief from pain.	☐ Pain prevents me from standing for more than 10 mins.
☐ Pain medication has no effect on the pain	☐ Pain prevents me from standing at all.

Section 2 – Personal Care (Washing, Dressing, etc.)	Section 7 – Sleeping
☐ I can take care of myself normally without causing increased pain.	☐ Pain does not prevent me from sleeping well.
☒ I can take care of myself normally but it increases my pain.	☒ I can sleep well only by using pain medication.
☐ It is painful to take care of myself and I am slow and careful.	☐ Even when I take pain medication, I sleep less than 6 hours.
☐ I need help but I am able to manage most of my personal care.	☐ Even when I take pain medication, I sleep less than 4 hours.
☐ I need help every day in most aspects of my care.	☐ Even when I take pain medication, I sleep less than 2 hours.
☐ I do not get dressed, wash with difficulty and stay in bed.	☐ Pain prevents me from sleeping at all

Section 3 – Lifting	Section 8 – Social Life
☐ I can lift heavy weights without increased pain.	☐ My social life is normal and does not increase my pain.
☐ I can lift heavy weights but it causes increased pain.	☐ My social life is normal, but it increases my level of pain.
☐ Pain prevents me from lifting heavy weights off the floor, but I can manage if weights are conveniently positioned, e.g. on a table.	☒ Pain prevents me from participating in more energetic activities (ex sports, dancing, etc.
☒ Pain prevents me from lifting heavy weights but I can manage light to medium weights if they are conveniently positioned.	☐ Pain prevents me from going out very often.
☐ I can lift only very light weights.	☐ Pain has restricted my social life to my home.
☐ I cannot lift or carry anything at all.	☐ I have hardly any social life because of my pain.

Section 4 - Walking	Section 9 – Traveling
☐ Pain does not prevent me walking any distance.	☐ I can travel anywhere without increased pain.
☐ Pain prevents me walking more than 1 mile.	☐ I can travel anywhere but it increases my pain.
☐ Pain prevents me walking more than ½ mile	☐ Pain restricts travel over 2 hours.
☒ Pain prevents me walking more than ¼ mile	☒ Pain restricts travel over 1 hour.
☐ I can only walk using crutches or a cane.	☐ Pain restricts my travel to short necessary journeys under ½ hour.
☐ I am in bed most of the time and have to crawl to the toilet.	☐ Pain prevents all travel except for visits to the doctor/therapist or hospital.

Section 5 - Sitting	Section 10 – Employment/Homemaking
☐ I can it in any chair as long as I like.	☐ My normal homemaking/job activities do not cause pain.
☐ I can only sit in my favorite chair as long as I like.	☐ My normal homemaking/job activities increase my pain, but I can still perform all that is required of me.
☒ Pain prevents me sitting more than 1 hour.	☒ I can perform most of my homemaking/job duties, but pain prevents me from performing more physically stressful activities (ex. Lifting, vacuuming).
☐ Pain prevents me from sitting more than ½ hour.	☐ Pain prevents me from doing anything but light duties.
☐ Pain prevents me from sitting more than 10 mins.	☐ Pain prevents me from doing even light duties.
☐ Pain prevents me from sitting at all.	☐ Pain prevents me from performing any job/homemaking chores.

23/50 = 46%

Fig. 19.2 The Modified Oswestry Disability Index (ODI) is a self-reported outcome tool that can be used to measure or quantify a patient's perceived disability due to low back pain. The patient selects one statement from each section that closest matches their current situation. The score is then summed and converted into an index score. This patient scored a 46%, which would be interpreted as "severe disability."

Bloom's Taxonomy Level	Case 19.B Questions
Create	1. Synthesizing the medical data and physical examination findings, develop an appropriate physical therapy assessment of the patient. 2. Develop two short-term physical therapy goals, including an appropriate timeframe. 3. Develop two long-term physical therapy goals, including an appropriate timeframe.
Evaluate	4. What are possible reasons for the lateral hip pain? 5. How should a physical therapist explain to the patient the risks of violating the postoperative precautions?
Analyze	6. What is purpose of testing both light touch and sharp/dull sensation? 7. If a loss or diminishment in light touch sensation is detected, in what way can this information be corroborated?
Apply	8. What are appropriate exercises to prescribe for the patient following today's examination? 9. In what ways can the patient's functional progress be assessed and determined?
Understand	10. If the patient does not improve his ability to perform repetitions during the 30-Second Sit to Stand Test, what should be reexamined?
Remember	11. What are the cardinal signs of infection? 12. When the L5 nerve root has been damaged, which muscles might be weak upon testing?

Bloom's Taxonomy Level	Case 19.B Answers

Create	1. The patient is a 51-year-old man who presents ~6 weeks after lumbar spinal fusion seeking guidance in recovery. Prior to surgery, he was independent with functional mobility and activities of daily living (ADLs). He currently requires a rolling walker and adaptive equipment for mobility and bathing. Upon physical examination, he exhibits limited RLE strength and motion, which has negatively affected his mobility, including ambulation and ascending/descending stairs. He also demonstrates impaired RLE sensation and increased right lateral hip pain. He would benefit from supervised physical therapy to improve his mobility and independence. Will continue to follow.
	2. Short-term goals:
	  • Patient will perform > 15 repetitions during 30-Second Sit to Stand Test within 6 weeks to improve lower extremity strength.
	  • Patient will perform TUG in < 12 seconds within 6 weeks to improve standing balance.
	  • Patient will perform 40-Meter Fast-Paced Walk Test in < 21 seconds within 6 weeks to improve endurance.
	3. Long-term goals:
	  • Patient will independently ambulate × 30 minutes continuously and with minimal adverse symptoms within 12 weeks to improve functional mobility.
	  • Patient will ascend/descend a flight of stairs, demonstrating reciprocal pattern and without a handrail, within 12 weeks to improve functional mobility.

Evaluate	4. Possible reasons for lateral hip pain include greater trochanteric pain syndrome, referred pain from lumbar spine, gluteal tendinopathy, and/or ecchymosis/tenderness from lying on side. 5. Potential risks of violating the post-op precautions include loosening of hardware, soft-tissue damage, and/or injury superior/inferior to the site of fusion. The patient should be made aware of these risks to maximize his safety and prevent adverse reactions.
Analyze	6. The purpose of testing light touch and sharp/dull sensation is to identify potential deficits in different pathways within the neural complex. 7. Ways to identify a deficit to light touch sensation are through testing of vibration via tuning fork or testing temperature.

Apply	8. Following today's physical examination, appropriate exercises to prescribe are:
	  • Strengthening: bridging, sit to stands, mini-squats, quadruped activities, standing hip flexion/extension/abduction/adduction.
	  • Aerobic: walking
	  • Stretching: gastrocnemius/soleus, and gentle hamstring while maintaining precautions.

(Continued)

(Continued)

Bloom's Taxonomy Level	Case 19.B Answers
	9. The patient's functional progression can be assessed and determined through the use of outcome measures. Examples include the 30-Second Sit to Stand, TUG, 40-Meter Fast-Faced Walk Test, and self-reported questionnaires.
Understand	10. If a patient does not improve his ability to perform repetitions during the 30-Second Sit to Stand Test, the patient's hip and knee strength and ROM, and cardiovascular endurance should be reassessed. Additionally, the physical therapist should follow up on the patient's carryover of the home exercise program.
Remember	11. Signs of infection include colored discharge at site of incision, erythema, and/or recent fever/illness. 12. When the L5 nerve root has been damaged, the gluteus medius (hip abduction) and tibialis anterior (ankle dorsiflexion) may exhibit weakness.

Key points
1. Red flags continue to require vigorous monitoring.
2. Functional ability and assessment are vital to prove efficacy of interventions.
3. Regular reassessment of limitations and deficits is crucial to justify interventions.

General Information	
Case no.	19.C
Authors	Josh Fede, PT, DPT, MTC, CSCS, USATF-L1 Brian Goonan, PT, DPT, Board Certified Clinical Specialist in Orthopaedic Physical Therapy Scott Siverling, PT, DPT, Board Certified Clinical Specialist in Orthopaedic Physical Therapy, Fellow of the American Academy of Orthopedic Physical Therapy
Diagnosis	Lower back, right lateral hip and foot pain
Setting	Outpatient clinic
Learner expectations	☐ Initial evaluation ☑ Re-evaluation ☐ Treatment session
Learner objectives	1. To assess the patient's functional progression. 2. To assess the patient's remaining physical deficits. 3. To assess the patient's readiness for return to work.

Medical	
Chief complaint	Right-sided lower back pain, lateral hip pain, and foot pain
History of Present Illness	The patient is a 51-year-old man who reports approximately 2.5-year history of progressive lower back pain and right-sided radiculopathy. He underwent an L5–S1 microdiscectomy approximately 1 year ago. During recovery, the patient began to have difficulty lifting his R foot while walking and his dorsal foot pain advanced to an "unbearable" level. He underwent a posterior lumbar spinal fusion (L4–L5/L5–S1) 12 weeks ago to resolve the ongoing neurological symptoms.
Past medical history.	Hypertension, hypercholesterolemia, gastroesophageal reflux disease.
Past surgical history	L5–S1 discectomy, cholecystectomy, appendectomy, L4–L5/L5–S1 fusion.
Allergies	None
Medications	Lisinopril, Lipitor, Omeprazole
Precautions/orders	Spinal precautions lifted Activity as tolerated

Social history	
Home setup	• Lives in a two-story home with his wife and three children. • Bedroom is on the second floor. • Has a guest bedroom and half bath on the first floor.
Occupation	• Financial advisor
Prior level of function	• Independent with functional mobility and ADLs. • Married father of three children. • (+) driver
Recreational activities	Prior to surgery: • Occasionally plays basketball in the summer. • Works out at the gym once or twice a week but has not exercised in over 1 year.

Medical management	Surgeon's office, 2 days ago
Follow-up	• Review of the patient's postoperative computed tomography (CT) scan shows that he underwent an L4–L5/L5–S1 fusion, posterior approach 12 weeks ago. • Patient reports surgeon saying pre-op that "Once I was in there, I could see what was wrong." Post-op, surgeon reported that "he was pleased with how everything looked." Patient also recalls the surgeon sharing some photographs from the procedure to illustrate the conditions from before the surgery and after it was complete. • Surgeon's formal report to follow.

Pause points
Based on the above information, what are the priorities for red flag screening? • Screening infection (fever, sensitivity along incision)? • Active straight leg raise (SLR) versus passive SLR? • Assessment of vital signs? • Outcome measures?

Physical Therapy Examination
Subjective
"I am finally sleeping 7 hours without waking up. I took only Tylenol with codeine for 2 days. I can now get by with just 1 naproxen before bed and 2600 mg ibuprofen throughout the day. I really want to start walking more for exercise, but my hip hurts when I push it past 5 blocks. I can feel more of my leg, it just kind of gets itchy sometimes, but that's no big deal." Patient also expresses a desire to start using a smoker he got as an anniversary present a few years ago but has been unable to secondary to pain.

Objective		
Vital signs	**Pre-treatment**	
Blood pressure (mmHg)	125/72	
Heart rate (beats/min)	65	
Respiratory rate (breaths/min)	18	
Pulse oximetry on room air (SpO_2)	99%	
Pain	0/10 at rest 4/10, right lateral hip, at worst, occurs after walking × 5 blocks.	
General	Observation	• Appears less irritable than he was on the initial evaluation and less distressed. This is thought to be due to increased sleep quality and quantity.

(Continued)

(Continued)

Physical Therapy Examination			
Musculoskeletal	Range of motion (ROM)	• Bilateral upper extremity (BUE): within functional limit (WFL). • Bilateral lower extremity (BLE): WFL • Lumbar extension: 50% (no pain) • Lumbar flexion: 80% (no pain, able to reach mid shin) • Lumbar rotation, left: 100% (no pain) • Lumbar rotation, right: 100% (no pain)	
	Strength	Right	Left
		• Hip extension: 5/5 • Hip abduction: 4+/5 • Knee extension: 5/5 • Knee flexion: 5/5 • Ankle dorsiflexion: 5/5 • Ankle eversion: 5/5 • Ankle plantar flexion: 4+/5 (18 single leg heel raises) • Great toe extension: 4/5	• Hip extension: 5/5 • Hip abduction: 5/5 • Knee extension: 5/5 • Knee flexion: 5/5 • Ankle dorsiflexion: 5/5 • Ankle eversion: 5/5 • Ankle plantar flexion: 5/5 • Great toe extension: 5/5
		• 30-Second Sit to Stand = 16 repetitions	
	Aerobic	• Able to complete 10 minutes on the bicycle with moderate resistance (level 3). • Heart rate: 117–122 beats/min • Borg Scale: 11–12/20	
	Flexibility	• (+) passive SLR for stiffness of right lower extremity (RLE) at 52 degrees, but no pain in calf, only in proximal hamstring. • (+) Thomas Test on RLE (30-degree hip flexion, 90-degree knee flexion).	
Neurological	Balance	• Sitting, static: independent • Sitting, dynamic: independent • Standing, static: independent • Standing, dynamic: independent • Single limb stance: left = 20 seconds, right 15 seconds • Timed Up and Go (TUG): 7.8 seconds	
	Cognition	• Alert and oriented × 4	
	Coordination	• Finger to nose: intact bilaterally • Heel to shin: intact bilaterally	
	Cranial nerves	• II–XII: intact	
	Reflexes	• Patellar: 2+ bilaterally • Achilles: 2+ bilaterally	
	Sensation	• LLE: intact to light touch. • RLE: diminished to light touch and pinprick at L5 and S1 dermatome levels.	
	Tone	• BUE and BLE: normal	
	Other	• Averaging 5,603 steps per day over the last 7 days, as measured by his wearable device.	
Integumentary	Skin integrity	• Unremarkable, incisions well healed, some hypomobility superior and to the right.	
Functional status			
Bed mobility	• Rolling either direction: independent • Supine to/from sit: independent		
Transfers	• Sit to/from stand: independent		
Ambulation	• Ambulated > 500 feet independently • Gait deviations notable for slight right heel whip in early swing phase of gait; normal gait speed.		

(Continued)

(Continued)

Physical Therapy Examination	
	• Tolerating walking 20 minutes of continuous community ambulation
Stairs	• Ascend/descend 12 steps independently • Demonstrated step-over pattern
Task specific	• Able to sit for 60 minutes at a time with "tolerable" symptoms
Sport specific	• Can shoot a basketball for 15 minutes with son in the backyard but has not been able to participate in competition due to doctor's orders.
Other	• 40-Minute Fast-Paced Walk Test: 19.8 seconds • Functional Movement Screen (FMS) = 14 No painful movements: 1 on deep squat (poor form with heel elevation) (► Fig. 19.3a, ► Fig. 19.3b). 1 on inline lunge each side due to loss of balance. 2 on hurdle step each side. 2 on rotary stability. 3 on trunk stability pushup. 2 on right SLR, 3 on left. 3 on shoulder mobility.

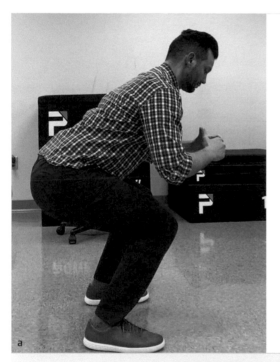 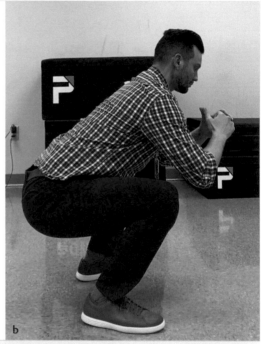

Fig. 19.3 Deep squat assessment as part of the functional movement screen. **(a)** The patient is demonstrating poor form and inability to perform a deep squat. If the patient were to move further into the squat, heel elevation would be noted. **(b)** Proper deep squat technique. (Adapted from Cook G, Burton L, Hoogenboom BJ, Voight M. Functional movement screening: the use of fundamental movements as an assessment of function—part 1. Int J Sports Phys Ther 2014;9(3):396–409)

Assessment	
☑ Physical therapist's	*Assessment left blank for learner to develop*
Goals	
Patient's	"I just want to get back to my normal activity."
Short term	1. *Goals left blank for learner to develop* 2.
Long term	1. *Goals left blank for learner to develop* 2.

Plan	
☑ Physical therapist's	1. Restore SLR via progressive weights on SLR flexion. 2. Restore calf strength via progressive weights on calf raises. 3. Progress lunge pattern from half kneeling to split squats. 4. Progress squat pattern from double leg box squat to single leg box squat. 5. Progress walking distance with monitoring wearable. Will continue to follow once a week×6 weeks.

Bloom's Taxonomy Level	Case 19.C Questions
Create	1. Synthesizing the medical data and physical examination findings, develop an appropriate physical therapy assessment of the patient. 2. Develop two short-term physical therapy goals, including an appropriate timeframe. 3. Develop two long-term physical therapy goals, including an appropriate timeframe.
Evaluate	4. What is a passing Thomas Test score? 5. What is more helpful in determining a plan of action—the overall score on a Functional Movement Screen or a low score (0 or 1) on an individual pattern?
Analyze	6. How would a positive Thomas Test affect kneeling ability? 7. What information can you glean from a half kneeling position?
Apply	8. How would mastering the kneeling position help this patient reach his short-term goals?
Understand	9. Why is hip mobility important after a lumbar fusion?
Remember	10. What are the three basic lower extremity movement patterns expressed in the Functional Movement Screen?

Bloom's Taxonomy Level	Case 19.C Answers
Create	1. The patient is 51-year-old man 12 weeks status post L4–L5/L5–S1 fusion. He is tolerating treatment well, with no adverse reactions. He has some remaining neurological signs on SLR, myotome, and sensation testing; however, his function is in line with what would be expected at this point of rehabilitation. He is sleeping through the night without the use of opioids and has made good progress toward his goals from initial evaluation. New goals were discussed with the patient and designed to help him return to normal function and activity. Will continue to follow. 2. Short-term goals (from initial evaluation): • Patient will perform > 15 repetitions during 30-Second Sit to Stand Test within 6 weeks to improve lower extremity strength: **MET**. • Patient will perform TUG in < 12 seconds within 6 weeks to improve standing balance: **MET**. • Patient will perform 40-Meter Fast-Paced Walk Test in < 21 seconds within 6 weeks to improve endurance: **MET**.

(Continued)

(Continued)

Bloom's Taxonomy Level	Case 19.C Answers
	Short-term goals (re-evaluation):
	• Patient will independently assume a kneeling position without symptoms within 3 weeks to allow him to use his new smoker.
	• Patient will independently walk × 30 minutes without symptoms within 3 weeks to improve endurance and functional mobility.
	3. Long-term goals (from initial evaluation):
	• Patient will independently ambulate × 30 minutes continuously and with minimal adverse symptoms within 12 weeks to improve functional mobility: ***PARTIALLY MET***.
	• Patient will ascend/descend a flight of stairs, demonstrating reciprocal pattern and without a handrail, within 12 weeks to improve functional mobility: ***MET***.
	Long-term goals (re-evaluation):
	• Patient will independently walk × 60 minutes without symptoms within 6 weeks to successfully complete his work commute.
	• Patient will return to previous level of activity, including shooting around basketball, within 6 weeks to maximize quality of life.
Evaluate	4. A passing score on the Thomas Test includes < 10 degree hip flexion and < 90 degree knee flexion.
	5. On the Functional Movement Screen, a low score on an individual pattern is more helpful in determining a plan of action. Understanding the patient's movement pattern can maximize therapeutic prescription to optimize outcomes.
Analyze	6. A (+) Thomas Test represents a mobility issue, which will prevent the patient from being able to get into a half kneeling position.
	7. In half kneeling, the physical therapist can assess the patient's ability to balance hip and core musculature in an upright position, and in particular, without challenging the muscles of L5/S1 myotome.
Apply	8. By mastering the half kneeling position, the patient can utilize that position to manipulate objects required for operating a smoker. Additionally, practicing static half kneeling is a great way to challenge the hip and core with very light loads (under 10 lb).
Understand	9. As lumbar ROM is now restricted mechanically at two levels, any motor programs that utilize lumbar movement (i.e., deep squat, forward bending) will be compromised. Furthermore, a hypomobile hip joint will present an obstacle for acquiring new motor programs that preserve the integrity of the surgery.
Remember	10. The three basic lower extremity movement patterns expressed in the Functional Movement Screen are as follows:
	• Deep squat: bilateral stance
	• Inline lunge: tandem stance
	• Hurdle step: single limb stance

Key points

1. When performing a 6-week re-evaluation, make sure to share the functional measurements with the operating surgeon. This information is essential for the surgeon to understand how the patient is progressing and/or regressing in physical therapy.

2. When designing interventions, make sure they are relevant and applicable to the patient's goals. Try to maintain a daily home exercise program of no more than three exercises that are safe yet challenging.

3. Physical therapy sessions are an ideal time to assess patient progress and see if the patient can handle the next progression of an exercise. Knowing the progressions and regressions of exercises is where a physical therapist provides a significant value to both the client and the surgeon.

Suggested Readings

30 second chair stand. Available at: https://www.cdc.gov/steadi/pdf/STEADI-Assessment-30Sec-508.pdf. Accessed May 1, 2020

Academy of Acute Care Physical Therapy. Laboratory Values Interpretation Resource. Available at: http://c.ymcdn.com/sites/www.acutept.org/resource/resmgr/docs/2017-Lab-Values-Resource.pdf. Accessed May 1, 2020

Altschul D, Kobets A, Nakhla J, et al. Postoperative urinary retention in patients undergoing elective spinal surgery. J Neurosurg Spine. 2017; 26(2):229–234

Chopko B, Liu JC, Khan MK. Anatomic surgical management of chronic low back pain. Neuromodulation. 2014; 17 Suppl 2: 46–51

Cook G, Burton L, Hoogenboom BJ, Voight M. Functional movement screening: the use of fundamental movements as an assessment of function—part 1. Int J Sports Phys Ther. 2014; 9(3): 396–409

Cook G, Burton L, Hoogenboom BJ, Voight M. Functional movement screening: the use of fundamental movements as an assessment of function—part 2. Int J Sports Phys Ther. 2014; 9(4):549–563

Five Times Sit to Stand. Available at: https://www.sralab.org/rehabilitation-measures/five-times-sit-stand-test. Accessed May 1, 2020

Goodman CC, Fuller KS. Pathology: Implications for the Physical Therapist. 4th ed. St. Louis, MO: Saunders Elsevier; 2015

Greenwood J, McGregor A, Jones F, Mullane J, Hurley M. Rehabilitation following lumbar fusion surgery: a systematic review and meta-analysis. Spine. 2016; 41(1):E28–E36

Greenwood J, McGregor A, Jones F, Hurley M. Evaluating rehabilitation following lumbar fusion surgery (REFS): study protocol for a randomised controlled trial. Trials. 2015; 16:251

Hillegass E, Puthoff M, Frese EM, Thigpen M, Sobush DC, Auten B, Guideline Development Group. Role of physical therapists in the management of individuals at risk for or diagnosed with venous thromboembolism: evidence-based clinical practice guideline. Phys Ther. 2016; 96(2):143–166

Madera M, Brady J, Deily S, et al. for the Seton Spine Rehabilitation Study Group. The role of physical therapy and rehabilitation after lumbar fusion surgery for degenerative disease: a systematic review. J Neurosurg Spine. 2017; 26(6):694–704

McGirt MJ, Parker SL, Chotai S, et al. Predictors of extended length of stay, discharge to inpatient rehab, and hospital readmission following elective lumbar spine surgery: introduction of the Carolina-Semmes Grading Scale. J Neurosurg Spine. 2017; 27(4):382–390

Osteoarthritis Research Society International. Recommended performance-based tests to assess physical function in people diagnosed with hip or knee osteoarthritis. Available at: https://www.oarsi.org/sites/default/files/docs/2013/manual.pdf. Accessed May 1, 2020

Timed Up and Go. Available at: https://www.sralab.org/rehabilitation-measures/timed-and-go. Accessed May 1, 2020

Yin D, Liu B, Chang Y, Gu H, Zheng X. Management of late-onset deep surgical site infection after instrumented spinal surgery. BMC Surg. 2018; 18(1):121

Zaina F, Tomkins-Lane C, Carragee E, Negrini S. Surgical versus nonsurgical treatment for lumbar spinal stenosis. Cochrane Database Syst Rev. 2016(1):CD010264

20 Vestibular Dysfunction

General Information	
Case no.	20.A Vestibular Dysfunction
Authors	Carolyn Haggerty, PT, DPT Sean F. Griech, PT, DPT, PhD, COMT, Board Certified Clinical Specialist in Orthopaedic Physical Therapy
Diagnosis	Vestibular dysfunction
Setting	Emergency Department Observation Unit
Learner expectations	☑ Initial evaluation ☐ Re-evaluation ☐ Treatment session
Learner objectives	1. Explain the pathophysiology of the patient's diagnosis. 2. Understand the medical management of patient's diagnosis and how it influences the physical therapy plan of care. 3. Select, implement, and interpret physical therapy interventions based on the medical examination findings. 4. Develop and implement a physical therapy plan of care to treat a patient with vestibular dysfunction in the emergency department setting.

Medical	
Chief complaint	Dizzy status post fall
History of present illness	The patient is a 69-year-old woman who presents to the emergency department with a 3- to 4-day history of dizziness. Upon waking on morning of emergency department observation unit admission, she is now status post fall out of bed. Patient presents status post fall out of bed upon waking on morning of admission to emergency department observation unit. **Duration of symptoms:** dizziness worsens with movement, did not quantify. Patient does not quantify duration of symptoms. She only reports her symptoms worsen with movement. **Recurrence of episodes:** dizziness occurs multiple times a day since onset. Symptoms occur with any movement. **Worse:** dizziness is worse with any movement, most notably waking up in the morning, and driving. Patient has been unable to drive to volunteer job. **Relief:** sitting resting, "not moving my head" **Endorses:** nausea, one episode of vomiting, feeling unbalanced, room-spinning, blurred vision "when I move my head," intermittent episodes of tinnitus in right ear, headache. **Denies:** changes in speech or swallow, photosensitivity, sensitivity to sound or smells, double vision, alcohol, tobacco use, exertion-induced symptoms.
Past medical history	Chronic otitis media, osteopenia, hypercholesterolemia, Vitamin D deficiency, hearing loss
Past surgical history	Appendectomy in 1963.
Allergies	Cats
Medications	Atorvastatin, Aspirin, Vitamin D, Calcium
Precautions/orders	Ambulate with assistance Fall risk

Social history	
Home setup	• Lives with her husband. • Two-story home; second floor bedroom and bathroom. • Half bath and kitchen on the first floor. • Laundry in basement. • Five steps to enter with L handrail ascending. • Full flight of steps to the second floor with L handrail ascending.
Occupation	• Retired; formerly an elementary education teacher. • Volunteers as a lunch aide at a local elementary school.

(Continued)

(Continued)

Social history	
Prior level of function	• Independent with mobility, activities of daily living (ADLs), instrumental ADLs (iADLs), driving. • Wears hearing aides.
Recreational activities	• Gardening, going to church, volunteer work, dinner dates with her husband and their friends.

Vital signs	Hospital day 0: emergency department
Blood pressure (mmHg)	118/78
Heart rate (beats/min)	80
Respiratory rate (breaths/min)	17
Pulse oximetry on room air (SpO$_2$)	97%
Temperature (°F)	96.9

Imaging/diagnostic test	Hospital day 0: emergency department
Pelvic X-ray	1. No fracture/acute abnormality observed.
Cervical/thoracic/lumbar X-ray	1. No fracture/acute abnormality observed; chronic age-related changes.
Head computed tomography (CT)	▶ Fig. 20.1 1. No acute intracranial abnormality observed.
Brain magnetic resonance imaging (MRI)	1. No acute intracranial abnormality.
Head/neck magnetic resonance angiography (MRA)	1. No acute abnormality or stenosis observed.
Electrocardiogram (ECG)	1. Normal sinus rhythm and rate ▶ Fig. 20.2. 2. No cardiac arrhythmias or abnormalities observed.
CT abdomen/pelvis	1. No acute abnormalities observed.

Medical management	Hospital day 0: emergency department
Medications	1. Intravenous (IV) fluids 2. Zofran 3. Valium 4. Tylenol 5. Meclizine
Tests/procedures	1. Placed on telemetry monitoring. 2. Monitor for orthostatic hypotension. 3. Physical therapy consultation ordered.

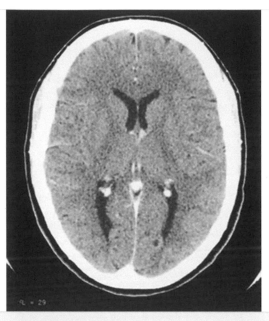

Fig. 20.1 Normal CT of the head, no evidence for acute intracranial abnormalities. (Adapted from Mattle H, Mumenthaler M, Taub E, eds. Fundamentals of Neurology: An Illustrated Guide. 2nd ed. New York, NY: Thieme; 2017.)

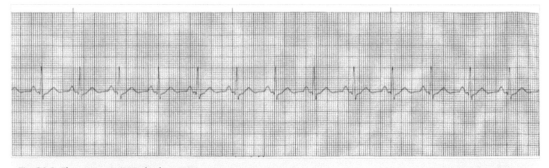

Fig. 20.2 The patient's ECG rhythm strip.

	Labs	Reference range	Hospital day 0: emergency department
Electrolytes	Calcium	8.6–10.3 mg/dL	8.6 mg/dL
	Chloride	98–108 mEq/L	100 mEq/L
	Magnesium	1.2–1.9 mEq/L	1.3 mEq/L
	Phosphate	2.3–4.1 mg/dL	3.0 mg/dL
	Potassium	3.7–5.1 mEq/L	3.8 mEq/L
	Sodium	134–142 mEq/L	137 mEq/L
Other	Troponin	<0.03 ng/mL	Negative
	Glucose	60–110 mg/dL	80 mg/dL

Pause points

Based on the above information, what are the priority
- Diagnostic tests and measures?
- Outcome measures?
- Treatment interventions?

Hospital Day 0, Emergency Department: Physical Therapy Examination				
Subjective				
"The room is moving around me when I get up."				
Objective				

Vital signs	Pre-treatment			Post-treatment
	Supine	Sitting	Standing	
Blood pressure (mmHg)	110/60	115/62	120/60	112/63
Heart rate (beats/min)	78	85	88	80
Respiratory rate (breaths/min)	12	15	15	15
Pulse oximetry on room air (SpO_2)	96	96	99	99
Pain	2/10 headache	2/10 headache	3/10 headache	2/10 headache

General		• Presents supine with head of bed elevated 20 degrees on litter in Emergency Department Observation Unit. • Brow furrowing, eyes open on visual observation. • Lines notable for peripheral IV in R radial aspect of wrist and telemetry monitor.
Cardiovascular and pulmonary		• Telemetry monitor reading normal sinus rhythm. • No adventitious lung sounds.
Gastrointestinal		• No distention or abdominal discomfort/pain reported. Eating normal diet.
Genitourinary		• Voiding without issue.
Musculoskeletal	Range of motion (ROM)	• Bilateral upper extremities (BUEs): within functional limit(s) (WFLs.) • Bilateral lower extremities (BLEs): WFL • Cervical active ROM (AROM): WFL, but endorses dizziness in all planes of motion.
	Strength	• BUE: grossly 4/5 throughout, decreased effort, appearing guarded. • BLE: grossly 4/5 throughout, decreased effort, appearing guarded.
	Aerobic	• Not tested
	Flexibility	• Mild thoracic kyphosis with forward head posture and rounded shoulders.
Neurological	Balance	• Sitting: independent in unsupported sitting with use of BUEs for support. • Standing eyes open: supervision with BUEs in high guard position, minimally increased sway observed. • Standing eyes closed: unable to tolerate due to fear of falling.
	Cognition	• Alert and oriented × 4
	Coordination	• Finger to nose: intact bilaterally • Heel to shin: intact bilaterally
	Cranial nerves	• I–XII: intact
	Reflexes	• Patellar: 2 + bilaterally
	Sensation	• Normal to light touch throughout.
	Tone	• Normal throughout BUEs and BLEs.
Vestibular	Saccades	• WNL
	Spontaneous Nystagmus	• None observed
	Smooth pursuits	• Within normal limits (WNL) in horizontal and vertical planes.

(Continued)

(Continued)

	Hospital Day 0, Emergency Department: Physical Therapy Examination	
	Gaze-evoked nystagmus with fixation	• Increased nystagmus observed with upward gaze to the left, decreased with gaze to the right.
	Gaze-evoked nystagmus without fixation	• Unable to assess, gaze fixation removing goggles unavailable at time of examination.
	Weber's Test	• Not tested; tuning fork not available in examination room.
	Head Thrust Test (Head Impulse Test)	• Positive, corrective saccade observed with testing to R.
	Vertebral Artery Test	• Negative bilaterally
	R Dix–Hallpike Test	• Positive, right posterior canal with nystagmus observed and reproduction of "spinning" symptoms, onset after 5 seconds, duration 30 seconds.
	L Dix–Hallpike Test	• Negative
	Roll Test	• Negative bilaterally
	Dynamic visual acuity	• Not tested; Snellen chart not available in examination room.
	Functional status	
Bed mobility	• Supine to/from sit: minimal assistance × 1 person, head of bed elevated ~45 degrees, guarding of movement observed. • Symptoms were reproduced, but patient's eyes were closed initially. Unable to observe for nystagmus due to eyes closed. The patient was able to open her eyes after a few seconds when sitting on the edge of the bed. It is unclear whether nystagmus is present due to tester's poor visualization of eye movements.	
Transfers	• Sit to/from stand: contact guard assistance	
Ambulation	• Ambulated 50 feet with contact guard, trunk sway observed. • Patient demonstrates improved trunk sway and was able to progress to supervision when provided rolling walker.	
Stairs	• Ascend/descend three steps with contact guard assistance and unilateral handrail, demonstrating step-to pattern.	

Assessment	
☑ Physical therapist's	*Assessment left blank for learner to develop*
Goals	
Patient's	"I want to go home. I want to feel less dizzy."
Short term	1. *Goals left blank for learner to develop* 2.
Long term	1. *Goals left blank for learner to develop* 2.

Plan	
☐ Physician's ☑ Physical therapist's ☐ Other's	Will follow for one to two additional sessions during emergency department observation admission. Refer to home physical therapy services for safety assessment in home and continued balance training. Recommend use of rolling walker for all upright mobility. Recommend transition from home physical therapy services to outpatient physical therapy for vestibular rehabilitation.

Bloom's Taxonomy Level	Case 20.A Questions
Create	1. Synthesizing the medical data and physical examination findings, develop an appropriate physical therapy assessment of the patient. 2. Develop two short-term physical therapy goals, including an appropriate timeframe. 3. Develop two long-term physical therapy goals, including an appropriate timeframe.
Evaluate	4. Concisely explain the physical therapy examination findings to the emergency resident physician.
Analyze	5. Relate how does the patient's subjective report relate to what a physical therapist may expect to see during the objective examination. 6. Distinguish what factors decrease concern for central causes of dizziness. 7. Differentiate which vestibular deficit a physical therapist would treat first based on the findings.
Apply	8. Describe the implementation of an appropriate intervention for this patient. 9. Determine the education a physical therapist would provide to a patient based on any intervention performed.
Understand	10. Explain the patient's risk factors associated for developing benign paroxysmal positional vertigo (BPPV) and unilateral vestibular hypofunction. 11. What are the physical therapy implications for some of the patient's home and/or hospital medications? 12. This therapist was unable to formally assess for presence of nystagmus with supine to sit transfers. Based on the patient's presentation, describe the direction (right vs. left) and type of nystagmus (horizontal, torsional, vertical) a physical therapist may expect to see with this change in position. 13. Explain why the patient demonstrates what may be considered "direction changing" nystagmus on the physical therapy evaluation.
Remember	14. Explain the difference in pathophysiology of BPPV and vestibular hypofunction. 15. What test is used as the standard of care prior to performing canalith repositioning maneuvers?

Bloom's Taxonomy Level	Case 20.A Answers
Create	1. The patient is a 69-year-old woman who presents to the emergency department with position changing dizziness and a fall out of bed. The patient presents with impaired balance and dizziness likely in the setting of vestibular dysfunction. She requires use of an assistive device for balance with ambulation and transfers. She demonstrates unilateral vestibular hypofunction involving the R peripheral vestibular system and R posterior canal BPPV based on the physical therapy examination findings. Her vestibular examination is notable for a impaired saccades with corrective saccade observed to the right during the Head Thrust Test and increased nystagmus with upward gaze to the left which is concerning for unilateral vestibular hypofunction. She additionally demonstrates a positive Dix–Hallpike Test for R posterior canal BPPV. At this time, she would greatly benefit from physical therapy services in the home setting post hospital discharge for continued balance training, vestibular training, and home modification to optimize her level of independence in her home setting. Recommend discharge home with use of a rolling walker for mobility on level surfaces and assist from husband for stair negotiation and iADLs as needed. Will continue to follow during emergency department stay to progress activity as tolerated. 2. Short-term goals: • Patient will perform sit to/from stand transfer with supervision in 1-2 sessions. • Patient will be able to independently recall and implement home modifications in 1-2 sessions physical therapy sessions. 3. Long-term goals: • Patient will perform all mobility and ADLs without a subjective report of increase in dizziness within 7 weeks. • Patient will independently ascend/descend a full flight of stairs with a railing as needed in 7 weeks.
Evaluate	4. Based on the patient's history and subjective report on evaluation, it appears that she has impaired vestibular function. Her examination is remarkable for impaired balance, gaze-evoked nystagmus, and a positive Head Thrust Test. This is strongly indicative of

(Continued)

(Continued)

Bloom's Taxonomy Level	Case 20.A Answers
	a unilateral vestibular hypofunction affecting the patient's right ear. Additionally, the patient also demonstrates a positive R Dix–Hallpike Test, which is indicative of right posterior canal BPPV. It is recommended that the patient receive home physical therapy services to progress her to becoming more independent with her balance in the home setting as she currently requires use of an assistive device to ambulate household distances. Once she is discharged from home physical therapy, it is recommended she pursue physical therapy services in the outpatient setting. She would benefit from outpatient vestibular rehabilitation for continued management and for continued management of her unilateral vestibular hypofunction and BPPV.
Analyze	5. Although not an exhaustive list, patients with a diagnosis of unilateral vestibular hypofunction may report any of the following: tinnitus, headache, difficulty focusing on moving targets during activites such as driving, watching traffic, or reports a duration of symptoms lasting a few days. These symptoms may be more indicative of an impaired vestibular ocular reflex (VOR), making head movements in a vertical or horizontal plane uncomfortable for the patient. On objective examination, the patient described in this case would likely demonstrate the following if they have a diagnosis of unilateral vestibular hypofunction: presence of gaze-evoked nystagmus, positive Head Thrust Test, and impaired standing and dynamic balance with eyes open or closed. Patients with a diagnosis of BPPV may subjectively report any of the following: room-spinning dizziness, onset or exacerbation of symptoms may be reported with positional change, many times upon waking in the morning, and a duration of a few seconds to minutes. These symptoms are more indicative of a dislodging of the otoconia in the semicircular canals. For a patient with a diagnosis of BPPV, they may demonstrate any of the following on objective examination: a positive Dix–Hallpike Test and spontaneous nystagmus at rest during an acute episode or acute exacerbation for patients with a history of BPPV.
	6. The following factors may reduce a physical therapist's concern for central causes of dizziness on evaluation: Equal and symmetrical strength and sensory testing, intact coordination and proprioception, absence of spontaneous nystagmus observed, gaze-evoked nystagmus that is not direction changing, intact saccades, negative vertebral artery testing, and nystagmus on positional testing that fatigues over time.
	7. The patient's symptoms of BPPV should be treated first prior to management of the patient's unilateral vestibular hypofunction.
Apply	8. The follow canalith repositioning techniques (CRTs) may be appropriate to be used with this patient to manage their symptoms of BPPV: Semont liberatory maneuver or Epley's maneuver. Semont liberatory maneuver, although originally developed to treat posterior canal cupulolithiasis, has been shown to be effective for treating posterior canalithiasis as well. Of note, cupulolithiasis and canalithiasis are considered different mechanical causes of BPPV. Cupulolithiasis is theorized to result from otoconia that become adherent to the cupula of the affected semicircular canal. This change results in displacement of the cupula. Canalithiasis is thought to be caused by free-floating otoconia in the semicircular canals. The free-floating otoconia within the viscous endolymph creates a pressure current following a change in position of the canal relative to gravity. There is mixed evidence as to whether one maneuver is preferred over the other. Some studies show both the Epley maneuver and Semont liberatory maneuver are equally effective in treatment of posterior canal BPPV. Other studies demonstrate that the Epley maneuver is more effective in treatment of posterior canal BPPV than the Semont liberatory maneuver. Nevertheless, the Semont liberatory maneuver may be appropriate when there are ROM restrictions or environmental limitations to performing the Epley maneuver. In the acute care setting, for example, there may be limited space in the environment to effectively perform the Epley maneuver. Therefore, the Semont liberatory maneuver may be an appropriate choice. It should be noted that if there are no environmental or physiologic restrictions, then the Epley maneuver should be the treatment of choice for patients with a positive Dix–Hallpike Test for BPPV. These treatments are recommended to be performed no more than three times on the affected ear in the context of a single treatment session.
	9. The patient may experience mild headache or "fogginess" the day after the repositioning maneuvers are performed. Some subjects also report episodes of losses of balance 1 day

(Continued)

(Continued)

Bloom's Taxonomy Level	Case 20.A Answers
	post maneuver. There is limited evidence to support post repositioning restrictions for most patients with BPPV. Postcanalith repositioning restrictions that were previously part of BPPV treatment include avoidance of head pitch for 24 hours, sleeping in a semireclined position with head elevated 30 degrees, and avoidance of sleeping on involved side for 2 to 3 days. Some patients may benefit from implementation of these behaviors if they have a history of recurrence of BPPV or demonstrate impulsivity in their movement that may cause a recurrence of their symptoms.
Understand	10. This patient has multiple risk factors for developing BPPV including age, gender, past medical history of osteopenia, and vitamin D deficiency. The patient has multiple risk factors for developing unilateral vestibular hypofunction including history of chronic otitis media, hearing loss, and tinnitus.
	11. Based on the patient's home medications, the administration of vitamin D and calcium may reduce this patient's risk of recurrence for BPPV. Based on the patient's hospital administered medications, Zofran, valium, and meclizine are helpful in symptom management to allow prior patient to tolerate participating in a physical therapy examination. However, the use of meclizine (an antihistamine) is a central nervous system (CNS) suppressant. As a result, some of the patient's symptoms of unilateral vestibular hypofunction may be skewed or masked due to meclizine's inhibitory effects on the CNS.
	12. There may be a misconception for clinicians based on examination findings that this patient demonstrates direction-changing nystagmus. This may be based on the positive findings for increased nystagmus with upward gaze to the left and a positive right Dix–Hallpike testing with R beating nystagmus observed. The findings on each of these tests would not be considered direction-changing nystagmus. That is because gaze-evoked nystagmus and the Dix–Hallpike Test assess two different components of the peripheral vestibular system. Gaze-evoked nystagmus is meant to examine the VOR or the otolith organs that detect horizontal and vertical acceleration, whereas Dix–Hallpike Tests the semicircular canals that help detect angular acceleration of the head.
	13. Based on patient presentation, a physical therapist may expect to see right beating torsional nystagmus on transfer from supine to sitting as this positional change may evoke the BPPV component of this patient's symptoms.
Remember	14. BPPV: There is a dislodgement of otoconia from the otolith organs into the semicircular canals. Otoconia have a greater relative gravity compared to endolymph that exist within the semicircular canals of the peripheral vestibular system. The otoconia floating in the endolymph of the semicircular canals causes a misfiring of the cupula that sits at the base of the semicircular canals. The cupula sends messages to the CNS regarding angular accelerations of the head ("pitch, yaw, roll"). Although this part of the organ is typically insensitive to gravity, the presence of the otoconia renders this part of the organ gravity sensitive. This creates a room-spinning sensation for the patient as the dislodged otoconia travels through the semicircular canal with any positional change in head position until it settles at the base of the canal or moves out of the canal. Hypofunction: Due to the presence of a unilateral vestibulopathy, there is a decrease in firing rates between the otolith organs. Because of the decrease in firing rate unilaterally, this creates a disruption in gaze stabilization or VOR since the vestibular system is sending inappropriate feedback to the oculomotor centers. This may cause a patient to experience oscillopsia or blurred vision with any vertical or horizontal head movement.
	15. The Vertebral Artery Test is still used as the standard of care prior to initiation of canalith repositioning maneuvers to rule out concern for vertebral artery insufficiency. However, due to poor validity studies, it is suggested that any risk of vertebrobasilar artery insufficiency may be obtained in the physical therapy history-taking through a thorough review of past medical history and identification of any red flags.

Key points

1. Use the physical therapy examination and evaluation tools to rule in or out central causes of vestibular dysfunction.

2. When able, track patient's progression across settings with similar outcome measures.

3. Develop a working physical therapy diagnosis that can be tested and retested after intervention is performed to determine the effectiveness of treatment.

General Information

Case no.	20.B
Authors	Carolyn Haggerty, PT, DPT Sean F. Griech, PT, DPT, PhD, COMT, Board Certified Clinical Specialist in Orthopaedic Physical Therapy
Diagnosis	Benign paroxysmal positional vertigo (BPPV)
Setting	Home
Learner expectations	☑ Initial evaluation ☐ Re-evaluation ☐ Treatment session
Learner objectives	1. List potential environmental factors or behaviors that may increase a patient's risk of falls. 2. Select appropriate outcome measures to be utilized in the home setting to measure patient progress. 3. Develop and implement a physical therapy plan of care to treat a patient with BPPV and hypofunction in the home setting. 4. Educate the patient and family on strategies to improve a patient's ability to perform activities of daily living (ADLs) and instrumental ADLs (iADLs) independently without an exacerbation of their symptoms.

Medical

Chief complaint	Dizziness
History of present illness	The patient is a 69-year-old woman 2 days after recent hospital discharge for dizziness and fall out of bed. **Duration of symptoms:** Patient does not quantify duration of symptoms but reports it worsens with movement. **Recurrence of episodes:** dizziness occurs multiple times daily since onset, reports symptoms are not as severe as they were prior to her emergency department observation unit admission. **Worse:** dizziness worsens with watching traffic and walking. Patient reports she has been unable to drive. **Relief:** dizziness is relieved with sitting at rest, "not moving my head". **Endorses:** Feels unbalanced, continues to require use of walker. Patient reports one episode of room spinning when sitting up out of bed one morning. Patient reports one loss of balance 1 day after emergency department admission where she "fell to the side," onto her couch. Patient also reports blurred vision "when I move my head," intermittent episodes of tinnitus in R ear, and headache that is improved with Tylenol. **Denies:** changes in speech or swallow, photosensitivity, sensitivity to sound or smells, double vision, alcohol, tobacco use, exertion-induced symptoms, nausea, vomiting.
Past medical history	Chronic otitis media, osteopenia, hypercholesterolemia, vitamin D deficiency
Past surgical history	Appendectomy in 1963
Allergies	Cats
Medications	Atorvastatin, Aspirin, Vitamin D, Calcium, Meclizine, Tylenol
Precautions/orders	Physical therapy home evaluation and treatment

Social history

Home setup	• Lives with her husband. • Two-story home; second floor bedroom and bathroom. • Half bath and kitchen on the first floor. • Laundry in basement. • Five steps to enter with L handrail ascending. • Full flight of steps to the second floor with L handrail ascending.
Occupation	• Retired, formerly an elementary education teacher. • Volunteers as a lunch aide at a local elementary school.

(Continued)

(Continued)

Social history	
Prior level of function	Prior to recent emergency department admission: • Independent with mobility, ADLs, iADLs, driving. • Wears hearing aides Upon emergency department discharge: • Uses rolling walker for upright mobility. • Spouse provides assistance for stair negotiation and household management tasks, particularly laundry, loading dishwasher, grocery shopping, and driving. • Uses a sock aid and shoe horn for donning socks/shoes, uses a shower chair for bathing, is able to make microwaveable meals.
Recreational activities	• Prior to emergency department admission was Gardening, going to church, volunteer work, dinner dates with her husband and their friends.

Pause points
Based on the above information, what are the priority • Diagnostic tests and measures? • Outcome measures? • Treatment interventions?

Physical Therapy Examination		
Subjective		
"I feel better, but I still get dizzy."		
Objective		
Vital signs	Pre-treatment	Post-treatment
Blood pressure (mmHg)	118/72	125/75
Heart rate (beats/min)	80	85
Respiratory rate (breaths/min)	14	16
Pulse oximetry on room air (SpO$_2$)	98%	97%
Borg scale	1	3
Pain	0	1–2 headache
General	• Husband greeted physical therapist at entrance to home. Patient found seated in recliner chair in living room. Rolling walker found positioned to side of patient's recliner chair.	
Cardiovascular and pulmonary	• Normal rate at radial pulse • No adventitious lung sounds heard • Pulses: 2 + bilateral dorsalis pedis and posterior tibialis • No lower extremity (LE) edema observed	
Gastrointestinal	• No distention or abdominal discomfort observed. No pain reported. • Eating a normal diet.	
Genitourinary	• Voiding without issue.	
Musculoskeletal	Range of motion (ROM)	• Bilateral UEs (BUEs): within functional limits (WFLs) • Bilateral LEs (BLEs): WFL • Cervical AROM: WFL, moves slowly with muscle guarding observed through full ROM
	Strength	• BUEs: grossly 5/5 throughout • BLEs: grossly 5/5 throughout
	Aerobic	• 30-Second Sit to Stand Test: able to perform 10 repetitions, slocut off score is 15. Patient moves slowly with guarded movement observed. Demonstrates minimal head and neck movement. Patient requires the use of BUEs on armrests for support.

(Continued)

(Continued)

		Physical Therapy Examination
		Rolling walker maintained in front of patient for balance. Dizziness is reported with position change.
	Flexibility	• Mild thoracic kyphosis with forward head posture and rounded shoulders
Neurological	Balance	• Sitting: independent in unsupported sitting without use of BUEs for support on edge of recliner chair • Standing eyes open, firm surface: supervision, minimally increased sway observed • Standing eyes closed firm surface: supervision, worsening trunk sway, tolerates × 5 seconds.
	Cognition	• Alert and oriented × 4
	Coordination	• Finger to nose: intact bilaterally • Heel to shin: intact bilaterally
	Cranial nerves	• I–XII: intact
	Reflexes	• Patellar: 2 + bilaterally
	Sensation	• Normal to light touch throughout
	Tone	• Normal throughout BUEs and BLEs
Vestibular	Spontaneous nystagmus	• None observed
	Smooth pursuits	• Within normal limits (WNLs)
	Gaze-evoked nystagmus with fixation	• Increased nystagmus observed with upward gaze to the left, decreased with gaze to the right.
	Gaze-evoked nystagmus without fixation	• Unable to remove fixation at time of evaluation
	Weber's Test	• Tuning fork not available at time of examination
	Head Thrust Test	• Positive, corrective saccade observed with testing to R
	Vertebral Artery Test	• Negative bilaterally
	R Dix–Hallpike Test	• Positive, R posterior canal, reproduction of symptoms reported, onset after 3 seconds, duration 15 seconds
	L Dix–Hallpike Test	• Negative
	Roll Test	• Negative bilaterally
	Dynamic visual acuity	• Snellen chart unavailable at time of examination

	Functional status
Bed mobility	• Rolling either direction: independent • Supine to/from sit: supervision, increased time to perform, appears guarded with movement, mild dizziness reported
Transfers	• Sit to/from stand: supervision without an assistive device, modified independence with rolling walker
Ambulation	• Ambulated × 40 feet from living room to kitchen with supervision and no assistive device • Gait deviations without an assistive device notable for guarded posture with BUEs in high guard posture, occasionally increased trunk sway, wide base of support, decreased limb clearance, and occasionally reaching for furniture/walls to maintain balance. • Ambulated × 40 feet from kitchen to living room with supervision and rolling walker • Gait deviations with an assistive device notable for no loss of balance, and improved cadence and gait speed grossly compared to ambulation without an assistive device.
Stairs	• Ascends/descends a flight of stairs with bilateral hands on unilateral handrail and supervision. Demonstrates side-stepping technique.
Task specific	• Supervision to wash dishes at kitchen sink and place in drying rack in standing

Assessment	
☑ Physical therapist's	*Assessment left blank for learner to develop*

Goals	
Patient's	"To feel less dizzy"
Short term	1.
	Goals left blank for learner to develop
	2.
Long term	1.
	Goals left blank for learner to develop
	2.

Plan	
☐ Physician's ☑ Physical therapist's ☐ Other's	Recommend continued home physical therapy services with a plan of care to be seen for treatment three times a week for 2 weeks. Upon achievement of home physical therapy goals, recommend continued physical therapy in an outpatient setting with concentration in vestibular rehab.

Bloom's Taxonomy Level	Case 20.B Questions
Create	1. Synthesizing the medical data and physical examination findings, develop an appropriate physical therapy assessment of the patient. 2. Develop two short-term physical therapy goals, including an appropriate timeframe. 3. Develop two long-term physical therapy goals, including an appropriate timeframe.
Evaluate	4. What are clinical signs and symptoms that this patient is having an exacerbation of her vestibular dysfunction? Support the answer.
Analyze	5. Differentiate which vestibular deficit a physical therapist should treat first based on the findings.
Apply	6. Determine an appropriate intervention to implement for this patient. 7. Explain how to determine the effectiveness of interventions for this patient. 8. Demonstrate education that should be provided to a patient based on any intervention performed.
Understand	9. Based on the findings, is this patient a falls risk? Which of the findings indicate this?
Remember	10. Name two other outcome measures this therapist can utilize with this patient to measure their progress.

Bloom's Taxonomy Level	Case 20.B Answers

Create	1. The patient is a 69-year-old woman who presents after an emergency department admission for dizziness status post fall now discharged to home setting. She currently demonstrates supervision level of assistance with a rolling walker for all upright mobility on a level surface. She requires increased time to perform all mobility with guarded posture observed likely in setting of report of increased dizziness with movement. She has been requiring assistance from her husband to perform iADLs. Prior to emergency department admission, she was functionally independent and socially active in her community. She reports she has been unable to drive or participate in her volunteer work since the onset of her symptoms of dizziness. Her examination findings are indicative of a diagnosis of R unilateral vestibular hypofunction and R posterior canal BPPV. She would benefit from home physical therapy services at this time with focus on mobility and balance training, activity modification to reduce risk of falls, and canalith repositioning testing to facilitate resolution of this patient's R posterior canal BPPV. Plan for Epley maneuver, gait training, and education on activity modification in the home to promote return to prior level of function in follow-up treatment session.
	2. Short-term goals:
	  • Patient will independently ambulate greater than 150 feet on a level surface within 2 weeks.
	  • Patient will demonstrate a negative R Dix–Hallpike Test on formal testing in 2-4 physical therapy sessions.

(Continued)

Bloom's Taxonomy Level	Case 20.B Answers
	3. Long-term goals: • Patient will perform all designated iADLs in her home setting independently without report of dizziness within 7 weeks. • Patient will return to driving independently in 8-10 weeks.
Evaluate	4. Hypofunction symptoms that may indicate worsening symptoms/exacerbation may include an acute recurrence of patient's chronic otitis media, worsening tinnitus, worsening hearing loss unilaterally, and decreased ability to perform functional mobility or ADL tasks. BPPV symptoms that may indicate worsening symptoms/exacerbation may include episodes of room-spinning dizziness with an increased severity of symptoms reported and/or an increased duration of nystagmus observed by examiner with position changes.
Analyze	5. Based on these findings, addressing the patient's symptoms of R posterior canal BPPV first would be most important. It will be necessary to determine resolution of BPPV prior to introduction of vestibular ocular reflex exercise testing to address this patient's vestibular hypofunction increased severity of symptoms reports or increased duration of nystagmus.
Apply	6. To address patient's R posterior canal BPPV, any of the following canalith repositioning maneuvers may be effective: Epley's maneuver, Semont's liberatory maneuver, or Gans' maneuver. Based on the most evidence, Epley's maneuver has been shown in studies to be the most effective technique to address posterior canal BPPV and should be the first choice of treatment. The Semont liberatory maneuver or Gans maneuver may be other positions to consider if there are any limitations to performing Epley's maneuver in the home setting. Special considerations should be taken into account if these alternative maneuvers are employed in treatment management including psychosocial factors, environmental restrictions, and any physiologic restrictions of the patient or clinician. To address this patient's impaired functional mobility, progressing gait training from use of an assistive device to trials without an assistive device would be an effective treatment of choice in the home setting. It is especially important to continuously monitor the patient for any reports of an exacerbation of their symptoms. Gradually increasing this patient's exposure to a more challenging stimulus in their environment with gait training such as incorporation of either horizontal or vertical head turns during ambulation in a straight path would be beneficial in improving their functional independence increased severity of symptoms reports or increased duration of nystagmus. 7. To determine the effectiveness of the canalith repositioning maneuvers, reassessment of either Dix–Hallpike or modified Dix–Hallpike testing to determine if there is a presence of nystagmus with a subjective report of a decrease in reproduction or severity of patient's symptoms is most effective. Improvement in symptoms can be monitored during reassessment via patient's subjective report as well as duration of nystagmus and symptoms. The effectiveness of mobility and ADL/iADL interventions can be determined by reassessing balance with mobility using the Clinical Test for Sensory Interaction and Balance (CTSIB) or another balance measure such as the 30-Second Sit to Stand Test. Additionally, a physical therapist can also incorporate a self-assessment tool such as the Dizziness Handicap Inventory (DHI) or the Motion Sensitivity Index to determine a patient's progress over time increased severity of symptoms reports or increased duration of nystagmus. 8. For canalith repositioning maneuvers, a physical therapist may focus on education on postmaneuver restrictions if the patient demonstrates high anxiety, poor postural awareness with mobility, or has demonstrated an exacerbation or recurrence of their symptoms during care. However, based on most evidence this may not be appropriate for most patients. A physical therapist may also consider educating the patient on reporting post maneuver symptoms such as increased headache, fogginess, or loss of balance that can typically occur 1 day after repositioning maneuvers are performed. The focus of the educational component of the intervention for this patient should be on home modifications to facilitate patient's ability to perform mobility, ADLs, and iADLs more independently without a severe exacerbation of their symptoms. For example, a physical therapist may want to educate the patient on use of squatting (▶ Fig. 20.3a) compared to bending at the waist (▶ Fig. 20.3b) to avoid excessive flexion of the head that may potentially dislodge otoconia into the posterior semicircular canals. Another example would be education on body mechanics with reaching activity. These strategies can be incorporated into functional tasks such as placing items in or out of the patient's

(Continued)

(Continued)

Bloom's Taxonomy Level	Case 20.B Answers
	dishwasher, washing machine, laundry, or placing clean dishes in their cabinets. Additionally, if the patient typically reports needing to void during the evening, the physical therapist may also want to educate patient on use of night lights to improve vision at night when ambulating in room or hallway of home. It is also imperative to educate this patient on resting in between any position changes. You may want to educate this particular patient on resting in between supine to sit transfers, as this patient reports this activity exacerbates their symptoms of room spinning. These accommodations are just a few examples that can be incorporated in this patient's daily routine to reduce their risk of falls increased severity of symptoms reports or increased duration of nystagmus. In addition to education on body mechanics and activity modification it is important to emphasize to a patient, particularly to those who are fearful of movement, that general mobility is safe and should be encouraged. This will help to challenge the patient's body to accommodate to the changes that have occurred to their peripheral vestibular system through compensation and habituation.
Understand	9. This patient would be considered a falls risk for a number of reasons based on examination findings. The patient currently requires use of an assistive device and supervision based on assessment for upright mobility. The patient's performance on the CTSIB including their inability to tolerate standing on a level surface with eyes closed may also put them at increased risk for falls.
Remember	10. As mentioned previously, incorporation of the CTSIB, Motion Sensitivity Index, or DHI may all be applicable outcome measures the physical therapist can use to measure a patient's progress during physical therapy course of care.

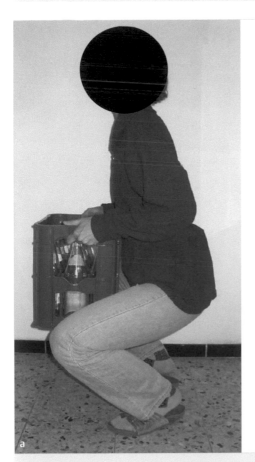 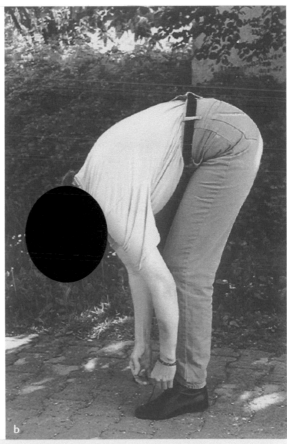

Fig. 20.3 Example of post-maneuver education that a physical therapist may provide on to avoid excessive flexion of the head that may potentially dislodge otoconia into the posterior semicircular canals. **(a)** Demonstrates a proper technique of using a squatting compared to **(b)** which is bending at the waist leading to a head down position. (Adapted from Brötz D, Weller M, eds. Lifting. In: Physical Therapy for Intervertebral Disk Disease: A Practical Guide to Diagnosis and Treatment. 1st ed. New York, NY: Thieme; 2016.)

Key points	
1. Lifestyle and home modifications based on physical therapy assessment can reduce a patient's risk for falls.	
2. Resolution of BPPV is important prior to initiation of vestibular rehabilitation for hypofunction.	
3. Identification of psychosocial factors is important to reduce risk of chronicity of symptoms and development of other vestibular disorders including persistent postural-perceptual dizziness.	

General Information	
Case no.	20.C
Authors	Carolyn Haggerty, PT, DPT Sean F. Griech, PT, DPT, PhD, COMT, Board Certified Clinical Specialist in Orthopaedic Physical Therapy
Diagnosis	Benign paroxysmal positional vertigo (BPPV)
Setting	Outpatient clinic
Learner expectations	☑ Initial evaluation ☐ Re-evaluation ☐ Treatment session
Learner objectives	1. Integrate information obtained from a medical history and physical with physical therapist patient history-taking to develop a hypothesis/differential diagnosis of BPPV versus vestibular hypofunction. 2. Select an appropriate battery of Physical Therapy Tests and measures to determine a differential diagnosis of hypofunction. 3. Develop and implement a physical therapy plan of care to treat a patient with vestibular hypofunction in the outpatient setting. 4. Determine the appropriate outcome measure to determine effectiveness of intervention.

Medical	
Chief complaint	Dizziness
History of present illness	The patient is a 69-year-old woman who presents 2 weeks posthospital discharge for a history of dizziness with concurrent fall out of bed upon waking. Referred from home physical therapy for continued outpatient vestibular therapy. **Duration of symptoms:** Patient did not quantify. She reports her dizziness worsens with movement and lasts until she rests. **Recurrence of episodes:** dizziness occurs once or twice daily **Worse:** dizziness worsens with watching traffic, reading, walking, has been unable to drive **Relief:** dizziness is relieved with sitting at rest, standing in place, "not moving my head" **Endorses:** Patient reports she has progressed to ambulating without use of walker, but reports occasionally feeling unbalanced and needing to catch herself on furniture. Occasional headache is reported after exercises provided by her home physical therapist. **Denies:** changes in speech or swallow, photosensitivity, sensitivity to sound or smells, double vision, alcohol, tobacco use, exertion-induced symptoms, nausea, vomiting
Past medical history	Chronic otitis media, osteopenia, hypercholesterolemia, vitamin D deficiency
Past surgical history	Appendectomy in 1963
Allergies	Cats
Medications	Atorvastatin, Aspirin, Vitamin D, Calcium, Meclizine prn, Tylenol prn
Precautions/orders	Outpatient vestibular evaluation and treatment

Social history	
Home setup	• Lives with her husband. • Two-story home; second floor bedroom and bathroom. • Half bath and kitchen on the first floor. • Laundry in basement. • Five steps to enter with L handrail ascending. • Full flight of steps to the second floor with L handrail ascending.
Occupation	• Retired; formerly an elementary education teacher. • Volunteers as a lunch aide at a local elementary school.
Prior level of function	Prior to recent emergency department admission patient reports she was • Independent with mobility, activities of daily living (ADLs), instrumental ADLs (iADLs); driving. • Wears hearing aides. Upon emergency department discharge patient reports she. • Uses a rolling walker for upright mobility. • Spouse provides supervision for stair negotiation and household management tasks, particularly laundry, loading dishwasher, grocery shopping, and driving. • Uses a sock aid and shoehorn for donning socks/shoes, uses a shower chair for bathing, is able to make microwaveable meals. Since home physical therapy discharge patient reports. • She no longer uses durable medical equipment for mobility • She Uses the following adaptive equipment: a sock aid and shoehorn for donning socks/shoes, and a shower chair for bathing • Patient Can independently make microwavable meals • Spouse continues to provide assist with supervision for stair negotiation • Spouse continues to assist with household management tasks including laundry, loading dishwasher, grocery shopping and driving
Recreational activities	• Patient enjoys gardening, going to church, volunteer work, dinner dates with her husband and their friends. She has not been able to participate in these activities since her emergency department visit."

Pause points
Based on the above information, what are the priority • Diagnostic tests and measures? • Outcome measures? • Treatment interventions?

Physical Therapy Examination
Subjective
"My husband drove me here. I had to keep my eyes closed the whole time because I felt so dizzy."
Objective

Vital signs	Pre-treatment	Post-treatment
Blood pressure (mmHg)	118/72	125/75
Heart rate (beats/min)	80	85
Respiratory rate (breaths/min)	14	16
Pulse oximetry on room air (SpO$_2$)	98%	97%
Borg scale	1	3
Pain	0	1–2 headache

(Continued)

(Continued)

Physical Therapy Examination		
General		• Patient presents seated in clinic waiting room, appearing in no acute distress. • Patient observed to demonstrate guarded posture with limited head movement when greeting the physical therapist. • She reports mild nausea with driving to the clinic.
Cardiovascular and pulmonary		• Normal rate at radial pulse. • No adventitious lung sounds heard. • Pulses: 2 + bilateral dorsalis pedis and posterior tibialis. • No lower extremity (LE) edema observed.
Gastrointestinal		• Mild nausea that patient attributes to the car ride to clinic. No distention or abdominal discomfort observed. No pain reported. • Reports eating a normal diet.
Genitourinary		• Voiding without issue
Musculoskeletal	Range of motion (ROM)	• Bilateral upper extremities (BUEs): within functional limit (WFL) • Bilateral lower extremities (BLEs): WFL • Cervical active ROM (AROM): WFL, moves slowly with muscle guarding observed through full ROM
	Strength	• BUE: grossly 5/5 throughout • BLE: grossly 5/5 throughout
	Aerobic	• 30-Second Sit to Stand Test: able to perform 13 repetitions (cutoff score: 15), with guarded movement observed, minimal head and neck movement observed. Patient is able to perform without use of BUEs on arm rests of chair. mild dizziness is reported with position change.
	Flexibility	• Mild thoracic kyphosis with forward head posture and rounded shoulders
Neurological	Balance	• Please refer to Clinical Test for Sensory Interaction and Balance (CTSIB) results below
	Cognition	• Alert and oriented × 4
	Coordination	• Finger to nose: intact bilaterally • Heel to shin: intact bilaterally
	Cranial nerves	• I–XII: grossly intact
	Reflexes	• Patellar: 2 + bilaterally
	Sensation	• Normal to light touch throughout
	Tone	• Normal throughout BUEs and BLEs
Vestibular	Spontaneous nystagmus	• None observed with and without fixation
	Smooth pursuits	• Within normal limit (WNL)
	Gaze-evoked nystagmus with fixation	• None observed
	Gaze-evoked nystagmus without fixation	• Increased left beating nystagmus observed with upward gaze to left and decreased with gaze to the right while using Frenzel lenses to suppress fixation
	Weber's Test	• Negative
	Head Thrust Test	• Positive, corrective saccade observed with testing to R
	Head Shake Test	• Five beat nystagmus observed to the left
	Vertebral Artery Test	• Negative bilaterally
	R Dix–Hallpike Test	• Negative

(Continued)

(Continued)

Physical Therapy Examination		
	L Dix–Hallpike Test	• Negative
	Roll Test	• Negative bilaterally
	Dynamic visual acuity	• Three-line loss of visual acuity compared to static visual acuity using standard Snellen chart
	CTSIB	• Normal except for sway with condition 4 (eyes closed, foam surface) and loss of balance to the right.
	Fukuda Step Test	• Positive with fall to the right
	Dizziness Handicap Inventory	• 64/100; considered severe handicap • ▶ Fig. 20.4
Functional status		
Bed mobility		• Rolling either direction: independent • Supine to/from sit: independent, increased time to perform, appears guarded with movement, no dizziness reported
Transfers		• Sit to/from stand: independent
Ambulation		• Ambulates × 150 feet independently with no assistive device • Gait deviations notable for guarded posture with decreased reciprocal arm swing, occasionally increased trunk sway, wide base of support, decreased limb clearance, occasionally reaching for walls to maintain balance.
Stairs		• Ascends/descends a full flight of stairs with modified independence and BUEs on a unilateral handrail, demonstrates side-stepping technique
Task specific		• Sit and watch traffic outside clinic window: unable to tolerate > 2 minutes

Assessment	
☑ Physical therapist's	*Assessment left blank for learner to develop*
Goals	
Patient's	"I want to be able to drive myself."
Short term	1. *Goals left blank for learner to develop* 2.
Long term	1. *Goals left blank for learner to develop* 2.

Plan	
☐ Physician's ☑ Physical therapist's ☐ Other's	Plan to follow patient for vestibular rehabilitation therapy for a frequency of two to three times a week for a total of 8 to 10 weeks in addition to establishment of a home exercise program to be performed 5 days a week.

Dizziness Handicap Inventory

Instructions: The purpose of this scale is to identify difficulties that you may be experiencing because of your dizziness. Please check "always", _or_ "no" _or_ "sometimes" to each question. Answer each question only as it pertains to your dizziness problem.

	Questions	Always	Sometimes	No
P1	Does looking up increase your problem?	☐	☒	☐
E2	Because of your problem, do you feel frustrated?	☒	☐	☐
F3	Because of your problem, do you restrict your travel for business or pleasure?	☒	☐	☐
P4	Does walking down the aisle of a supermarket increase your problem?	☒	☐	☐
F5	Because of your problem, do you have difficulty getting into or out of bed?	☐	☒	☐
F6	Does your problem significantly restrict your participation in social activities, such as going out to dinner, going to movies, dancing or to parties?	☒	☐	☐
F7	Because of your problem, do you have difficulty reading?	☐	☒	☐
F8	Does performing more ambitious activities like sports, dancing, and household chores, such as sweeping or putting dishes away; increase your problem?	☒	☐	☐
E9	Because of your problem, are you afraid to leave your home without having someone accompany you?	☒	☐	☐
E10	Because of your problem, have you been embarrassed in front of others?	☐	☒	☐
P11	Do quick movements of your head increase your problem?	☒	☐	☐
F12	Because of your problem, do you avoid heights?	☐	☐	☒
P13	Does turning over in bed increase your problem?	☐	☒	☐
F14	Because of your problem, is it difficult for you to do strenuous housework or yard work?	☐	☒	☐
E15	Because of your problem, are you afraid people may think that you are intoxicated?	☐	☐	☒
F16	Because of your problem, is it difficult for you to go for a walk by yourself?	☐	☒	☐
P17	Does walking down a sidewalk increase your problem?	☐	☒	☐
E18	Because of your problem, is it difficult for you to concentrate?	☐	☒	☐
F19	Because of your problem, is it difficult for you to walk around your house in the dark?	☒	☐	☐
E20	Because of your problem, are you afraid to stay home alone?	☐	☒	☐
E21	Because of your problem, do you feel handicapped?	☒	☐	☐
E22	Has your problem placed stress on your relationship with members of your family or friends?	☐	☒	☐
E23	Because of your problem, are you depressed?	☐	☒	☐
F24	Does your problem interfere with your job or household responsibilities?	☐	☒	☐
P25	Does bending over increase your problem?	☐	☒	☐

Fig. 20.4 Dizziness Handicap Inventory.

Bloom's Taxonomy Level	Case 20.C Questions
Create	1. Synthesizing the medical data and physical examination findings, develop an appropriate physical therapy assessment of the patient.
	2. Develop two short-term physical therapy goals, including an appropriate timeframe for outpatient care.
	3. Develop two long-term physical therapy goals, including an appropriate timeframe for outpatient care.
Evaluate	4. This patient previously had symptoms of gaze-evoked nystagmus with fixation. Provide support as to why this might be absent on the physical therapy examination today.
	5. Which components of the physical therapy examination not previously tested support or contribute to the differential diagnosis of unilateral vestibular hypofunction for this patient?
Analyze	6. Describe the relationship between impaired balance and vestibular hypofunction in a patient.
	7. Analyze the patient's posture at rest and with gait. What other interventions can be incorporated to address these deficits?
	8. Can a patient's posture influence symptoms of dizziness?
Apply	9. Determine an intervention to address the patient's impaired vestibular dysfunction.
	10. Determine an intervention to address the patient's impaired balance.
Understand	11. Explain how to determine the effectiveness of the intervention for this patient.
	12. Describe the education a physical therapist would provide to a patient based on any intervention performed.
Remember	13. What is the role of cognition in vestibular therapy intervention?

Bloom's Taxonomy Level	Case 20.C Answers
Create	1. The patient is a 69-year-old woman who presents after discharge from home physical therapy with persistent report of dizziness and impaired balance. The patient's examination findings are consistent with unilateral vestibular hypofunction affecting the right peripheral vestibular system with findings significant for positive Head Thrust Test to the right, gaze-evoked nystagmus that is increased with gaze to the left without fixation, and positive Head Shake Test. She demonstrates guarded posture with all mobility. Her gait is remarkable for decreased cadence, narrow base of support, and decreased reciprocal arm swing. She reports she was functionally independent and active in her community prior to emergency department visit 2 weeks ago. She will benefit from outpatient vestibular rehabilitation to decrease symptoms of dizziness with movement and promote return to prior level of function. Plan to progress VOR exercises initiated in patient's home physical therapy treatment plan in follow-up session.
	2. Short-term goals:
	• Patient will be independent in recall and implementation of home exercise program in three physical therapy sessions.
	• Patient will report a 10-point improvement on her score for the Dizziness Handicap Inventory in 2 weeks.
	3. Long-term goals:
	• Patient will report a 20-point improvement on their score for the Dizziness Handicap Inventory within 6 weeks.
	• Patient will demonstrate normal dynamic visual acuity on formal testing within 8 weeks.
	• Patient will return to to her volunteer job without a report of an increase in her symptoms in 10 weeks.
	• Patient will return to driving in 8-10 weeks.
Evaluate	4. Due to the subacute nature of this patient's vestibular dysfunction, many times it is expected that nystagmus may only be visible in the absence of fixation.
	5. Gaze-evoked nystagmus without fixation, a positive Head Shake Test without fixation, and a loss of balance on condition 4 of the CTSIB all support a differential diagnosis of R unilateral vestibular hypofunction.

(Continued)

429

(Continued)

Bloom's Taxonomy Level	Case 20.C Answers
Analyze	6. With an impaired right peripheral vestibular system, the patient is more closely relying on the somatosensory system and visual system to maintain balance. Having an impairment of one of these three components of a patient's balance center will impact their performance with mobility and task specific activities. These impairments can also increase a patient's risk for falls.
	7. manual therapy, postural muscle stretching, and proprioceptive exercises may be beneficial to incorporate in your treatment plan to address postural deficits of forward head posture and increased thoracic kyphosis. there is evidence that this can be an effective treatment for cervical dizziness.
	8. Patients with dizziness may also be at risk for developing cervicogenic dizziness, which can sometimes be described as an "internal dizziness." This is more commonly seen in patients with whiplash-associated disorders (WAD). This was not confirmed during the patient's emergency department evaluation. Therefore, it is unclear if there is a component of WAD to this patient's injury. Cervicogenic dizziness can be confirmed on differential diagnosis with cervical dizziness testing including the Head–Neck differentiation Test, Smooth Pursuit Neck Torsion Test, and joint position sense testing.
Apply	9. VOR exercise are the intervention of choice for this patient. In vestibular rehabilitation, these are typically initiated in sitting, performing VOR × 1, then progressing to VOR × 2. The therapist The Physical Therapist may also consider incorporating a cognitive task to progress this exercise. Providing a visual target with text on the target and asking the patient to read aloud while performing the VOR × 1 or VOR × 2 exercises is an example of incorporating a cognitive task.
	10. Substitution exercises should be incorporated into a vestibular treatment program for the patient to address this patient's impairments. Substitution exercises involve changing the variables and measures of a task for a patient. For example, a patient may be asked to perform a task with eyes open versus closed on an even versus uneven surface. Another example of a substitution exercise may include walking on an uneven sidewalk to challenge the patient's vestibular system. In order to progress a patient using substitution exercises, it is suggested that the therapist start by having the patient perform the exercises in a static standing position first. As the patient's symptoms improve with performing the tasks provided by the therapist in static standing that they can progress to dynamic standing activity. ▶ Fig. 20.5
Understand	11. Effectiveness of therapy intervention should be through reassessment of all examination measures performed on initial evaluation, particularly CTSIB, functional mobility, and DHI to track progress.
	12. It is important to explain to the patient that some of the exercises you are asking them to perform may provoke their symptoms. Education should help the patient to understand that provocation promotes central compensation, and ultimately, a reduction in severity of symptoms.
Remember	13. Cognition can be incorporated into adaptation and habituation exercises as a patient's symptoms improve. Examples of cognitive tasks that cane be incorporated into a treatment program include but are not limited to use of Stroop tasks, short- or long-term memory recall tasks, questions/answers during a tasks, or mathematical questions.

Key points

1. During the subacute phase of vestibular dysfunction, clinicians may only be able to elicit symptoms of nystagmus in the absence of fixation.

2. Incorporation of cognition into a vestibular rehabilitation program will improve effectiveness and efficacy of a patient's rehabilitation program.

3. Provocation of symptoms to achieve central compensation is necessary in order to improve a patient's symptoms.

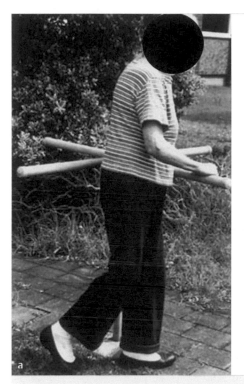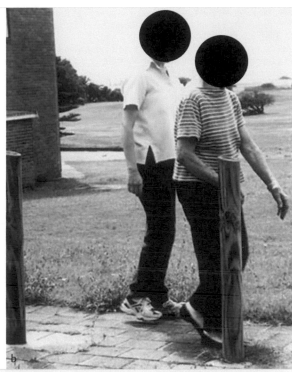

Fig. 20.5 Example of a progression of performing substitution exercises first in a static standing position (a) to dynamic standing activity (b). (Adapted from Mehrholz J, ed. Maximizing muscle endurance and physical fitness. In: Physical Therapy for the Stroke Patient. Early Stage Rehabilitation, 1st ed. New York, NY: Thieme; 2012.)

Suggested Readings

30 Second Sit to Stand Test. Shirley Ryan AbilityLab. Available at: www.sralab.org/rehabilitation-measures/30-second-sit-stand-test

Anagnostou E, Stamboulis E, Kararizou E. Canal conversion after repositioning procedures: comparison of Semont and Epley maneuver. J Neurol. 2014; 261(5):866–869

Ajayan PV, Aleena PF, Anju MJ. Epley's maneuver versus Semont's maneuver in treatment of posterior canal benign positional paroxysmal vertigo. Int J Res Med Sci. 2017; 5(7):2854–2860

Alshahrani A, Johnson EG, Cordett TK. Vertebral artery testing and differential diagnosis in dizzy patients. Physical Therapy and Rehabilitation. 2014; 1(1):3

Bernhardt J, Ellis P, Denisenko S, Hill K. Changes in balance and locomotion measures during rehabilitation following stroke. Physiother Res Int. 1998; 3(2):109–122

Black RA, Halmagyi GM, Thurtell MJ, Todd MJ, Curthoys IS. The active head-impulse test in unilateral peripheral vestibulopathy. Arch Neurol. 2005; 62(2):290–293

Cohen HS, Kimball KT. Treatment variations on the Epley maneuver for benign paroxysmal positional vertigo. Am J Otolaryngol. 2004; 25(1):33–37

Corallo G, Versino M, Mandalà M, Colnaghi S, Ramat S. The functional head impulse test: preliminary data. J Neurol. 2018; 265 Suppl 1:35–39

Ding J, Liu L, Kong WK, Chen XB, Liu X. Serum levels of 25-hydroxy vitamin D correlate with idiopathic benign paroxysmal positional vertigo. Biosci Rep. 2019; 39(4):BSR20190142

Dizziness Handicap Inventory. Shirley Ryan AbilityLab. Available at: www.sralab.org/rehabilitation-measures/dizziness-handicap-inventory. Accessed April 1, 2020

Dynamic Visual Acuity Test: Non-Instrumented. Shirley Ryan AbilityLab. Available at: www.sralab.org/rehabilitation-measures/dynamic-visual-acuity-test-non-instrumented. Accessed April 1, 2020

Emri M, Kisely M, Lengyel Z, et al. Cortical projection of peripheral vestibular signaling. J Neurophysiol. 2003; 89(5):2639–2646

Ertugrul S, Soylemez E. Investigation of the relationship between posterior semicircular canal benign paroxysmal positional vertigo and sleep quality. Annals of Medical Research. 2019; 26 (10):2359–2363

Grande-Alonso M, Moral Saiz B, Mínguez Zuazo A, Lerma Lara S, La Touche R. Biobehavioural analysis of the vestibular system and posture control in patients with cervicogenic dizziness. A cross-sectional study. Neurologia. 2018; 33(2):98–106

Guerra-Jiménez G, Domènech-Vadillo E, Álvarez-Morujo de Sande MG, et al. Healing criteria: How should an episode of benign paroxistic positional vertigo of posterior semicircular canal's resolution be defined? Prospective observational study. Clin Otolaryngol. 2019; 44(3):219–226

Gupta AK, Sharma KG, Sharma P. Effect of Epley, Semont maneuvers and Brandt–Daroff exercise on quality of life in patients with posterior semicircular canal benign paroxysmal positional vertigo (PSCBPPV). Indian J Otolaryngol Head Neck Surg. 2019; 71 (1):99–103

Hain TC, Fetter M, Zee DS. Head-shaking nystagmus in patients with unilateral peripheral vestibular lesions. Am J Otolaryngol. 1987; 8(1):36–47

Hall CD, Herdman SJ. Reliability of clinical measures used to assess patients with peripheral vestibular disorders. J Neurol Phys Ther. 2006; 30(2):74–81

Hall CD, Herdman SJ, Whitney SL, et al. Vestibular rehabilitation for peripheral vestibular hypofunction: an evidence-based clinical practice guideline: from the American Physical Therapy Association Neurology Section. J Neurol Phys Ther. 2016; 40(2):124–155

Haynes DS, Resser JR, Labadie RF, et al. Treatment of benign positional vertigo using the Semont maneuver: efficacy in patients presenting without nystagmus. Laryngoscope. 2002; 112(5):796–801

Honaker JA, Boismier TE, Shepard NP, Shepard NT. Fukuda stepping test: sensitivity and specificity. J Am Acad Audiol. 2009; 20(5):311–314, quiz 335

Horn LB, Rice T, Stoskus JL, Lambert KH, Dannenbaum E, Scherer MR. Measurement characteristics and clinical utility of the clinical test of sensory interaction on balance (CTSIB) and Modified CTSIB in individuals with vestibular dysfunction. Arch Phys Med Rehabil. 2015; 96(9):1747–1748

Jacobson GP, Newman CW. The development of the dizziness handicap inventory. Arch Otolaryngol Head Neck Surg. 1990; 116(4):424–427

Jeong SH, Choi SH, Kim JY, Koo JW, Kim HJ, Kim JS. Osteopenia and osteoporosis in idiopathic benign positional vertigo. Neurology. 2009; 72(12):1069–1076

Jeong SH, Kim JS. Impaired calcium metabolism in benign paroxysmal positional vertigo: a topical review. J Neurol Phys Ther. 2019; 43 Suppl 2:S37–S41

Kao WT, Parnes LS, Chole RA. Otoconia and otolithic membrane fragments within the posterior semicircular canal in benign paroxysmal positional vertigo. Laryngoscope. 2017; 127(3):709–714

Kinne BL, Perla MJ, Weber DT. Semont maneuver vs. Epley maneuver for canalithiasis of the posterior semicircular canal: a systematic review. Phys Ther Rev. 2016; 21(2):102–108

Koo JW, Kim JS, Hong SK. Vibration-induced nystagmus after acute peripheral vestibular loss: comparative study with other vestibule-ocular reflex tests in the yaw plane. Otol Neurotol. 2011; 32(3):466–471

Liu Y, Wang W, Zhang AB, Bai X, Zhang S. Epley and Semont maneuvers for posterior canal benign paroxysmal positional vertigo: a network meta-analysis. Laryngoscope. 2016; 126(4):951–955

Martellucci S, Attanasio G, Ralli M, et al. Does cervical range of motion affect the outcomes of canalith repositioning procedures for posterior canal benign positional paroxysmal vertigo? Am J Otolaryngol. 2019; 40(4):494–498

Martens C, Goplen FK, Aasen T, Nordfalk KF, Nordahl SHG. Dizziness handicap and clinical characteristics of posterior and lateral canal BPPV. Eur Arch Otorhinolaryngol. 2019; 276(8):2181–2189

Mostafa BE, Shafik AG, El Makhzangy AM, Taha H, Abdel Mageed HM. Evaluation of vestibular function in patients with chronic suppurative otitis media. ORL J Otorhinolaryngol Relat Spec. 2013; 75(6):357–360

Obrist D, Nienhaus A, Zamaro E, Kalla R, Mantokoudis G, Strupp M. Determinants for a successful Sémont maneuver: an in vitro study with a semicircular canal model. Front Neurol. 2016; 7(7):150

Reid SA, Rivett DA. Manual therapy treatment of cervicogenic dizziness: a systematic review. Man Ther. 2005; 10(1):4–13

Schubert MC, Herdman SJ, Tusa RJ. Vertical dynamic visual acuity in normal subjects and patients with vestibular hypofunction. Otol Neurotol. 2002; 23(3):372–377

Schuknecht HF. Cupulolithiasis. Arch Otolaryngol. 1969; 90(6):765–778

Son EJ, Lee DH, Oh JH, Seo JH, Jeon EJ. Correlation between the dizziness handicap inventory and balance performance during the acute phase of unilateral vestibulopathy. Am J Otolaryngol. 2015; 36(6):823–827

Sugaya N, Arai M, Goto F. Changes in cognitive function in patients with intractable dizziness following vestibular rehabilitation. Sci Rep. 2018; 8(1):9984

Trinidade A, Goebel JA. Persistent postural-perceptual dizziness: a systematic review of the literature for the balance specialist. Otol Neurotol. 2018; 39(10):1291–1303

Uz U, Uz D, Akdal G, Çelik O. Efficacy of Epley maneuver on quality of life of elderly patients with subjective BPPV. J Int Adv Otol. 2019; 15(3):420–424

Yang TH, Lee JH, Oh SY, Kang JJ, Kim JS, Dieterich M. Clinical implications of head-shaking nystagmus in central and peripheral vestibular disorders: is perverted head-shaking nystagmus specific for central vestibular pathology? Eur J Neurol. 2020; 27(7):1296–1303

Zhang YB, Wang WQ. Reliability of the Fukuda stepping test to determine the side of vestibular dysfunction. J Int Med Res. 2011; 39(4):1432–1437

Whitney SL, Sparto PJ, Furman JM. Vestibular Rehabilitation and Factors That Can Affect Outcome. Semin Neurol. 2020;40(1):165-172

Ellis AW, Schöne CG, Vibert D, Caversaccio MD, Mast FW. Cognitive Rehabilitation in Bilateral Vestibular Patients: A Computational Perspective. Front Neurol. 2018;9:286. Published 2018 Apr 27

Index

Note: Page numbers set **bold** or *italic* indicate headings or figures, respectively.